D0772451

Carpal Tunnel Syndrome and Other Disorders of the Median Nerve

Carpal Tunnel Syndrome and Other Disorders of the Median Nerve

Second Edition

Richard B. Rosenbaum, M.D.

Neurology Division, The Oregon Clinic; Clinical Professor of Neurology, Oregon Health and Sciences University, Portland, Oregon

José L. Ochoa, M.D., Ph.D., D.Sc.

Oregon Nerve Center at Good Samaritan Hospital; Clinical Professor of Neurology and Neurosurgery, Oregon Health and Sciences University, Portland, Oregon

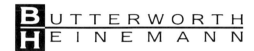

BUTTERWORTH
HEINEMANN

An Imprint of Elsevier Science

Amsterdam • Boston • London • Oxford • New York • Paris
San Diego • San Francisco • Singapore • Sydney • Tokyo

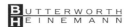

An Imprint of Elsevier Science

225 Wildwood Avenue
Woburn, MA 01801

Copyright © 2002 by Elsevier Science Inc. All rights reserved.

No part of this publication may be reproduced, stored in a retrieval system, or transmitted in any form or by any means, electronic, mechanical, photocopying, recording, or otherwise, without the prior written permission of the publisher (Butterworth–Heinemann, 225 Wildwood Avenue, Woburn, MA 01801).

Notice

Neurology is an ever-changing field. Standard safety precautions must be followed, but as new research and clinical experience broaden our knowledge, changes in treatment and drug therapy may become necessary or appropriate. Readers are advised to check the most current product information provided by the manufacturer of each drug to be administered to verify the recommended dose, the method and duration of administration, and contraindications. It is the responsibility of the treating physician, relying on experience and knowledge of the patient, to determine dosages and the best treatment for each individual patient. Neither the Publisher nor the author assume any liability for any injury and/or damage to persons or property arising from this publication.

The Publisher

First Edition 1993.

Library of Congress Cataloging-in-Publication Data
Rosenbaum, Richard B.,
  Carpal tunnel syndrome and other disorders of the median nerve / Richard B.
 Rosenbaum, José L. Ochoa.—2nd ed.
   p. ; cm.
  Includes bibliographical references and index.
  ISBN 0-7506-7314-1
   1. Carpal tunnel syndrome. 2. Median nerve—Diseases. I. Ochoa, José L. II. Title.
   [DNLM: 1. Carpal Tunnel Syndrome. 2. Median Nerve—pathology.]
RC422.C26 R67 2002
616.8′7—dc21

                                                      2001056694

Publisher: Susan F. Pioli
Editorial Assistant: Joan Ryan

SSC/MVY

Printed in the United States of America

Last digit is the print number: 9 8 7 6 5 4 3 2 1

To our wives, children, and parents

Contents

Foreword

Roger Gilliatt was preparing a foreword to the first edition of this book just before his untimely death. We miss his wisdom and example.

Preface

A decade ago, in the first edition of this book, we asked: "Has medicine become so complex that we need a separate text for each nerve in the body?"

Median nerve compression at the wrist is an archetype for other focal compression neuropathies. It also has unique features that distinguish it from other focal nerve compressions, such as the anatomic interrelationships of the nerve within the bony carpal canal and the effects of wrist posture and tendon movement on the median nerve.

Long before carpal tunnel syndrome began to draw attention in the media, at social gatherings, and in factories and offices around the country, physicians had been regularly attentive to it in their patients. As neurologists, we see hundreds of cases each year. There are approximately 4,000 articles indexed in Medline to the subject heading *carpal tunnel syndrome*. Nearly one-half of them have been published in the decade since our first edition. Despite this ever-growing scientific literature and clinical experience, we repeatedly find that patients with carpal tunnel syndrome can be a challenge to diagnose and treat. Behind the genesis of this book was a desire to synthesize the recorded knowledge about this prevalent syndrome and to answer some of the questions raised by our patients and colleagues.

Carpal tunnel syndrome is, by definition, a clinical condition manifest by signs and symptoms. Many people, if investigated in detail, have subclinical evidence of median nerve dysfunction in the carpal tunnel. The clinician must be wary of relying on diagnostic tests that demonstrate subclinical pathology and that potentially lead to overdiagnosis and overtreatment.

The excellent clinical description by Kremer, Gilliatt, Golding, and Wilson (1953) has not been surpassed:

> The usual complaint is then of attacks of painful tingling in one or both hands at night, sufficient to wake the sufferer after a few hours' sleep. The pain and paraesthesiae are usually described as "burning" or "agonising," and a deep-seated ache may spread up the forearm to the elbow. The ache is severest on the inner aspect of the forearm and more rarely may be felt in muscles as high as the shoulder. With the pain and tingling there is a subjective feeling of uselessness in the fingers, which are sometimes described as swollen; yet on inspection little or no swelling is apparent. Relief may be obtained by hanging the arm out of bed or shaking or rubbing the hand; but, as symptoms increase, the patients often get out of bed and walk about until eased.

Recent studies have shown the high prevalence of mild acroparesthesia in the population, expanding our sense of the spectrum of carpal tunnel syndrome, emphasizing instances when the syndrome never comes to medical attention or maintains a mild course (Chapter 3). There is still no substitute for evaluating patients with a careful history and physical examination. The clinician must attend carefully to the timing, location, and nature of symptoms, distinguishing pain, paraesthesias, and motor phenomena. Separation of carpal tunnel syndrome from other neurologic conditions and differential diagnosis in relation to other musculoskeletal disorders start with a thorough clinical evaluation (Chapter 4). Most cases of carpal tunnel syndrome are idiopathic or occupational; the patient's history and physical examination are the most important tools to explore alternative causes of the syndrome and to consider personal risk factors, such as obesity, in the genesis of the syndrome (Chapters 5 and 6).

Often, the clinical examination is sufficient to yield a confident diagnosis of carpal tunnel syndrome and to guide initial conservative treatment without further laboratory, electrophysiologic, or imaging evaluation. There is a continued search for better electrodiagnostic tests for carpal tunnel syndrome, but there still is no gold standard for the diagnosis (Rosenbaum, 1999) (Chapters 7 and 8). Methods for neurophysiologic investigation of carpal tunnel syndrome have become more and more sensitive and may detect abnormalities in large-caliber myelinated fibers before symptoms develop. Nerve conduction techniques will necessarily show occasional false-negative and false-positive results. Nerve conduction testing is a key diagnostic aid but cannot replace clinical diagnostic judgment. Attributing an atypical assortment of sensorimotor symptoms in the upper limb to carpal tunnel syndrome based on nerve conduction tests without appropriate clinical evidence of the syndrome remains, however, a common error. There is increased interest in imaging the carpal tunnel, but no imaging is necessary for most patient evaluations (Chapter 11).

Occupational carpal tunnel syndrome is widespread and has extensive legal and economic implications. The relationship between occupation and carpal tunnel syndrome has been widely debated. In the last decade, the literature on occupational carpal tunnel syndrome has been supplemented with a number of cross-sectional, case-controlled, and longitudinal studies, which have clarified the causal role of occupation, yet questions persist regarding optimal evaluation and management of workers who develop carpal tunnel syndrome (Chapter 13).

Carpal tunnel syndrome is a focal, usually chronic, compression neuropathy. The pathophysiology of carpal tunnel syndrome is intriguingly complex (Chapter 12). Important determinants include:

1. Individual variation in size and contents of the carpal tunnel;
2. Pathologic change that occurs in connective tissue within the carpal tunnel, such as edema and fibrosis of flexor synovium;
3. Variable pressure within the carpal tunnel, affected steadily by canal anatomy and connective tissue pathology and dynamically by changes in wrist posture and hand use and by shifts in distribution of body fluid;
4. Eventual chronic focal mechanical compression of the median nerve, leading first to damage in the myelin of large caliber fibers;
5. Transient episodes of compression and ischemia of the median nerve, resulting in spontaneous firing of sensory fibers and producing the intermittent paresthesias that are so characteristic of the syndrome; and
6. Variable susceptibility to compression of individual fibers within the median nerve based on nerve fiber diameter and myelination and also, to some extent, on

fascicular arrangement of the nerve. In myelinated fibers, conduction block occurs earlier than axonal interruption. Small-caliber nerve fibers are relatively resistant to compression and ischemia. In every patient, it is helpful to attempt to clarify which of these mechanisms is operative and to determine which portions of the patient's median nerve are responsible for symptoms.

A syndrome is, by definition, a collection of signs and symptoms. Strictly speaking, symptomatic carpal tunnel syndrome is redundant, and asymptomatic carpal tunnel syndrome is nearly nonexistent, referring only to that small group of patients who develop physical evidence of median neuropathy without ever being aware of the symptoms. Yet, the pathogenesis that leads to carpal tunnel syndrome starts before any symptoms develop. We have very little information about the range of carpal tunnel sizes in the population and about whether the risk of developing carpal tunnel syndrome varies with canal size. We know little about the cause or reversibility of pathology in the flexor tendon synovium.

The early pathologic changes in large myelinated fibers are often asymptomatic. Physiologic dysfunction of a portion of these fibers is often clinically undetectable. In many individuals, median nerve compression apparently may reach this stage and then never go on to become a clinical problem.

Understanding the pathophysiology of carpal tunnel syndrome helps in planning treatment and in evaluating the results of carpal tunnel surgery. Many individuals with intermittent or mild symptoms can forego treatment or be treated with simple nonoperative approaches. Nonoperative therapy has been studied more intensively in the last decade, including controlled studies of steroids, either injected into the carpal tunnel or taken orally, and several imaginative new approaches to treatment (Chapter 14).

In some patients, the appearance of symptoms, especially the paresthesias from ectopic nerve impulse generation, announces that the underlying pathology has reached a symptomatic stage, and surgical treatment eventually becomes necessary. Carpal tunnel endoscopy has fostered great interest in choosing appropriate surgical therapy; the debate between advocates of endoscopic and open surgery has generated more sophisticated methods of outcome assessment (Chapter 15). In most patients who undergo carpal tunnel surgery, the symptoms are completely relieved after section of the flexor retinaculum, even though some asymptomatic pathologic changes in the median nerve may remain.

Evidence of interruption of the axons of myelinated fibers or of dysfunction of small-caliber fibers is an indication for more aggressive therapy and also an indication that recovery of neuronal function may be slow or incomplete after successful therapy.

We have emphasized both pathophysiology and clinical findings. Analysis of patients from both a clinical and pathophysiologic viewpoint often helps in diagnosis of difficult cases and in planning therapy.

References

Kremer M, Gilliatt RW, Golding JSR, Wilson TG. Acroparaesthesiae in the carpal-tunnel syndrome. Lancet 1953;2:595.

Rosenbaum RB. Carpal tunnel syndrome and the myth of El Dorado. Muscle Nerve 1999;22:1165–67.

Acknowledgments

Eugenia Vásquez Bermudez was the illustrator for the first edition. Douglas Katagiri provided additional illustrations for the second edition.

We thank the following colleagues for their invaluable support, encouragement, and suggestions: Peggy Burrill, Morris Button, Mario Campero, Catherine Ellison, Gary Franklin, George Goodman, Gary Howell, Charles Jablecki, Paul Kohnen, Atiya Mansoor, Paolo Marchettini, Christopher J. Morgan, Peter Nathan, Beverly Phillipson, Stephen F. Quinn, Patrick Radecki, James T. Rosenbaum, Lois O. Rosenbaum, Robert A. Rosenbaum, Thomas J. Rosenbaum, Amy Roth, Jay Sonnad, Renato Verdugo, Richard Wernick, Asa Wilbourn, and David Yarnitsky.

Our thanks also to our office staffs for their long hours of assistance.

Susan Pioli, our editor at Butterworth–Heinemann, has long been our friend and support.

Chapter 1
Anatomy of the Median Nerve

Thorough understanding of median neuropathies requires a detailed awareness of the anatomy of the median nerve. Figure 1-1 schematically depicts formation, course, and branching of the median nerve. Knowledge of the relationships between nerve and surrounding bone and connective tissues is important to the study of entrapment neuropathies. Imaging techniques such as computed tomography, ultrasound, and magnetic resonance imaging (MRI) allow noninvasive study of median nerve topographical relationships. Anomalous nerve courses and patterns of innervation sometimes cause atypical clinical presentations and can often be demonstrated by combining anatomic knowledge with clinical and laboratory testing. The intraneural topography of nerve fascicles can account for the clinical presentation of partial nerve injuries.

Sunderland (1978) reviews the anatomy of the nerve in exquisite detail, based on dissection of 200 arms.

Median Nerve Formation

The median nerve is formed from nerve roots C5 to T1 as shown in Figure 1-2. The C5, C6, and C7 roots contribute to the lateral cord of the brachial plexus. The C8 and T1 roots contribute to the medial cord of the brachial plexus. Components from the medial and lateral cords of the plexus join to form the median nerve.

Table 1-1 summarizes the contribution of individual cervical nerve roots to the innervation of each muscle supplied by the median nerve. The contributions vary, of course, from individual to individual. Kendall and colleagues (1993) discuss some of the disagreements among different authorities regarding the radicular supply of each muscle. For example, C7 is often listed as contributing to flexor pollicis longus; however, in one series of 28 patients with surgically confirmed C7 radiculopathy severe enough to cause fibrillations in triceps, flexor carpi radialis, or pronator teres, not one of the patients had fibrillations in flexor pollicis longus (Levin, Maggiano & Wilbourn, 1996). Another area of debate is the major root contribution to median-innervated thenar muscles, which at times are spared in C8 radiculopathy. Correlations of electromyography and surgical findings imply that abductor pollicis brevis is often predominately supplied by the T1 root (Levin et al., 1996). However, some authorities list these thenar muscles as innervated by C6 or C7 (Mumenthaler & Schliak, 1991; Kendall, 1993).

The medial cord of the brachial plexus from the C8 and T1 roots provides the motor supply of the thenar hand muscles and most of the motor supply to the anterior interosseus nerve. In contrast, the lateral cord of the brachial plexus, from the C5, C6, and C7 roots, provides motor fibers to pronator teres and flexor carpi radialis, and part of the motor supply to palmaris longus and finger flexors. The lateral cord is the usual pathway for median nerve sensory fibers supplying the skin of the hand.

There are a number of uncommon anomalies that can affect the nerve roots and proximal median nerve (Kerr, 1918; Kaplan & Spinner, 1980). For example

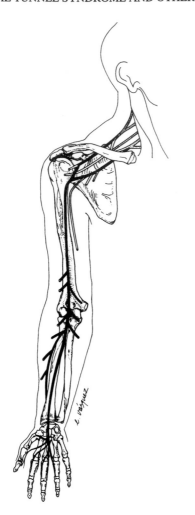

Figure 1-1. The median nerve.

1. The median nerve can lack fibers from the C5 or T1 roots.
2. The median nerve and lateral and medial cords can follow a variety of patterns in relation to the axillary artery.
3. The connection from the lateral cord to the median nerve can consist of one or multiple discrete bundles (Sargon, Uslu, Celik & Aksit, 1995).
4. The median and musculocutaneous nerves can connect by proximal anastomoses or even be fused (Le Minor, 1990; Kaus & Wotowicz, 1995; Eglseder & Goldman, 1997; Venieratos & Anagnostopoulou, 1998; Basar, Aldur, Celik, Yuksel & Tascioglu, 2000; Jakubowicz & Ratajczak, 2000).

5. The musculocutaneous nerve can be absent, so that proximal median nerve branches supply the usual musculocutaneous motor and sensory innervation (Ihunwo, Osinde & Mukhtar, 1997; Gumusburun & Adiguzel, 2000).

Median Nerve Branches

The median nerve gives off a number of motor branches in the forearm, as illustrated in Figure 1-3. Often more than one branch goes to an individual muscle. The number of branches per muscle can vary, and the order of branching is not constant (Sunderland, 1978; Canovas, Mouilleron & Bonnel, 1998; Chantelot, Feugas, Guillem, Chapnikoff, Remy & Fontaine, 1999). Typically, the initial branches, usually two to four, are to the pronator teres. Subsequent branches are to flexor carpi radialis, palmaris longus (this muscle is not always present), and flexor digitorum superficialis. In the antecubital space and forearm, nerve branches also supply elbow and radioulnar joints and the brachial artery.

Anterior Interosseous Nerve

The anterior interosseous nerve branches from the median nerve distal to the muscular branches in the forearm (Figure 1-4). The anterior interosseous nerve is a predominantly motor nerve that innervates the flexor pollicis longus, pronator quadratus, and part of the flexor digitorum profundus (FDP) muscles. The anterior interosseous nerve innervates the FDP for the index finger almost always, the FDP for the middle finger approximately half the time, and the FDP to the ring or little fingers rarely (Sunderland, 1978). The ulnar nerve provides the remainder of the FDP innervation. The anterior interosseous nerve carries no cutaneous innervation; its deep sensory branches supply the radiocarpal and carpal-carpal joints and probably those forearm muscles to which it provides motor innervation.

Palmar Cutaneous Branch of the Median Nerve

The median palmar cutaneous nerve is purely sensory, innervating the skin of the proximal palm and

Figure 1-2. Formation of the median nerve.

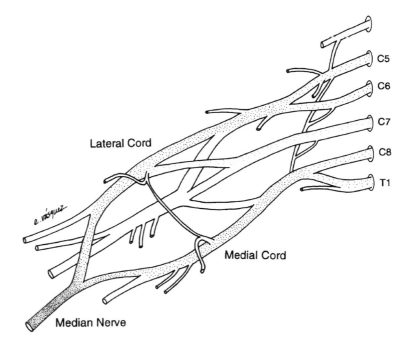

thenar eminence. The nerve originates from the median nerve 3 to 22 cm proximal to the distal wrist crease (Hobbs, Magnussen & Tonkin, 1990; al-Qattan, 1997). However, it does not separate from the median nerve immediately, branching usually from the radial side of the nerve an average of 4 to 6 cm proximal to distal wrist crease (range, 27 to 78 mm) (Martin, Seiler & Lesesne, 1996; Watchmaker, Weber & Mackinnon, 1996). It usually runs in the radial direction, but an ulnar-

Table 1-1. Nerve Root Contributions to the Median Nerve

Lateral Cord			Medial Cord	
C6 Root	C7 Root	Muscle	C8 Root	T1 Root
		Muscular branches in the forearm		
x	X	Pronator teres		
x	X	Flexor carpi radialis	x	
	x	Palmaris longus	X	x
	x	Flexor digitorum sublimis	X	X
		Anterior interosseous nerve branches		
	x	Flexor pollicis longus	X	X
	x	Flexor digitorum profundus	X	X
	x	Pronator quadratus	X	X
		Hand intrinsic muscles		
		Abductor pollicis brevis	X	x
		Opponens pollicis	X	x
		Flexor pollicis brevis	X	X
	x	Lumbricals	X	X

X = major contributing roots; x = minor contributing roots.
Adapted from W Haymaker, B Woodhall. Peripheral Nerve Injuries (2nd ed). Philadelphia: Saunders, 1953.

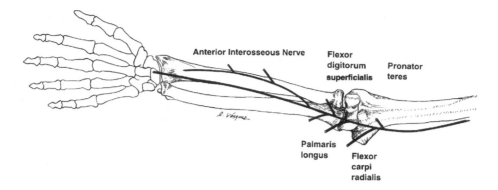

Figure 1-3. Motor branches of the median nerve in the forearm.

directed course occurs in a few individuals (Figure 1-5) (Das & Brown, 1976; Siegel, Davlin & Aulicino, 1993). The nerve typically travels under the radial margin of the flexor digitorum superficialis, deep to the antebrachial fascia, in the fascial sheath and synovium along the ulnar margin of the flexor carpi radialis. Next, the nerve becomes increasingly superficial, traveling through a tunnel 3 to 15 mm long in the antebrachial fascia and flexor retinaculum (Naff, Dellon & Mackinnon, 1993). Occasionally, the nerve branches proximal to the distal wrist crease (DaSilva, Moore, Weiss, Akelman & Sikirica, 1996). In the palm distal to its tunnel, the nerve is often adjacent to the distal palmaris longus tendon [and on rare occasions can run through the palmaris longus tendon (Dowdy, Richards & McFarlane, 1994)], then takes a subcutaneous course, forming its terminal cutaneous sensory branches. It can also send sensory branches to portions of the flexor retinaculum and carpal bones (Ferreres, Suso, Ordi, Llusa & Ruano, 1995; DaSilva et al., 1996). Figure 1-6 shows the typical extent of the terminal branches of the median palmar cutaneous nerve, but there is significant variation in the terminal branch patterns with

medial branches rarer than lateral branches (Bezerra, Carvalho & Nucci, 1986).

In addition to innervation by the median palmar cutaneous nerve, the palm can receive overlapping innervation from the digital branches of the median nerve, the anterior branch of the lateral cutaneous nerve of the forearm, the superficial radial nerve, the medial cutaneous nerve of the forearm, and the ulnar nerve. Variations in ulnar innervation of the palm are discussed in Chapter 15. Interruption of the median palmar cutaneous branch does not always cause discernible sensory loss because of overlap with these other nerves.

Terminal Branches of the Median Nerve

The terminal trifurcation of the median nerve occurs near the distal edge of the carpal tunnel. The radial branch becomes the common digital nerve to the thumb and index finger. The recurrent thenar motor branch can derive from this radial branch or more proximally from the median nerve. The central and ulnar branches become the other two common digital nerves.

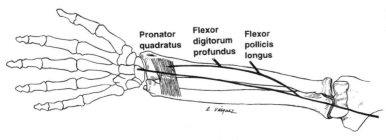

Figure 1-4. Motor branches of the anterior interosseous nerve.

Figure 1-5. The palmar cutaneous branch of the median nerve follows a variety of courses. (Reproduced with permission from SK Das, HG Brown. In search of complications in carpal tunnel decompression. Hand 1976;8: 243–49.)

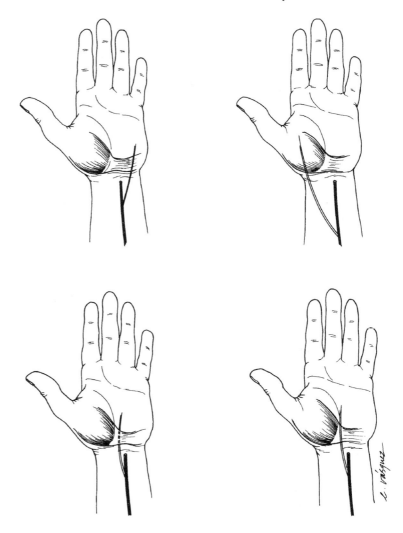

Recurrent Thenar Motor Branch of the Median Nerve

Nerve Supply of the Thenar Muscles

The recurrent thenar motor branch supplies the median-innervated thenar muscles. The typical pattern is that the recurrent motor branch supplies the abductor pollicis brevis, opponens pollicis, and the flexor pollicis brevis. There are a number of terminal branching variations (Olave, Prates, Del Sol, Sarmento & Gabrielli, 1995; Olave, Prates, Gabrielli & Pardi, 1996). In fact, the typical pattern occurs in only approximately one-third of hands (Rowntree, 1949). Figure 1-7 shows the distribution of the variations on this pattern. The most common variation is supply of flexor pollicis brevis by the ulnar nerve or by both the median

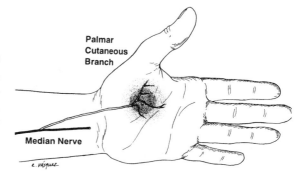

Figure 1-6. The median palmar cutaneous nerve. The shaded area shows the typical distribution of sensory cutaneous innervation. (Redrawn with permission from RE Carroll, DP Green. The significance of the palmar cutaneous nerve at the wrist. Clin. Orthop. 1972;83:24–28.)

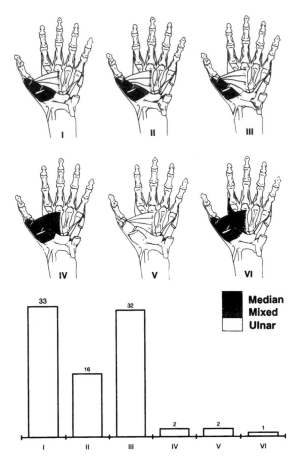

Some of the variations can be explained by communications (Riche-Cannieu anastomosis) in the palm between the deep branch of the ulnar nerve and the median nerve and its branches (Figure 1-8) (Sunderland, 1978; Kaplan & Spinner, 1980). Mannerfelt (1966) and Falconer and Spinner (1985) dissected 19 hands and found 6 instances of the Riche-Cannieu anastomosis. Harness and Sekeles (1971) found ulnar-median anastomoses in 27 of 35 hands and described a number of variations in the connections. Electrodiagnostic studies comparing the size of the compound muscle action potential recorded over the abductor pollicis brevis muscle to median and ulnar stimulation at the wrist also give evidence of a high incidence of ulnar to median motor communication in the hand (Kimura, Ayyar & Lippmann, 1983).

Very rarely, an anastomotic branch from the radial nerve to the median nerve can innervate the abductor pollicis brevis. Contribution of musculocutaneous nerve fibers to muscles also innervated by the median nerve is another rarity (Marinacci, 1964b; Schultz & Kaplan, 1984).

Figure 1-7. Variations in supply of the thenar muscles by the median and ulnar nerves. As shown by the bar graph, the classic pattern of median innervation of abductor pollicis brevis, opponens pollicis, and flexor pollicis brevis is present in only approximately one-third of hands. (Redrawn with permission from T Rowntree. Anomalous innervation of the hand muscles. J. Bone Joint Surg. 1949;31B:505–10.)

and the ulnar nerves (Forrest, 1967; Ajmani, 1996). The extremes of variation include ulnar supply of every thenar muscle or median supply of all hand intrinsic muscles. In the latter case, the rare all median hand, the innervation of those hand intrinsics that are normally ulnar-innervated is usually via the Martin-Gruber anastomosis (Marinacci, 1964a). An extraordinary pattern is for the median nerve to innervate the hypothenar muscles via an anomalous branch that arises from the median nerve in the carpal tunnel (Seradge & Seradge, 1990).

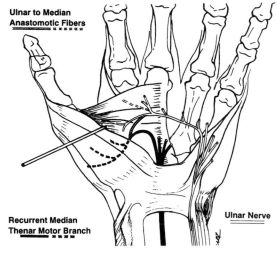

Figure 1-8. Fibers can pass from the ulnar to the median nerve in the palm via the Riche-Cannieu anastomosis. (Redrawn with permission from EB Kaplan, M Spinner. Normal and Anomalous Innervation Patterns in the Upper Extremity. In GE Omer Jr., M Spinner [eds], Management of Peripheral Nerve Problems. Philadelphia: Saunders, 1980;75–99.)

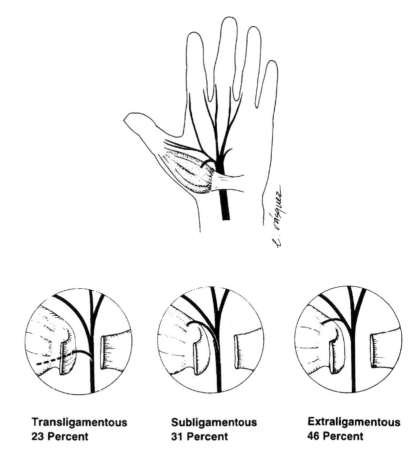

Figure 1-9. The recurrent thenar motor branch varies in its course. The three most common patterns are shown. (Redrawn with permission from U Lanz. Anatomical variations of the median nerve in the carpal tunnel. J. Hand Surg. 1977;2:44-53; incidence data from S Poisel. Ursprung und verlaf des ramus muscularis des nervus digitalis palmaris communis I [N. medianus]. Chir. Praxis 1974;18: 471–74.)

Transligamentous 23 Percent   **Subligamentous 31 Percent**   **Extraligamentous 46 Percent**

Course of the Recurrent Thenar Motor Branch

The recurrent motor branch to the thenar muscles varies in its departure from the median nerve and in its relationship to the flexor retinaculum (Figure 1-9) (Poisel, 1974; Lanz, 1977; Falconer & Spinner, 1985). The recurrent motor branch typically leaves the radial side of median nerve distal to the flexor retinaculum and then curves back to reach the thenar muscles. However, the recurrent motor branch can leave the median nerve within the carpal tunnel then either pierce the flexor retinaculum (transligamentous course) or cross the distal edge of the flexor retinaculum before curving back to the muscles (subligamentous course). The reported incidence of a transligamentous course of the nerve varies from as high as 80% to as low as 7% of anatomic dissections, with at least part of the variations attributable to disagreement among anatomists on the location of the distal border of the transverse carpal liga-

ment (Johnson & Shrewsbury, 1970; Kozin, 1998).

At times, an anomalous hypertrophic muscle lies on the volar surface of the flexor retinaculum, and the recurrent thenar branch can originate in a transligamentous or subligamentous fashion and then continue its course buried in this muscle (Hurwitz, 1996). Commonly, a single recurrent motor branch divides into three terminal branches to the abductor pollicis brevis, opponens pollicis, and flexor pollicis brevis; however, a number of variations are known (Lanz, 1977; Mumford, Morecraft & Blair, 1987; Hurwitz, 1996). Examples of rare anomalies are two or even three motor branches, departure of the recurrent motor branch from the ulnar side of the median nerve, a proximal accessory motor branch originating from the median nerve proximal to the carpal tunnel, or accessory thenar motor branches arising distally in the tunnel (Figure 1-10).

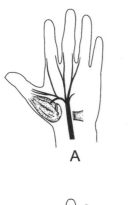
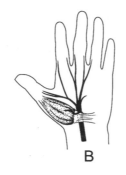
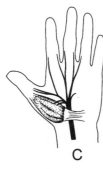
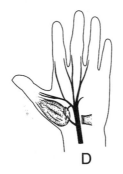

Figure 1-10. Unusual anomalies of the recurrent thenar motor branch. **(A)** Thenar branch leaving the median nerve on its ulnar aspect (Entin, 1968). **(B)** Thenar branch superficial to the flexor retinaculum (Mannerfelt & Hybbinette, 1972). **(C)** Double thenar motor branch. **(D)** Accessory branch proximal to the carpal tunnel running directly into the thenar musculature (Linburg & Albright, 1970). (Redrawn with permission of the publisher from U Lanz. The Carpal Tunnel Syndrome. In R Tubiana [ed], The Hand. Philadelphia: Saunders, 1993;463–86.)

Digital Nerves

Figure 1-11 illustrates the usual pattern of the digital branches of the median nerve. The radial side of each finger is supplied by a "radial" proper digital nerve; the ulnar side of each finger by an "ulnar" proper digital nerve. The terminology is confusing here because *ulnar* and *radial* in this context refer to the medial and lateral sides of the finger in these branches of the *median* nerve. The proper digital nerves have a variable number of terminal branches (Zenn, Hoffman, Latrenta & Hotchkiss, 1992). At each web space, the proper digital nerves for adjacent fingers usually join to form a common digital nerve in the palm. Typically, the radial and ulnar proper digital nerves of the thumb and first three common digital nerves arise from the median nerve.

There are at least three variations in branching of the proper digital nerves of the thumb and lateral index finger (Jolley, Stern & Starling, 1997) (Figure 1-12):

Type I. The first common digital nerve divides to form proper digital nerves to the lateral index finger and medial thumb; a separate proper digital nerve arises from the median nerve to supply the lateral thumb (69% of hands per Jolley et al., 1997).

Type II. The first common digital nerve gives off proper digital nerves to the lateral index finger, and then divides into the proper digital nerves of the medial and lateral thumb (6% of hands).

Type III. The first common digital nerve trifurcates to form proper digital nerves to the lateral index finger, medial thumb, and lateral thumb (25% of hands).

Each proper digital nerve carries cutaneous sensory fibers from the volar fingertip and from the ipsilateral half of the volar and lateral finger and distal dorsal finger. Those fibers from the dorsal aspect of the finger usually join the proper digital nerves proximal to the proximal interphalangeal joint, often

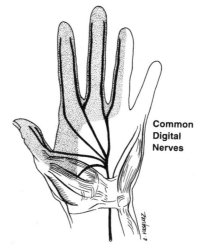

Figure 1-11. The common digital nerves in the palm divide to form the proper digital nerves to each finger. The shaded area represents the usual area of median cutaneous sensory innervation. The recurrent motor branch of the median nerve is also shown in the diagram.

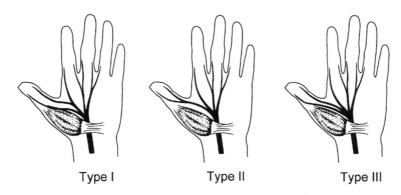

Type I   Type II   Type III

Figure 1-12. Variations of the digital nerves to the thumb. Type I: common digital nerve to thumb and index finger with proper digital nerve to radial side of the thumb. Type II: common digital nerve to thumb and radial digital nerve to index finger. Type III: trifurcation pattern with proper digital nerves to radial and ulnar aspects of thumb and radial side of index finger. (Redrawn with permission from BJ Jolley, PJ Stern, T Starling. Patterns of median nerve sensory innervation to the thumb and index finger: an anatomic study. J. Hand Surg. 1997;22A:228–31.)

proximal to the metacarpal-phalangeal joint; in the thumb, the distal dorsal sensory fibers usually join the superficial radial nerve (Wallace & Coupland, 1975; Bas & Kleinert, 1999). The digital nerves also carry sensory fibers from the finger joints and flexor tendons (Schultz, Krishnamurthy & Johnston, 1984; Pesson, Finney, Depaolo, Dabezies & Zimny, 1991).

Sensory innervation of the dorsal distal digits can show significant overlap with innervation both by branches of the median digital nerves and by distal extensions of the superficial radial nerve or the dorsal ulnar cutaneous nerve (Bas & Kleinert, 1999). Connections of the median to radial or ulnar fibers often occur on the dorsum of the digits (Bas & Kleinert, 1999).

Sensory integrity of the tip of the thumb is very important to hand function, and surgeons have studied the anatomy of the digital nerves to the thumb in detail to facilitate microscopic repair (Hirasawa, Sakakida, Tokioka & Ohta, 1985). In the distal phalanx of the thumb, each proper digital nerve divides into three terminal branches, which are protected under subcutaneous tissue (Chow, 1980).

Fibers from the ulnar and radial digital nerves can overlap at the finger tip so that damage to a single proper digital nerve can cause ipsilateral sensory loss on one side of the proximal finger but spare sensation on the finger tip (Dellon, 1981).

The median cutaneous sensory patterns have been mapped in humans by careful study of patients with median, ulnar, or radial nerve injuries using a camel hair brush to find the areas of sensory loss (Stopford, 1918). Figure 1-13 shows the usual pattern and the limits of variation. The typical pattern is present in about three-fourths of patients: The median digital nerves supply the palmar surfaces of the thumb, index, middle, and lateral one-half of the ring fingers; the digital nerves also supply the dorsal tips of the index, middle, and lateral side of the ring finger at least as far proximally as the distal interphalangeal joints and sometimes over the more proximal phalanges.

Many individuals have variations from the usual sensory pattern. Frequently areas of innervation overlap so that injury to an individual nerve causes a smaller area of sensory loss than predicted by classical anatomic charts. Crossover with the cutaneous innervation of the ulnar and superficial radial nerves is common.

The most common variation is supply of the lateral aspect of the ring finger by the ulnar nerve. At times this area has both median and ulnar innervation. In one group of cadavers, 80% to 90% of palms showed a communication—the so-called Berrettini branch—between the ulnar nerve and median-innervated digital nerves to either the radial proper digital nerve to the ring finger or the third common digital nerve (Figure 1-14) (Meals & Shaner, 1983; Ferrari & Gilbert, 1991; Stancic, Micovic & Potocnjak, 1999). In another cadaver survey, two-thirds of hands showed median-ulnar or ulnar-median communi-

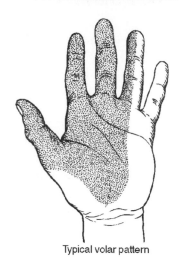

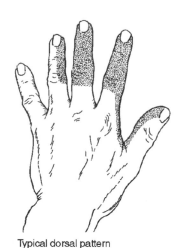

Figure 1-13. Variations of median sensory innervation of the hands. (Redrawn with permission from JSB Stopford. The variation in the distribution of the cutaneous nerves of the hands and digits. J. Anat. 1918;53:14–25.)

Typical volar pattern   Typical dorsal pattern

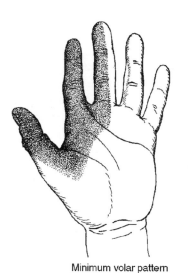

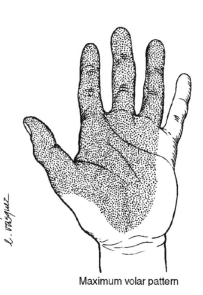

Minimum volar pattern   Maximum volar pattern

cating branches in the palm (Bas & Kleinert, 1999). Rarely, fibers from the radial proper digital nerve of the middle finger travel to the ulnar nerve via this communication. This anastomosis explains the ulnar innervation of the lateral ring finger or even the medial middle finger in some individuals. These anastomotic fibers are often near the distal medial margin of the transverse carpal ligament, can be anywhere in the middle three-fifths of the ulnar palm, and must be protected at the time of carpal tunnel surgery (Ferrari & Gilbert, 1991; Don Griot, Zuidam, van Kooten, Prose & Hage, 2000).

Another area of variation is the volar thumb where radial overlap of the usual median territory is common (Fetrow, 1970). Sensory innervation of the volar surface of the other digits via the superficial radial nerve is exceedingly rare (Bergman, Blom & Senström, 1970).

In the average median nerve, two-thirds of the fascicular cross-sectional area is destined for the digital nerves (Sunderland, 1978). On average a proper digital nerve is composed of 9 to 15 fascicles and contains 1,500 to 3,000 or more myelinated fibers (Bonnel, Foucher & Saint-Andre, 1989).

Figure 1-14. Anastomotic fibers often communicate between median and ulnar digital nerves. Examples of some variations are shown. (Reproduced with permission from RA Meals, M Shaner. Variations in digital sensory patterns: a study of the ulnar nerve-median nerve palmar communicating branch. J. Hand Surg. 1983;8: 411–14.)

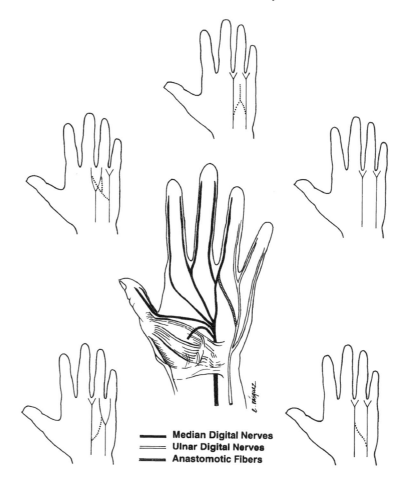

■■■ **Median Digital Nerves**
═══ **Ulnar Digital Nerves**
▬▬▬ **Anastomotic Fibers**

Median Nerve Branches to the Lumbricals

The terminal motor branches of the median nerve typically innervate the lumbricals of the index and middle fingers, whereas the ulnar nerve innervates the lumbricals of the ring and little fingers (Sunderland, 1978). The motor branch to the first lumbrical usually arises from the radial proper digital nerve of the index finger, whereas the motor branch to the second lumbrical usually arises from the common digital nerve of the second intermetacarpal space (Schultz & Kaplan, 1984; Lauritzen, Szabo & Lauritzen, 1996). This pattern is found in about one-half of hands. The most common variation is partial median-innervation of the lumbrical of the ring finger. Rarer variations are median-innervation of the lumbrical of the little finger or ulnar-innervation of the lumbrical of the index finger.

Median Nerve Autonomic Innervation

The digital nerves also carry sudomotor and vasomotor sympathetic fibers to skin and blood vessels. There is a wide variation in the relative contributions of ulnar and median nerves to the sympathetic supply of the superficial arterial arch of the palm (Meals & Shaner, 1983). On the palmar surface of the hand, the cutaneous sensory distribution of the median nerve matches the cutaneous vasomotor distribution of median sympathetic fibers (Woollard & Phillips, 1932). The median sympathetic vasomotor pattern can be documented by thermography after local anesthetic nerve blocks. Color Plates 10.1A, 16.2D, and 16.4D are hand thermograms obtained after local anesthetic block of the median nerve. On the dorsum of the hand, the pattern of warming demonstrated by thermography after median or ulnar nerve block matches the median or ulnar volar cutaneous sensory pattern; the thermogram of the dorsum of the hand is unaffected by radial nerve block. The median nerve is the usual source of vasomotor innervation of the dorsal lateral hand, even though the sensory and sudomotor innervation of this territory is usually by the superficial radial nerve (Campero, Verdugo & Ochoa, 1993).

Sweat glands are supplied by sympathetic sudomotor fibers that accompany sensory fibers. Fingerprinting followed by ninhydrin staining can be used to document cutaneous sympathetic sudomotor supply to the fingers. This technique can be combined with local anesthetic nerve blocks to document variations in cutaneous innervation. The results parallel those found by examining sensation in patients after nerve injuries (Fetrow, 1970).

Topographic Relationships

Upper Arm

In the upper arm the median nerve travels with the brachial artery in a neurovascular bundle. The median nerve usually passes over (ventral to), rather than under, the brachial artery (Eglseder & Goldman, 1997). The course is along the medial aspect of the arm and is relatively superficial, particularly as the bundle leaves the axilla, and again in the antecubital fossa. In the axilla the median nerve is near the ulnar and musculocutaneous nerves and the medial cutaneous nerves of the arm and forearm. By mid-humerus the median-brachial artery bundle is well separated from these other nerves.

Antecubital Space and Proximal Forearm

The median nerve crosses the antecubital fossa to enter the proximal forearm. In doing so it can pass under one or two fibrous arches, which are potential sites of nerve compression (see Figure 17-5) (Dellon, 1986). Johnson and colleagues (Johnson, Spinner & Shrewsbury, 1979) found at least one fibrous arch in 75% of cadaver arms. These relationships, discussed in more detail in the following paragraphs, are of particular interest in considering the pronator syndrome and other forms of median nerve compression in the forearm (see Chapter 17).

Ligament of Struthers

In approximately 1% of the population, the median nerve enters the antecubital space by passing under a ligament running from the medial epicondyle and medial intermuscular septum to the distal anterior medial humerus (see Figure 17-7). When this ligament (ligament of Struthers) is present, it usually attaches proximally to the humerus at an anomalous bony supracondylar spur, up to 2 cm long, located 1 to 6 cm above the elbow. The supracondylar spur is present in less than 4% of the population and can vary in prominence (Kessel & Rang, 1966). At times the spur is easily palpable; at the other extreme, the ligament can arise from the humerus without a visible spur (Suranyi, 1983). Alternatively, the supracondylar spur can be present without a corresponding ligament (Dellon & Mackinnon, 1987). When the ligament is present, the median nerve runs beneath it in a neurovascular bundle. The brachial artery can run within the bundle; alternatively, the brachial artery can divide proximal to the bundle so that only the ulnar artery runs with the median nerve under the ligament (Gessini, Jandolo & Pietrangeli, 1983). Presence of the ligament of Struthers can be associated with unusually proximal branching of the anterior interosseous nerve and of the muscular branches to pronator teres and other forearm muscles; an anomalous head of pronator teres can originate from the ligament (Gunther, DiPasquale & Martin, 1993).

Lacertus Fibrosus

The median nerve passes through the antecubital space beneath the lacertus fibrosus (also called the aponeurosis of the biceps brachii), a fascial band that runs from the biceps tendon medially toward the proximal ulna (see Figure 17-6) (Martinelli, Gabellini, Poppi, Gallassi & Pozzati, 1982). The lacertus fibrosus is continuous with the origin of the humeral head of the pronator teres muscle.

Humeral Origin of Pronator Teres

The relationship of the median nerve to the pronator teres muscle is variable (Beaton & Anson, 1939; Dellon, 1986; Dellon & Mackinnon, 1987; Nebot-Cegarra, Perez-Berruezo & Reina de la Torre, 1991). One source of variation depends on whether the humeral head of the pronator teres originates at the medial humeral epicondyle or more proximally. In the common pattern the pronator teres originates at the medial epicondyle or within 2 cm of it, and the median nerve remains uniformly cylindrical as it passes beneath the humeral head of the pronator.

One variant is origin of the pronator teres 2 cm or more proximal to the epicondyle (Dellon & Mackinnon, 1987). In this configuration the fascial edge of the pronator teres crosses the antecubital space proximal to the elbow flexion crease so that the nerve is potentially compressed with elbow extension or forearm pronation. Dellon (1986) found this variant in 11 of the 64 cadavers studied; when this variant was present, there was often a groove or segmental narrowing in the median nerves where the pronator mass crossed.

Heads of Pronator Teres

Typically, the median nerve passes between the deep (ulnar) head and superficial (humeral) head of the pronator teres. Possible variations include absence of the deep head, passage of the nerve deep to both heads, and penetration of the nerve through the superficial head. In one series only 83% of cadaver arms showed the typical pattern (Beaton & Anson, 1939).

Flexor Digitorum Superficialis

Once past the pronator teres, the median nerve courses deep to the flexor digitorum superficialis, which also can vary in its origin. Along this course many individuals have an idiosyncratic arrangement of fibrous bands that can arise from the pronator teres, flexor carpi radialis, and flexor digitorum superficialis muscles and that have the potential for nerve compression (see Figure 17-5) (Johnson & Spinner, 1989).

Forearm—Anterior Interosseous Nerve

The anterior interosseous nerve branches from the median nerve. In more than 90% of people this branching occurs distal to the pronator teres, 5 to 8 cm distal to the lateral epicondyle (Spinner, 1970; Chidgey & Szabo, 1989). If the branching occurs proximal to pronator teres, the anterior interosseous and median nerves usually remain parallel in their course past the heads of pronator teres (Megele, 1988).

The anterior interosseous nerve can be crossed in the forearm by several anatomic structures: an accessory head of the flexor pollicis longus (Gantzer's muscle; see Figure 17-3), ulnar collateral vessels, flexor digitorum superficialis to the flexor pollicis longus, the deep tendinous head of the pronator teres, or a fibrous arch (Spinner & Schreiber, 1969; al-Qattan, 1996). The anterior interosseous nerve can originate from the posterior, ulnar, or radial aspect of the median nerve and seems to be more susceptible to compression when originating from the radial aspect (Dellon, 1986; Shirali, Hanson, Branovacki & Gonzalcz, 1998).

Distal Forearm

In the forearm the median nerve is sheltered by the flexor digitorum superficialis until the nerve is about 5 cm proximal to the wrist (Sunderland, 1978).

Carpal Tunnel

Robbins (1963) reviewed the anatomy of the carpal tunnel in detail based on dissection of seven cadavers. In vivo evaluation of carpal tunnel anatomy is now possible with computed tomography studies (Zucker-Pinchoff, Hermann & Srinivasan, 1981; Cone, Sabo, Resnick, Gelberman, Taleisnik & Gilula, 1983; Jessurun, Hillen, Zonneveld, Huffstadt, Beks & Overbeek, 1987) and MRI (Middleton, Kneeland, Kellman, Cates, Sanger, Jesmanowicz & Froncisz, 1987; Mesgarzadeh, Schneck & Bonakdarpour, 1989; Zeiss, Skie, Ebraheim & Jackson, 1989) (Figures 1-15 and 1-16).

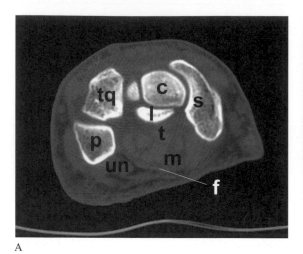

A

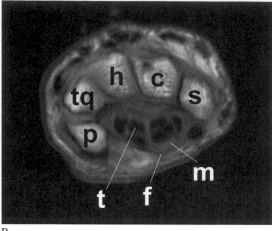

B

Figure 1-15. Normal computed tomography **(A)** and magnetic resonance image **(B)** of the proximal carpal tunnel (right hand, palm down, thumb to the right). (c = capitate; f = flexor retinaculum; h = hamate; l = lunate; m = median nerve; p = pisiform; s = scaphoid; t = flexor tendons; tq = triquetrum; un = ulnar nerve.) (Images courtesy of Gary Howell, M.D.)

Carpal Bones

The tunnel is formed dorsally and laterally by the eight carpal bones and volarly by the transverse carpal ligament. The bones form a roughly C-shaped arcade in two sets of four bones. Proximally, the four bones—naming from radial side to ulnar side—are the scaphoid (navicular), lunate, triquetrum, and pisiform. The volar portion of the lunate projects into the tunnel. The distal four bones—from radial to ulnar—are the trapezium and trapezoid (alternative names: greater and lesser multangular), capitate, and hamate. The bones are covered and joined by ligaments on their dorsal and volar surfaces. The carpal tunnel is open at its distal and proximal borders; radio-

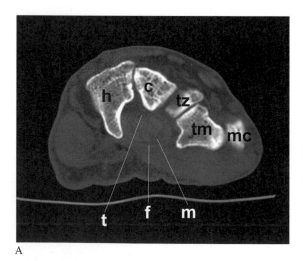

A

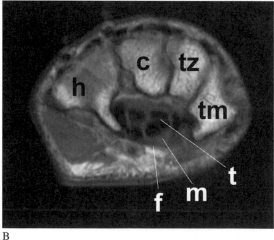

B

Figure 1-16. Normal computed tomography **(A)** and magnetic resonance image **(B)** of the distal carpal tunnel (right hand, palm down, thumb to the right). (c = capitate; f = flexor retinaculum; h = hamate; m = median nerve; mc = first metacarpal; t = flexor tendons; tm = trapezium; tz = trapezoid.) (Images courtesy of Gary Howell, M.D.)

contrast injected into the carpal tunnel flows freely into the palmar compartment of the hand and the flexor compartment of the forearm (Figure 1-17) (Cobb, Dalley, Posteraro & Lewis, 1992).

Cailliet (1994) provides a clear discussion of the anatomy of hand and wrist bones and ligaments that is important to understanding hand disorders other than median neuropathies.

Terminology: Flexor Retinaculum or Transverse Carpal Ligament?

The transverse carpal ligament attaches to the hook of the hamate and the pisiform on the ulnar side of the hand, and to the scaphoid tubercle, trapezium, and sometimes the radial styloid on the radial side to close the oval-shaped tunnel. The width of the carpal tunnel is minimal (mean, 20 mm) at the level of the hook of the hamate (Cobb, Dalley, Posteraro & Lewis, 1993). The proximal border of the transverse carpal ligament aligns roughly with the distal wrist crease. The transverse carpal ligament ranges from 1 to 2 mm in thickness. Its greatest thickness is over the distal two-thirds of the capitate. At this point, 20 to 25 mm from its proximal origin, the tunnel has its smallest cross-sectional area. Proximally, the attachment of the transverse carpal ligament to the pisiform allows for intermittent laxity of the ligament because the pisiform is a mobile, sesamoid bone (Cailliet, 1994). The pisiform becomes fixed when the flexor carpi ulnaris tendon is taut. Distally the transverse carpal ligament maintains more constant tension.

Traditionally, the terms *transverse carpal ligament* and *flexor retinaculum* have been used synonymously. More recently, Cobb and colleagues (1993) have proposed that the flexor retinaculum includes not only the transverse carpal ligament but also the distal portion of the deep investing fascia of the forearm and palmar aponeurosis between the thenar and hypothenar muscles. Although these fascial structures are thinner than the transverse carpal ligament, they do enclose the tendons and median nerve that run in the carpal tunnel and consist of transversely oriented collagen fibers running parallel to those in the transverse carpal ligament. Histologically, they can be distinguished from the more superfi-

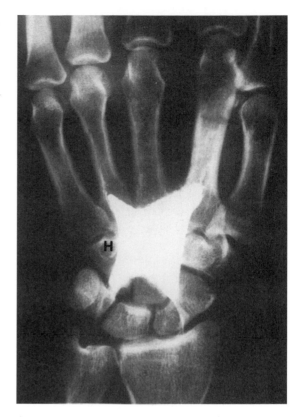

Figure 1-17. Anteroposterior radiograph of the right hand of a cadaver with radiopaque material in the classic carpal tunnel. (H = hook of the hamate.) (Reprinted with permission from TK Cobb, BL Dalley, RH Posteraro, RC Lewis. Anatomy of the flexor retinaculum. J. Hand Surg. 1993;18A:91–99.)

cial palmar fascia, which is continuous with the antebrachial fascia and has longitudinally oriented collagen fibers. Zbrodowski and Gajisin (1988) describe additional details of the anatomy and blood supply of the flexor retinaculum.

Flexor Tendons

Dorsally, the four tendons of the FDP overlie the carpal bones. The four tendons of the flexor digitorum superficialis occupy the volar, medial portion of the tunnel. The sheaths of these eight flexor tendons join to form the ulnar bursa, which extends both proximally and distally to the flexor retinaculum. The flexor pollicis longus tendon is in the volar, lateral position and is contained in a separate radial bursa. The tendon of the flexor carpi radialis adjoins the dorsal lateral

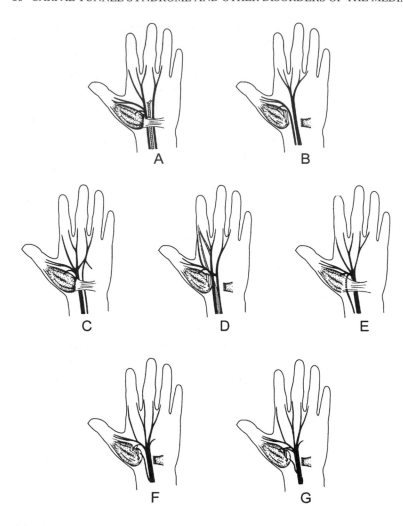

Figure 1-18. Anomalous median nerve variations within the carpal tunnel. **(A)** High division of the median nerve with median artery. **(B)** High division of the median nerve with larger ulnar portion (Kessler, 1969). **(C)** High division of the median nerve with smaller ulnar portion (Winkelman & Spinner, 1973). **(D)** High division of the median nerve with accessory lumbrical muscle between the two branches (Schultz, Endler & Huddleston, 1973). **(E)** Accessory branch proximal to the carpal tunnel (Ogden, 1972). **(F)** Accessory branch proximal to the carpal tunnel perforating the transverse carpal ligament. **(G)** Accessory branch from the ulnar aspect of the median nerve proximal to the carpal tunnel. (Redrawn with permission from U Lanz. The Carpal Tunnel Syndrome. In R Tubiana [ed], The Hand. Philadelphia: Saunders, 1993;463–86.)

border of the tunnel; the flexor retinaculum divides as it makes its radial attachments to form a separate passage outside the carpal tunnel for this tendon.

Median Nerve in the Carpal Tunnel

The median nerve is normally just dorsal to the flexor retinaculum, superficial to the flexor pollicis longus tendon laterally and the flexor digitorum superficialis tendons medially. The tendons of flexor digitorum superficialis to the index and middle fingers are the tendons closest to the median nerve and can indent its dorsal surface (Lanz, 1993). As the nerve enters the tunnel, it is shaped as a flattened ellipse with its anterior-posterior diameter roughly one-half of its medial-lateral diameter (Tanzer, 1959; Middleton et al., 1987). Its dimensions can increase slightly between the proximal and distal ends of the tunnel.

There are many known patterns of median nerve branching within or just proximal or distal to the carpal tunnel (Figure 1-18; see also Figures 1-9, 1-10). Lanz (1977) divided these into four groups:

1. Variations of the recurrent motor branch. (These have been discussed in the section on the recurrent thenar motor branch; see Figures 1-9 and 1-10.)
2. Accessory branches in or just beyond the distal carpal tunnel (see Figure 1-10).

3. High division of the median nerve (see Figure 1-18).
4. Accessory branches proximal to the carpal tunnel (see Figure 1-18).

The multiple complex anomalies can combine; an example is a median nerve that divided in the forearm around a median artery, gave off the palmar cutaneous branch more proximally than normal, gave off the medial common digital nerve in the forearm, rejoined in a ring around the median artery, then distally had a double recurrent thenar branch (Sañudo, Chikwe & Evans, 1994). The prevalences vary depending on whether the data comes from cadaver dissections or surgical series, on the care of the dissector, and on the definitions used for anatomic structures. For example, a recent series found that more than 20% of hands had a sensory branch arising from the nerve in the carpal tunnel, piercing the flexor retinaculum, and apparently innervating carpal bones and joints; yet this variation had not been described in numerous other studies of median nerve anatomy (Steinberg, Luger, Taitz & Arensburg, 1998). These minor anatomic details are highly important to the surgeon who wishes to avoid inadvertent nerve injury.

Variations in Canal Contents

A number of anatomic variations of the carpal tunnel contents are known (Tountas, Bihrle, MacDonald & Bergman, 1987). The incidence of these variations differs from series to series, and is, as expected, higher in cadaver studies than in surgical series, because the former allow a more thorough search for variations. At times the anomalies are visible by wrist MRI (Pierre-Jerome, Bekkelund, Husby, Mellgren, Osteaux & Nordstrom, 1996).

Extra structures within the tunnel, or anomalous arrangements of normal structures, can decrease volume available for the median nerve and increase the possibility of nerve compression. A persistent median artery can enter the tunnel with the median nerve. At times the nerve divides around the artery. The superficial palmar branch of the radial artery rarely runs through the carpal tunnel (Olave, Prates, Gabrielli, Del Sol & Mandiola, 1996). The lumbrical muscles typically originate off the FDP tendons distal to the tunnel but, on occasion, lumbrical muscles can originate within the tunnel (Siegel, Kuzma & Eakins, 1995). The distal muscle bellies of flexor digitorum superficialis or profundus can extend into the proximal portion of the tunnel; this occurs more often in women than in men (Holtzhausen, Constant & de Jager, 1998). Tendons of flexor digitorum superficialis or flexor pollicis longus occasionally interpose between the median nerve and flexor retinaculum. Presence of both the median and ulnar nerves within the carpal tunnel is a very unusual anomaly (Eskesen, Rosenrn & Osgaard, 1981; Galzio, Magliani, Lucantoni & D'Arrigo, 1987; Tyrdal, Solheim & Alho, 1997). Chapter 6 reviews anomalous contents of the carpal canal that have been reported in patients with carpal tunnel syndrome.

Digital Nerve Relationships

Sunderland (1978) and Schultz and Kaplan (1984) provide detailed descriptions of the courses of the digital nerves. The two medial common digital branches of the median nerve travel into the palm between metacarpals accompanied by flexor tendons and blood vessels. At the metacarpal heads, a "digital tunnel" is formed by deep and superficial metacarpal ligaments connecting adjoining metacarpals. The digital nerves are particularly vulnerable to entrapment or traumatic injury at this point.

In the fingers each proper digital nerve runs in a neurovascular bundle with the digital artery and a small venous plexus lateral to the tendon sheath (Eaton, 1968).

Intraneural Anatomy

The median nerve has the histologic arrangement typical of a peripheral nerve (Figure 1-19) (Sunderland, 1991). The nerve consists of multiple nerve fiber fascicles surrounded by connective tissue or epineurium. The fascicles are loosely bound by the collagenous epineurium. An extensive network of arterioles, venules, and lymphatics provides circulation within the epineurium. In the median nerve the ratio of connective tissue to neuronal tissue varies so that the fascicles can occupy 25% to 71% percent of the cross-sectional area of

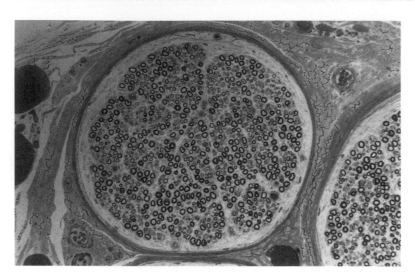

Figure 1-19. Cross-sectional photomicrograph of normal human nerve trunk, showing abundant large- and small-caliber myelinated fibers scattered randomly in the endoneurium. Unmyelinated fibers are not discerned by optic microscopy. The structure of endoneurial capillaries appears normal. A perineurial sheath defines the fascicle. Maximum diameter of myelinated fibers is 15 μm.

the nerve (Sunderland, 1978). This ratio changes from person to person and also along the course of an individual nerve.

Each fascicle is encased in a tighter cellular and connective tissue sheath, the perineurium. Capillaries are the chief blood vessels within the perineurium. Sunderland (1945, 1978) provides extensive data on the intraneural topography of median nerve fascicles. Figure 1-20 is an example of the fascicular anatomy of the nerve shortly before its terminal branching. Sunderland (1945, 1978) and Bonnel and colleagues

(1980, 1981) found abundant intermingling of fascicles as the nerve courses from neck to hand and variation in the number of fascicles along the course of the nerve. Sunderland assumed that these fascicular changes implied extensive nerve fiber crossover.

Sunderland's description of intraneural anatomy is based on serial sections of a single median nerve and does not allow tracing of individual nerve fibers along the fascicles. A computer-aided study of serial sections of 30 median nerves suggests that fascicular integrity is maintained over

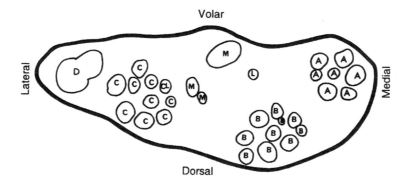

Figure 1-20. Fascicular anatomy of the median nerve at the distal end of the carpal tunnel. (A = cutaneous fibers from the third interspace; B = cutaneous fibers from the second interspace; C = cutaneous fibers from the first interspace; D = cutaneous fibers from the radial side of the thumb; L = lumbrical fibers; M = thenar muscle fibers.) (Reprinted with permission from S Sunderland. The intraneural topography of the radial, median and ulnar nerves. Brain 1945;68:243–98; and S Sunderland. The Median Nerve. Anatomical and Physiological Considerations. In Nerves and Nerve Injuries [2nd ed]. Edinburgh U.K.: Churchill Livingstone, 1978;674.)

long portions of the nerve (Watchmaker, Gumucio, Crandall, Vannier & Weeks, 1991). Microelectrode studies of median and ulnar nerve function suggest that despite interfascicular connections, each fascicle maintains a substantial degree of independence in fiber contents. Tactile stimulation of the fingers elicits electrical responses in individual fascicles at the wrist corresponding to the sensory distribution of single or adjacent digital nerves (Hagbarth, Hongell, Hallin & Torebjörk, 1970). Microstimulation of nerve fascicles in the distal upper arm shows that most of the cutaneous sensory fibers within a fascicle at this level innervate the cutaneous territory of a single digital nerve (Schady, Ochoa, Torebjörk & Chen, 1983; Marchettini, Cline & Ochoa, 1990). Much of the organization of the nerve into distinct motor and sensory territories occurs at the level of the brachial plexus, rather than through interfascicular connections.

The fascicles destined for a nerve branch are distinctly separate from other fascicles for some distance before the actual branching occurs. For example, the fascicles containing fibers for the anterior interosseous nerve are distinct from the rest of the median nerve at the level of the cords of the brachial plexus (Sunderland, 1945). The fascicles destined for the anterior interosseous nerve run on the dorsal medial aspect of median nerve as it travels through the antecubital space, and these fascicles can be microdissected free as a nerve bundle with its own epineurium separate from the remainder of the median nerve 93 mm or more proximal to the medial humeral epicondyle (Jabaley, Wallace & Heckler, 1980). The fascicles destined for the common digital nerve to the third web space run on the medial aspect of the median nerve (see Figure 1-20); when dissected free as high as 21 cm proximal to the radial styloid, the fascicle for the common digital nerve has only a few interconnections with the remainder of the median nerve (Ross, Mackinnon & Chang, 1992).

Analysis of distal partial nerve injuries supports the anatomic and microelectrode data on fascicular arrangement (Perotto & Delagi, 1979). There is great individual variation in the arrangement of fascicles within the nerve, so it is difficult to predict the nature of the neurologic deficit caused by injury to only a portion of the nerve (Bonnel et al., 1980). For example, in partial nerve injuries at the wrist studied by Perotto and Delagi (1979), fascicles to the lumbricales appeared more dorsally located than Sunderland predicted.

At first glance, this intraneural detail seems of little practical import; however, variations in fascicular anatomy are among the factors that determine the probability of neural regeneration after transection and suture. A practical application is harvest of individual nerve fascicles which form the common digital nerve to the third web space as a donor nerve graft (Ross et al., 1992). In theory, the arrangement of fascicles and connective tissue within the nerve might affect the susceptibility of the nerve to compression, but we are unaware of data linking individual variations in intraneural topography to the risk of developing carpal tunnel syndrome or other compression neuropathies in humans.

Vascular Supply of the Median Nerve

In the axilla and upper arm, the median nerve receives its blood supply from the accompanying axillary and brachial arteries. In the forearm and hand, the vascular supply is variable but fits into three basic patterns (Pecket, Gloobe & Nathan, 1973). The common pattern, found in 70% of cadavers studied, is for the radial and ulnar arteries to supply the median nerve via multiple anastomotic branches that feed a small artery adjoining the anterior surface of the nerve. In the palm, the nerve and its branches receive blood from the superficial arterial arch (Gajisin & Zbrodowski, 1993).

In 10% of cadavers, a persistent median artery arises from the brachial artery and accompanies the median nerve in the forearm and through the carpal tunnel. The median artery is usually present only in the fetus. When a well-developed median artery persists, anastomoses between the radial and ulnar arteries are poorly developed, and the superficial palmar arterial arch is absent.

Twenty percent of cadavers exhibit an intermediate pattern: The median artery is present but often incompletely developed, and the superficial palmar arch and other contributions from the radial and ulnar arteries are also present.

Variations of Median Nerve Branching

Tountas and Bergman (1993) have provided an elegant compilation of anatomic variations of the upper extremity. A number of variations in median nerve anatomy are clinically important (all of these, except the first two, have been discussed previously):

1. Median-ulnar communications in the forearm
2. The all-ulnar hand without communications in the forearm
3. Variations in the course of the palmar cutaneous nerve
4. Anomalous patterns within the carpal tunnel
5. Median-ulnar sensory connections in the hand
6. Variable courses of the recurrent thenar motor branch
7. Variations in median and ulnar innervation of the hand intrinsic muscles
8. Anomalous structures crossing the median nerve in the antecubital space and forearm
9. Musculocutaneous nerve–median nerve connections

Median-Ulnar Communications in the Forearm

Martin-Gruber Anastomosis

The most common clinically relevant variation in hand and forearm innervation is the crossing of motor nerve fibers from the median nerve to the ulnar nerve in the forearm (Figures 1-21 and 1-22). This variation is known as the *Martin-Gruber anastomosis*. The incidence has been reported to be 10% to 40% percent of median nerves (Thomson, 1893; Mannerfelt, 1966; Amoiridis, 1992; Taams, 1997; Shu, Chantelot, Oberlin, Alnot & Shao, 1999). The anastomosis was present in 15% of normal fetuses (Srinivasan & Rhodes, 1981). The crossing fibers can supply hypothenar, thenar, or interosseous muscles; the adductor pollicis and first dorsal interosseous are the mus-

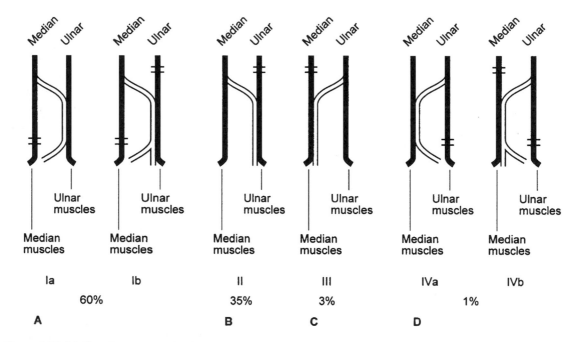

Figure 1-21. Median-ulnar communications in the forearm. Types I and II **(A,B)** are traditional forms of Martin-Gruber anastomosis. Types III and IV **(C,D)** are variants of ulnar to median communications in the forearm. The percentages show the relative prevalence of these anomalies but do not include the majority pattern of nonanomalous innervation. (Adapted with permission from SJ Leibovic, H Hastings II. Martin-Gruber revisited. J. Hand Surg. 1992;17A:47–53; as drawn in CP Tountas, RA Bergman. Anatomic Variations of the Upper Extremity. New York: Churchill Livingstone, 1993.)

Figure 1-22. The fibers of the Martin-Gruber anastomosis carry fibers from the median nerve to the ulnar nerve in the forearm. In the most common pattern, the median nerve fibers travel with the anterior interosseous nerve. A number of other variations are shown. (Redrawn with permission from R Srinivasan, J Rhodes. The median-ulnar anastomosis [Martin-Gruber] in normal and congenitally abnormal fetuses. Arch. Neurol. 1981;38:418–19.)

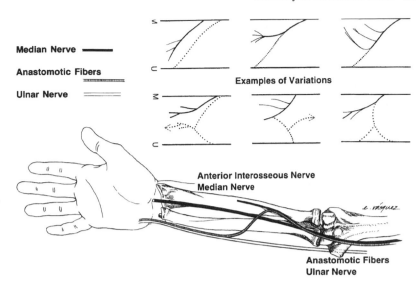

cles most likely to receive innervation via a Martin-Gruber anastomosis (see Table 7-8) (Spinner, 1978; Sun & Streib, 1983). Leibovic and Hastings (1992) classify Martin-Gruber anastomoses as category Ia when the anastomotic fibers supply only muscles normally innervated by the median nerve, as category Ib when the anastomotic fibers supply both traditional median and ulnar muscles, and as category II when the anastomotic fibers supply only muscles normally innervated by the ulnar nerve. Usually the crossing fibers originate from the distal anterior interosseus nerve rather than from the median nerve proper, but a number of other branching patterns are described (Shu et al., 1999):

1. Branching from the proximal anterior interosseous nerve to the ulnar nerve
2. Branching directly from median to ulnar nerve
3. Branching from the median branch to flexor digitorum superficialis
4. Branching from the anterior interosseous nerve to the branch of the ulnar nerve innervating FDP (Nakashima, 1993)
5. Branching from the anterior interosseous nerve then bifurcating to join the ulnar nerve at more than one site (Thomson, 1893; Srinivasan & Rhodes, 1981)

A survey of the incidence of the Martin-Gruber anastomosis using nerve conduction tests suggests

that the anomaly is inherited as an autosomal dominant pattern in some families (Crutchfield & Gutmann, 1980). The Martin-Gruber anastomosis can lead to unusual sparing of muscles after proximal ulnar nerve injuries or, conversely, to unexpectedly widespread denervation after proximal median nerve injuries (Lum & Kanakamedala, 1986). For example, a patient with leprosy developed a combination of complete distal median and proximal ulnar neuropathies (Brandsma, Birke & Sims, 1986). Median-innervated thenar muscles and ulnar-innervated forearm muscles were paretic, but because of a Martin-Gruber anastomosis, there was sparing of some intrinsic hand muscles, the nerve fibers of which crossed the antecubital space with the median nerve and then crossed the wrist with the ulnar nerve.

Electromyographic detection of the Martin-Gruber anastomosis and its potential effects in the presence of carpal tunnel syndrome are covered in Chapter 7.

Median-to-Ulnar Sensory Crossovers in the Forearm

Median-to-ulnar sensory crossover proximal to the wrist is extremely rare. In one reported case, fibers left the median nerve proximal to the wrist, passed to the ulnar nerve, and appeared to carry sensory fibers for cutaneous sensation of the little finger (Saeed & Davies, 1995).

The Martin-Gruber anastomosis usually carries motor but not sensory fibers (Valls-Solé, 1991). However, there are least two examples of Martin-Gruber anastomosis in which sensory fibers from the middle or little fingers leave the hand with the ulnar nerve and cross to the median nerve in the forearm (Santoro, Rosato & Caruso, 1983; Claussen, Ahmad, Sunwoo & Oh, 1996). Another patient had carpal tunnel syndrome, Martin-Gruber anastomosis, and sensory fibers from the middle finger traveling with the ulnar nerve across the wrist and elbow (Simonetti & Krarup, 2000).

Ulnar-to-Median Crossovers in the Forearm

Ulnar-to-median crossovers in the forearm are also very rare. Marinacci (1964b) described a case of median nerve transection in the forearm with denervation of median-innervated forearm muscles but preservation of all hand intrinsic muscles. Nerve stimulation showed that nerve fibers destined for thenar muscles traveled with the ulnar nerve at the elbow but crossed the wrist at the usual location for the median nerve. Ulnar-to-median anastomosis in the forearm can be discovered as an incidental finding on nerve conduction studies or during forearm surgery (Streib, 1979; Stancic, Burgic & Micovic, 2000).

At times, ulnar-to-median connections are an incidental anatomic finding of unknown functional import. An example is an instance of fibers running from the ulnar nerve and from its dorsal cutaneous branch to the median nerve (Hoogbergen & Kauer, 1992). However, if noted during life, minor anomalies can be clarified by clever use of nerve blocks and nerve conduction testing. Hopf (1990) reported a case of ulnar-to-median sensory crossover in the forearm. After ulnar nerve block at the elbow, the patient had sensory loss not only in the little finger and ulnar side of the ring finger, but also in the radial side of the ring finger and ulnar side of the middle finger. Electrical stimulation of the digital nerves on the radial side of the ring finger or ulnar side of the middle finger elicited a sensory nerve action potential over the median nerve at the wrist (but not in the antecubital space) and over the ulnar nerve at the elbow (but not at the wrist). The patient had no evidence of crossover of motor fibers.

Collision studies of sensory conduction in another patient with the same anomalous sensory pattern suggested that in some patients the nerve fibers to the radial side of the ring finger and ulnar side of the middle finger took a different anomalous course, traveling with the ulnar nerve across the wrist and through the forearm (Valls-Solé, 1991).

All-Ulnar Motor Hand without Martin-Gruber Anastomosis

There a few reported instances of an *all-ulnar hand* demonstrated by nerve conduction studies (Ganes, 1992; Rao, LaMarche, Gutmann & Gutmann, 1995; Sachs, Raynor & Shefner, 1995). These individuals have no motor responses in any hand intrinsic muscles to median nerve stimulation in the wrist or antecubital space. Stimulation of the ulnar nerve anywhere along its course activates all hand intrinsic muscles. A variation on this theme is ulnar supply of all thenar muscles, while the median nerve still supplies the first lumbrical (LoMonaco, Padua, Gregori, Valente & Tonali, 1997). Ulnar and median sensory studies are normal. The implication is that motor fibers that would normally travel in the median nerve instead run from the medial cord of the brachial plexus with the ulnar nerve. Theoretically, once the ulnar nerve enters the hand, the motor fibers for the thenar muscles could rejoin the median nerve via a Riche-Cannieu anastomosis or travel directly to the thenar muscles. Because some degree of Riche-Cannieu anastomosis is a frequent occurrence, whereas direct innervation of thenar muscle by the deep branch of the ulnar nerve is unreported, the former hypothesis is more plausible.

References

Ajmani ML. Variations in the motor nerve supply of the thenar and hypothenar muscles of the hand. J. Anat. 1996;189: 145–50.

al-Qattan MM. Gantzer's muscle. J. Hand Surg. 1996; 21B:269–70.

al-Qattan MM. Anatomical classification of sites of compression of the palmar cutaneous branch of the median nerve. J. Hand Surg. 1997;22B:48–49.

Amoiridis G. Median-ulnar nerve communications and anomalous innervation of the intrinsic hand muscles: an electrophysiological study. Muscle Nerve 1992;15:576–79.

Bas H, Kleinert JM. Anatomic variations in sensory innervation of the hand and digits. J. Hand Surg. 1999;24A:1171–84.

Basar R, Aldur MM, Celik HH, Yuksel M, Tascioglu AB. A connecting branch between the musculocutaneous nerve and the median nerve. Morphologie 2000;84:25–27.

Beaton LE, Anson BJ. The relation of the median nerve to the pronator teres muscle. Anat. Rec. 1939;7:23–26.

Bergman FO, Blom SEG, Senström SJ. Radical excision of a fibro-fatty proliferation of the median nerve, with no neurological loss symptoms. Plast. Reconstr. Surg. 1970;46:375–80.

Bezerra AJ, Carvalho VC, Nucci A. An anatomical study of the palmar cutaneous branch of the median nerve, including a description of its own unique tunnel. J. Hand Surg. 1986;18B:316–17.

Bonnel F. Fascicular organization of the peripheral nerves. Int. J. Microsurg. 1981;3:85–92.

Bonnel F, Foucher G, Saint-Andre J-M. Histologic structure of the palmar digital nerves of the hand and its application to nerve grafting. J. Hand Surg. 1989;14A:874–81.

Bonnel F, Mailhe P, Allieu Y, Rabischong P. Bases anatomiques de la chirurgie fasciculaire du nerf médian au poignet. Ann. Chir. 1980;9:707–10.

Brandsma JW, Birke JA, Sims J D.S. The Martin-Gruber innervated hand. J. Hand Surg. 1986;11A:536–39.

Cailliet R. Hand Pain and Impairment (4th ed). Philadelphia: F. A. Davis, 1994.

Campero M, Verdugo RJ, Ochoa JL. Vasomotor innervation of the skin of the hand: a contribution to the study of human anatomy. J. Anat. 1993;182:361–68.

Canovas F, Mouilleron P, Bonnel F. Biometry of the muscular branches of the median nerve to the forearm. Clin. Anat. 1998;11:239–45.

Chantelot C, Feugas C, Guillem P, Chapnikoff D, Remy F, Fontaine C. Innervation of the medial epicondylar muscles: an anatomic study in 50 cases. Surg. Radiol. Anat. 1999;21:165–68.

Chidgey LK, Szabo RM. Anterior Interosseous Nerve Palsy. In RM Szabo (ed), Nerve Compression Syndromes: Diagnosis and Treatment. Thorofare, NJ: SLACK Inc., 1989;153–62.

Chow SP. Digital nerves in the terminal phalangeal region of the thumb. Hand 1980;12:193–96.

Claussen GC, Ahmad BK, Sunwoo IN, Oh SJ. Combined motor and sensory median-ulnar anastomosis: report of an electrophysiologically proven case. Muscle Nerve 1996;19:231–33.

Cobb TK, Dalley BK, Posteraro RH, Lewis RC. The carpal tunnel as a compartment. An anatomic perspective. Ortho. Rev. 1992;21:451–53.

Cobb TK, Dalley BK, Posteraro RH, Lewis RC. Anatomy of the flexor retinaculum. J. Hand Surg. 1993;18A:91–99.

Cone RO, Sabo R, Resnick D, Gelberman R, Taleisnik J, Gilula LA. Computed tomography of the normal soft tissues of the wrist. Invest. Radiol. 1983;18:546–51.

Crutchfield CA, Gutmann L. Hereditary aspects of median-ulnar nerve communications. J. Neurol. Neurosurg. Psychiatry 1980;43:53–55.

Das SK, Brown HG. In search of complications in carpal tunnel decompression. Hand 1976;8:243–49.

DaSilva MF, Moore DC, Weiss AP, Akelman E, Sikirica M. Anatomy of the palmar cutaneous branch of the median nerve: clinical significance. J. Hand Surg. 1996;21A:639–43.

Dellon AL. Evaluation of Sensibility and Re-Education of Sensation in the Hand. Baltimore: Williams & Wilkins, 1981.

Dellon AL. Musculotendinous variations about the medial humeral epicondyle. J. Hand Surg. 1986;11B:175–81.

Dellon AL, Mackinnon SE. Musculoaponeurotic variations along the course of the median nerve in the proximal forearm. J. Hand Surg. 1987;12B:359–63.

Don Griot JPW, Zuidam JM, van Kooten EO, Prose LP, Hage JJ. Anatomic study of the ramus communicans between the ulnar and median nerves. J. Hand Surg. 2000;25A:948–54.

Dowdy PA, Richards RS, McFarlane RM. The palmar cutaneous branch of the median nerve and the palmaris longus tendon: a cadaveric study. J. Hand Surg. 1994;19A:199–202.

Eaton RG. The digital neurovascular bundle. Clin. Orthop. 1968;61:176–85.

Eglseder WA Jr, Goldman M. Anatomic variations of the musculocutaneous nerve in the arm. Am. J. Orthop. 1997;26:777–80.

Entin MA. Carpal tunnel syndrome and its variants. Surg. Clin. North Am. 1968;48:1097–1112.

Eskesen V, Rosenrn J, Osgaard O. Atypical carpal tunnel syndrome with compression of the ulnar and median nerves. Case report. J. Neurosurg. 1981;54:668–69.

Falconer D, Spinner M. Anatomic variations in the motor and sensory supply of the thumb. Clin. Orthop. 1985;195:83–96.

Ferrari GP, Gilbert A. The superficial anastomosis on the palm of the hand between the ulnar and median nerves. J. Hand Surg. 1991;16B:511–14.

Ferreres A, Suso S, Ordi J, Llusa M, Ruano D. Wrist denervation. Anatomical considerations. J. Hand Surg. 1995;20B:761–68.

Fetrow KO. Practical and important variations in sensory nerve supply to the hand. Hand 1970;2:178–84.

Forrest WJ. Motor innervation of human thenar and hypothenar muscles in 25 hands: a study combining electromyography and percutaneous nerve stimulation. Can. J. Surg. 1967;10:196–99.

Gajisin S, Zbrodowski A. Local vascular contribution of the superficial palmar arch. Acta Anat. (Basel) 1993;147:248–51.

Galzio RJ, Magliani V, Lucantoni D, D'Arrigo C. Bilateral anomalous course of the ulnar nerve at the wrist causing ulnar and median nerve compression syndromes. J. Neurosurg. 1987;67:754–56.

Ganes T. Complete ulnar innervation of the thenar muscles combined with normal sensory fibres in a subject with no peripheral nerve lesion. Electromyogr. Clin. Neurophysiol. 1992;32:559–63.

Gessini L, Jandolo B, Pietrangeli A. Entrapment neuropathies of the median nerve at and above the elbow. Surg. Neurol. 1983;19:112–16.

Gumusburun E, Adiguzel E. A variation of the brachial plexus characterized by the absence of the musculocutaneous nerve: a case report. Surg. Radiol. Anat. 2000;22:63–65.

Gunther SF, DiPasquale D, Martin R. Struthers' ligament and associated median nerve variations in a cadaveric specimen. Yale J. Biol. Med. 1993;66:203–8.

Hagbarth K-E, Hongell A, Hallin RG, Torebjörk HE. Afferent impulses in median nerve fascicles evoked by tactile stimuli of the human hand. Brain Res. 1970;24:423–42.

Harness D, Sekeles E. The double anastomotic innervation of thenar muscles. J. Anat. 1971;109:461–66.

Hirasawa Y, Sakakida K, Tokioka T, Ohta Y. An investigation of the digital nerves of the thumb. Clin. Orthop. 1985;198: 191–96.

Hobbs RA, Magnussen PA, Tonkin MA. Palmar cutaneous branch of the median nerve. J. Hand Surg. 1990;15A:38–43.

Holtzhausen LM, Constant D, de Jager W. The prevalence of flexor digitorum superficialis and profundus muscle bellies beyond the proximal limit of the carpal tunnel: a cadaveric study. J. Hand Surg. 1998;23A:32–37.

Hoogbergen MM, Kauer JM. An unusual ulnar nerve-median nerve communicating branch. J. Anat. 1992;181(3):513–16.

Hopf HC. Forearm ulnar-to-median nerve anastomosis of sensory axons. Muscle Nerve 1990;13:654–6.

Hurwitz PJ. Variations in the course of the thenar motor branch of the median nerve. J. Hand Surg. 1996;21B:344–46.

Ihunwo AO, Osinde SP, Mukhtar AU. Distribution of median nerve to muscles of the anterior compartment of the arm. Cent. Afr. J. Med. 1997;43:359–60.

Jabaley ME, Wallace WH, Heckler FR. Internal topography of major nerves of the forearm and hand: a current view. J. Hand Surg. 1980;5:1–18.

Jakubowicz M, Ratajczak W. Variation in morphology of the biceps brachii and coracobrachialis muscles associated with abnormal course of blood vessels and nerves. Folia Morphol. (Warsz.) 2000;58:255–58.

Jessurun W, Hillen B, Zonneveld F, Huffstadt AJ, Beks JW, Overbeek W. Anatomical relations in the carpal tunnel: a computed tomographic study. J. Hand Surg. 1987;12B:64–67.

Johnson RK, Shrewsbury MM. Anatomical course of the thenar branch of the median nerve–usually in a separate tunnel through the transverse carpal ligament. J. Bone Joint Surg. 1970;52A:269–73.

Johnson RK, Spinner M. Median Nerve Compression in the Forearm: The Pronator Tunnel Syndrome. In RM Szabo (ed), Nerve Compression Syndromes: Diagnosis and Treatment. Thorofare, NJ: SLACK Inc., 1989;137–52.

Johnson RK, Spinner M, Shrewsbury MM. Median nerve entrapment syndrome in the proximal forearm. J. Hand Surg. 1979;4:48–51.

Jolley BJ, Stern PJ, Starling T. Patterns of median nerve sensory innervation to the thumb and index finger: an anatomic study. J. Hand Surg. 1997;22A:228–31.

Kaplan EB, Spinner M. Normal and Anomalous Innervation Patterns in the Upper Extremity. In GE Omer Jr, M Spinner (eds), Management of Peripheral Nerve Problems. Philadelphia: Saunders, 1980;75–99.

Kaus M, Wotowicz Z. Communicating branch between the musculocutaneous and median nerves in human. Folia Morphol. (Warsz.) 1995;54:273–77.

Kendall FP, McCreary EK, Provance PG. Muscles: Testing and Function (4th ed). Baltimore: Williams & Wilkins, 1993.

Kerr AT. The brachial plexus of nerves in man, the variations in its formation and branches. Am. J. Anat. 1918;23:285–395.

Kessel L, Rang M. Supracondylar spur of the humerus. J. Bone Joint Surg. 1966;48:765–69.

Kessler I. Unusual distribution of the median nerve at the wrist. Clin. Orthop. 1969;67:124–26.

Kimura I, Ayyar DR, Lippmann SM. Electrophysiological verification of the ulnar to median nerve communications in the hand and forearm. Tohoku J. Exp. Med. 1983; 141:269–74.

Kozin SH. The anatomy of the recurrent branch of the median nerve. J. Hand Surg. 1998;23A:852–58.

Lanz U. Anatomical variations of the median nerve in the carpal tunnel. J. Hand. Surg 1977;2:44–53.

Lanz U. The Carpal Tunnel Syndrome. In R Tubiana (ed), The Hand. Philadelphia: Saunders, 1993;463–86.

Lauritzen RS, Szabo RM, Lauritzen DB. Innervation of the lumbrical muscles. J. Hand Surg. 1996;21B:57–58.

Leibovic SJ, Hastings II H. Martin-Gruber revisited. J. Hand Surg. 1992;17A:47–53.

Le Minor JM. A rare variation of the median and musculocutaneous nerves in man. Arch. Anat. Histol. Embryol. 1990;73: 33–42.

Levin KH, Maggiano HJ, Wilbourn AJ. Cervical radiculopathies: comparison of surgical and EMG localization of single-root lesions. Neurology 1996;46:1022–25.

Linburg RM, Albright JA. An anomalous branch of the median nerve. A case report. J. Bone Joint Surg. 1970;52:182–83.

LoMonaco M, Padua L, Gregori B, Valente EM, Tonali P. Ulnar innervation of the thenar eminence with preservation of median innervation of first lumbrical muscle. Muscle Nerve 1997;20:629–30.

Lum PB, Kanakamedala R. Conduction of the palmar cutaneous branch of the median nerve. Arch. Phys. Med. Rehabil. 1986;67:805–6.

Mannerfelt L. Studies on the hand in ulnar nerve paralysis. Acta. Orthop. Scand. 1966;S87:1–176.

Mannerfelt L, Hybbinette CH. Important anomaly of the thenar motor branch of the median nerve. A clinical and anatomical report. Bull. Hosp. Joint Dis. 1972;33:15–21.

Marchettini P, Cline M, Ochoa JL. Innervation territories for touch and pain afferents of single fascicles of the human ulnar nerve. Brain 1990;113:1491–1500.

Marinacci AA. Diagnosis of "all median hand." Bull. L. A. Neur. Soc. 1964a;29:191–97.

Marinacci AA. The problem of unusual anomalous innervation of hand muscles. Bull. L. A. Neur. Soc. 1964b;29:133–42.

Martin CH, Seiler JG 3rd, Lesesne JS. The cutaneous innervation of the palm: an anatomic study of the ulnar and median nerves. J. Hand Surg. 1996;21A:634–38.

Martinelli P, Gabellini AS, Poppi M, Gallassi R, Pozzati E. Pronator syndrome due to thickened bicipital aponeurosis. J. Neurol. Neurosurg. Psychiatry 1982;45:181–82.

Meals RA, Shaner M. Variations in digital sensory patterns: a study of the ulnar nerve-median nerve palmar communicating branch. J. Hand Surg. 1983;8:411–14.

Megele R. Anterior interosseous nerve syndrome with atypical nerve course in relation to the pronator teres. Acta. Neurochir. (Wien). 1988;91:144–46.

Mesgarzadeh M, Schneck CD, Bonakdarpour A. Carpal tunnel: MR imaging part I. Normal anatomy. Radiology 1989;171: 743–48.

Middleton WD, Kneeland JB, Kellman GM, Cates JD, Sanger JR, Jesmanowicz A, Froncisz W, Hyde JS. MR imaging of the carpal tunnel: normal anatomy and preliminary findings in the carpal tunnel syndrome. AJR. Am. J. Roentgenol. 1987;148:307–16.

Mumenthaler M, Schliak H (eds). Peripheral Nerve Lesions. New York: Thieme, 1991.

Mumford J, Morecraft R, Blair WF. Anatomy of the thenar branch of the median nerve. J. Hand Surg. 1987;12A:361–65.

Naff N, Dellon AL, Mackinnon SE. The anatomical course of the palmar cutaneous branch of the median nerve, including a description of its own unique tunnel. J. Hand Surg. 1993;18B:316–17.

Nakashima T. An anatomic study on the Martin-Gruber anastomosis. Surg. Radiol. Anat. 1993;15:193–95.

Nebot-Cegarra J, Perez-Berruezo J, Reina de la Torre F. Variations of the pronator teres muscle: predispositional role to median nerve entrapment. Archives d'Anatomie, d'Histologie et d'Embryologie 1991–92;74:35–45.

Ogden JA. An unusual branch of the median nerve. J. Bone Joint Surg. 1972;54:1779–81.

Olave E, Prates JC, Del Sol M, Sarmento A, Gabrielli C. Distribution patterns of the muscular branch of the median nerve in the thenar region. J. Anat. 1995;186:441–46.

Olave E, Prates JC, Gabrielli C, Del Sol M, Mandiola E. Abnormal course of the superficial palmar branch of the radial artery. Surg. Radiol. Anat. 1996;18:151–53.

Olave E, Prates JC, Gabrielli C, Pardi P. Morphometric studies of the muscular branch of the median nerve. J. Anat. 1996;189:445–49.

Pecket P, Gloobe H, Nathan H. Variations in the arteries of the median nerve. With special considerations on the ischemic factor in the carpal tunnel syndrome (CTS). Clin. Orthop. 1973;97:144–47.

Perotto AO, Delagi EF. Funicular localization in partial median nerve injury at the wrists. Arch. Phys. Med. Rehabil. 1979;60:165–69.

Pesson CM, Finney TP, Depaolo CJ, Dabezies EJ, Zimny ML. Anatomical demonstration of the nerve-supply to the flexor tendon. J. Hand Surg. 1991;16B:92–93.

Pierre-Jerome C, Bekkelund SI, Husby G, Mellgren SI, Osteaux M, Nordstrom R. MRI of anatomical variants of the wrist in women. Surg. Radiol. Anat. 1996;18:37–41.

Poisel S. Ursprung und verlauf des ramus muscularis des nervus digitalis palmaris communis I (N. medianus). Chir. Praxis 1974;18:471–74.

Rao N, LaMarche D, Gutmann L, Gutmann L. Further observations on all ulnar motor hand due to anomalous routing at the brachial plexus. Muscle Nerve 1995;18:1353.

Robbins H. Anatomical study of the median nerve in the carpal tunnel and etiologies of the carpal-tunnel syndrome. J. Bone Joint Surg. 1963;45A:953–66.

Ross D, Mackinnon SE, Chang YL. Intraneural anatomy of the median nerve provides "third web space" donor nerve graft. J. Reconstr. Microsurg. 1992;8:225–32.

Rowntree T. Anomalous innervation of the hand muscles. J. Bone Joint Surg. 1949;31B:505–10.

Sachs GM, Raynor EM, Shefner JM. The all ulnar motor hand with forearm anastomosis. Muscle Nerve 1995;18: 309–13.

Saeed WR, Davies DM. Sensory innervation of the little finger by an anomalous branch of the median nerve associated with recurrent, atypical carpal tunnel syndrome. J. Hand Surg. 1995;20B:42–43.

Santoro L, Rosato R, Caruso G. Median-ulnar nerve communications: electrophysiological demonstration of motor and sensory fibre cross-over. J. Neurol. 1983;229:227–35.

Sañudo JR, Chikwe J, Evans SE. Anomalous median nerve associated with persistent median artery. J. Anat. 1994;185:447–51.

Sargon MF, Uslu SS, Celik HH, Aksit D. A variation of the median nerve at the level of brachial plexus. Bull. Assoc. Anat. 1995;79:25–26.

Schady W, Ochoa JL, Torebjörk HE, Chen LS. Peripheral projections of fascicles in the human median nerve. Brain 1983;106:745–60.

Schultz RJ, Endler PM, Huddleston HD. Anomalous median nerve and an anomalous muscle belly of the first lumbrical associated with carpal-tunnel syndrome. J. Bone Joint Surg. 1973;55:1744–46.

Schultz RJ, Kaplan EB. Nerve Supply to the Muscles and Skin of the Hand. In M Spinner (ed), Kaplan's Functional and Surgical Anatomy of the Hand (3rd ed). Philadelphia: Lippincott, 1984;222–43.

Schultz RJ, Krishnamurthy S, Johnston AD. A gross anatomic and histologic study of the innervation of the proximal interphalangeal joint. J. Hand Surg. 1984;9A:669–74.

Seradge H, Seradge E. Median innervated hypothenar muscle: anomalous branch of median nerve in the carpal tunnel. J. Hand Surg. 1990;15A:356–59.

Shirali S, Hanson M, Branovacki G, Gonzalez M. The flexor pollicis longus and its relation to the anterior and posterior interosseous nerves. J. Hand Surg. 1998;23B:170–72.

Shu HS, Chantelot C, Oberlin C, Alnot JY, Shao H. Martin-Gruber communicating branch: anatomical and histological study. Surg. Radiol. Anat. 1999;21(2):115–8.

Siegel DB, Kuzma G, Eakins D. Anatomic investigation of the role of the lumbrical muscles in carpal tunnel syndrome. J. Hand Surg. 1995;20A:860–63.

Siegel JL, Davlin LB, Aulicino PL. An anatomical variation of the palmar cutaneous branch of the median nerve. J. Hand Surg. 1993;18B:182–83.

Simonetti S, Krarup C. Unusual ulnar sensory innervation and Martin-Gruber anastomosis in a patient with a carpal tunnel syndrome. J. Neurol. 2000;247:141–42.

Spinner M. The anterior interosseous-nerve syndrome, with special attention to its variations. J. Bone Joint Surg. 1970;52A:84–94.

Spinner M. Injuries to the Major Branches of Peripheral Nerves of the Forearm (2nd ed). Philadelphia: Saunders, 1978.

Spinner M, Schreiber SN. Anterior interosseous-nerve paralysis as a complication of supracondylar fractures of the humerus in children. J. Bone Joint Surg. 1969;51A:1584–90.

Srinivasan R, Rhodes J. The median-ulnar anastomosis (Martin-Gruber) in normal and congenitally abnormal fetuses. Arch. Neurol. 1981;38:418–19.

Stancic MF, Burgic N, Micovic V. Marinacci communication. Case report. J. Neurosurg. 2000;92:860–62.

Stancic MF, Micovic V, Potocnjak M. The anatomy of the Berrettini branch: implications for carpal tunnel release. J. Neurosurg. 1999;91:1027–30.

Steinberg EL, Luger E, Taitz C, Arensburg B. Anatomic variant of the median nerve in the carpal tunnel. Clin. Orthop. 1998;352:128–30.

Stopford JSB. The variation in distribution of the cutaneous nerves of the hand and digits. J. Anat. 1918;53:14–25.

Streib EW. Ulnar-to-median nerve anastomosis in the forearm: electromyographic studies. Neurology 1979;29: 1534–37.

Sun SF, Streib EW. Martin-Gruber anastomosis: electromyographic studies. Electromyogr. Clin. Neurophysiol. 1983;23: 271–85.

Sunderland S. The intraneural topography of the radial, median and ulnar nerves. Brain 1945;68:243–98.

Sunderland S. The Median Nerve. Anatomical and Physiological Considerations. In Nerves and Nerve Injuries (2nd ed). Edinburgh U.K.: Churchill Livingstone, 1978;656–90.

Sunderland S. Nerve Injuries and Their Repair. Edinburgh: Churchill Livingstone, 1991.

Suranyi L. Median nerve compression by Struther's ligament. J. Neurol. Neurosurg. Psychiatry 1983;46:1047–49.

Taams KO. Martin-Gruber connections in South Africa. An anatomical study. J. Hand Surg. 1997;22B:328–30.

Tanzer RC. The carpal-tunnel syndrome. J. Bone Joint Surg. 1959;41A:626–34.

Thomson A. Third annual report of the committee of collective investigation of the anatomical society of Great Britain and Ireland for the year 1891-92. J. Anat. Physiol. 1893;27:192–94.

Tountas CP, Bergman RA. Anatomic Variations of the Upper Extremity. New York: Churchill Livingstone, 1993.

Tountas CP, Bihrle DM, MacDonald CJ, Bergman RA. Variations of the median nerve in the carpal canal. J. Hand Surg. 1987;12A:708–12.

Tyrdal S, Solheim LF, Alho A. Anomalous nerve anatomy at the wrist? Annales Chir. Gynaecol. 1997;86:79–83.

Valls-Solé J. Martin-Gruber anastomosis and unusual sensory innervation of the fingers: report of a case. Muscle Nerve 1991;14:1099–1102.

Venieratos D, Anagnostopoulou S. Classification of communications between the musculocutaneous and median nerves. Clin Anat 1998;11:327–31.

Wallace WA, Coupland RE. Variations in the nerves of the thumb and index finger. J. Bone Joint Surg. 1975;57A: 491–94.

Watchmaker GP, Gumucio CA, Crandall RE, Vannier MA, Weeks PM. Fascicular topography of the median nerve: a computer based study to identify branching patterns. J. Hand Surg. 1991;16A:53–59.

Watchmaker GP, Weber D, Mackinnon SE. Avoidance of transection of the palmar cutaneous branch of the median nerve in carpal tunnel release. J. Hand Surg. 1996; 21A:644–50.

Winkelman NZ, Spinner M. A variant high sensory branch of the median nerve to the third web space. Bull. Hosp. Joint Dis. 1973;34:161–63.

Woollard HH, Phillips R. The distribution of sympathetic fibres in the extremities. J. Anat. 1932;67:18–26.

Zbrodowski A, Gajisin S. The blood supply of the flexor retinaculum. J. Hand Surg. 1988;13B:35–39.

Zeiss J, Skie M, Ebraheim N, Jackson WT. Anatomic relations between the median nerve and flexor tendons in the carpal tunnel: MR evaluation in normal volunteers. AJR. Am. J. Roentgenol. 1989;153:533–36.

Zenn MR, Hoffman L, Latrenta G, Hotchkiss R. Variations in digital nerve anatomy. J. Hand Surg. 1992; 17A:1033–36.

Zucker-Pinchoff B, Hermann G, Srinivasan R. Computed tomography of the carpal tunnel: a radioanatomical Study. J. Comput. Assist. Tomogr. 1981;5:525–28.

Chapter 2

Historical Understanding of Carpal Tunnel Syndrome

Modern understanding of carpal tunnel syndrome has evolved from a variety of clinical and pathologic observations on median nerve injury after wrist trauma, on thenar atrophy as a consequence of median neuropathy, and on the results of surgical decompression of the median nerve in the carpal tunnel. A unifying insight was the recognition that acroparesthesia, a common, well-known symptom, was often the first manifestation of median nerve compression and could be relieved by carpal tunnel surgery.

Median Neuropathy after Wrist Fracture

In the nineteenth and early twentieth centuries, case reports described median neuropathy caused by nerve compression at the wrist as a complication of distal radial fracture (Blecher 1908, Lewis & Miller, 1922). Paget (1865; p. 50) is frequently credited with one of the first English descriptions:

> A man was at Guy's Hospital, who, in consequence of a fracture at the lower end of the radius, repaired by an excessive quantity of new bone, suffered compression of the median nerve. He had ulceration of the thumb, and fore and middle fingers, which resisted various treatment, and was cured only by so binding the wrist that the parts of the palmar aspect being relaxed, the pressure on the nerve was removed. So long as this was done, the ulcers became and remained well; but as soon as the man was allowed to use his hand, the pressure on the nerves was renewed, and the ulceration of the parts supplied by them returned.

Lewis and Miller (1922) reported an extensive series of traumatic nerve injuries. They included one case of distal median neuropathy, with thenar atrophy and median-distribution hypesthesia, becoming symptomatic 18 years after a reverse Colles' fracture. The distal radial fragment was displaced anteriorly. In 1924, Galloway explored the median nerve in the wrist and proximal palm for a patient who had developed median neuropathy as a delayed sequel of hand trauma (Amadio, 1995).

Abbott and Saunders (1933) classified the types of median nerve injuries that may be associated with distal radial fractures. Type 1, direct injury to the median nerve in the forearm by fractured bone, was very rare. The more common problem was type 2, secondary compression of the median nerve against the proximal edge of the flexor retinaculum by the displaced fracture. Type 3 was delayed median neuropathy appearing as a late sequel after distal radial fracture. Type 4 was median nerve compression exacerbated by treatment of the radial fracture by fixation in palmar flexion.

Zachary (1945) described two patients who developed median neuropathy as a late sequel of fractures. One patient had had a scaphoid fracture; the other patient had a malunited Colles' fracture. Both presented with partial thenar atrophy with minimal median sensory disturbance. In both cases median nerve compression in the carpal tunnel was identified as the cause, and both patients were treated with section of the flexor retinaculum. Zachary explained the sparing of flexor pollicis brevis in his patients by the ulnar innervation of this muscle in some individuals and the paucity of sensory findings by selective vulnerability of different median nerve fibers to trauma. He noted that motor recovery after surgery (done by Professor Herbert Seddon) occurred in the patient who had had symptoms for 15 months but not in the patient who had had thenar paralysis for 14 years.

Thenar Atrophy

Hunt (1911) described a case of thenar atrophy to the American Neurological Association in 1909 and published this case with two others. His patients had atrophy of thenar muscles innervated by the median nerve and no abnormalities on sensory examination. Each patient had done repetitive gripping, and Hunt hypothesized damage to the recurrent motor branch of the median nerve. Today, noting that at least two of his patients went through a period of intermittent hand paresthesia before developing motor signs, we would probably diagnose these patients as having severe carpal tunnel syndrome.

Marie and Foix (1913) described the autopsy results in an 80-year-old woman with bilateral isolated thenar atrophy. They noted normal bulk of the ulnar-innervated thumb adductor and thinning of the median nerve beneath the flexor retinaculum (*ligament annulaire*) with thickening of the median nerve in the distal forearm proximal to the site of constriction. With myelin stains, they demonstrated attenuation of the myelin sheath in the constricted portion of the nerve, suggesting that transection of the flexor retinaculum might have been appropriate treatment if the diagnosis had been made in life. Mumenthaler (1984) has provided an English translation of this paper.

Brouwer (1920) described 15 patients with isolated partial atrophy of thenar muscles. He attributed the localized atrophy to phylogenetic congenital "inferiority" of the thenar muscles with a possible causative role of overuse of the affected muscles.

Moersch (1938) reported a woman with bilateral progressive thenar wasting. He hypothesized damage to the recurrent thenar motor nerve by direct trauma or irritation. He noted that some patients with thenar atrophy also had median sensory symptoms, and he suggested that the median nerve in these patients might be compressed by the flexor retinaculum.

Wartenberg (1939) provided an extensive review of early theories on isolated thenar atrophy, including contributions by Harris (1911), Lhermitte and deMassary (1930), and Dorndorf (1931). He cited the work of Marie and Foix (1913) and Moersch (1938) on the possible pathogenic import of the flexor retinaculum, and he was aware that patients with thenar atrophy might have sensory complaints. Despite his scholarship, he sided with Brouwer (1920), concluding that partial thenar atrophy resulted from "abiotrophy" rather than from median neuropathy.

Acroparesthesias

A distinctive clinical syndrome of periodic hand paresthesias has been recognized for well over a century, even though understanding of its relation to the median nerve is a more recent development. Mitchell (1881), in a chapter on sleep disorders, described transient nocturnal hand paresthesias as "night palsy" or "brachial monoplegia," but included descriptions of patients with more widespread "nocturnal hemiplegia."

Putnam (1880) reported a number of patients with periodically recurring paresthesias of their hands. His clinical description clearly fits that of carpal tunnel syndrome: Hand paresthesias or numbness occurred especially at night or in the early morning, often with associated arm pain. Numbness most prominently affected fingers innervated by the median nerve. The fingers felt stiff at times. Symptoms improved with hanging or shaking the hand. One patient and the mother of another patient noted exacerbation of symptoms during pregnancy. The hands often felt swollen to the patient, but objective swelling was rarely evident. Women were affected much more commonly than were men. Putnam hypothesized that the syndrome was caused by alterations of the distal blood supply of nerves.

Ormerod (1883) in his report, "On a peculiar numbness and paresis of the hands," described 12 women who had intermittent nocturnal hand paresthesias. He recognized that his patients' symptoms were different than those of Raynaud's phenomenon and mentioned the relationship between symptoms and daily hand activities. Sinkler (1884) reported nine similar cases.

Saundby (1885) described some patients who had nocturnal hand paresthesias and other patients who had paresthesias in hands and feet. He attributed the cause to a stomach disorder and ascribed successful treatment to rhubarb powder, peppermint water, subchloride of mercury, and bromide of potassium. He credited Handfield Jones—who in 1870 diagnosed the syndrome as brachial neuralgia—among his predecessors who had considered this disorder.

Schultze (1893) is credited with introducing the term *acroparesthesia* for this syndrome (cited in Kremer, Gilliatt, Golding & Wilson, 1953).

Wartenberg (1944) described *brachialgia statica paresthetica* as a syndrome of nocturnal hand pain and paresthesias waking patients from sleep. He emphasized the absence of objective physical signs and the long, benign, waxing and waning course of the condition. His patients were mostly women aged 40 to 55 years, who tended to describe their paresthesias as ulnar in distribution. Wartenberg thought that the cause was transient compression of the lower brachial plexus during sleep. Behrman (1945) also attributed acroparesthesia to brachial plexopathy.

Walshe (1945) commented on seeing an increased number of cases of acroparesthesia in women during the World War II, which he attributed to women's increased manual activities in wartime. His patients clearly had the characteristics that are now recognized as carpal tunnel syndrome, including nocturnal paresthesias and generally normal physical examinations. He hypothesized that the cause was pressure on the brachial plexus by a normal first rib.

McArdle, in a lecture in 1949 to the Association of British Neurologists, articulated the relationship between acroparesthesias and median nerve compression in the carpal tunnel (cited in Kremer et al., 1953).

Surgery for Carpal Tunnel Syndrome

Learmonth (1933) reported that he had sectioned the transverse carpal ligament of a 71-year-old woman with severe median neuropathy complicated by ulcerations of the tips of the index and middle fingers. At surgery the median nerve appeared compressed between the ligament and osteophytes arising from the carpal bones. The ulcers healed postoperatively. Amadio (1992) has reviewed patient records from the Mayo Clinic and traces the clinical experiences that preceded the publication of this case.

Cannon and Love (1946) reported 38 cases with what they termed *tardy median palsy*, insidious and progressive median neuropathy. In nine of these cases, they decompressed the median nerve by section of the transverse carpal ligament. They also made transverse incisions in the epineurium. Four of their cases had wrist deformities secondary to old fractures, one had acromegaly, one had a median neuroma in the carpal tunnel, and three had no clear cause of their carpal tunnel syndrome.

Brain, Wright, and Wilkinson (1947) reported six women with typical motor and sensory symptoms of carpal tunnel syndrome. All six underwent section of the transverse carpal ligament with rapid relief of pain and paresthesia. Phalen and colleagues (1950) described three successful carpal tunnel decompressions. Kremer and colleagues (1953) confirmed the relationship between acroparesthesia and carpal tunnel syndrome by successful relief of acroparesthesia after surgical section of the flexor retinaculum.

Interest in carpal tunnel syndrome has been growing over the last five decades. Subsequent chapters cover current knowledge of carpal tunnel syndrome and include references to the evolution of this knowledge. For example, the history of electrodiagnosis of carpal tunnel syndrome is included in Chapter 7, and the history of the understanding of the effect of activity on carpal tunnel syndrome appears in Chapter 13.

References

Abbott LC, Saunders JBdeCM. Injuries of the median nerve in fractures of the lower end of the radius. Surg. Gynecol. Obstet. 1933;57:507–16.

Amadio PC. The Mayo Clinic and carpal tunnel syndrome. Mayo Clin. Proc. 1992;67:42–48.

Amadio PC. The first carpal tunnel release? J. Hand Surg. 1995;20B:40–41.

Behrman S. Acroparaesthesia. Proc. R. Soc. Med. 1945;38: 600–1.

Blecher DR. Die schädigung des Nervus medianus also Komplikation des typischen Radiusbruches Deutsche. Ztschr. Z. Chir. 1908;93:34–45.

Brain WR, Wright AD, Wilkinson M. Spontaneous compression of both median nerves in the carpal tunnel. Lancet 1947; 1:277–82.

Brouwer B. The significance of phylogenetic and ontogenetic studies for the neuropathologist. J. Nerv. Ment. Dis. 1920; 51:113–37.

Cannon BW, Love JG. Tardy median palsy; median neuritis; median thenar neuritis amenable to surgery. Surgery 1946;20:210–16.

Hunt JR. The thenar and hypothenar types of neural atrophy of the hand. Am. J. Med. Sci. 1911;141:224–41.

Kremer M, Gilliatt RW, Golding JSR, Wilson TG. Acroparaesthesiae in the carpal-tunnel syndrome. Lancet 1953;2:595.

Learmonth JR. Treatment of diseases of peripheral nerves. Surg. Clin. North Am. 1933;13:905–13.

Lewis D, Miller EM. Peripheral nerve injuries associated with fractures. Trans. Am. Surg. Assoc. 1922;40:489–580.

Marie P, Foix C. Atrophie isolée de l'éminence thénar d'origine névritique: rôle du ligament annulaire antérieur du carpe dans la pathogénie de la lésion. Rev. Neurol. (Paris) 1913;26:647–49.

Mitchell SW. Lectures on Diseases of the Nervous System. Philadelphia: Lea, 1881.

Moersch FP. Median thenar neuritis. Proc. Staff Mtgs. Mayo Clin. 1938;13:220–22.

Mumenthaler M. Carpal tunnel syndrome: First description. Neurology 1984;34:921.

Ormerod JA. On a peculiar numbness and paresis of the hands. St. Barts. Hosp. Rep. 1883;19:17–26.

Paget J. Lectures on surgical pathology. Philadelphia: Lindsay & Blakiston; 1865.

Phalen GS, Gardner WJ, La Londe AA. Neuropathy of the median nerve due to compression beneath the transverse carpal ligament. J. Bone Joint Surg. 1950;32A:109–12.

Putnam JJ. A series of cases of paraesthesia, mainly of the hands, of periodical recurrence and possibly of vaso-motor origin. Arch. Med. 1880;4:147–62.

Saundby R. On a special form of numbness of the extremities. Lancet 1885;2:422–23.

Sinkler W. On a form of numbness of the upper extremities. N. Y. Med. J. 1884;40:107–8.

Walshe FMR. On "acroparaesthesia" and so-called "neuritis" of the hands and arms in women. BMJ. 1945;2:596–98.

Wartenberg R. Partial thenar atrophy. Arch. Neurol. Psychiat. (Chicago) 1939;42:373–93.

Wartenberg R. Brachialgia statica paresthetica. J. Nerv. Ment. Dis. 1944;99:877–87.

Zachary RB. Thenar palsy due to compression of the median nerve. Surg. Gynecol. Obstet. 1945;81:213–17.

Chapter 3
Carpal Tunnel Syndrome: Clinical Presentation

The *definition* of carpal tunnel syndrome is relatively easy: a constellation of symptoms and signs due to median nerve compression in the carpal canal. The *identification* of patients with carpal tunnel syndrome is routine for skilled clinicians. The *specification* of diagnostic criteria for carpal tunnel syndrome is challenging. There are a variety of possible clinical presentations: The most common is chronic median nerve compression presenting as acroparesthesias, but other uncommon variants include thenar atrophy without sensory symptoms, acute carpal tunnel syndrome, and atypical descriptions of nerve compressive symptoms, particularly in children or the elderly (Spinner, Bachman & Amadio, 1989).

There is no absolute clinical standard or definitive test for carpal tunnel syndrome. Histopathologic proof of local median nerve disease is unavailable as a diagnostic resource. Many published series discuss the findings in hundreds of patients with carpal tunnel syndrome without offering a precise criterion standard for the patients eligible for the diagnosis (Yamaguchi, Lipscomb & Soule, 1965; Phalen, 1972; Maxwell, Clough, Reckling & Kelly, 1973; Hybbinette & Mannerfelt, 1975; Gainer & Nugent, 1977; Paine & Polyzoidis, 1983). Here we discuss the symptoms and physical findings in carpal tunnel syndrome before struggling with more rigorous clinical criteria for making the diagnosis.

Symptoms

A careful history is the first step toward diagnosis of carpal tunnel syndrome. Without strong histori-cal support for the diagnosis, reliance on physical examination or on tests such as nerve conduction studies invites error.

Acroparesthesias of the hands are the most common presenting symptoms of carpal tunnel syndrome. A clinical description by Kremer and colleagues (1953) is quoted in the introduction to this text. Important historic points are the nature, location, and timing of both paresthesias and pain.

Paresthesias

Today patients with carpal tunnel syndrome often come to medical attention early in their illness, when intermittent hand paresthesias are the predominant symptoms. At this early stage, pain can be absent or trivial.

Early in the syndrome, sensory symptoms are intermittent (Table 3-1). Patients frequently characterize the paresthesias as their hand "going to sleep" and often attribute the symptoms to "cutting off circulation." They can sometimes identify arm postures in sleep that seem to incite symptoms. Paresthesias, sometimes accompanied by pain, characteristically interrupt sleep and also can be present on awakening in the morning or recur at rest during the day. Particularly common times of occurrence are while driving a car, reading, or holding a telephone receiver. The paresthesias characteristically are relieved when the patient shakes the affected hand (Gunnarsson, Amilon, Hellstrand, Leissner & Philipson, 1997). Patients can note that certain hand activities, such as pro-

Table 3-1. Timing of Symptoms in 100 Patients with Clinically and Electrodiagnostically Verified Carpal Tunnel Syndrome

Timing of Symptoms	Percent of Patients
Awaken from sleep by pain or paresthesias	63
Hand numb on awakening in the morning	61
Paresthesias when driving	58
Paresthesias when reading	70
Relief of symptoms by shaking the hands	68

Data from JC Stevens, BE Smith, AL Weaver, EP Bosch, HG Deen Jr., JA Wilkins. Symptoms of 100 patients with electromyographically verified carpal tunnel syndrome. Muscle Nerve 1999;22:1448–56.

longed gripping, cause symptoms, which usually abate shortly after the activity is stopped. In some patients, paresthesias—and pain when present—are most prominent during repetitive wrist use, and nocturnal hand symptoms are absent or less bothersome (Braun, Davidson & Doehr, 1989).

The nocturnal paresthetic symptoms of carpal tunnel syndrome can cause poor sleep quality, fragmented sleep, and excessive daytime sleepiness (Lehtinen, Kirjavainen, Hurme, Lauerma, Martikainen & Rauhala, 1996). Polysomnography in patients with this nocturnal symptom pattern can show increased body and hand movement during sleep.

Distribution of the paresthesias is variable, not always clearly following the sensory field of the median nerve; even anatomically sophisticated patients can report that paresthesias include all the digits or even seem to favor ulnar-innervated digits (Figure 3-1) (Oswald, Wertsch, Vennix, Brooks & Spreitzer, 1994; Gupta & Benstead, 1997). Paresthesias can spread to the palm or even more proximally (Figure 3-2) (Stevens, Smith, Weaver, Bosch, Deen Jr. & Wilkens, 1999). Unusual sensory patterns, reported by less than 10% of patients with carpal tunnel syndrome, are limitation of the paresthesias to the dorsum of the hand, to a single median-innervated finger, or to the ring and little fingers (Stevens et al., 1999). The diagnosis is more likely to be carpal tunnel syndrome when the sensory changes are limited to, or at least include, two or three median-innervated digits (Katz & Stirrat, 1990). In patients who have had traumatic finger amputations and later develop carpal tunnel syndrome, phantom paresthesias can radiate to the amputated fingers (Braverman & Root, 1997).

Symptoms characteristically develop insidiously. Figure 3-3 shows the duration of symptoms before the diagnosis was made in one series (Phalen, 1966). By the time the patient comes to the physician, the frequency of nocturnal awakening has gradually increased. The patient can identify a change in hand activities temporally related to the development of symptoms and even note relief of symptoms on vacations or weekends. The white-collar home handyman might report a reverse pattern with symptoms only occurring after weekends of work around the house.

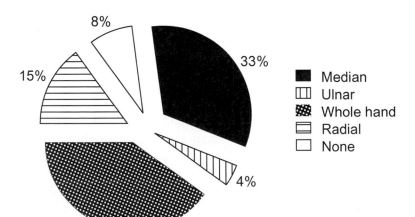

Figure 3-1. Distribution of tingling and numbness in hands with carpal tunnel syndrome and with no clinical findings or electrodiagnostic abnormalities beyond the median nerve. (Data from SK Gupta, TJ Benstead. Symptoms experienced by patients with carpal tunnel syndrome. Can. J. Neurol. Sci. 1997;24:338–42.)

Figure 3-2. Proximal spread of paresthesias in hands with carpal tunnel syndrome and with no clinical findings or electrodiagnostic abnormalities beyond the median nerve. (Data from JC Stevens, BE Smith, AL Weaver, EP Bosch, HG Deen Jr., JA Wilkins. Symptoms of 100 patients with electromyographically verified carpal tunnel syndrome. Muscle Nerve 1999; 22:1448–56.)

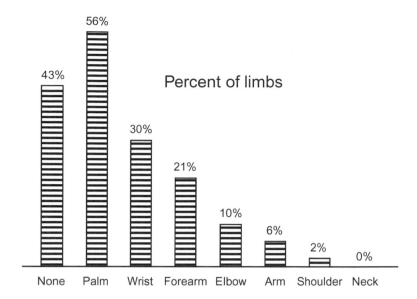

In some patients, symptoms are preceded by a change in health such as development of rheumatoid arthritis, appearance of other symptoms of hypothyroidism or diabetes, or pregnancy. In the majority of patients, however, the symptoms arise in an otherwise healthy body. Often no recent change in a lifelong pattern of hand and arm use is evident.

With time, sensory symptoms can become constant during the day. In patients who have developed a fixed sensory loss, anatomical reliability of sensory assessment is increased, and the initial nocturnal pattern of positive sensory symptoms can abate.

Hand and Arm Pain

Hand and arm pain usually accompanies the paresthesias of carpal tunnel syndrome; however, painless paresthesias do occur, particularly early in the evolution of symptoms. The pain is rarely severe; in one

Figure 3-3. Duration of symptoms (years) of carpal tunnel syndrome before diagnosis. (Duration was not recorded for 5% of hands.) (Data from GS Phalen. The carpal-tunnel syndrome. Seventeen years' experience in diagnosis and treatment of six hundred fifty-four hands. J. Bone Joint Surg. 1966;48A:211–28.)

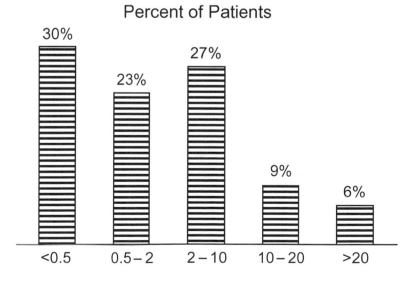

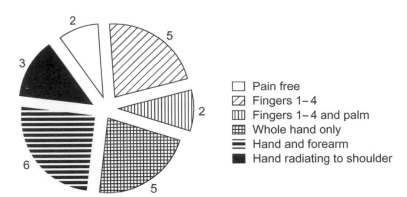

Figure 3-4. Location of hand and arm pain in patients with carpal tunnel syndrome. (Data from E Lang, D Claus, B Neundorfer, HO Handwerker. Parameters of thick and thin nerve-fiber functions as predictors of pain in carpal tunnel syndrome. Pain 1995;60:295–302.)

group of patients with symptoms severe enough to warrant carpal tunnel surgery, the average pain rating was 40% of a visual analogue pain scale (Lang, Claus, Neundorfer & Handwerker, 1995). The pain occurs periodically, accompanying the intermittent paresthesias and resolving when the patient changes posture or activity or shakes out the hand.

Whereas patients typically perceive the paresthesias as localized below the wrist, the pain or paresthesias often radiate into the forearm, and pain is more likely than paresthesias to spread as proximally as the shoulder (Figure 3-4). From 5% to 40% of patients with carpal tunnel syndrome report pain referred to the ipsilateral shoulder (Cherington, 1974). In rare instances the shoulder pain can be the predominant symptom (Kummel & Zazanis, 1973). If the patient's sole problem is carpal tunnel syndrome, the pain will appear and disappear along with the paresthesias. Continuous arm pain, or arm pain that occurs independent of episodes of paresthesias, signals the possibility of an alternative or additional cause of arm symptoms.

The intraneural stimulation studies of Torebjörk and colleagues (1984) provide an experimental parallel for proximal referral of pain in carpal tunnel syndrome. Stimulation of median nerve cutaneous sensory fascicles with a microelectrode elicited cutaneous pain in the median-innervated sensory territory. In contrast, stimulation of median nerve motor fascicles elicited deep pain projected to median-innervated muscles. In approximately one-fourth of motor fascicles, stimulation also elicited deep pain referred to the upper arm, axilla, or pectoral regions. Studies of the human ulnar nerve give comparable results (Marchettini, Cline & Ochoa, 1990).

Two series emphasize the clinical clues that are helpful in assessing the possibility of carpal tunnel

syndrome in patients with proximal upper extremity pain. LaBan and colleagues (1975) described 22 patients who presented with neck and shoulder pain and who had improvement of these symptoms after carpal tunnel release. Invariably, these patients had physical signs of carpal tunnel syndrome, including thenar weakness, and their proximal symptoms often worsened with wrist hyperextension or flexion.

Crymble (1968) described 21 patients who had prominent proximal arm pain that led to initial diagnoses such as cervical radiculopathy or brachial plexopathy. The diagnosis of carpal tunnel syndrome was often delayed in these patients, yet they responded well to carpal tunnel surgery. Crymble emphasized that patients' proximal pain might be more severe than their distal pain. The important diagnostic details were that in each case the pain did extend distally to the hand and forearm, and the patients' distal arm symptoms were, in character and timing, typical for carpal tunnel syndrome. One of us has described a personal experience with an analogous presentation of ulnar neuropathy with proximal symptoms (Ochoa, 1990).

In summary, neck, shoulder, or proximal arm pain that is separable from associated distal arm pain and hand paresthesias is rarely, if ever, a symptom of carpal tunnel syndrome. When carpal tunnel syndrome does cause proximal pain, the patient will have accompanying distal arm symptoms and signs.

Hand Symptom Diagram

Katz and Stirrat (1990) emphasize the importance of a careful clinical history for establishing the diagnosis of carpal tunnel syndrome, and they recommend inviting patients to fill out a hand symptom diagram, recording their areas of pain, tingling, numbness, and decreased sensation. In Katz and Stirrat's series, if patients had a classic sensory pattern with sensory symptoms limited to at least two of the thumb, index finger, and middle finger, the diagnosis, when established, was invariably carpal tunnel syndrome. The probability of the diagnosis decreased the further the patient's sensory diagram strayed from the classic pattern (Table 3-2). The hand symptom diagram had an average sensitivity of 71% and a specificity of 66% when physicians studied diagrams from patients with carpal tunnel syndrome or other causes of upper extremity pain or paresthesias and tried, without interviewing or examining the patients, to predict which had electrodiagnostically and clinically confirmed carpal tunnel syndrome (Stevens et al., 1999). When additional data about precipitating and relieving factors, obtained from a hand symptom questionnaire, was provided to the physicians, average diagnostic sensitivity increased to 88% but specificity fell to 51%. Sensitivity and specificity varied markedly from one physician to the next.

Regression Model Based on History

A regression model, derived from a symptom questionnaire, can be used to predict whether an individual will have carpal tunnel syndrome confirmed by nerve conduction abnormalities. The questionnaire has a sensitivity of 79% and a specificity of 55% (Bland, 2000). The strongest weight is given to nocturnal exacerbation of symptoms and to distribution of sensory complaints to the thumb, index finger, and middle finger or to the middle and ring fingers. Morning symptoms, exacerbation while driving, and relief by shaking the hand are also significant historic clues in this model.

"Autonomic" Symptoms

Symptoms potentially attributable to autonomic dysfunction, such as subjective finger swelling, dry palms, Raynaud's phenomenon, and finger blanching, occur in a significant minority of patients with carpal tunnel syndrome (Table 3-3) (Verghese, Gala-

Table 3-2. Classification of Symptom Quality and Location for Use with Hand Diagrams or Focused Questions

Symptom	Description
Classic/ probable	Numbness, tingling, burning, or pain in at least two of digits 1, 2, or 3. Palm pain, wrist pain, or radiation proximal to the wrist is allowed.
Possible	Numbness, tingling, burning, or pain in at least one of digits 1, 2, or 3.
Unlikely	No symptoms in digits 1, 2, or 3.

Reprinted with permission from D Rempel, B Evanoff, PC Amadio, M de Krom, G Franklin, A Franzblau, R Gray, F Gerr, M Hagberg, T Hales, JN Katz, G Pransky. Consensus criteria for the classification of carpal tunnel syndrome in epidemiologic studies. Am. J. Public Health 1998;88:1447–51.

nopoulou & Herskovitz, 2000). The incidence of these symptoms in normal individuals and in patients with other arm conditions is not well defined, so these symptoms are of questionable diagnostic value. For example, among patients who had carpal tunnel syndrome confirmed by nerve conduction studies, just over one-half reported hand swelling, but among patients with hand symptoms and normal median nerve conduction, approximately two-thirds reported hand swelling (Burke, Burke, Bell, Stewart, Mehdi & Kim, 1999). The mechanism of these symptoms is also ill defined. Compression of median autonomic fibers might play a role; the sympathetic skin response in the symptomatic hand is abnormal in approximately one-third of hands of carpal tunnel syndrome patients that have these symptoms compared to approximately one-ninth of hands of carpal tunnel syndrome patients that do not have these symptoms.

Table 3-3. Incidence of "Autonomic" Symptoms in Hands with Carpal Tunnel Syndrome

Symptom	Percent of Limbs with Symptom
Finger swelling (subjective or visible)	32
Dry palms	22
Raynaud's phenomenon	18
Finger blanching	17

Data from J Verghese, AS Galanopoulou, S Herskovitz. Autonomic dysfunction in idiopathic carpal tunnel syndrome. Muscle Nerve 2000;23:1209–13.

Motor Symptoms

Patients with carpal tunnel syndrome commonly report stiffness, clumsiness, and even weakness of their hands, usually before they have developed any motor or sensory functional deficit detectable by formal neurologic examination. Testing using a repetitive pinch and release task confirms that the patients with carpal tunnel syndrome often have impaired manual speed and dexterity (Jeng, Radwin & Fryback, 1997). Although the severity of this deficit correlates somewhat with abnormalities of median motor and sensory conduction, manual dexterity is impaired in some patients who have normal nerve conduction studies (Jeng, Radwin, Moore, Roberts, Garrity & Oswald, 1997). Perhaps inhibited flexor tendon movement within the carpal tunnel, due to the flexor tendinopathy that often accompanies carpal tunnel syndrome, accounts for some of this loss of hand dexterity.

As median nerve damage progresses, thenar weakness can become more pronounced, and thenar atrophy can appear. On occasion patients present with severe thenar atrophy and weakness, with median sensory loss, or both, and deny passing through a stage of intermittent pain and paresthesias that preceded the development of fixed neurologic signs. This presentation is more common in patients aged 60 years or older. It is unclear whether these patients are heavy sleepers who have slept through the stage of nocturnal paresthesias, stoics who have ignored intermittent hand symptoms, or physiologically distinctive patients who have been spared the characteristic early symptoms.

Examination

Patients being evaluated for carpal tunnel syndrome should have a regional arm and neck examination and a neurologic examination that should include such details as pupils, strength and sensation in all extremities, gait, and tendon reflexes. The examination must be sufficiently thorough to clarify the differential diagnosis, look for causative medical or orthopedic disorders, and consider the possibility of coexisting conditions. Neurologic issues include existence of other mononeuropathies, brachial plexopathy, radiculopathy, myelopathy, or diffuse peripheral neuropathy. At times wrist and hand examination will give evidence of tenosynovitis, deformity, or injury. The adequacy of vascular supply and the possibility of autonomic, skin, or trophic changes are important.

In patients with carpal tunnel syndrome, physical findings are an indication of the severity of median nerve dysfunction. In early or mild cases, when symptoms are intermittent, neurologic deficit is usually absent; demonstration of neurologic deficits indicates that median nerve injury has passed the initial stages. The incidence of abnormal signs varies from series to series depending on the examination methods of the authors and the distribution of severity of cases in the series. Nonetheless, the *relative* sensitivity of signs follows a reliable pattern among series. Meta-analyses that limit consideration to series of patients who have electrodiagnostically confirmed carpal tunnel syndrome give a skewed impression of the value of physical examination techniques (D'Arcy & McGee, 2000).

Sensory Examination

The patient with carpal tunnel syndrome almost always describes paresthetic phenomena, yet the sensory examination is often normal despite the patient's sensory complaints. Although most patients have some disturbance of sensation by history, examination demonstrates hypesthesia in only approximately 70% of patients in older surgical series (Phalen, 1966, 1972; Maxwell et al., 1973; Hybbinette & Mannerfelt, 1975). A small number of patients describe "hyperesthesia." Loss of two-point discrimination is a rarer finding. The incidence of changes on sensory examination is lower now than in the past because patients are coming to medical attention earlier in the course of the syndrome.

Spindler and Dellon (1982) compared a variety of clinical sensory tests in 74 symptomatic hands with carpal tunnel syndrome. They tested pain sensitivity using a 25-gauge needle. Perception of vibration was measured by asking the patient to report the feeling of a 256-Hz tuning fork head touching the fingertip. Two-point discrimination was tested both to a static pressure at one application to the fingertip and as a "moving two-point

Figure 3-5. The sensitivity of sensory tests in patients with carpal tunnel syndrome. (Data from HA Spindler, AL Dellon. Nerve conduction studies and sensibility testing in carpal tunnel syndrome. J. Hand Surg. 1982;7:260–63.)

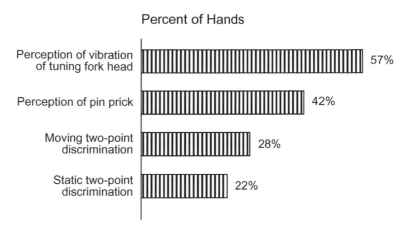

discrimination" test by dragging the stimuli along the surface of the fingertip. Figure 3-5 shows the sensitivity of the tests in this series. The order of sensitivity was not invariable so that a total of 66% of hands showed abnormality on some aspect of the sensory exam. In many cases with intermittent symptoms, the vibration perception test was the only abnormal test of sensation.

The relative sensitivities of sensory tests have a parallel in experimental subjects experiencing acute median nerve compression (Lundborg, Gelberman, Minteer-Convery, Lee & Hargens, 1982; Gelberman, Szabo, Williamson & Dimick, 1983). Pressure is applied to the volar wrist so that the median nerve is compressed without more generalized vascular compression. Usually paresthesias appear after a few minutes of compression at pressures greater than 30 mm Hg. The more sensitive sensory tests—monofilament testing or vibration perception threshold—can become abnormal about the time of perception of paresthesias or shortly after paresthesias appear. Abnormal two-point discrimination is a relatively late manifestation of acute nerve compression.

Sensory abnormalities, when present, do not always follow the traditional median sensory distribution (volar thumb, index, middle, and lateral half of the ring finger) because of the wide variety of anatomic variations (see Figure 1-13). Sensation on the volar hand is often blunted over callused skin; examination of sensation on the median-innervated dorsal distal digits can be particularly helpful (Dawson, Hallett & Wilbourn, 1999). A photograph of the mapped pattern of sensory abnormalities is useful for documenting consis-

tency of examinations and for following the patient's clinical course (Figure 3-6).

The skin of the thenar eminence receives its sensory innervation from the recurrent palmar branch of the median nerve. This branch typically leaves the median nerve proximal to the carpal tunnel, so thenar sensory loss might indicate a median neuropathy proximal to the carpal tunnel or an anomalous sensory pattern.

The diagnostic value of sensory testing can be improved by using quantitative sensory testing techniques as discussed in Chapter 9 (Szabo, Gelberman & Dimick, 1984; Borg & Lindblom, 1988). The sensitivity can be increased further by using provocative techniques to elicit the sensory abnormalities (Borg & Lindblom, 1986; Braun et al., 1989).

Motor Examination

In experimental acute median nerve compression, thenar weakness usually does not occur until sensory loss is marked (Lundborg et al., 1982; Gelberman et al., 1983). Clinically, in chronic median nerve compression, the same pattern is the norm: Thenar weakness is rarer than sensory loss, and thenar atrophy is even less common. The muscles that receive median innervation distal to the carpal tunnel are abductor pollicis brevis (APB), opponens pollicis, flexor pollicis brevis, and the lumbricals to the index and middle fingers. Figures 3-7, 3-8, and 3-9 illustrate examining the strength of the thenar muscles. Weakness of APB is the most sensitive motor sign of carpal tunnel syndrome. APB

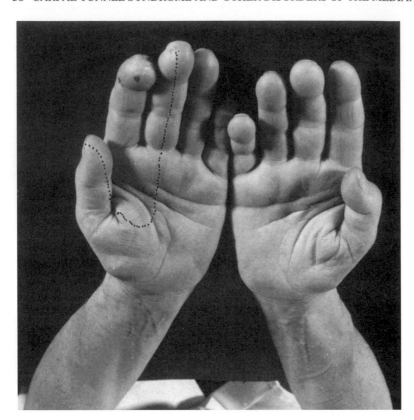

Figure 3-6. Photograph of the sensory deficit in a patient with severe bilateral carpal tunnel syndrome. Note the unusual finding of chronic trophic ulcers on the fingertips.

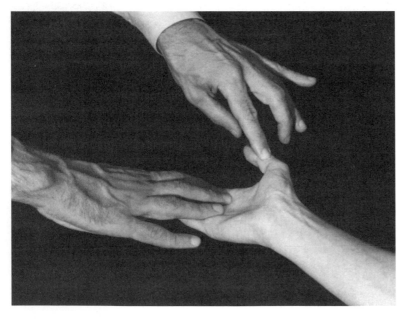

Figure 3-7. Abductor pollicis brevis is tested by assessing strength of thumb movement away from the palm in a plane perpendicular to the plane of the palm.

Figure 3-8. The opponens pollicis moves the metacarpal bone of the thumb to touch the little finger; the thumb is rotated so that the thumbnail becomes parallel to the palm.

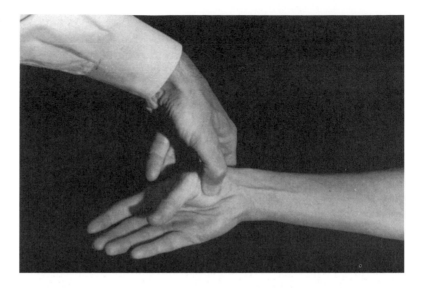

is the least likely of the thenar muscles to receive ulnar innervation. Care should be taken to examine APB strength in relative isolation by ensuring that the thumb is held parallel to the index finger while testing abduction up from the plane of the palm. Side-to-side confrontational testing of the APB is done by asking the subject to strongly press the lateral tips of the thumbs against each other while holding the palms parallel to each other. Subtle asymmetries of APB strength are visible as a decrease in the angle between the thumb and the plane of the palm on the weaker side (Busch-bacher, 1997). This confrontational test can be taught to patients so that they can monitor their own APB strength.

The opponens pollicis mediates rotation at the metacarpal-trapezial joint, swinging the thumb medially to meet the little finger. While testing this

Figure 3-9. The flexor pollicis brevis is tested by assessing the strength of flexion of the metacarpal-phalangeal joint of the thumb. Be wary of trick movements from action of the flexor pollicis longus or opponens pollicis.

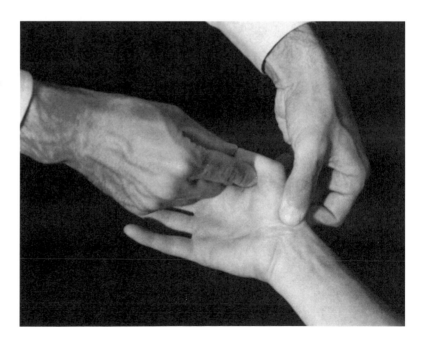

motion, be certain that the movement is occurring at the metacarpal-trapezial joint rather than through action of flexor pollicis brevis at the phalangeal-metacarpal joint. This is important because flexor pollicis brevis is more likely than opponens pollicis to receive innervation from the ulnar nerve and, hence, is more likely to be spared in a median neuropathy.

Lumbricals are difficult to test in isolation. One test for lumbrical weakness is to observe action at the distal interphalangeal joints while the metacarpal-phalangeal joints are voluntarily flexed to 90 degrees. If the lumbricals are weak, the distal interphalangeal joints will not be maintained in extension (Aiache & Delagi, 1974). Even if the lumbricals are examined with care, lumbrical strength is often relatively preserved in carpal tunnel syndrome until after thenar muscles are weakened (Desjacques, Egloff-Baer & Roth, 1980; Yates, Yaworski & Brown, 1981; Logigian, Busis, Berger, Bruyninckx, Khalil, Shahani & Young, 1987).

Motor examination in the patient with suspected carpal tunnel syndrome should exclude motor manifestations of more widespread neurologic dysfunction such as ulnar neuropathy, proximal median neuropathy, brachial plexopathy, or cervical radiculopathy.

Cutaneous Examination

Patients with carpal tunnel syndrome often describe their hands as swollen, particularly on arising from sleep. Nonetheless, Phalen (1966) detected hand swelling in only 51 of 654 hands with carpal tunnel syndrome. Even when hand volume is carefully measured, most patients with carpal tunnel syndrome show no significant swelling over the course of the day (Wilson-MacDonald, Caughey & Myers, 1984).

Phalen (1966) described isolated volar forearm swelling on the ulnar side of the palmaris longus tendon approximately 1 cm wide and extending approximately 2.5 cm proximally from the distal wrist crease in 11% of his patients. This physical finding, colloquially called *Phalen's volar hot dog*, is attributed to a swollen ulnar bursa compressed at the transverse carpal ligament (Figure 3-10) (Dorwart, 1983; Finger & Vogel, 1998).

Cutaneous manifestations of carpal tunnel syndrome are varied but quite uncommon. In severe cases, ulcerative, necrotic, or bullous lesions of the skin of the median-innervated fingertips can occur (see Figure 3-6) (Cox, Large, Paterson & Ive, 1992; Tosti, Morelli, D'Alessandro & Bassi, 1993; Fritz, Burg & Boni, 2000). Digital anhydrosis, dorsal digital alopecia, and nail changes have been described and can improve after carpal tunnel release (Aratari, Regesta & Rebora, 1984). A patient with carpal tunnel syndrome and hand exposure to detergents developed contact dermatitis limited to the median-innervated digits (Fast, Parikh & Ducommun, 1989). Trophic changes severe enough to lead to finger amputation are extremely rare (Quinlan, 1967).

Wrist Shape

A number of authors have debated whether wrist shape correlates with median nerve conduction latencies across the carpal; this debate is reviewed in detail in Chapter 8.

Provocative Tests

Patients with carpal tunnel syndrome typically appear in the physician's examining room with intermittent symptoms and no objective neurologic dysfunction. A number of provocative tests have been used to elicit or relieve symptoms or neurologic abnormalities. Invariably, initial descriptions of these tests are followed by reports showing that the tests have higher rates of false-positive and false-negative results than initially reported.

Systematic reviews of physical examination findings in patients with carpal tunnel syndrome discuss the methodologic deficits of many of the studies cited in the following paragraphs (D'Arcy & McGee, 2000; Massy-Westropp, Grimmer & Bain, 2000). The conclusions of these reviews are biased if they rely on studies that use a criterion standard for carpal tunnel syndrome that requires that the diagnosis be supported by abnormal nerve conduction studies. Among subjects with normal median nerve conduction, the "false-positive" rate for provocative tests is higher in subjects who have symptoms suggestive of carpal tunnel syn-

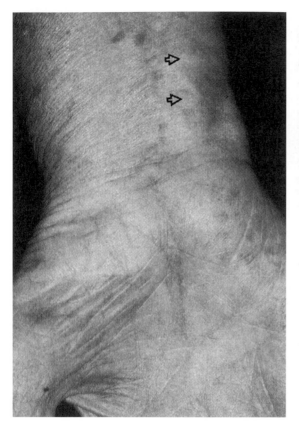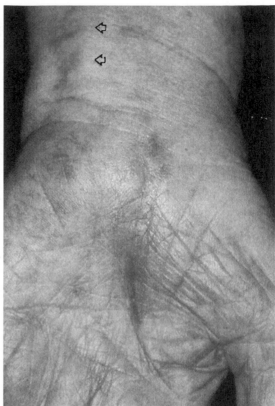

Figure 3-10. Phalen's "volar hot dog" is visible in both wrists (*arrows*) of this patient who has bilateral carpal tunnel syndrome. (Reprinted with permission from D Finger, P Vogel. Carpal tunnel syndrome. Arthritis Rheum. 1998;41:182.)

drome than in asymptomatic subjects (Gerr & Letz, 1998). Similarly, the specificity of provocative tests is lower in a group of patients with hand and arm symptoms not attributed to carpal tunnel syndrome than it is in a group of asymptomatic individuals (Szabo, Slater, Farver, Stanton & Sharman, 1999).

Phalen's Sign

Phalen (1966) described the "wrist flexion test": The patient is asked to hold the forearms vertically and to allow both hands to drop into complete flexion at the wrist for approximately one minute. The position is shown in Figure 3-11.

An individual who has a positive Phalen's sign reports numbness or paresthesias in the distribution of the median nerve within 1 minute of sustained wrist flexion. Reports of pain alone do not prove median compression, but the test is particularly helpful if the individual reports pain and paresthesias mimicking his or her typical intermittent symptoms. Phalen found the test positive in 74% of hands with carpal tunnel syndrome. He attributed some of the false-negative results to hands that already had "an advanced degree of sensory loss." Other series have found similar sensitivity of the test (Gellman, Gelberman, Tan & Botte, 1986; Seror, 1988; Novak, Mackinnon, Brownlee & Kelly, 1992). Perhaps, Phalen's sign is more often positive in women than in men who have carpal tunnel syndrome (Padua, Padua, Aprile & Tonali, 1999). Reliability of Phalen's test was "satisfactory" in one study and "modest" in another (Marx, Hudak, Bombardier, Graham, Goldsmith & Wright, 1998; Salerno, Franzblau, Werner, Chung, Schultz, Becker & Armstrong, 2000).

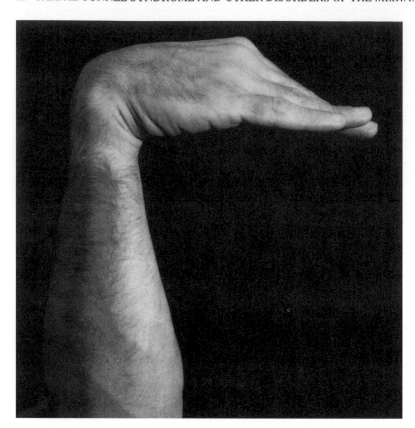

Figure 3-11. Phalen's test is performed by asking the patient to report any symptoms induced by 1 minute of sustained wrist flexion. This test relies on subjective reporting by the patient and is most helpful if the patient describes induction of paresthesias in the sensory distribution of the median nerve.

Phalen noted that median paresthesias occur in normal persons if wrist flexion is sustained long enough. False-positive results in Phalen's test are found in as many as 25% of normal hands (Gellman et al., 1986; Seror, 1988; Kuschner, Ebramzadeh, Johnson, Brien & Sherman, 1992). As with Tinel's sign, the diagnostic value of Phalen's test is diluted by the high incidence of false-positives in a condition with relatively low prevalence in the general population. The relationship of true-positive to false-positive results varies depending on how long wrist flexion is sustained; a receiver operating characteristic curve analysis (receiver operating characteristic curves are discussed in more detail in Chapter 8) suggested that 40 seconds of sustained wrist flexion offered the best discrimination between patients with carpal tunnel syndrome and control subjects (Tetro, Evanoff, Hollstien & Gelberman, 1998).

Phalen (1972) did not believe that wrist extension was a useful provocative maneuver; however, sometimes similar symptoms can be evoked by 1 minute of sustained full wrist extension, the "reverse Phalen's test" (Werner, Bir & Armstrong, 1994).

Tinel's Sign

Tinel (1915) reported that percussion over a post-traumatic neuroma often elicited tingling sensations (*fourmillement*) perceived in the distribution of the injured nerve. Hoffman also reported the phenomenon in 1915 (Alfonso & Dzwierzynski, 1998). The phenomenon is not limited to posttraumatic neuromas, and Phalen (1966) found this sign present with percussion over the median nerve at the wrist in 73% of his patients with carpal tunnel syndrome. The sign can be elicited over a variety of nerves and so is properly described by location: for example, "a positive Tinel's sign over the median nerve at the wrist." The test is only positive for carpal tunnel syndrome if the percussion over the median nerve at the wrist leads to paresthesias in a median distribution; it should not be confused with percussion tenderness of the wrist. Tinel's sign is more likely to be positive in patients with sensory deficit to two-point discrimination than in those with a normal sensory examination; in contrast, Phalen's test or the carpal compression test do not vary in sensitivity with variations in the sensory examination (Novak et al., 1992). Reliability of Tinel's sign was "satisfactory" in one study and "modest" in another (Marx et al., 1998; Salerno et al., 2000).

In different series the sensitivity of Tinel's sign in patients with carpal tunnel syndrome has ranged from 65% to 14% (Golding, Rose & Selvarajah, 1986; Daras, Tuchman, Spector, Zalzal & Rogoff, 1987; Kuschner et al., 1992; Buch-Jaeger & Foucher, 1994; Gunnarsson et al., 1997; Gerr & Letz, 1998). The high incidence of Tinel's sign in individuals without carpal tunnel syndrome is now widely recognized. The incidence of false-positives has been reported to be from 6% to 45% (Gelmers, 1979; Gellman et al., 1986; Golding et al., 1986; Seror, 1987b). The incidence of false-positives in these series increases parallel to the incidence of true-positives. For example, the incidence of positives, both true and false, can be increased by extending the wrist and using a "Queen Square" reflex hammer for the percussion (Mossman & Blau, 1987). In the general population, most individuals with a positive Tinel's sign over the median nerve at the wrist will not have other indicia of carpal tunnel syndrome.

Median Nerve Compression Test

Jungo (1969) elicited median distribution paresthesias in patients with carpal tunnel syndrome by applying pressure with the thumb over the transverse carpal ligament for 1 minute. To perform the median nerve compression test the examiner applies pressure directly over the volar wrist or carpal tunnel for 15 to 120 seconds (Paley & McMurtry, 1985; Durkan, 1991). Some examiners use a pressure approximating systolic arterial pressure (e.g., approximately 150 mm Hg or 2.9 psi); others use pressures as high as 12 to 15 psi (776 mm Hg) (Wainner, Boninger, Balu, Burdett & Helkowski, 2000). A gauge is available to apply a measured pressure (Durkan, 1994; Wainner et al., 2000). The test is positive if the patient reports paresthesias in the distribution of the median nerve; wrist pain or tenderness should not be interpreted as a positive test. Reported values for sensitivity of this test have ranged from 23% to 100% and reports of specificity have varied from 29% to 100% (Mossman & Blau, 1987; Wil-

liams, Mackinnon, Novak, McCabe & Kelly, 1992; De Smet, Steenwerckx, Van den Bogaert, Cnudde & Fabry, 1995; Ghavanini & Haghighat, 1998). The results of the median nerve compression test are reproducible (Marx et al., 1998; Salerno et al., 2000).

Closed Fist Test (Lumbrical Provocation Test)

The closed fist test is performed by asking the patient to maintain active fist closure with the wrist in neutral position for 30 to 60 seconds (Cobb, An, Cooney & Berger, 1994; Yii & Elliot, 1994; De Smet et al., 1995). The test is positive if the subject reports hand paresthesias by the end of the specified time. In a small series, the test was positive in 62% of patients with carpal tunnel syndrome confirmed by electrodiagnosis, but it was rarely positive in patients with hand paresthesias and normal electrodiagnostic studies (De Smet et al., 1995). However, sensitivity and specificity of the test were less impressive when they were evaluated in a series of patients who reported a broad range of symptom severity (Karl, Carney & Kaul, 2001).

Combined Wrist Flexion and Carpal Compression

A test combining the principles of Phalen's test and the carpal compression test can be performed by the examiner pressing his or her thumb firmly and evenly on the subject's median nerve at the volar wrist while the subject sustains 60-degree wrist flexion (Tetro et al., 1998). The subject's elbow is extended with the forearm supinated. The test is positive if the subject reports median-distribution numbness, pain, or paresthesias. In patients with carpal tunnel syndrome, 82% have a positive test after 20 seconds in this posture; 86% have a positive test after 30 seconds. A receiver operating characteristic curve analysis suggests that the best discrimination between normal subjects and patients with carpal tunnel syndrome is obtained when the test is performed for 20 seconds, and that this test provides better diagnostic discrimination than Phalen's test, Tinel's sign, or the carpal compression test. A variation on this approach is to perform Phalen's test for 1 minute followed by carpal compression for 30 seconds and to consider occurrence of paresthesias during either maneuver a positive response (Fertl, Wober & Zeitlhofer, 1998).

Tourniquet Test

Gilliatt and Wilson (1953, 1954) described the use of forearm ischemia to provoke the symptoms of carpal tunnel syndrome. They reported that after occlusion of forearm blood flow using a pneumatic cuff, patients with carpal tunnel syndrome experienced reproduction of their intermittent symptoms of hand paresthesias or experienced sensory loss in a median distribution. The paresthesias typically developed in 3 minutes or less; the sensory loss usually took 5 to 10 minutes to become established. Gilliatt and Wilson stressed that normal subjects often note acroparesthesias with forearm ischemia; distinguishing features in the carpal tunnel syndrome patients were the localization of the paresthesias or sensory loss to the median distribution and the development of the median sensory loss in less than 10 minutes. Patients with other focal neuropathies or radiculopathies can also respond to arm ischemia with sensory loss in a sensory pattern appropriate to their lesion.

In a controlled study using only 1 minute of forearm ischemia, a false-positive result was found in 40% of control subjects without carpal tunnel syndrome (Gellman et al., 1986). In comparison, 71% of carpal tunnel syndrome patient's had a true-positive test after 1 minute of ischemia.

"Flick" Sign

Pryse-Phillips (1984) noted that his patients often shook or "flicked" the wrist of the symptomatic hand when describing their attempts to alleviate carpal tunnel syndrome symptoms. He reported a 93% true-positive rate in patients with nerve conduction evidence supporting the diagnosis of carpal tunnel syndrome. The false-positive rate was 5% in patients with other neurogenic symptoms in the hand. Subsequent correspondents found that the sensitivity and specificity of this sign were disappointingly lower in their own patients (Krendel, Jobsis, Gaskell & Sanders, 1986; Seror, 1987a; Roquer & Herraiz, 1988).

Tethered Median Nerve Stress Test

The tethered median nerve stress test is performed by hyperextending the index finger at the distal interphalangeal joint with the wrist supinated (LaBan, Friedman & Zemenick, 1986; LaBan, MacKenzie & Zemenick, 1989). A positive test is production of volar forearm pain. In the small series in which this test was described, 18 of 20 patients with carpal tunnel syndrome had positive tests. Subsequent reports have found that this test has much lower sensitivity for carpal tunnel syndrome (43% to 50%), a relatively low specificity (59%), and little utility as a diagnostic aid (Kaul, Pagel & Dryden, 2000; Raudino, 2000).

Relief Maneuver

In patients who are symptomatic at the time of examination, the relief maneuver can be attempted (Manente, Torrieri, Pineto & Uncini, 1999). With the patient's palm up, the examiner gently squeezes the distal metacarpal heads, slightly adducting the index and little fingers. If this does not abolish or improve symptoms within 30 seconds, a second maneuver is for the examiner to pronate the patient's hand while gently pulling on the middle and ring fingers. According to this preliminary report, the initial maneuver relieved symptoms in 91% of hands with symptoms of carpal tunnel syndrome and the second maneuver relieved symptoms in the remaining 9% of patients.

Hand Elevation Test

In the hand elevation test, patients are asked to raise their hands over their heads and maintain that position until symptoms occur or, at most, for 2 minutes (Ahn, 2001). Among women who had symptoms of carpal tunnel syndrome and abnormal median nerve conduction, three-fourths reported developing symptoms during this maneuver. The test was positive in only 3 of 200 control women but has not been tested in larger populations.

Provocative Tests—Summary

On statistical grounds, based on specificity and sensitivity rates, the provocative tests cannot prove the diagnosis of carpal tunnel syndrome in patients with atypical symptomatic presentations. The ability of the provocative tests to improve diagnostic accuracy is dependent on the prevalence of carpal tunnel syndrome in the population being examined. The results of provocative tests must be interpreted with thoughtful suspicion in patients with varied or widespread somatic aches and pains or in patients who are suggestible. In an occasional instance, however, they can be especially helpful when a provocative maneuver replicates a patient's symptoms or allows a more accurate assessment of localization of sensory symptoms or signs.

The provocative tests often become positive early in the course of carpal tunnel syndrome (Novak et al., 1992). In patients with typical symptoms of carpal tunnel syndrome and normal median nerve conduction results, the provocative tests are positive nearly as often as they are in patients with carpal tunnel syndrome confirmed by nerve conduction results (Buch-Jaeger & Foucher, 1994; Gerr & Letz, 1998). Some authors classify provocative tests as "false-positive" when they are the only clinical abnormality in patients who have paresthetic hand symptoms and normal median nerve conduction. In many mild cases of carpal tunnel syndrome (classes 1A and 1B as defined in the section Clinical Classification of Carpal Tunnel Syndrome), however, the provocative tests are important indicators of median nerve irritability when other physical signs and diagnostic tests are negative.

Epidemiology

Clinical Series

Many large clinical series of patients with carpal tunnel syndrome provide a consistent description of the demographics of carpal tunnel syndrome patients (Yamaguchi, et al., 1965; Phalen, 1966; Maxwell et al., 1973; Birkbeck & Beer, 1975; Hybbinette & Mannerfelt, 1975; Gainer & Nugent, 1977; Tountas, MacDonald, Meyerhoff & Bihrle, 1983). Some 70%

of patients are women, and 30% are men. The proportion of male patients is higher in some work-related settings (Tountas et al., 1983; Franklin, Haug, Peck, Heyer & Checkoway, 1990). The clinical presentation is similar in men and women, but men are less likely than woman to complain of pain when symptomatic (Padua et al., 1999).

Over one-half of patients with carpal tunnel syndrome have symptoms of the syndrome in both hands. The prevalence of symptoms in the less symptomatic hand increases to more than 80% if patients are questioned closely and increases if symptoms have been present for more than 1 year (Padua, Padua, Nazzaro & Tonali, 1998). Of those with unilateral symptoms, the dominant hand is more frequently affected. For example, Gainer and Nugent (1977) found that the dominant hand was predominantly affected two-thirds of the time. Reinstein (1981) confirmed this in both right- and left-handed patients (Figure 3-12). In unusual industrial settings, when the nondominant hand is predominantly stressed, carpal tunnel syndrome can favor the nondominant hand (Falck & Aarnio, 1983).

Carpal tunnel syndrome has its highest incidence between 40 and 60 years of age. It is rare before age 20 years or after age 80 years. The age distribution of patients in a typical clinical series is shown in Figure 3-13 (Phalen, 1966).

Clinical Series with Population-Based Denominators

One retrospective epidemiological study ("Carpal tunnel syndrome in Rochester, Minnesota, 1961 to 1980") provides a population-based survey of carpal tunnel syndrome with care taken to ascertain cases that came to medical attention and to define the criteria for the diagnosis (Stevens, Sun, Beard, O'Fallon & Kurland, 1988). The results match those in the clinical series. Figure 3-14 shows the age distribution of the first episode of carpal tunnel syndrome in this population. Table 3-4 shows the incidence of carpal tunnel syndrome in the population.

A survey in Santa Clara County, California, suggests that carpal tunnel syndrome might be more common there than it was in Rochester, Minnesota, earlier (Anonymous, 1989). The California survey counted patients who came to medical attention dur-

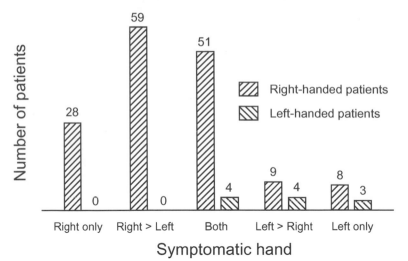

Figure 3-12. Relationship between hand dominance and symptomatic hand(s) of patients with carpal tunnel syndrome. (Data from L. Reinstein. Hand dominance in carpal tunnel syndrome. Arch. Phys. Med. Rehabil. 1981;62:202–3.)

ing 1988 for carpal tunnel syndrome in a county of 1.4 million people. Some 7,214 cases of carpal tunnel syndrome were reported (515 per 100,000 population) even though only 30% of physicians replied to the query. The study has incomplete case finding, however, and poor case definition.

Incidence data for carpal tunnel surgery are available for Ontario, Canada, in which the denominator is based on the number of residents covered by the Provincial Health Insurance Plan. For example, in 1988 the highest incidence of operations was 369 per 100,000 covered insureds among women aged 50 to 54 years (Liss, Armstrong, Kusiak & Galitis, 1992).

A study of primary care practices between 1988 and 1990 found that 0.1 % of new patient visits were for new onset of symptoms of carpal tunnel syndrome (Miller, Iverson, Fried, Green & Nutting, 1994). An epidemiological study in Marshfield, Wisconsin, found that between 1991 and 1993 the annual incidence of newly diagnosed probable or

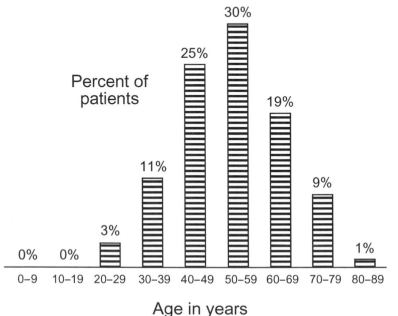

Figure 3-13. Age distribution of patients with carpal tunnel syndrome in a clinical series. (Data from GS Phalen. The carpal-tunnel syndrome. Seventeen years' experience in diagnosis and treatment of six hundred fifty-four hands. J. Bone Joint Surg. 1966;48A:211–28.)

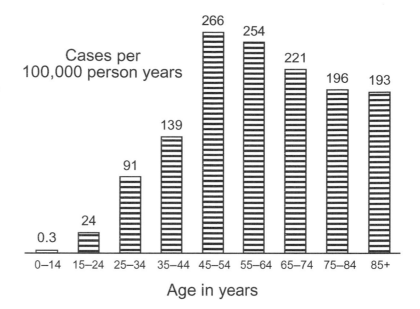

Figure 3-14. Age distribution of incidence of carpal tunnel syndrome in the citizens of Rochester, Minnesota. (Data from JC Stevens, S Sun, CM Beard, WM O'Fallon, LT Kurland. Carpal tunnel syndrome in Rochester, Minnesota, 1961 to 1980. Neurology 1988;38:134–38.)

definite carpal tunnel syndrome was 346 cases per 100,000 patient-years, nearly three times the highest incidence found in the earlier Rochester study (Nordstrom, DeStefano, Vierkant & Layde, 1998). The increasing incidence of carpal tunnel syndrome coming to clinical attention is probably caused by many factors, such as increased awareness of the syndrome by patients, increased diagnostic acumen of physicians, improved sensitivity of nerve conduction tests, changing case definitions, and variations in patient exposure to risk factors for development of carpal tunnel syndrome.

General Population Surveys

The studies mentioned in previous sections all deal with patients who have come to medical attention. Attempts to determine the prevalence of carpal tunnel syndrome in the general population are complicated by uncertain diagnostic accuracy. In the U.S. National Health Interview Survey for 1988, 1,550 respondents per 100,000 surveyed reported that in the previous year they had had hand symptoms that they believed were attributable to carpal tunnel syndrome. Among those who had been employed during the previous year, 530 per 100,000 reported that they had had hand symptoms that year that a medical professional had attributed to carpal tunnel syn-

drome (Tanaka, Wild, Seligman, Halperin, Behrens & Putz-Anderson, 1995).

An age- and sex-stratified randomized sample of the population of Maastricht, The Netherlands, was asked as part of a health survey whether they ever awoke at night with "unpleasant sensations" in their fingers (De Krom, Knipschild, Kester, Thijs, Boekkooi & Spaans, 1992). The surveyors termed these symptoms *brachialgia nocturna paraesthetica.* Among respondents not previously diagnosed as having carpal tunnel syndrome, brachialgia nocturna paraesthetica had occurred in 15% of women and 8% of men; an additional 4% of women had previ-

Table 3-4. Carpal Tunnel Syndrome in Rochester, Minnesota*

Years	Women	Men	Total
1961–1965	132	33	88
1966–1970	151	40	102
1971–1975	133	58	100
1976–1980	173	68	125
1961–1980	149	52	105

*Age-adjusted incidence per 100,000 patient-years.
Data from JC Stevens, S Sun, CM Beard, WM O'Fallon, LT Kurland. Carpal tunnel syndrome in Rochester, Minnesota, 1961 to 1980. Neurology 1988;38:134–38.

Table 3-5. Prevalence of Carpal Tunnel Syndrome in a General Population in Southern Sweden*

Prevalence Per 100,000 Subjects	Men	Women
Hand symptoms	10,400	17,300
Clinically certain carpal tunnel syndrome	2,800	4,600
Clinically certain carpal tunnel syndrome with abnormal median nerve conduction	2,100	3,000

*Hand symptoms were defined as pain, numbness, or tingling in two or more of the first four digits at least twice weekly in the 4 weeks before the survey. Clinically certain carpal tunnel syndrome was based on assessment of the history by a single experienced hand surgeon. Abnormal median nerve conduction was defined as a sensory latency difference of 0.8 msecs or more, subtracting the ulnar little finger-to-wrist latency from the median middle finger-to-wrist latency.

Data from I Atroshi, C Gummesson, R Johnsson, E Ornstein, J Ranstam, I Rosén. Prevalence of carpal tunnel syndrome in a general population. JAMA. 1999;282:153–58.

ously had carpal tunnel surgery or been diagnosed as having carpal tunnel syndrome. When the symptomatic respondents were studied with nerve conduction studies, 5,800 per 100,000 women and 600 per 100,000 men had electrically confirmed carpal tunnel syndrome. A population-based questionnaire survey with follow-up nerve conduction testing in a British general practice found similar orders of magnitude for symptomatic individuals and for abnormal median nerve conduction results (Ferry, Pritchard, Keenan, Croft & Silman, 1998). The results of a Swedish population survey are shown in Table 3-5. The U.S. National Health Interview Survey and these British, Swedish, and Dutch studies show that most individuals in the general population with hand paresthesias do not seek medical attention; a significant fraction of these would have diagnosable carpal tunnel syndrome if they were evaluated by physicians. We still know little of the long-term natural history of these nonpatients, but chronic mild carpal tunnel syndrome, not requiring formal treatment, is probably much more common than the more severe cases seen in physician's offices.

There is little cross-cultural data on the prevalence of carpal tunnel syndrome. A door-to-door survey among the Parsi population of Bombay, India, found that carpal tunnel syndrome, with a prevalence of 557 cases per 100,000 population, was the most common neurologic disorder in this community (Bharucha, Bharucha & Bharucha, 1991). A report of a low incidence of carpal tunnel syndrome in black South Africans makes no pretense of thorough case finding (Goga, 1990).

Definition and Diagnostic Criterion Standards for Carpal Tunnel Syndrome

Carpal tunnel syndrome is defined as compression of the median nerve in the carpal tunnel accompanied by clinical manifestations of nerve fiber dysfunction. The usual symptoms of pain and paresthesias are often not accompanied by abnormal findings on physical examination. An occasional patient with carpal tunnel syndrome has an asymptomatic neurologic deficit, such as thenar weakness and atrophy, due to the nerve compression.

Defining a syndrome is much simpler than stating diagnostic criteria for it. There is no gold standard for the diagnosis of carpal tunnel syndrome (Rempel, Evanoff, Amadio, de Krom, Franklin, Franzblau, Gray & Gerr, 1998; Franzblau & Werner, 1999; Rosenbaum, 1999). The absence of a gold standard is to be expected for a syndrome with varied clinical manifestations, varied causes, and incompletely understood pathophysiology. However, every research study of carpal tunnel syndrome needs to specify a working diagnostic criterion standard for carpal tunnel syndrome. The choice of the diagnostic standard depends on the aims of the research and influences the outcome of the study.

Some authors have used diagnostic standards based on electrodiagnostic criteria alone. These standards contradict the definition of carpal tunnel syndrome that specifically states that the syndrome includes clinical manifestations. Because of the high incidence of mild abnormalities of nerve conduction in the general asymptomatic population, diagnostic criteria that are solely electrodiagnostic are problematic (Atroshi, Gummesson, Johnsson, Ornstein, Ranstam & Rosén, 1999). To avoid circular reasoning, studies of electrodiagnostic sensitivity and specificity for carpal tunnel syndrome need to use diagnostic criteria that are independent of results of electrodiagnostic findings (Jablecki, Andary, So, Wilkins & Williams, 1993).

Studies that use both clinical and electrodiagnostic criteria for carpal tunnel syndrome are least likely to include patients with false-positive diagnoses. In some instances, this design is desirable. However, patients with mild carpal tunnel syndrome might be disproportionately excluded from these studies, resulting in an underestimate of the incidence or prevalence of carpal tunnel syndrome and a skewing of the clinical conception of the syndrome owing to overrepresentation of more severe cases.

Studies that use clinical criteria alone for the diagnosis of carpal tunnel syndrome probably overestimate the incidence of the syndrome. For example, some studies that base the diagnosis on hand pain without paresthesias can misconstrue a number of patients who have alternative causes of hand pain as examples of patients who have carpal tunnel syndrome.

A consensus committee has analyzed various diagnostic criteria for carpal tunnel syndrome, estimating the likelihood of a correct diagnosis of carpal tunnel syndrome for different case definitions (Table 3-6) (Rempel et al., 1998).

Table 3-6. Estimated Likelihood of Carpal Tunnel Syndrome for Case Definitions That Include Electrodiagnostic Studies

Symptom*	Electrodiagnosis	Ordinal Likelihood of Carpal Tunnel Syndrome
Classic/probable	Positive	+++
Possible	Positive	++
Classic/probable	Negative	+/–
Possible	Negative	–
Unlikely	Positive	–
Unlikely	Negative	– –

*Per Table 3-2.
The ordinal likelihood that a patient has carpal tunnel syndrome is indicated by the + (diagnosis is more likely) and – (diagnosis is less likely) symbols.
Modified with permission from D Rempel, B Evanoff, PC Amadio, M de Krom, G Franklin, A Franzblau, R Gray, F Gerr, M Hagberg, T Hales, JN Katz, G Pransky. Consensus criteria for the classification of carpal tunnel syndrome in epidemiologic studies. Am. J. Public Health 1998;88:1447–51.

Clinical Classification of Carpal Tunnel Syndrome

No criterion standard solves the problem of making a correct diagnosis in difficult clinical settings. Carpal tunnel syndrome is a diagnosis based on symptoms. In many patients with hand symptoms, we lack unequivocal diagnostic criteria to determine whether symptoms that might be those of carpal tunnel syndrome are indeed the consequence of focal dysfunction of the median nerve. The high incidence of asymptomatic nerve compression, the inaccuracies of diagnostic signs and tests, the possibility of multiple common conditions contributing to hand symptoms, and the natural variations in the ways patients experience and describe symptoms all contribute to diagnostic uncertainty. There will always be patients in whom carpal tunnel syndrome is a possible but unproved diagnosis. At times the most reliable diagnostic criterion is the opinion of an experienced clinician (Katz, Larson, Sabra, Krarup, Stirrat, Sethi, Eaton, Fossel & Liang, 1990).

Without doubt, in many cases the diagnosis of carpal tunnel syndrome is clear-cut. In other cases, particularly when clinical confirmation of the diagnosis is unavailable or when multiple conditions can be contributing to arm and hand symptoms and signs, the clinical diagnosis is less certain. When the diag-

nosis of carpal tunnel syndrome is uncertain, the clinician should use the *uncertainty* as a decision-making aid and be wary of unnecessarily aggressive therapy. An uncertain diagnosis implies that if carpal tunnel syndrome is present, any median nerve injury is likely to be mild. In this setting, observation over time or clinical trials of conservative therapies often provide the best diagnostic and therapeutic strategies.

Table 3-7 offers a clinical staging classification—based on symptoms and signs of carpal tunnel syndrome—which reflects escalating nerve fiber pathology. We believe that carpal tunnel syndrome has a very broad clinical spectrum, such that many individuals have symptoms that fulfill the definition of symptomatic median nerve compression at the wrist, but only a fraction of these individuals seek medical care and a even smaller fraction need surgical treatment. Many patients are on the border between one class and another. The scheme is offered to encourage clinicians to think about carpal tunnel syndrome pathophysiologically. Detailed discussion of the pathophysiologic concepts is found in subsequent chapters.

Class 0. *Asymptomatic median nerve pathology.* This is present in a large portion of the clinically normal population. In small series, abnormal nerve histology has been found in more than 40% of

Table 3-7. Classification of Median Neuropathies at the Carpal Tunnel

Class	Symptoms	Signs
0—Asymptomatic	None	None
1—Intermittently symptomatic	Intermittent positive symptoms	Provocative test often positive, but neurologic deficit usually absent
2—Persistently symptomatic	Continual positive or negative symptoms	Neurologic deficit sometimes present
3—Severe	Negative symptoms usually flagrant	Neurologic deficit present, can include evidence of axonal interruption

median nerves studied at autopsy. The more subtle tests of nerve conduction show abnormalities in approximately 20% of the population, so even the most sensitive available tests might not reveal all instances of mild pathologic change in the nerve.

Some individuals remain asymptomatic despite electrodiagnostic evidence of more severe dysfunction of median nerve myelinated fibers. These individuals can have clearly abnormal sensory and motor nerve conduction but have no symptoms or signs of carpal tunnel syndrome and require no specific treatment. One common example is abnormal nerve conduction in an asymptomatic hand, contralateral to a hand with carpal tunnel syndrome. Another example is the persistence of abnormal nerve conduction following carpal tunnel surgery that has successfully relieved all symptoms of the median neuropathy.

Class 1. *Intermittently symptomatic median nerve compression*. These individuals typically have intermittent hand paresthesias. Neurologic examination shows no sensory or motor deficit. In some, paresthesias can be reproduced by provocative tests.

The paresthesias result from ectopic nerve impulse activity, which can occur whether or not large myelinated nerve fibers have delayed conduction, so only some of these individuals have abnormalities on nerve conduction tests. There is a wide range of severity within this class.

Class 1A. *Subclinical median nerve irritability*. At the mildest extreme, ectopic neuronal firing occurs only with provocative tests—for example, a person has a positive Tinel's sign over the median nerve at the wrist or a positive Phalen's test. These individuals might not have any other symptoms of carpal tunnel syndrome; hence, the positive provocative tests are "false-positives" for the diagnosis of carpal tunnel syndrome.

Many people find that their hands "go to sleep" at one time or another. They have mild median nerve irritability that usually is not brought to medical attention and is insufficient to merit a diagnosis of carpal tunnel syndrome.

Class 1B. *Mild carpal tunnel syndrome*. At the next level of severity, many individuals in class 1 have transient symptoms of carpal tunnel syndrome, then return to an asymptomatic state. Examples are most women with carpal tunnel syndrome during pregnancy and some individuals who develop carpal tunnel syndrome after a few days or weeks of a particular activity, which they then stop. Symptoms can resolve completely; nerve conduction abnormalities can resolve completely or partially. Some individuals remain in this class for many years, experiencing symptoms from time to time, without progression to more serious nerve dysfunction. Some require no treatment; others respond well to nonoperative therapies such as change of activities or splinting.

Class 1C. *Moderate intermittent carpal tunnel syndrome*. The most severely affected individuals in class 1 have recurrent hand symptoms many times a week. At this stage they usually have local slowing of nerve conduction across the carpal tunnel. The neurologic examination usually shows no fixed neurologic deficit. Some benefit from conservative therapy and can be reclassified as 1B or better; in others, troublesome symptoms are eventually treated with surgery.

Class 2. *Persistently symptomatic carpal tunnel syndrome*. These individuals are much more likely than individuals in class 1 to have deficits on neurologic examination and usually have abnormal median nerve conduction reflecting substantial neuropathy. When sensory loss in the median distribution is present, symptoms and signs of ectopic neuronal firing such as paresthesias and Phalen's sign can become less prominent (Phalen, 1966). These patients rarely obtain lasting relief from nonsurgical therapy, but symptoms and signs are completely relieved by surgery in most patients in this class.

Figure 8-5 contrasts patients with intermittent and patients with persistent symptoms in regard to electrodiagnostic and clinical findings. Deciding whether an individual patient is in class 1 or class 2 can be difficult. Rarely, a patient with persistent symptoms despite conservative therapy has normal nerve conduction studies and a normal neurologic examination. Before subjecting these patients to surgery, the history and response to provocative tests should be extremely reliable.

Class 3. *Severe carpal tunnel syndrome with clinical evidence of median nerve axonal interruption.* These patients can have thenar atrophy, fibrillations or neuropathic motor units on electromyography, or evidence of small-fiber sensory or sympathetic dysfunction. Most are symptomatic, but an occasional patient is unaware of symptoms until physical signs are discovered. Most of these patients have some improvement after carpal tunnel surgery, but recovery of neurologic function can be delayed or incomplete.

References

Ahn DS. Hand elevation: a new test for carpal tunnel syndrome. Ann. Plast. Surg. 2001;46:120–24.

Aiache AE, Delagi EF. A pure sign of lumbrical function. Plast. Reconstr. Surg. 1974;54:312–15.

Alfonso MI, Dzwierzynski W. Hoffman-Tinel sign. The realities. Phys. Med. Rehabil. Clin. N. Am. 1998;9:721–36,v.

Anonymous. Occupational disease surveillance: carpal tunnel syndrome. MMWR. Morb. Mortal. Wkly. Rep. 1989;38(28):485–9.

Aratari E, Regesta G, Rebora A. Carpal tunnel syndrome appearing with prominent skin symptoms. Arch. Dermatol. 1984;120:517–19.

Atroshi I, Gummesson C, Johnsson R, Ornstein E, Ranstam J, Rosén I. Prevalence of carpal tunnel syndrome in a general population. JAMA. 1999;282:153–58.

Bharucha NE, Bharucha AE, Bharucha EP. Prevalence of peripheral neuropathy in the Parsi community of Bombay. Neurology 1991;41:1315–17.

Birkbeck MQ, Beer TC. Occupation in relation to the carpal tunnel syndrome. Rheumatol. Rehabil. 1975;14:218–21.

Bland JD. The value of the history in the diagnosis of carpal tunnel syndrome. J. Hand Surg. 2000;25B:445–50.

Borg K, Lindblom U. Increase of vibration threshold during wrist flexion in patients with carpal tunnel syndrome. Pain 1986;26:211–19.

Borg K, Lindblom U. Diagnostic value of quantitative sensory testing (QST) in carpal tunnel syndrome. Acta Neurol. Scand. 1988;78:537–41.

Braun RM, Davidson K, Doehr S. Provocative testing in the diagnosis of dynamic carpal tunnel syndrome. J. Hand Surg. 1989;14A:195–97.

Braverman DL, Root BC. "Phantom" carpal tunnel syndrome. Arch. Phys. Med. Rehabil. 1997;78:1157–59.

Buch-Jaeger N, Foucher G. Correlation of clinical signs with nerve conduction tests in the diagnosis of carpal tunnel syndrome. J. Hand Surg. 1994;19B:720–24.

Burke DT, Burke MA, Bell R, Stewart GW, Mehdi RS, Kim HJ. Subjective swelling: a new sign for carpal tunnel syndrome. Am. J. Phys. Med. Rehabil. 1999;78:504–8.

Buschbacher R. Side-to-side confrontational strength-testing for weakness of the intrinsic muscles of the hand. J. Bone Joint Surg. 1997;79A:401–5.

Cherington M. Proximal pain in carpal tunnel syndrome. Arch. Surg. 1974;108:69.

Cobb TK, An KN, Cooney WP, Berger RA. Lumbrical muscle incursion into the carpal tunnel during finger flexion. J. Hand Surg. 1994;19B:434–38.

Cox NH, Large DM, Paterson WD, Ive FA. Blisters, ulceration and autonomic neuropathy in carpal tunnel syndrome. Br. J. Dermatol. 1992;126:611–13.

Crymble B. Brachial neuralgia and the carpal tunnel syndrome. Br. Med. J. 1968;3:470–71.

Daras M, Tuchman AJ, Spector S, Zalzal P, Rogoff B. Tinel's sign. A reappraisal of its use. Presse Med. 1987;16:918.

D'Arcy CA, McGee S. Does this patient have carpal tunnel syndrome? JAMA. 2000;283:3110–17.

Dawson DM, Hallett M, Wilbourn AJ, eds. Entrapment Neuropathies, 3rd ed. Philadelphia: Lippincott–Raven, 1999.

De Krom MCTFM, Knipschild PG, Kester ADM, Thijs CT, Boekkooi PF, Spaans F. Carpal tunnel syndrome: prevalence in the general population. J. Clin. Epidemiol. 1992;45:373–76.

Desjacques P, Egloff-Baer S, Roth G. Lumbrical muscles and the carpal tunnel syndrome. Electromyogr. Clin. Neurophysiol. 1980;20:443–49.

De Smet L, Steenwerckx A, Van den Bogaert G, Cnudde P, Fabry G. Value of clinical provocative tests in carpal tunnel syndrome. Acta Orthop. Belg. 1995;61:177–82.

Dorwart BB. Volar "Hot Dog" at the wrist: a new sign in carpal tunnel syndrome. Clin. Res. 1983;31:649A.

Durkan JA. A new diagnostic test for carpal tunnel syndrome. J. Bone Joint Surg. 1991;73A:535–38.

Durkan JA. The carpal-compression test. An instrumented device for diagnosing carpal tunnel syndrome. Ortho. Rev. 1994;23:522–25.

Falck B, Aarnio P. Left-sided carpal tunnel syndrome in butchers. Scand. J. Work Environ. Health 1983;9:291–97.

Fast A, Parikh S, Ducommun EJ. Dermatitis-sympathetic dysfunction in carpal tunnel syndrome. A case report. Clin. Orthop. 1989:124–26.

Ferry S, Pritchard T, Keenan J, Croft P, Silman AJ. Estimating the prevalence of delayed median nerve conduction in the general population. Br. J. Rheumatol. 1998;37:630–35.

Fertl E, Wober C, Zeitlhofer J. The serial use of two provocative tests in the clinical diagnosis of carpal tunnel syndrome. Acta Neurol. Scand. 1998;98:328–32.

Finger D, Vogel P. Carpal tunnel syndrome. Arthritis Rheum. 1998;41:182.

Franklin GM, Haug JA, Peck NB, Heyer N, Checkoway H. Occupational carpal tunnel syndrome in Washington State, 1984–1987. Neurology 1990;40:420.

Franzblau A, Werner RA. What is carpal tunnel syndrome? JAMA. 1999;282:186–87.

Franzblau A, Werner R, Albers JW, et al. Workplace surveillance for carpal tunnel syndrome using hand diagrams. J. Occup. Rehabil. 1994;4:185–98.

Fritz TM, Burg G, Boni R. Carpal tunnel syndrome with ulcerous skin lesions. Dermatology 2000;201:165–67.

Gainer JV Jr., Nugent GR. Carpal tunnel syndrome: report of 430 operations. South. Med. J. 1977;70:325–28.

Gelberman RH, Szabo RM, Williamson RV, Dimick MP. Sensibility testing in peripheral-nerve compression syndromes. An experimental study in humans. J. Bone Joint Surg. 1983;65A:632–38.

Gellman H, Gelberman RH, Tan AM, Botte MJ. Carpal tunnel syndrome. An evaluation of the provocative diagnostic tests. J. Bone Joint Surg. 1986;68A:735–37.

Gelmers HJ. The significance of Tinel's sign in the diagnosis of carpal tunnel syndrome. Acta Neurochir. (Wien.) 1979;49: 255–58.

Gerr F, Letz R. The sensitivity and specificity of tests for carpal tunnel syndrome vary with the comparison subjects. J. Hand Surg. 1998;23B:151–55.

Ghavanini MR, Haghighat M. Carpal tunnel syndrome: reappraisal of five clinical tests. Electromyogr. Clin. Neurophysiol. 1998;38:437–41.

Gilliatt RW, Wilson TG. A pneumatic-tourniquet test in the carpal-tunnel syndrome. Lancet 1953;2:595–97.

Gilliatt RW, Wilson TG. Ischaemic sensory loss in patients with peripheral nerve lesions. J. Neurol. Neurosurg. Psychiatry 1954;17:104–14.

Goga IE. Carpal tunnel syndrome in black South Africans. J. Hand Surg. 1990;15B:96–99.

Golding DN, Rose DM, Selvarajah K. Clinical tests for carpal tunnel syndrome: an evaluation. Br. J. Rheumatol. 1986;25: 388–90.

Gunnarsson LG, Amilon A, Hellstrand P, Leissner P, Philipson L. The diagnosis of carpal tunnel syndrome. Sensitivity and specificity of some clinical and electrophysiological tests. J. Hand Surg. 1997;22B:34–37.

Gupta SK, Benstead TJ. Symptoms experienced by patients with carpal tunnel syndrome. Can. J. Neurol. Sci. 1997;24: 338–42.

Hybbinette CH, Mannerfelt L. The carpal tunnel syndrome. A retrospective study of 400 operated patients. Acta Orthop. Scand. 1975;46:610–20.

Jablecki CK, Andary MT, So YT, Wilkins DE, Williams FH. Literature review of the usefulness of nerve conduction studies and electromyography for the evaluation of patients with carpal tunnel syndrome. Muscle Nerve 1993;16:1392–1414.

Jeng OJ, Radwin RG, Fryback DG. Preliminary evaluation of a sensory and psychomotor functional test battery for carpal tunnel syndrome: Part 1—Confirmed cases and normal subjects. Am. Ind. Hyg. Assoc. J. 1997;58: 852–60.

Jeng OJ, Radwin RG, Moore JS, Roberts M, Garrity JM, Oswald T. Preliminary evaluation of a sensory and psycho-motor functional test battery for carpal tunnel syndrome: Part 2—Industrial subjects. Am. Ind. Hyg. Assoc. J. 1997;58:885–92.

Jungo O. Eine einfache Prüfung zum Nachweis des Karpaltunnelsyndroms. Manuelle Med. 1969;7:54–55.

Karl AI, Carney ML, Kaul MP. The lumbrical provocation test in subjects with median inclusive paresthesia. Arch. Phys. Med. Rehabil. 2001;82:935–37.

Katz JN, Larson MG, Sabra A, Krarup C, Stirrat CR, Sethi R, Eaton HM, Fossel AH, Liang MH. The carpal tunnel syndrome: diagnostic utility of the history and physical examination findings. Ann. Intern. Med. 1990; 112:321–27.

Katz JN, Stirrat CR. A self-administered hand diagram for the diagnosis of carpal tunnel syndrome. J. Hand Surg. 1990;15A:360–63.

Katz JN, Stirrat CR, Larson MG, Fossel AH, Eaton HM, Liang MH. A self-administered hand diagram for the diagnosis and epidemiologic study of carpal tunnel syndrome. J. Rheumatol. 1990;17:1495–98.

Kaul MP, Pagel KJ, Dryden JD. Lack of predictive power of the "tethered" median stress test in suspected carpal tunnel syndrome [see comments]. Arch. Phys. Med. Rehabil. 2000;81: 348–50.

Kremer M, Gilliatt RW, Golding JSR, Wilson TG. Acroparesthesia in the carpal tunnel syndrome. Lancet 1953;2:595.

Krendel DA, Jobsis M, Gaskell PC Jr, Sanders DB. The flick sign in carpal tunnel syndrome. J. Neurol. Neurosurg. Psychiatry 1986;49:220–21.

Kummel BM, Zazanis GA. Shoulder pain as the presenting complaint in carpal tunnel syndrome. Clin. Orthop. 1973;92:227–30.

Kuschner SH, Ebramzadeh E, Johnson D, Brien WW, Sherman R. Tinel's sign and Phalen's test in carpal tunnel syndrome. Orthopedics 1992;15:1297–1302.

LaBan MM, Friedman NA, Zemenick GA. "Tethered" median nerve stress test in chronic carpal tunnel syndrome. Arch. Phys. Med. Rehabil. 1986;67:803–4.

LaBan MM, MacKenzie JR, Zemenick GA. Anatomic observations in carpal tunnel syndrome as they relate to the tethered median nerve stress test. Arch. Phys. Med. Rehabil. 1989;70:44–46.

LaBan MM, Zemenick GA, Meerschaert JR. Neck and shoulder pain. Presenting symptoms of carpal tunnel syndrome. Mich. Med. 1975;74:549–50.

Lang E, Claus D, Neundorfer B, Handwerker HO. Parameters of thick and thin nerve-fiber functions as predictors of pain in carpal tunnel syndrome. Pain 1995;60:295–302.

Lehtinen I, Kirjavainen T, Hurme M, Lauerma H, Martikainen K, Rauhala E. Sleep-related disorders in carpal tunnel syndrome. Acta Neurol. Scand. 1996;93:360–65.

Liss GM, Armstrong C, Kusiak RA, Galitis MM. Use of provincial health insurance plan billing data to estimate carpal tunnel syndrome morbidity and surgery rates. Am. J. Ind. Med. 1992;22:395–409.

Logigian EL, Busis NA, Berger AR, Bruyninckx F, Khalil N, Shahani BT, Young RR. Lumbrical sparing in carpal tunnel syndrome: anatomic, physiologic, and diagnostic implications. Neurology 1987;37:1499–1505.

Lundborg G, Gelberman RH, Minteer-Convery M, Lee YF, Hargens AR. Median nerve compression in the carpal tunnel—

functional response to experimentally induced controlled pressure. J. Hand Surg. 1982;7:252–59.

Manente G, Torrieri F, Pineto F, Uncini A. A relief maneuver in carpal tunnel syndrome. Muscle Nerve 1999;22:1587–89.

Marchettini P, Cline M, Ochoa JL. Innervation territories for touch and pain afferents of single fascicles of the human ulnar nerve. Brain 1990;113:1491–1500.

Marx RG, Hudak PL, Bombardier C, Graham B, Goldsmith C, Wright JG. The reliability of physical examination for carpal tunnel syndrome. J. Hand Surg. 1998;23B:499–502.

Massy-Westropp N, Grimmer K, Bain G. A systematic review of the clinical diagnostic tests for carpal tunnel syndrome. J. Hand Surg. 2000;25A:120–27.

Maxwell JA, Clough CA, Reckling FW, Kelly CR. Carpal tunnel syndrome. A review of cases treated surgically. J. Kans. Med. Soc. 1973;74:190–93.

Miller RS, Iverson DC, Fried RA, Green LA, Nutting PA. Carpal tunnel syndrome in primary care: a report from ASPN. Ambulatory Sentinel Practice Network. J. Fam. Pract. 1994;38:337–44.

Mossman SS, Blau JN. Tinel's sign and the carpal tunnel syndrome. BMJ. 1987;294:680.

Nordstrom DL, DeStefano F, Vierkant RA, Layde PM. Incidence of diagnosed carpal tunnel syndrome in a general population. Epidemiology 1998;9:342–45.

Novak CB, Mackinnon SE, Brownlee R, Kelly L. Provocative sensory testing in carpal tunnel syndrome. J. Hand Surg. 1992;17B:204–8.

Ochoa JL. Neuropathic pains, from within: personal experiences, experiments, and reflections on mythology. In: Dimitrijevic M, Wall PD, Lindblom U, eds. Recent Achievements in Restorative Neurology 3: Altered Sensation and Pain. Basel, Switzerland: S. Karger, 1990;100–11.

Oswald TA, Wertsch JJ, Vennix MJ, Brooks LL, Spreitzer AM. Ulnar paresthesia as a presenting symptom of carpal tunnel "syndrome." Muscle Nerve 1994;17:1082.

Padua L, Padua R, Aprile I, Tonali P. Italian multicentre study of carpal tunnel syndrome. Differences in the clinical and neurophysiological features between male and female patients. J. Hand Surg. 1999;24B:579–82.

Padua L, Padua R, Nazzaro M, Tonali P. Incidence of bilateral symptoms in carpal tunnel syndrome. J. Hand Surg. 1998; 23B:603–6.

Paine KW, Polyzoidis KS. Carpal tunnel syndrome. Decompression using the Paine retinaculotome. J. Neurosurg. 1983;59:1031–36.

Paley D, McMurtry RY. Median nerve compression test in carpal tunnel syndrome diagnosis: reproduces signs and symptoms in affected wrist. Ortho. Rev. 1985;14:41–45.

Phalen GS. The carpal-tunnel syndrome. Seventeen years' experience in diagnosis and treatment of six hundred fifty-four hands. J. Bone Joint. Surg 1966;48A:211–28.

Phalen GS. The carpal-tunnel syndrome. Clinical evaluation of 598 hands. Clin. Orthop. 1972;83:29–40.

Pryse-Phillips WE. Validation of a diagnostic sign in carpal tunnel syndrome. J. Neurol. Neurosurg. Psychiatry 1984;47: 870–72.

Quinlan AG. Carpal tunnel syndrome presenting as a complete median-nerve palsy with trophic changes. BMJ. 1967;1:32.

Raudino F. Tethered median nerve stress test in the diagnosis of carpal tunnel syndrome. Electromyogr. Clin. Neurophysiol. 2000;40:57–60.

Reinstein L. Hand dominance in carpal tunnel syndrome. Arch. Phys. Med. Rehabil. 1981;62:202–3.

Rempel D, Evanoff B, Amadio PC, de Krom M, Franklin G, Franzblau A, Gray R, Gerr F, Hagberg M, Hales T, Katz JN, Pransky G. Consensus criteria for the classification of carpal tunnel syndrome in epidemiologic studies. Am. J. Public Health 1998;88:1447–51.

Roquer J, Herraiz J. Validity of Flick sign in CTS diagnosis. Acta. Neurol. Scand. 1988;78:351.

Rosenbaum RB. Carpal tunnel syndrome and the myth of El Dorado. Muscle Nerve 1999;22:1165–67.

Salerno DF, Franzblau A, Werner RA, Chung KC, Schultz JS, Becker MP, Armstrong TJ. Reliability of physical examination of the upper extremity among keyboard operators. Am. J. Ind. Med. 2000;37:423–30.

Seror P. Carpal tunnel syndrome. Value of a new diagnostic test. Presse Med. 1987a;16:914.

Seror P. Tinel's sign in the diagnosis of carpal tunnel syndrome. J. Hand Surg. 1987b;12B:364–65.

Seror P. Phalen's test in the diagnosis of carpal tunnel syndrome. J. Hand Surg. 1988;13B:383–85.

Spindler HA, Dellon AL. Nerve conduction studies and sensibility testing in carpal tunnel syndrome. J. Hand Surg. 1982;7:260–63.

Spinner RJ, Bachman JW, Amadio PC. The many faces of carpal tunnel syndrome. Mayo Clin. Proc. 1989;64:829–36.

Stevens JC, Smith BE, Weaver AL, Bosch EP, Deen Jr. HG, Wilkens JA. Symptoms of 100 patients with electromyographically verified carpal tunnel syndrome. Muscle Nerve 1999;22:1448–56.

Stevens JC, Sun S, Beard CM, O'Fallon WM, Kurland LT. Carpal tunnel syndrome in Rochester, Minnesota, 1961 to 1980. Neurology 1988;38:134–38.

Szabo RM, Gelberman RH, Dimick MP. Sensibility testing in patients with carpal tunnel syndrome. J. Bone Joint Surg. 1984;66A:60–64.

Szabo RM, Slater RR Jr, Farver TB, Stanton DB, Sharman WK. The value of diagnostic testing in carpal tunnel syndrome. J. Hand Surg. 1999;24A:704–14.

Tanaka S, Wild DK, Seligman PJ, Halperin WE, Behrens VJ, Putz-Anderson V. Prevalence and work-relatedness of self-reported carpal tunnel syndrome among U.S. workers: analysis of the Occupational Health Supplement data of 1988 National Health Interview Survey. Am. J. Ind. Med. 1995;27:451–70.

Tetro AM, Evanoff BA, Hollstien SB, Gelberman RH. A new provocative test for carpal tunnel syndrome. Assessment of wrist flexion and nerve compression. J. Bone Joint Surg. 1998;80B:493–98.

Tinel J. Le signe du "fourmillement" dans les lesions des nerfs peripheriques. Presse Med. 1915;47:388–89.

Torebjörk HE, Ochoa JL, Schady W. Referred pain from intraneural stimulation of muscle fascicles in the median nerve. Pain 1984;18:145–56.

Tosti A, Morelli R, D'Alessandro R, Bassi F. Carpal tunnel syndrome presenting with ischemic skin lesions, acroosteolysis, and nail changes. J. Am. Acad. Dermatol. 1993; 29:287–90.

Tountas CP, MacDonald CJ, Meyerhoff JD, Bihrle DM. Carpal tunnel syndrome. A review of 507 patients. Minn. Med. 1983;66:479–82.

Verghese J, Galanopoulou AS, Herskovitz S. Autonomic dysfunction in idiopathic carpal tunnel syndrome. Muscle Nerve 2000;23:1209–13.

Wainner RS, Boninger ML, Balu G, Burdett R, Helkowski W. Durkan gauge and carpal compression test: accuracy and diagnostic test properties. J. Orthop. Sports Phys. Ther. 2000;30:676–82.

Werner RA, Bir C, Armstrong TJ. Reverse Phalen's maneuver as an aid in diagnosing carpal tunnel syndrome. Arch. Phys. Med. Rehabil. 1994;75:783–86.

Williams TM, Mackinnon SE, Novak CB, McCabe S, Kelly L. Verification of the pressure provacative test in carpal tunnel syndrome. Ann. Plast. Surg. 1992;29:8–11.

Wilson-MacDonald J, Caughey MA, Myers DB. Diurnal variation in nerve conduction, hand volume, and grip strength in the carpal tunnel syndrome. BMJ. 1984;289:1042.

Yamaguchi D, Lipscomb P, Soule E. Carpal tunnel syndrome. Minn. Med. 1965;48:22–31.

Yates SK, Yaworski R, Brown WF. Relative preservation of lumbrical versus thenar motor fibres in neurogenic disorders. J. Neurol. Neurosurg. Psychiatry 1981;44:768–74.

Yii NW, Elliot D. A study of the dynamic relationship of the lumbrical muscles and the carpal tunnel. J. Hand Surg. 1994;19B:439–43.

Chapter 4
Differential Diagnosis of Carpal Tunnel Syndrome

The diagnosis of carpal tunnel syndrome merits consideration in patients with hand or arm pains, paresthesias, numbness, stiffness, weakness, or muscular atrophy. The differential diagnosis primarily includes other disorders of nerve including focal or diffuse diseases of peripheral nerves, brachial plexus, nerve roots, and cervical spinal cord. In patients who present with arm and hand pain or stiffness, disorders of joint, bone, tendon, and soft tissue are often at the forefront of the differential diagnosis. The diagnostic task is more complex if multiple conditions are contributing to limb symptoms, especially if one condition is causing limb symptoms and also contributing to the pathogenesis of carpal tunnel syndrome.

Introductory discussions of diseases of the hand and arm are available elsewhere (Cailliet, 1994; Lister, 1994; Lichtman & Alexander, 1997). Choosing the entities to include in this chapter has been a challenge. Is angina pectoris in the differential diagnosis because it can present with arm pain? Is hyperventilation in the differential diagnosis because it can cause acral paresthesias? The problem of proximal arm pain in carpal tunnel syndrome is reviewed in Chapter 3, yet diseases of the shoulder joint are rarely confused with carpal tunnel syndrome. This chapter focuses on the diagnosis of conditions that are most likely to be confused with carpal tunnel syndrome. Chapter 5 reviews the relation of carpal tunnel syndrome to other medical conditions.

Neurologic Differential Diagnosis

Hand paresthesias and hand, wrist, or forearm pain characterize a number of other upper extremity neuropathies. Other median neuropathies are discussed in detail in Chapters 17 and 18. Fully developed ulnar or radial neuropathies, brachial plexopathies, or cervical radiculopathies should be easily separable from carpal tunnel syndrome by findings on neurologic examination (Stewart, 2000; Dawson, Hallett & Wilbourn, 1999). The diagnosis is complicated when multiple neuropathic abnormalities coexist or when symptoms are atypical and unaccompanied by signs of nerve dysfunction. For example, among 400 patients operated on for carpal tunnel syndrome, Hybbinette and Mannerfelt (1975) identified seven patients who obtained no benefit from carpal tunnel surgery and in whom an alternative neurologic diagnosis was made postoperatively: cervical radiculopathy (4), syringomyelia (1), neurosarcoma of the brachial plexus (1), and post-radiation brachial plexopathy (1). Among 12 patients who had unsuccessful carpal tunnel surgery, eventual neurologic diagnoses included diffuse peripheral neuropathy, cervical radiculopathy or myelopathy, motor neuron disease, syringomyelia, and multiple sclerosis (Witt & Stevens, 2000).

Ulnar Neuropathy

Ulnar neuropathy, like carpal tunnel syndrome, can present with hand paresthesias, hand weakness, or upper extremity pain. In the fully developed case with nonanomalous anatomy, the differential diagnosis is simple: Sensory loss is usually limited to the little finger and ulnar half of the ring finger; motor loss affects the hand intrinsic muscles except for opponens pollicis, flexor pollicis brevis, abductor pollicis brevis, and the lateral lumbricals. Flexor carpi ulnaris and the ulnar-innervated finger flexors can be weak with more proximal lesions. The diagnostic complexity increases when evaluating mild cases without objective signs, cases with simultaneous disease of median and ulnar nerves, or cases with anomalous patterns of innervation.

Chapter 1 discusses the anomalies of motor and sensory innervation, such as the "all-median hand" or ulnar innervation of thenar muscles (Rowntree, 1949). Chapter 7 includes a discussion of use of nerve conduction studies to clarify anomalous innervation.

Many patients with carpal tunnel syndrome report paresthesias or have sensory loss that includes the medial ring finger or even the little finger (Stevens, Smith, Weaver, Bosch, Deen & Wilkens, 1999). In a sample of 52 hands with clinical and electrodiagnostic evidence of carpal tunnel syndrome and with normal ulnar nerve conduction, 40% of patients reported numbness or tingling in the whole hand, and 4% reported numbness and tingling limited to the ulnar distribution (Gupta & Benstead, 1997). Hands affected by carpal tunnel syndrome, but without clinical evidence of ulnar neuropathy, are more likely than control hands to have abnormal thresholds for vibration perception in the little finger (Imai, Matsumoto & Minami, 1990). In one series, more than one-fourth of hands with carpal syndrome had abnormalities by monofilament or two-point discrimination sensory testing in the little finger (Silver, Gelberman, Gellman & Rhoades, 1985). Most of these abnormalities improved after carpal tunnel release surgery without surgery on Guyon's canal. This observation might be explained by anomalous patterns of innervation or by imprecise sensory mapping, but the incidence exceeds that usually reported for median innervation of the little finger (Stopford, 1918). Silver and colleagues (1985) speculate that ulnar nerve compression at Guyon's canal often coexists with carpal tunnel syndrome and that section of the flexor retinaculum might rearrange wrist anatomy enough to decrease the nerve compression in Guyon's canal.

Electrodiagnostic testing of patients with carpal tunnel syndrome should include median nerve conduction studies and studies of at least one other nerve in the symptomatic arm (Anonymous, 1993).

If the patient has sensory symptoms or other clinical findings that might be explained by ulnar neuropathy, the ulnar nerve should be one of the nerves studied. Interpretation of the results is complicated by conflicting reports on the incidence of ulnar nerve conduction test abnormalities in patients with carpal tunnel syndrome, which is discussed in more detail in Chapter 7.

Radial Neuropathy

A complete radial neuropathy with wrist drop is not mistakable for carpal tunnel syndrome. Isolated neuropathy of the superficial branch of the radial nerve is also distinctive; patients have no weakness but do have paresthesias, numbness, and sometimes pain or hyperpathia localized to the dorsal lateral aspect of the forearm and wrist. A potential point of confusion is that as many as 10% of patients with carpal tunnel syndrome describe their paresthesias as predominantly on the dorsums of their hands and fingers (Stevens et al., 1999).

The posterior interosseous nerve is the terminal motor branch of the radial nerve; posterior interosseous neuropathy causes weakness of finger and thumb extension without paresthesias or sensory loss. The extensor carpi radialis is innervated by the radial nerve proper, but extensor carpi ulnaris is innervated by the posterior interosseous nerve, so patients with posterior interosseous neuropathy do not have wrist drop but often deviate the hand radially during wrist extension.

Some authors use *radial tunnel syndrome* to describe a condition of lateral proximal forearm pain and tenderness over the radial tunnel, at which point the radial nerve or its posterior interosseous branch travel between the heads of the supinator muscle. The pain is typically increased by resisted middle finger extension or supination with the elbow extended. The syndrome is not accompanied by focal muscle weakness. In some of these patients, nocturnal awakening with arm pain is purportedly a prominent symptom (Carfi & Ma, 1985). If hand paresthesias occur, they are usually not prominent. Whether this type of radial tunnel syndrome is neurogenic is disputed (Rosenbaum, 1999). Whatever its pathogenesis, this syndrome of pain and tenderness over the extensor mass of the forearm, distal to the lateral epicondyle, is easily

Figure 4-1. Pattern of sensory deficit in a patient who has brachial plexopathy. This 36-year-old woman was initially thought to have a median neuropathy based on progressive sensory loss in the pattern shown (**A, B**). Evolution of her findings over years eventually led to the diagnosis of brachial plexopathy. Brachial plexus exploration confirmed this diagnosis with pathologic evidence of localized hypertrophic demyelination.

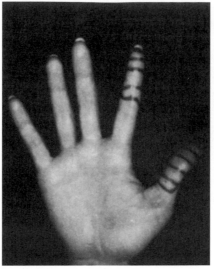

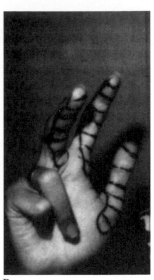

A

B

distinguishable from carpal tunnel syndrome, in which pain, when it includes the forearm, is more ventral and unaccompanied by proximal lateral forearm tenderness.

Brachial Plexopathy

The symptomatic presentation of an abnormality in the brachial plexus varies both with the portion of the plexus affected and with the cause of the plexopathy. In most cases, the extent of neurologic signs clearly distinguishes a brachial plexopathy from carpal tunnel syndrome. The distinction between neuralgic amyotrophy and proximal median neuropathies is discussed in Chapter 17.

The sensory changes of upper brachial plexopathies can overlap the median cutaneous sensory distribution. Patients with these upper plexopathies often have abnormal median distal sensory nerve conduction tests, even though the pathology is much more proximal than the carpal tunnel; an abnormal median distal sensory latency in these cases is not necessarily evidence of coexistent carpal tunnel syndrome. Figure 4-1 illustrates the pattern of sensory loss in a patient with brachial plexopathy who was initially thought to have a median neuropathy.

Patients with lower brachial plexopathies can develop weakness and atrophy in hand intrinsic muscles. When the cause of the lower brachial plexopathy is compression of the brachial plexus by the anatomic structures of the neck and axilla, the condition is termed *true neurogenic thoracic outlet syndrome*. These patients should be distinguishable from those with carpal tunnel syndrome by weakness in ulnar-innervated hand intrinsic muscles. They should differ from patients with combined ulnar and median neuropathies by the preservation of sensation in the median distribution. In patients with lower brachial plexopathies, nerve conduction studies can also be helpful by showing normal median motor and sensory conduction, whereas ulnar or medial antebrachial cutaneous sensory action potentials are abnormal (Gilliatt, Willison, Dietz & Williams, 1978; Nishida, Price & Minieka, 1993; Le Forestier, Moulonguet, Maisonobe, Léger & Bouche, 1998). If the thenar muscles are severely atrophied, the median thenar compound muscle action potential amplitude is, of course, decreased, and the median motor nerve conduction velocity can be slowed. The differential diagnosis of patients with lower brachial plexopathy includes Pancoast's syndrome caused by tumors at the lung apex, so patients with lower brachial plexopathy should be examined carefully for hoarseness caused by involvement of the recurrent laryngeal nerve and for Horner's syndrome caused by involvement of the cervical sympathetic ganglion.

Compression of the subclavian artery in the thoracic outlet (arterial thoracic outlet syndrome) is a rare condition that can cause forearm pain and paresthesias accompanied by signs of unilateral arterial insufficiency such as Raynaud's phenomenon, ischemic finger tip ulcers, or other signs of arm ischemia (Dawson et al., 1999). Venous thoracic outlet syndrome, also rare, can cause arm pain, swelling, and discoloration accompanied by dilatation of peripheral arm veins.

There is an ongoing debate on the role of brachial plexus compression in causing arm pain and paresthesia in patients with normal neurologic examinations and normal electrodiagnostic evaluations. The terms *nonspecific thoracic outlet syndrome* and *disputed thoracic outlet syndrome* have been applied to a heterogeneous group of patients. Some have posterior neck pain with radiation down the medial arm and medial hand paresthesias. Others have more proximal arm or shoulder girdle pain. Many have ipsilateral headaches (Dawson et al., 1999; Roos & Wilbourn, 1999). In some of these patients, abnormality of the thoracic outlet is considered because of reproduction of symptoms or impairment of arterial pulses by certain positions that alter the configuration of the thoracic outlet. These maneuvers (Adson's test, arm hyperabduction, the military brace position, hand exercise with arms up in the surrender position) are so frequently abnormal in asymptomatic individuals, however, that they have little value as diagnostic tests. Both compression neuropathies, such as carpal tunnel syndrome, and cervical radiculopathies can cause upper extremity pain and paresthesias before nerve compression is advanced enough to cause objective neurologic deficit or electrodiagnostic abnormalities. Theoretically, this could also occur with brachial plexus compression at the thoracic outlet; practically, we find that it is rarely, if ever, reasonable to diagnosis thoracic outlet syndrome with enough confidence to recommend thoracic outlet surgery unless the patient has objective confirmation of brachial plexus compression or of vascular compromise.

Cervical Radiculopathy

The neurologic signs and symptoms of cervical radiculopathies can overlap those of carpal tunnel syndrome. Forearm and upper arm pain can be a feature of either disorder, but neck pain is more characteristic of cervical radiculopathy. In addition to neck and arm pain, cervical radiculopathy can cause referred pain in the pectoral or interscapular areas. The location of the pain is of relatively little value in predicting which cervical root is generating the pain. Radiculopathic pain has protean qualities: deep, superficial, aching, gnawing, steady, fleeting, electrical, stabbing, or dysesthetic. A key historical point of differentiation from carpal tunnel syndrome is the timing of symptoms: Radiculopathies usually have steady rather than inter-mittent, nocturnal or rest-induced paresthesias. The pain of radiculopathies can be persistent even when the paresthesias are intermittent. The symptoms of radiculopathy can often be increased by neck turning, Valsalva's maneuver, local pressure in the area of pain, or arm stretching. Sometimes the pain can be decreased by gentle manual neck traction or by the patient reaching over the head toward the contralateral ear. Spurling's sign (induction of arm pain and paresthesias by turning the head toward the symptomatic side and extending the neck) is indicative of radiculopathy.

C-6 radiculopathy can cause cutaneous sensory symptoms on the lateral hand, typically most noticeable on the dorsum of the hand, particularly on the thumb, index finger, and web space between them. Motor changes, such as deltoid or biceps weakness, and depression of the biceps reflex, when present, clearly indicate a radiculopathy or other proximal abnormality rather than a median neuropathy.

The sensory symptoms of a C-7 radiculopathy center on the middle finger and its neighbors. The prominence of sensory symptoms on the dorsum of the hand is atypical for carpal tunnel syndrome. When weakness is present, forearm muscles innervated by the median nerve, especially the pronators, can be weak, but triceps will also be weak, and thenar muscles will be spared. A depressed triceps jerk clearly favors a radiculopathy.

Radiculopathy is much rarer at C-8 than at C-7 or C-6. Weakness, when present, includes not only median-innervated thenar muscles but also ulnar-innervated hand intrinsic muscles and distal radial-innervated muscles such as extensor indicis proprius. The sensory changes are in the ulnar, rather than the median, territory.

Patients with radiculopathy alone should have normal nerve conduction studies. Sensory nerve action potential amplitude should be normal in radiculopathy even from digits with well-established sensory loss (Wilbourn & Aminoff, 1988).

Diseases of the Central Nervous System

Many diseases of the brain and cervical spinal cord can cause characteristic hand syndromes. Rondot (1993) offers a thorough review of the hand postures and other hand findings specific to a wide variety of central nervous system diseases. The neurologist rarely has trouble separating carpal tunnel syndrome from central nervous system causes of focal arm symptoms. Every patient with suspected carpal tunnel syndrome should have a screening neurologic history and examination without shortsighted limitation of the evaluation to the patient's arm. For example, patients with multiple sclerosis sometimes experience focal hand paresthesias. A man who had sharp pains radiating from his right elbow to his hand, hand weakness, and paresthesia in his right middle and ring fingers underwent carpal tunnel surgery but remained symptomatic; he was later found to have tabes dorsalis (Gorsche & Verstraten, 1996). Syringomyelia or tumors of the cervical spinal cord can cause sensory and motor deficits limited to the hand. Transient ischemic attacks or focal sensory seizures can cause intermittent hand symptoms.

Small lesions in the thalamus, such as lacunar strokes, can on rare occasion cause contralateral motor and sensory deficits limited to the distribution of a single peripheral nerve, such as the median or ulnar (Lampl, Gilad, Eshel & Sarova-Pinhas, 1995). The localization of the pathology to the central nervous system is usually evident by associated signs such as more diffuse arm clumsiness than expected with a peripheral nerve lesion, hyperreflexia ipsilateral to the hand deficit, or an accompanying Babinski's sign.

Patients with cervical myelopathies can present with hand sensory symptoms and weakness of hand intrinsic muscles. Usually the extent of neu-rologic abnormality, often including the legs, make the diagnosis clear. The diagnosis is more difficult when cervical myelopathy and carpal tunnel syndrome coexist (Epstein, Epstein & Carras, 1989). At times the diagnosis of myelopathy is aided by spinal imaging, such as magnetic resonance imaging, and electrophysiologic investigation of spinal cord conduction, such as somatosensory evoked responses or transcranial magnetic motor stimulation (Subramaniam, de la Harpe & Corlett, 1997); in some patients the coexisting diagnoses are clarified by operating on the more pressing problem, then reevaluating residual symptoms and signs.

Lesions of the upper cervical cord at the level of the foramen magnum can be particularly challenging when hand numbness and clumsiness develop insidiously, and hand intrinsic weakness precedes other neurologic signs. In one series of 57 patients with extramedullary foramen magnum tumors, three were initially misdiagnosed as having carpal tunnel syndrome (Yasuoka, Okazaki, Daube & MacCarty, 1978).

Patients with motor neuron disease occasionally have striking weakness and atrophy of thenar muscles, but a careful examination reveals more widespread motor dysfunction and absence of median sensory abnormalities. Monomelic amyotrophy is a form of motor neuron diseases that differs from amyotrophic lateral sclerosis by having atrophy and weakness limited to a single limb, lack of upper motor neuron signs, and relatively benign course; in some cases it preferentially involves hand intrinsic or forearm flexor muscles (Donofrio, 1994).

Patients using canes or crutches are vulnerable to development of carpal tunnel syndrome. This is well described in paraplegics and has also been noted in patients with residual weakness from polio (see Table 13-2 for references).

Thenar Hypoplasia

Congenital thenar hypoplasia is a rare condition, which can present with bilateral or unilateral "atrophy" (really hypotrophy) localized to thenar muscles without pain or sensory abnormalities. Although presumably present from birth, it can escape recognition until mid-childhood or even adulthood. Cavanagh (1979) reported a woman who first became symptomatic in her late 40s and who was initially misdiagnosed as having carpal tunnel syndrome. The patients have strikingly weak, atrophic thenar muscles. Neurologic examination is otherwise normal. Median nerve conduction studies show normal sensory conduction; motor conduction studies show a small or absent thenar compound muscle action potential, but electromyographic needle examination of the atrophic muscles shows no evidence of neuropathic abnormalities. Further support for the diagnosis of congenital thenar hypoplasia is finding bony malformations of the carpals, first metacarpal, or thumb phalanges on wrist and hand radiographs.

Su and colleagues (1972) reported a 33-year-old woman who had unilateral congenital absence of the opponens pollicis, abductor pollicis brevis, superficial head of the flexor pollicis brevis, and recurrent thenar motor branch of the median nerve. The patient had a normal adductor pollicis and deep head of the flexor pollicis brevis and no skeletal deformities of her hand.

Non-Neurologic Differential Diagnosis

Tenosynovitis

Tenosynovitis (Lister, 1994; Amadio, 1995), or inflammation of the synovial tendon sheaths, is characterized by pain elicited by tendon movement or by increased tendon load during muscle contraction. Typically joint movement that stretches the tendon causes pain; in contrast, the pain of arthritis occurs with any movement of the joint. Tenderness over the tendon is more common than other manifestations of inflammation, such as warmth, heat, or swelling. Tenosynovitis can be localized to one or a few tendons or be more generalized. It can be secondary to an inflammatory process, such as rheumatoid arthritis, gout, or focal infection. More commonly tenosynovitis is localized to a single tendon and either is caused by strain or overuse or is idiopathic.

de Quervain's tenosynovitis is a common localized tenosynovitis that affects the extensor pollicis brevis and abductor pollicis longus tendons. Patients with de Quervain's tenosynovitis typically describe aching discomfort over the radial styloid that increases with wrist or thumb movement. Pain can spread into the forearm or hand. A classic sign is increase in pain when the thumb is held in flexion while the wrist is deviated ulnarly (Finkelstein's sign).

Intersection syndrome is another painful condition of the radial forearm. It is distinguishable from de Quervain's tenosynovitis because the tenderness in intersection syndrome is located about 4 to 10 cm proximal to the wrist and more ulnarward than the usual site of tenderness in de Quervain's. The cause is inflammation of the bursa at the intersection of the muscle bellies of abductor pollicis longus and extensor pollicis brevis passing over the wrist extensor tendons. Patients with intersection syndrome often have crepitus at the point of intersection and sometimes have a Finkelstein's sign.

Linburg's syndrome (Linburg & Comstock, 1979) presents with volar distal forearm tenderness. The discomfort increases with passive index finger extension with the thumb actively flexed. Patients often have an anomalous tendinous band connecting the tendons of flexor pollicis longus and flexor digitorum profundus to the index finger, an anomaly that is present in about 15% of arms. In other patients, hypertrophy of the adjacent tendons of the two muscles accounts for the clinical findings. Some patients have median distribution paresthesias (Lombardi, Wood & Linscheid, 1988; Amadio, 1995).

Lateral epicondylitis or *tennis elbow*, another common tenosynovitis in the forearm, involves the extensor muscles that arise from the lateral humeral epicondyle. The characteristics are focal tenderness near the lateral epicondyle and increase in the pain with wrist extension against resistance.

Medial epicondylitis (golfer's elbow) is less common than lateral epicondylitis. As the name implies, pain and tenderness typically involve any of the five muscle-tendon units that originate from the medial epicondyle. Pain is increased by wrist flexion against resistance.

Tendinitis can be localized to other forearm tendons such as those of the biceps, extensor carpi radialis, extensor carpi ulnaris, extensor digitorum, extensor pollicis longus, flexor carpi radialis, or flexor carpi ulnar (Brooker, 1977; Amadio, 1995).

Some patients describe forearm pain induced by forearm use. Many of these patients have nonspecific clinical findings, and terms like *tendinitis* or *chronic muscular strain* are applied loosely for want of a more specific diagnostic term.

Tenosynovitis can affect the flexor digitorum superficialis or flexor digitorum profundus tendons in the palm. Patients who have this condition typically describe pain in the palm or dorsum of the hand, induced or increased by finger flexion (Lapedus & Guidotti, 1972; Gottlieb, 1991). Patients can have local swelling of the tendon in the palm or more diffuse palmar swelling. The digital flexor tenosynovitis can cause trigger finger, a finger suddenly snapping or catching during flexion so that reextension is prohibited. Trigger finger most commonly occurs in the thumb, middle, or ring fingers. On examination a nodule is sometimes palpable on the affected tendon proximal to the metacarpal-phalangeal joint. There is an increased incidence of digital flexor tenosynovitis in patients with rheumatoid arthritis, diabetes mellitus, myxedema, amyloidosis, or hand trauma.

These focal tendon problems are usually clearly separable from carpal tunnel syndrome by history and physical examination. Diagnosis is more difficult, however, when tenosynovitis coexists with carpal tunnel syndrome. For example, Phalen (1972) found de Quervain's tenosynovitis in four, tennis elbow in 15, and trigger finger or thumb in 32 of 384 patients with carpal tunnel syndrome. Recent series show similar experience (Table 4-1). It is unclear whether these associations reflect coincident occurrence of common conditions, increased detection of a second condition once symptoms of the first draw attention to the arm, or a pathogenic link between two conditions.

Osteoarthritis

Osteoarthritis (Lister, 1994) of the finger joints most commonly involves the distal interphalangeal joints. It presents with joint stiffness and deformity (Heberden's nodes at the distal or, less commonly, Bouchard's nodes at the proximal interphalangeal joints). Finger pain can be prominent, particularly with finger use; the pain of finger joint osteoarthritis is further characterized by relief at rest, little pain at night, and little associated morning stiffness. The lack of paresthesias and the presence of focal deformities and tender-

Table 4-1. Incidence of Trigger Digit or de Quervain's Synovitis among 1,310 Patients with Carpal Tunnel Syndrome*

Condition	Number of Hands
Trigger digit	205
Thumb	47
Index finger	16
Middle finger	75
Ring finger	50
Little finger	17
de Quervain's tenosynovitis	18

*Overall, 10.2 % of patients or 16.7% of hands had trigger digit or de Quervain's tenosynovitis.
Data from H Assmus. Tendovaginitis stenosans: a frequent complication of carpal tunnel syndrome. Nervenarzt 2000; 71:474–76.

ness should make osteoarthritis hard to confuse with carpal tunnel syndrome.

The trapezio-metacarpal joint, commonly called the *basal joint of the thumb*, is the most common site of osteoarthritis in the hand. Osteoarthritis of the basal joint of the thumb presents with wrist pain localized to the base of the thumb. The pain increases with thumb use so that the hand can have a dull ache after use or by the end of the day. The pain might interfere with sleep but will rarely appear anew during sleep or be most troublesome on arising. Physical examination shows tenderness localized to the base of the metacarpal of the thumb. Pain can often be reproduced by rotation and compression of the metacarpal at this joint. Joint crepitus and instability are late findings.

Osteoarthritis of the trapezio-metacarpal joint, particularly in more advanced cases, is often accompanied by other joint or tendon involvement (Melone, Beavers & Isani, 1987). Examples are scapho-trapezial-trapezoidal arthritis, deformity of the metacarpo-phalangeal joint of the thumb, trigger digits, or tenosynovitis of the wrist. Scapho-trapezial arthritis can cause tenderness in the anatomic snuffbox or over the thenar eminence distal to the scaphoid tubercle. Patients with scapho-trapezial arthritis or trapezio-metacarpal arthritis have an increased incidence of carpal tunnel syndrome (Sarkin, 1975; Crosby, Linscheid & Dobyns, 1978).

Other osteoarthritic syndromes that can present with wrist pain include piso-triquetral joint arthritis, which typically causes focal and tenderness directly over pisiform bone and which is occasionally associated with ulnar neuropathy, and isolated carpal bone cysts, which are likely to cause pain only if they have radiographic sclerotic margins or communicate with a joint space.

Inflammatory Arthropathies

Patients with inflammatory arthropathies in the hand have focal joint warmth, tenderness, swelling, and redness. In contrast, carpal tunnel syndrome by itself causes no more than occasional, mild diffuse hand swelling without localized signs of inflammation. When paresthesias or signs of median neuropathy accompany inflammatory signs, carpal tunnel syndrome and arthritis are sometimes both present. Rheumatoid arthritis, gout, pseudogout, and other inflammatory arthropathies of the wrist and hand as causes of carpal tunnel syndrome are discussed in Chapter 6.

Hand Infection

An infection in the thenar or deep palmar spaces can present with palm or wrist pain but should be distinguishable from acute carpal tunnel syndrome by classic local signs of inflammation—warmth, swelling, redness, and tenderness. A deep palmar space infection, when fully developed, presents with swelling that is prominent on the dorsal aspect of the hand with some loss of palmar concavity and fixed finger posture. The tenderness is present day or night, but throbbing, nocturnal pain can become prominent as the pressure of pus develops in the closed space. When these infections have a fulminant course, they are rarely confused with carpal tunnel syndrome; however, as pressure increases in the carpal canal, acute carpal tunnel syndrome can develop as a secondary manifestation of the infection.

When the carpal canal or deep palmar space is infected with indolent organisms such as mycobacteria or fungi, the symptoms of carpal tunnel syndrome can precede the physical evidence of inflammation by months. A more detailed discussion of carpal tunnel syndrome complicating granulomatous infections is in Chapter 6.

Hand Stiffness

Patients with carpal tunnel syndrome frequently complain of hand or finger tightness or resistance to motion. On rare occasion, a carpal tunnel syndrome patient describes the stiffness as the most troublesome symptom. When hand stiffness is prominent, the differential diagnosis includes the stiffness of rheumatoid or osteoarthritis. Both rheumatoid stiffness and carpal tunnel stiffness are often prominent on awakening. Patients with scleroderma describe stiff hands or fingers because of skin tightness.

Patients with Dupuytren's contracture have abnormal palmar fascia that is thickened and distorted by fibrous bands. The contracture pulls the affected fingers, most commonly the ring or little fingers, into flexion, and advanced cases are easily identified by the presence of contracture on examination. Both Phalen (1966) and Yamaguchi (1965) found that approximately 2% of their patients with carpal tunnel syndrome also had Dupuytren's contracture, but the prevalence of Dupuytren's increases with increasing age, so these cases might represent chance concurrence of common conditions.

Diabetics can develop painless limitation of finger joint motion. Diabetic limited finger joint mobility can occur in young insulin-dependent diabetics before they develop neuropathy or carpal tunnel syndrome (Rosenbloom, 1989). The patient's inability to fully extend the distal and proximal interphalangeal joints is evident when the patient tries unsuccessfully to place the palm flat on a table. Older diabetics with limited finger joint mobility are more likely than other diabetics to have carpal tunnel syndrome or to have abnormal distal median nerve conduction without typical symptoms of carpal tunnel syndrome (Chaudhuri, Davidson & Morris, 1989).

Two neurologic syndromes enter into the differential diagnosis of hand stiffness. Writer's cramp is a focal dystonia characterized by recurring hand or forearm cramping with use. Even when the dystonia is uncomfortable, pain is rarely a prominent feature, and paresthesias are absent. Myotonia can also present with hand cramping and stiffness. In patients with myotonic dystrophy, weakness and atrophy of hand intrinsic muscles might complicate the diagnosis.

Ganglions and Hand Tumors

Ganglions are the most common soft tissue masses in the hand or wrist. They are fibrous cysts filled with clear mucinous fluid that arise from the synovium of joints or tendons. A minority of the cysts is posttraumatic. In most cases they present as painless masses and offer little diagnostic challenge. They can cause chronic wrist pain. The most common location is the dorsum of the wrist.

On rare occasions, ganglions occur in the carpal canal. In one series of 89 hand ganglions, two were in the carpal canal and were associated with carpal tunnel syndrome (Hvid-Hansen, 1970). When in the carpal canal, they are palpable intermittently or not at all.

A large variety of other hand tumors can occur (Johnson, Kilgore & Newmeyer, 1985). On occasion, hand tumors compress the median nerve and cause carpal tunnel syndrome as the presenting feature. Table 6-4 lists hand masses that have been reported in patients with carpal tunnel syndrome. When hand tumors such as osteoid osteoma involve bone, night pain can be a prominent symptom. Chapter 19 discusses tumors of the median nerve.

Raynaud's Phenomenon

Raynaud's phenomenon is blanching or cyanosis of digits precipitated by cold or emotional stress (Blunt & Porter, 1981). Blanching is reversible, episodic, and often followed by red fingers from reactive hyperemia. One or more digits of hands or feet can be involved. The digits often feel painful, numb, or heavy during an episode of Raynaud's phenomenon. An occasional patient with carpal tunnel syndrome will note finger blanching coincident with occurrence of hand pain and paresthesia (Garland, Bradshaw & Clark, 1957). Nonetheless, it is rarely difficult to distinguish Raynaud's phe-

nomenon from carpal tunnel syndrome based on the patient's description of symptoms.

The conditions sometimes coexist. In a population survey in which 8% of men and 10% of women had Raynaud's phenomenon, approximately 2% of those with Raynaud's also reported having carpal tunnel syndrome (Brand, Larson, Kannel & McGuirk, 1997). At the Mayo Clinic, approximately 1% of patients seen with carpal tunnel syndrome also had Raynaud's (Linscheid, Peterson & Juergens, 1967). In most of these patients with both conditions, an underlying collagen disease was the common cause. A typical example is scleroderma, which is commonly accompanied by Raynaud's and which can also cause carpal tunnel syndrome (Sukenik, Abarbanel, Buskila, Potashnik & Horowitz, 1987). Rheumatoid arthritis, systemic lupus erythematosus, or systemic vasculitis can also cause both syndromes. Raynaud's and carpal tunnel syndrome also coexist in some chronic renal failure patients on hemodialysis (Schwarz, Keller, Seyfert, Poll, Molzahn & Distler, 1984). Other potential causes of both syndromes include myxedema, trauma, and hand-arm vibration syndrome (discussed in Chapter 13). Unilateral Raynaud's phenomenon is rarely caused by arterial compression at the thoracic outlet; if the lower brachial plexus is simultaneously compressed, cutaneous paresthesias are more likely to be in the little and ring fingers rather than in a classic median nerve distribution.

Loebe and Heidrich (1988) found subtle laboratory evidence of cold-induced digital artery vasospasm in 4 of 40 patients with carpal tunnel syndrome. Their technique showed a similar incidence of arterial abnormalities in patients without carpal tunnel syndrome, supporting their conclusion that carpal tunnel syndrome is unimportant in the pathogenesis of Raynaud's phenomenon.

In contrast to the above results, two studies of patients with clinical and electrodiagnostically definite carpal tunnel syndrome have supported an association between idiopathic carpal tunnel syndrome and Raynaud's phenomenon. Among patients with carpal tunnel syndrome, 36% were diagnosed as having Raynaud's phenomenon compared to 12% of controls; the results are biased, however, because the pain and paresthesia of carpal tunnel syndrome were among the diagnostic criteria for Raynaud's (Pal, Keenan,

Table 4-2. Causes of Wrist Pain

Avascular necrosis of the lunate (Kienböck's disease)
Bone cysts
Carpal instability
Congenital deformities
Fracture (apparent, occult, nonunited)
Ganglions
Infections of bone, joint, or tendon
Neoplasms
Neurologic causes
Neuromas
Osteoarthritis
Scapholunate advanced collapse (SLAC wrist)
Tendinitis
Tenosynovial inflammatory diseases

For more details, see R Cailliet. Hand Pain and Impairment (4th ed). Philadelphia: FA Davis, 1994; and DM Lichtman, AH Alexander (eds). The Wrist and Its Disorders (2nd ed). Philadelphia: Saunders, 1997.

Misra, Moussa & Morris, 1996). In another group of patients with definite carpal tunnel syndrome, 60% had Raynaud's phenomenon based on symptoms and on objective diminution of the arterial pulse in the thumb or index finger after 1 minute immersion in cold water (Chung, Gong & Baek, 1999).

In patients with both conditions, release of the flexor retinaculum usually relieves symptoms of carpal tunnel syndrome but might not alleviate the symptom's of Raynaud's (Linscheid et al., 1967). However, Waller and Dathan (1985) reported amelioration of Raynaud's after carpal tunnel surgery, and Chung and colleagues (2000) found that among 18 patients who had both carpal tunnel syndrome and Raynaud's phenomenon, over one-half had improvement in the Raynaud's after carpal tunnel surgery.

Chronic Wrist Pain

The orthopedic causes of chronic wrist pain are extensive, and evaluation of wrist pain is often difficult (Lichtman & Alexander, 1997). In addition to neurologic and inflammatory conditions discussed above, the differential diagnosis includes numerous disorders of bone and connective tissue (Table 4-2).

Avascular lunate necrosis (Kienböck's disease) is particularly important in this regard

because it can cause insidious development of pain without preceding trauma (Gelberman & Szabo, 1984). Pain in Kienböck's disease can be prominent at night. In early cases, wrist radiographs can be normal. Clues favoring avascular lunate necrosis rather than carpal tunnel syndrome are absence of paresthesias, presence of pain on wrist movement, and compromise of wrist range of motion.

Summary

This chapter reviews some of the conditions that might initially be mistaken for carpal tunnel syndrome or conditions that carpal tunnel syndrome might mimic by presenting with atypical symptoms. Chapter 3 on clinical presentation, Chapters 17 and 18 on median neuropathies outside the carpal tunnel, and Chapters 5 and 6 on carpal tunnel syndrome and other medical conditions cover additional topics on the diagnosis of carpal tunnel syndrome.

References

Amadio PC. De Quervain's Disease and Tenosynovitis. In SL Gordon, SJ Blair, LJ Fine (eds), Repetitive Motion Disorders of the Upper Extremity. Rosemont, IL: American Academy of Orthopedic Surgeons, 1995;435–48.

Anonymous. Practice parameter for electrodiagnostic studies in carpal tunnel syndrome: summary statement. American Association of Electrodiagnostic Medicine, American Academy of Neurology, American Academy of Physical Medicine and Rehabilitation. Muscle Nerve 1993;16: 1390–91.

Blunt RJ, Porter JM. Raynaud's syndrome. Semin. Arthritis Rheum. 1981;10:282.

Brand FN, Larson MG, Kannel WB, McGuirk JM. The occurrence of Raynaud's phenomenon in a general population: the Framingham Study. Vascular Med. 1997;2: 296–301.

Brooker AF. Extensor carpi radialis tenosynovitis. Ortho. Rev. 1977;5:99–100.

Cailliet R. Hand Pain and Impairment (4th ed). Philadelphia: F. A. Davis, 1994.

Carfi J, Ma DM. Posterior interosseous syndrome revisited. Muscle Nerve 1985;8:499–502.

Cavanagh NP, Yates DA, Sutcliffe J. Thenar hypoplasia with associated radiologic abnormalities. Muscle Nerve 1979;2:431–36.

Chaudhuri KR, Davidson AR, Morris IM. Limited joint mobility and carpal tunnel syndrome in insulin-dependent diabetes. Br. J. Rheumatol. 1989;28:191–94.

Chung MS, Gong HS, Baek GH. Prevalence of Raynaud's phenomenon in patients with idiopathic carpal tunnel syndrome. J. Bone Joint Surg. 1999;81B:1017–19.

Chung MS, Gong HS, Baek GH. Raynaud's phenomenon in idiopathic carpal tunnel syndrome: postoperative alteration in its prevalence. J. Bone Joint Surg. 2000;82B: 818–19.

Crosby EB, Linscheid RL, Dobyns JH. Scaphotrapezial trapezoidal arthrosis. J. Hand Surg. 1978;3:223–34.

Dawson DM, Hallett M, Wilbourn AJ (eds). Entrapment Neuropathies (3rd ed). Philadelphia: Lippincott–Raven, 1999.

Donofrio PD. AAEM case report: 28: monomelic amyotrophy. Muscle Nerve 1994;17:1129–34.

Epstein NE, Epstein JA, Carras R. Coexisting cervical spondylotic myelopathy and bilateral carpal tunnel syndromes. J. Spinal Disord. 1989;2:36–42.

Garland H, Bradshaw JP, Clark JM. Compression of the median nerve in the carpal tunnel and its relation to acroparaesthesiae. BMJ. 1957;1:730.

Gelberman RH, Szabo RM. Kienbock's disease. Orthop. Clin. North Am. 1984;15:355–67.

Gilliatt RW, Willison RG, Dietz V, Williams IR. Peripheral nerve conduction in patients with a cervical rib and band. Ann. Neurol. 1978;4:124–29.

Gorsche RG, Verstraten KLK. A butcher with sharp pains in his arms. Lancet 1996;348:862.

Gottlieb NL. Digital flexor tenosynovitis: diagnosis and clinical significance. J. Rheumatol. 1991;18:954–55.

Gupta SK, Benstead TJ. Symptoms experienced by patients with carpal tunnel syndrome. Can. J. Neurol. Sci. 1997;24:338–42.

Hvid-Hansen O. On the treatment of ganglia. Acta Chir. Scand. 1970;136:471–76.

Hybbinette CH, Mannerfelt L. The carpal tunnel syndrome. A retrospective study of 400 operated patients. Acta. Orthop. Scand. 1975;46:610–20.

Imai T, Matsumoto H, Minami R. Asymptomatic ulnar neuropathy in carpal tunnel syndrome. Arch. Phys. Med. Rehabil. 1990;71:992–94.

Johnson J, Kilgore E, Newmeyer W. Tumorous lesions of the hand. J. Hand Surg. 1985;10A:284–86.

Lampl Y, Gilad R, Eshel Y, Sarova-Pinhas I. Strokes mimicking peripheral nerve lesions. Clin. Neurol. Neurosurg. 1995;97:203–7.

Lapedus PW, Guidotti FP. Stenosing tenovaginitis of the wrist and fingers. Clin. Orthop. 1972;83:87–90.

Le Forestier N, Moulonguet A, Maisonobe T, Léger J-M, Bouche P. True neurogenic thoracic outlet syndrome: electrophysiological diagnosis in six cases. Muscle Nerve 1998;21:1129–34.

Lichtman DM, Alexander AH, eds. The Wrist and Its Disorders, 2nd ed. Philadelphia: Saunders, 1997.

Linburg RM, Comstock BE. Anomalous tendon slips from the flexor pollicis longus to the flexor digitorum profundus. J. Hand Surg. 1979;4A:79–83.

Linscheid RL, Peterson LF, Juergens JL. Carpal-tunnel syndrome associated with vasospasm. J. Bone Joint Surg. 1967;49A:1141–46.

Lister G. The Hand: Diagnosis and Indications (3rd ed). Edinburgh, U.K.: Churchill Livingstone, 1994.

Loebe M, Heidrich H. The carpal tunnel syndrome—a disease underlying Raynaud's phenomenon? Angiology 1988;39:891–901.

Lombardi RM, Wood MB, Linscheid RL. Symptomatic restrictive thumb-index flexor tenosynovitis: incidence of musculotendinous anomalies and results of treatment. J. Hand Surg. 1988;13A:325–28.

Melone CP Jr, Beavers B, Isani A. The basal joint pain syndrome. Clin. Orthop. 1987;220:58–67.

Nishida T, Price SJ, Minieka MM. Medial antebrachial cutaneous nerve conduction in true neurogenic thoracic outlet syndrome. Electromyogr. Clin. Neurophysiol. 1993;33:285–88.

Pal B, Keenan J, Misra HN, Moussa K, Morris J. Raynaud's phenomenon in idiopathic carpal tunnel syndrome. Scand. J. Rheumatol. 1996;25:143–45.

Phalen GS. The carpal-tunnel syndrome. Seventeen years' experience in diagnosis and treatment of six hundred fifty-four hands. J. Bone Joint Surg. 1966;48A:211–28.

Phalen GS. The carpal-tunnel syndrome. Clinical evaluation of 598 hands. Clin. Orthop. 1972;83:29–40.

Rondot P. The Hand in Diseases of the Nervous System. In R Tubiana (ed), The Hand. Philadelphia: Saunders, 1993;23–39.

Roos DB, Wilbourn AJ. Issues and Opinions. Thoracic outlet syndrome. Muscle Nerve 1999;22:126–38.

Rosenbaum RB. Disputed radial tunnel syndrome. Muscle Nerve 1999;22:960–67.

Rosenbloom AL. Limitation of finger joint mobility in diabetes mellitus. J. Diabet. Complications. 1989;3:77–87.

Rowntree T. Anomalous innervation of the hand muscles. J. Bone Joint Surg. 1949;31B:505–10.

Sarkin TL. Osteoarthritis of the trapeziometacarpal joint. S. Afr. Med. J. 1975;49:392–94.

Schwarz A, Keller F, Seyfert S, Poll W, Molzahn M, Distler A. Carpal tunnel syndrome: a major complication in long-term hemodialysis patients. Clin. Nephrol. 1984;22:133–37.

Silver MA, Gelberman RH, Gellman H, Rhoades CE. Carpal tunnel syndrome: associated abnormalities in ulnar nerve function and the effect of carpal tunnel release on these abnormalities. J. Hand Surg. 1985;10A:710–13.

Stevens JC, Smith BE, Weaver AL, Bosch EP, Deen HG Jr, Wilkens JA. Symptoms of 100 patients with electromyographically verified carpal tunnel syndrome. Muscle Nerve 1999;22:1448–56.

Stewart JD. Focal Peripheral Neuropathies (3rd ed). Philadelphia: Lippincott Williams & Wilkins, 2000.

Stopford JSB. The variation in distribution of the cutaneous nerves of the hand and digits. J. Anat. 1918;53:14–25.

Su CT, Hoopes JE, Daniel R. Congenital absence of the thenar muscles innervated by the median nerve. Report of a case. J. Bone Joint Surg. 1972;54A:1087–90.

Subramaniam P, de la Harpe D, Corlett RJ. Focal tenosynovial amyloid deposition as a rare cause of median nerve compression at the wrist. Aust. N. Z. J. Surg. 1997;67:138–39.

Sukenik S, Abarbanel JM, Buskila D, Potashnik G, Horowitz J. Impotence, carpal tunnel syndrome and peripheral neuropathy as presenting symptoms in progressive systemic sclerosis. J. Rheumatol. 1987;14:641–43.

Waller DG, Dathan JR. Raynaud's syndrome and carpal tunnel syndrome. Postgrad. Med. J. 1985;61:161–62.

Wilbourn AJ, Aminoff MJ. AAEE Minimonograph #32: the electrophysiologic examination in patients with radiculopathies. Muscle Nerve 1988;11:1099–1114.

Witt JC, Stevens JC. Neurologic disorders masquerading as carpal tunnel syndrome: 12 cases of failed carpal tunnel release. Mayo. Clin. Proc. 2000;75:409–13.

Yamaguchi D, Lipscomb P, Soule E. Carpal tunnel syndrome. Minn. Med. 1965;48:22–31.

Yasuoka S, Okazaki H, Daube JR, MacCarty CS. Foramen magnum tumors. Analysis of 57 cases of benign extramedullary tumors. J. Neurosurg. 1978;49:828–38.

Chapter 5

Carpal Tunnel Syndrome with Other Medical Conditions: Part I

Compression of the median nerve in the carpal canal is the primary pathologic process underlying carpal tunnel syndrome. For a given wrist position, the capacity of the canal is fixed; any expansion of a portion of its contents increases the pressure in the canal and compresses the median nerve. The pressure in the carpal canal varies with wrist position. Chapter 12 discusses changes of canal pressure with wrist motion and the relation between canal pressure and median nerve compression. Chapter 13 reviews the role of wrist motion and use in the development of carpal tunnel syndrome.

The contents of the carpal canal might expand from edema, inflammation, hemorrhage, abnormal deposits such as calcium or uric acid, neoplasm, or infiltrative diseases such as amyloidosis. Anomalous canal contents can decrease the space available for normal structures. A canal that is smaller than average, whether from congenital variation or acquired deformity, develops a proportionately larger increase in pressure for a given expansion of canal contents. Associated pathology of the median nerve, such as a diffuse peripheral neuropathy or a more proximal nerve injury or compression, can increase its likelihood of becoming symptomatic when compressed.

Most cases of carpal tunnel syndrome are unrelated to a canal anomaly or systemic illness. The most commonly associated systemic illnesses are diabetes mellitus, rheumatoid arthritis, and hypothyroidism. Carpal tunnel syndrome can complicate pregnancy or occur with other hormonal changes. Collagen diseases or acromegaly are rarer causes. Some patients have a history of prior wrist fracture or blunt trauma. Some have other coincident musculoskeletal conditions, including de Quervain's tenosynovitis, trigger finger or thumb, Raynaud's phenomenon, lateral humeral epicondylitis (tennis elbow), or disease of the shoulder.

Table 5-1 and Figure 5-1 provide estimates of the incidence of various diseases associated with carpal tunnel syndrome based on the combined results of some of the larger clinical series (Yamaguchi, Lipscomb & Soule, 1965; Phalen, 1966; Maxwell, Clough, Reckling & Kelly, 1973; Hybbinette & Mannerfelt, 1975; Gainer & Nugent, 1977; Loong, 1977). The diagnostic criteria for carpal tunnel syndrome and for associated conditions, the rigor with which associated conditions were sought, and the referral patterns vary from series to series, so these incidences are approximations at best. Figure 5-1 shows the frequency of the most common associations found in these series.

Table 5-1 lists some of the rarer associations. The list does not discriminate between chance and pathogenic associations.

Most instances of carpal tunnel syndrome are occupational (see Chapter 13) or idiopathic. Phillips (1967) followed 41 patients with idiopathic carpal tunnel syndrome for 7 years; during that period, no systemic diseases were recognized that contributed to the development of carpal tunnel syndrome.

Lists such as those in Table 5-1 and Figure 5-1 are relatively easy to produce but leave a number of questions unanswered:

1. If a patient has disease X, what is his or her risk of developing carpal tunnel syndrome?

Table 5-1. Diagnoses Found in 2,705 Carpal Tunnel Syndrome Patients

Amyloidosis (12)	Gout (10)	Neurofibromatosis (1)
Anomalous muscles (3)	Herpes zoster at T-1 (1)	Peripheral neuropathy (14)
Asthma (2)	Hodgkin's disease (1)	Pernicious anemia (1)
Brain tumor (2)	Hurler's syndrome (3)	Plantar fasciitis (2)
Carcinoma (2)	Hypertension (7)	Polycythemia (1)
Carpal tunnel lipoma (1)	Leukemia (1)	Psoriasis (3)
Collagen disease (12)	Median artery thrombosis (1)	Raynaud's phenomenon (12)
Dyschondroplasia (2)	Mononeuropathy multiplex (3)	Sarcoidosis (3)
Emphysema (2)	Multiple myeloma (4)	Tietse's syndrome (2)
Epilepsy (1)	Multiple sclerosis (1)	Tuberculosis (6)
Ganglion (9)	Mycosis fungoides (1)	

2. Should a patient with carpal tunnel syndrome be tested for previously undiagnosed disease Y?
3. If a patient has carpal tunnel syndrome and disease Z, is treatment of disease Z likely to lead to improvement in the carpal tunnel syndrome?

Wherever possible, the following discussion tries to address these issues.

Carpal Canal Stenosis

Small canal size is not listed in Table 5-1 or Figure 5-1, yet a *mismatch* between canal size and size of canal contents must be part of the compressive process. The cross-sectional area of the carpal canal can be estimated from plain radiographs, computed tomography scans, or magnetic resonance imaging (MRI) scans. More detail is provided in Chapter 11. Some authors have suggested that small canal size or "carpal canal stenosis" explains the vulnerability of some patients to development of carpal tunnel syndrome (Dekel, Papaioannou, Rushworth & Coates, 1980; Gelmers, 1981; Bleecker, Bohlman, Moreland & Tipton, 1985). Although this hypothesis is intuitively attractive, other studies of carpal canal size have not confirmed it (Winn & Habes, 1990; Cobb, Bond, Cooney & Metcalf, 1997). The imaging analysis of the carpal tunnel can be refined by using wrist MRI to compare the cross-sectional area of the canal to the cross-sectional areas of the median nerve and flexor tendons within the canal (Cobb et al., 1997). As a group, patients with definite carpal tunnel syndrome had a higher ratio of the area of canal contents to

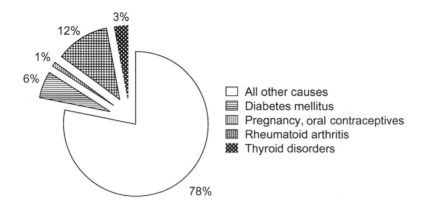

Legend:
- ☐ All other causes
- ☰ Diabetes mellitus
- ▥ Pregnancy, oral contraceptives
- ▦ Rheumatoid arthritis
- ▓ Thyroid disorders

3%
12%
1%
6%
78%

Figure 5-1. The four most common diagnostic associations among 2,705 patients with carpal tunnel syndrome were rheumatoid arthritis, diabetes mellitus, thyroid disorders, and pregnancy or use of oral contraceptives.

canal cross-sectional area than did control subjects; however, there was great overlap among the ratios for the patient and control groups, so this analysis is useful neither as a diagnostic test nor as a full explanation for individual susceptibility to carpal tunnel syndrome.

Some studies suggest a correlation between wrist shape and median nerve conduction. These studies, reviewed in Chapter 8, provide insufficient clinical data to examine whether variations in wrist shape should be counted among the causes of carpal tunnel syndrome.

Deformities of the Carpal Canal

Bony anomalies or deformities can reduce the cross-sectional area of the canal. Carpal tunnel syndrome can develop as a late sequel of deformities caused by carpal or radial fractures or other wrist trauma (Lewis & Miller, 1922; Abbott & Saunders, 1933; Cannon & Love, 1946). Congenital anomalies causing carpal tunnel syndrome include a hypoplastic scaphoid with dysplastic radius, anomalous distal radius projecting into the canal, or anterior subluxation of carpal bones (Madelung's deformity) (Izhar-ul-Haque, 1982; Radford & Matthewson, 1987; Luchetti, Mingione, Monteleone & Cristiani, 1988). A patient with carpal osteopetrosis presented with carpal tunnel syndrome (Rakic, Elhosseiny, Ramadan, Iyer, Howard & Gross, 1986).

Connective Tissue Diseases

Tenosynovitis

Swelling of the tenosynovium of the finger flexors contributes to the median nerve compression in many cases of carpal tunnel syndrome. The pathogenesis is discussed in more detail in Chapter 12. In a case-control epidemiologic study, patients with lateral epicondylitis (tennis elbow), another form of upper extremity tenosynovitis, were at increased risk of having carpal tunnel syndrome (Ferry, Hannaford, Warskyj, Lewis & Croft, 2000).

Osteoarthritis

Osteoarthritis of the fingers most commonly affects the distal or proximal interphalangeal joints causing Heberden's (distal) or Bouchard's (proximal) nodes. Disease of these joints has not been associated with an increased incidence of carpal tunnel syndrome; however, we are unaware of a study that specifically addresses this question. The basal thumb joint is another joint that is commonly affected by osteoarthritis. When patients with basal thumb joint arthritis that was severe enough to require surgical therapy were surveyed carefully, 43% were found to have carpal tunnel syndrome (Florack, Miller, Pellegrini, Burton & Dunn, 1992). Patients with advanced degenerative arthritis of the carpal bones often also have carpal tunnel syndrome (Fassler, Stern & Kiefhaber, 1993). In a rare patient, the carpal tunnel syndrome can be directly attributed to a carpal osteophyte protruding directly into the carpal tunnel (Engel, Zinneman, Tsur & Farin, 1978).

Rheumatoid Arthritis

Rheumatoid arthritis is the systemic inflammatory disease most commonly associated with carpal tunnel syndrome, and carpal tunnel syndrome is the most common entrapment neuropathy occurring in patients with rheumatoid arthritis. In the combined series of carpal tunnel patients, 12% had rheumatoid arthritis. The prevalence of rheumatoid arthritis was 9% in another group of patients with carpal tunnel syndrome (Crow, 1960).

Carpal tunnel syndrome has been reported to occur in one-fifth or more of patients with rheumatoid arthritis, but reported incidences vary greatly with the severity of the rheumatoid arthritis and the diagnostic criteria used for carpal tunnel syndrome (Wells & Johnson, 1962; Smukler, Patterson, Lorenz & Weiner, 1963; Chamberlain & Corbett, 1970; Moran, Chen, Muirden, Jiang, Gu, Hopper, Jiang, Lawler & Chen, 1986). For example, a Chinese series found carpal tunnel syndrome in only 2% of patients with rheumatoid arthritis. Fleming and colleagues (1976), inquiring carefully for early extraarticular symptoms in rheumatoid patients, found median sensory symptoms in more than one-

Table 5-2. Carpal Tunnel Syndrome and Median Nerve Conduction in 45 Patients with Rheumatoid Arthritis

	Median Nerve Conduction	
	Abnormal*	Normal
Patients with signs or symptoms of carpal tunnel syndrome	15	9
Patients without signs or symptoms of carpal tunnel syndrome	7	14

*Median distal motor latency greater than 5.0 msecs or a distal sensory latency greater than 4.0 msecs. Thus, incidence of abnormal tests is undoubtedly low by current standards.
Data from CG Barnes, HL Currey. Carpal tunnel syndrome in rheumatoid arthritis. A clinical and electrodiagnostic survey. Ann. Rheum. Dis. 1967;26:226–33.

half of patients within 1 year of onset of rheumatoid arthritis. Patients with rheumatoid arthritis who are older than 40 years are three times more likely than age-matched controls to develop carpal tunnel syndrome (42% versus 13%) (Herbison, Teng, Martin & Ditunno, 1973).

Patients with rheumatoid arthritis frequently have signs of tenosynovitis of hand and forearm flexors, manifested by focal tendon tenderness or swelling, loss of finger range of motion, or digital triggering. Among patients with rheumatoid arthritis, 47% of those with flexor tenosynovitis had carpal tunnel syndrome, compared to 13% of those without clinical evidence of flexor synovitis (Gray & Gottlieb, 1977).

In advanced rheumatoid disease, carpal deformities can contribute to median nerve compression. For example, in a case of dorsal carpal dislocation with flexor tendon rupture, the distal ulna was displaced into the carpal canal and compressed the median nerve (Craig & House, 1984).

Early in the course of rheumatoid arthritis, many patients who have symptoms suggesting carpal tunnel syndrome have normal distal motor and sensory latencies (Chamberlain & Corbett, 1970). Conversely, occasional patients with rheumatoid arthritis have abnormal median nerve conduction studies but no symptoms of carpal tunnel

syndrome (Lanzillo, Pappone, Crisci, di Girolamo, Massini & Caruso, 1998; Sivri & Guler-Uysal, 1999). Table 5-2 shows the correlation between nerve conduction results and symptoms in one series of rheumatoid patients (Barnes & Currey, 1967).

Successful medical treatment of rheumatoid arthritis often relieves the symptoms of carpal tunnel syndrome. With treatment, reduced symptoms of median nerve irritation parallel reduction of the inflammatory disease in hand joints and tendons. Nerve conduction abnormalities often also improve (Vemireddi, Redford & PombeJara, 1979). When symptoms persist despite medical therapy, carpal tunnel surgery is often successful. In some cases, flexor synovectomy is performed after division of the flexor retinaculum (Ostroumova, 1969; Ranawat & Straub, 1970; Hooper, 1972; Ferlic, 1996). When synovitis is not aggressive, simple section of the flexor retinaculum, even endoscopically, can relieve carpal tunnel symptoms (Belcher, Varma & Schonauer, 2000).

Carpal tunnel syndrome can complicate wrist arthroplasty performed for treatment of rheumatoid carpal disease (Lamberta, Ferlic & Clayton, 1980).

Progressive Systemic Sclerosis and Related Disorders

Progressive systemic sclerosis (PSS) accounts for only a small number of carpal tunnel syndrome patients, both because PSS is much rarer than rheumatoid arthritis and because carpal tunnel syndrome is an infrequent complication of PSS. One small series found that one-fourth of 16 patients with PSS had carpal tunnel syndrome (Machet, Vaillant, Machet, Esteve, Muller, Khallouf & Lorette, 1992). Patients with PSS who have no symptoms of carpal tunnel syndrome can have minor abnormalities of median transcarpal nerve conduction (Lori, Matucci-Cerinic, Casale, Generini, Lombardi, Pignone, Scaletti & Gangemi, 1996). However, of 125 patients with PSS questioned yearly for neurologic symptoms, only four were found to have carpal tunnel syndrome (Lee, Bruni & Sukenik, 1984). If the carpal tunnel syndrome develops before any of the classic manifestations of PSS, the pathologic relation between the two conditions is uncertain (Sukenik, Abarbanel, Buskila, Potashnik & Horowitz, 1987; Barr & Blair, 1988; Berth-Jones, Coates, Graham-Brown & Burns, 1990). Some cases of carpal tunnel syndrome in patients with PSS might reflect coincidence rather than a pathologic link; however, in one patient with carpal tunnel syndrome and PSS, histology of flexor tendon sheath showed a polymorphous inflammatory infiltrate in small vessels, distinct from the chronic fibrotic changes typical of idiopathic carpal tunnel syndrome (Machet et al., 1992). In another patient with PSS and a clinical presentation similar to carpal tunnel syndrome, the median nerve compression was caused by sclerodermatous change in the antebrachial fascia of the distal forearm rather than by compression in the carpal tunnel (Ko, Jones & Steen, 1996).

Carpal tunnel syndrome can complicate the sclerodermatous syndrome caused by vinyl chloride toxicity. Similar to patients with PSS, workers exposed to vinyl chloride sometimes develop Raynaud's phenomenon and skin thickening. The syndrome is sometimes called *occupational acroosteolysis* because radiographs sometimes show resorption of the distal phalanges. In small series, these patients have had a high incidence of acroparesthesias and of carpal tunnel syndrome (Veltman, Lange, Jühe, Stein & Bachner, 1975; Gama & Meira, 1978).

Toxic oil syndrome, an inflammatory illness caused by ingesting adulterated rapeseed oil, has clinical features overlapping those of PSS (Alonso-Ruiz, Zea-Mendoza, Salazar-Vallinas, Rocamora-Ripoll & Beltrán-Gutierrez, 1986). Among 214 patients with toxic oil syndrome, 31 had symptoms suggestive of carpal tunnel syndrome. Symptoms evolved from 1 to 17 months after onset of toxic oil syndrome. Abnormal nerve conduction studies in 11 cases supported the diagnosis of carpal tunnel syndrome (Olmedo-Garzon, Leiva-Santana, Alonso-Ruiz & Riva-Meana, 1983).

Carpal tunnel syndrome is a common complication of eosinophilic fasciitis, a rare inflammatory condition of subcutaneous fascia. Superficially, eosinophilic fasciitis resembles scleroderma because both cause stiffening and thickening of soft tissue of the extremities. Unlike scleroderma, it predominantly inflames subcutaneous fascia and spares dermis and viscera. The wrist and forearms are often sites of this inflammation. Physical findings include focal induration and loss of joint range of motion. Hand involvement and Raynaud's phenomenon, both common features of scleroderma, are atypical in eosinophilic fasciitis. In small series of patients with eosinophilic fasciitis, between one-fourth and three-fourths of patients had carpal tunnel syndrome (Barnes, Rodnan, Medsger & Short, 1979; Jones, Beetham, Silverman & Margles, 1986; Lakhanpal, Ginsburg, Michet, Doyle & Moore, 1988; McGrory, Schmidt, Wold & Amadio, 1998).

Both carpal tunnel syndrome and mononeuropathy multiplex with median nerve involvement have been reported in patients with the eosinophilia-myalgia syndrome due to L-tryptophan ingestion (Selwa, Feldman & Blaivas, 1990; Shulman, 1990).

Polymyalgia Rheumatica

Carpal tunnel syndrome is the most common neuropathic complication of polymyalgia rheumatica (PMR) (Miller & Stevens, 1978; Richards, 1980). Patients with giant cell arteritis sometimes develop carpal tunnel syndrome or, less commonly, a vasculitic median neuropathy as one manifestation of mononeuritis multiplex (Caselli, Daube, Hunder & Whisnant, 1988). The symptoms of carpal tunnel syndrome can precede other symptoms of PMR (Chan & Kaye, 1982; Herrera, Sanmarti, Ponce, Lopez-Soto & Munoz-Gomez, 1997). A prospective survey of 177 patients with PMR found that 14% had carpal tunnel syndrome, which in three-fourths of the cases was among the presenting symptoms of the PMR (Salvarani, Cantini, Macchioni, Olivieri, Niccoli, Padula & Boiardi, 1998). In a population-based survey of patients with temporal arteritis, however, less than 2% had carpal tunnel syndrome, even though more than 40% had manifestations of PMR (Salvarani & Hunder, 1999). Nearly one-half of patients with PMR have some manifestation of peripheral musculoskeletal inflammation, so the differential diagnosis of hand symptoms in these patients includes carpal tunnel syndrome, peripheral arthritis, distal tenosynovitis, and the syndrome of distal extremity swelling with pitting edema. These conditions often coexist: A radionuclide bone scan study found evidence of wrist synovitis in 11 of 25 patients with PMR; two of these patients had clinical evidence of carpal tunnel syndrome (O'Duffy, Hunder & Wahner, 1980). The differential diagnosis of the combination of wrist pitting edema and carpal tunnel syndrome includes both PMR and chondrocalcinosis. Uncommonly, both occur in the same patient (Richards, 1981).

In patients with PMR and carpal tunnel syndrome, the symptoms of carpal tunnel syndrome usually improve with steroid therapy (Ahmed & Braun, 1978; Salvarani et al., 1998). If the patients do undergo carpal tunnel surgery, histopathology of synovial tissue sometimes shows lymphocytic synovitis (Salvarani et al., 1998). In extraordinary cases, patients with symptoms of carpal tunnel syndrome have had giant cell arteritis of a persistent median artery (Merianos, Smyrnis, Tsomy & Hager, 1983; Dennis & Ransome, 1996).

Systemic Lupus Erythematosus

Carpal tunnel syndrome is the most common peripheral nerve complication of systemic lupus erythematosus. At times, carpal tunnel syndrome precedes any systemic symptoms, and the association might be fortuitous (Sidiq, Kirsner & Sheon, 1972). In a survey of neuromuscular complications in 30 patients with systemic lupus, however, 10 had symptoms of carpal tunnel syndrome, and seven of these had nerve conduction abnormalities supporting the diagnosis (Omdal, Mellgren & Husby, 1988).

Fibromyalgia

Fibromyalgia is a condition that generates controversy (Bohr, 1996). In one study, approximately 30% of patients labeled with fibromyalgia had paresthesias in a median distribution, and more than one-half of these had the diagnosis of carpal tunnel syndrome supported by nerve conduction studies (Perez-Ruiz, Calabozo, Alonso-Ruiz, Herrero, Ruiz-Lucea & Otermin, 1995). Whether carpal tunnel syndrome is more common in patients diagnosed with fibromyalgia than it is in the general population is one more controversy (Cimmino, Parisi, Moggiana & Accardo, 1996; Perez-Ruiz, Calabozo, Alonso-Ruiz & Ruiz-Lucea, 1997).

Gout

Gout of the hand or wrist is an infrequent cause of either acute or chronic carpal tunnel syndrome (Champion, 1969; Pai & Tseng, 1993). Of 2,705 patients with carpal tunnel syndrome, three had gout. Conversely, of 10 patients with gout of the hand, four had carpal tunnel syndrome (Moore & Weiland, 1985). The typical gouty patient with carpal tunnel syndrome has tophi on the flexor tendon synovium in the carpal canal (Akizuki & Matsui, 1984; Hoyt, 1986; Janssen & Rayan, 1987; Weinzweig, Fletcher & Linburg, 2000). Either computed tomography or MRI of the wrist will usually show abnormalities if tophi are present (Chen, Chung, Yeh, Pan, Yang, Lai, Liang & Resnick, 2000). Carpal tunnel syndrome due to gouty tophi is occasionally bilateral (Pledger, Hirsch & Freiberg, 1976; Green, Dilworth & Levitin, 1977; Tsai, Yu & Tsai, 1996; Ali, Hofford, Mohammed, Maharaj, Sookhoo & van Velzen, 1999). Rarely, tophi can cause both carpal tunnel syndrome and ulnar nerve compression at the elbow (Jacoulet, 1994). Patients usually get symptomatic relief of the symptoms of carpal tunnel syndrome after carpal tunnel surgery. In one case, tophi oozing from the wound delayed healing (Lianga, Waslen & Penney, 1986).

Chondrocalcinosis

Patients with chondrocalcinosis of the wrists sometimes have either symptoms of carpal tunnel syndrome or asymptomatic slowing of median transcarpal nerve conduction (Gerster, Lagier, Boivin & Schneider, 1980; Lagier, Boivin & Gerster, 1984; Binder, Sheppard & Paice, 1989). Among 22 patients with evidence of chondrocalcinosis on wrist radiographs, 14 had prolonged median distal motor latencies, and eight of these had clinical carpal tunnel syndrome. The calcification is usually not grossly evident at surgery. At times, chondrocalcinosis presents with acute wrist inflammation, or pseudogout, confirmed by wrist radiograph or demonstration of calcium pyrophosphate crystals in the carpal canal. The pseudogout can cause acute carpal tunnel syndrome (Spiegel, Ginsberg, Skosey & Kwong, 1976; Lewis & Fiddian, 1982; Goodwin & Arbel, 1985; Chiu, Wong, Choi & Chow, 1992; Rate, Parkinson, Meadows & Freemont, 1992). A report of a patient who had chondrocalcinosis, PMR, and carpal tunnel syndrome is mentioned previously in the section Polymyalgia Rheumatica; a report of a patient with carpal tunnel syndrome, chondrocalcinosis, and hyperparathyroidism is mentioned later in the section Disorders of Calcium Metabolism.

Miscellaneous Connective Tissue or Dermatologic Diseases

Any illness that causes carpal synovial inflammation, infiltration, or edema can lead to median nerve compression. Small series or case reports link other rheumatic conditions and carpal tunnel syndrome. Three percent to 6% of patients with primary Sjögren's syndrome have carpal tunnel syndrome (Binder, Snaith & Isenberg, 1988; Andonopoulos, Lagos, Drosos & Moutsopoulos, 1990). Among 28 patients with Sjögren's syndrome and peripheral nerve disease, 10 had carpal tunnel syndrome (Molina, Provost & Alexander, 1985).

Winkelmann and colleagues (1982) reported five patients with carpal tunnel syndrome accompanying a cutaneous connective tissue disease. Skin manifestations included generalized morphea, lichen scleroses, fasciitis, discoid lupus, and lupus panniculitis. In two patients, synovial biopsy showed lymphoproliferative changes. Both the carpal tunnel syndrome and the skin disease can improve with chloroquine therapy.

Of six patients with palmar fasciitis and polyarthritis, two had carpal tunnel syndrome (Medsger, Dixon & Garwood, 1982). This syndrome can be a harbinger of carcinoma of the ovary.

A patient with mixed connective tissue syndrome had bilateral carpal tunnel syndrome and bilateral trigeminal sensory neuropathies (Vincent & Van Houzen, 1980). Prednisone therapy gave symptomatic improvement of the carpal tunnel syndrome and the systemic inflammatory disease.

Benign joint hypermobility is manifested by increased joint range of motion. Often, patients with this condition can hyperflex at the wrists and hyperabduct at the thumbs to touch the thumbs to their ipsilateral forearm. March and colleagues (1988) described four patients with benign joint hypermobility who developed symptoms of carpal tunnel syndrome from sleeping with their wrists habitually hyperflexed; symptoms resolved with change of sleep postures.

Granuloma annulare causes nonscaly, annular palpable plaques with indurated borders, usually on the extremities. In addition, patients can have subcutaneous and soft tissue inflammation. In a patient who had carpal tunnel syndrome and granuloma annulare in both arms, successful treatment of the granuloma annulare with chlorambucil was accompanied by resolution of the symptoms and nerve conduction manifestations of the carpal tunnel syndrome (Winkelmann & Stevens, 1994).

Acrokeratosis paraneoplastica (Bazex's syndrome) is a paraneoplastic complication of squamous cell carcinoma of the gastrointestinal or upper respiratory tracts. In a patient who presented with acrokeratosis of the nose, ears, fingers, and toes, hand symptoms suggested carpal tunnel syndrome and finger abnormalities included mild swelling, cyanosis, scaling, and abnormal nails. The acrokeratosis and the carpal tunnel syndrome improved after radiotherapy of squamous cell carcinoma of his nasopharynx (Poskitt & Duffill, 1992).

Other case reports link carpal tunnel syndrome to cases of dermatomyositis/polymyositis, multicentric reticulohistiocytois, sarcoidosis of the flexor tenosynovium, papular mucinosis of the fingers, or lymphoma (Quinones, Perry & Rushton, 1966; Miller, 1967; Flam, Ryan, Mah-Poy, Jacobs & Neldner, 1972; Stephens, Ross, Charles-Holmes, McKee & Black, 1993; Kersting-Sommerhoff, Hof, Golder, Becker & Werber, 1995).

Endocrinopathies

Diabetes Mellitus

Diabetes mellitus is one of the most common systemic illnesses found in association with carpal tunnel syndrome. The prevalence of diabetes in reported series of patients who have carpal tunnel syndrome varies from about 3% to 20%, reflecting variations in factors such as referral patterns and diagnostic criteria; the weighted average from a

Table 5-3. Prevalence of Neuropathies in Patients with Diabetes Mellitus

	Insulin-Dependent Diabetics (%)	Non–Insulin-Dependent Diabetics (%)
Prevalence of generalized neuropathy	54	45
Prevalence of symptomatic carpal tunnel syndrome	11	6
Prevalence of asymptomatic slowing of median conduction across the carpal tunnel	22	29

Data from PJ Dyck, KM Kratz, JL Karnes, WJ Litchy, R Klein, JM Pach, DM Wilson, PC O'Brien, LJ Melton. The prevalence by staged severity of various types of diabetic neuropathy, retinopathy, and nephropathy in a population-based cohort: the Rochester Diabetic Neuropathy Study. Neurology 1993;43:817.

number of series is that approximately 7% of patients who have carpal tunnel syndrome also have diabetes mellitus (Wilbourn, 1999). In a combined series of 2,705 patients with carpal tunnel syndrome, 166 were diabetic. Dieck and Kelsey (1985) examined 40 women with carpal tunnel syndrome, aged 45 to 74 years, in a hospital-based case-control study. Patients with carpal tunnel syndrome had a history of diabetes nearly three times (95% confidence interval: 1.3 to 6.5) more frequently than did controls. A prevalence study in a French diabetes clinic found that 26% of insulin-dependent diabetics and 15% of non–insulin-dependent diabetics but only 3% to 5% of age- and sex-matched controls had carpal tunnel syndrome (Renard, Jacques, Chammas, Poirier, Bonifacj, Jaffiol, Simon & Allieu, 1994).

Nerve entrapment in the carpal tunnel is only one of many peripheral neuropathic complications of diabetes (Dyck & Thomas, 1999). In groups of diabetics, the reported prevalence of symptomatic carpal tunnel syndrome varies from 1% to 21%, reflecting variations in diagnostic criteria and severity and duration of diabetes; the weighted average from a number of series is that nearly 6% of patients who have diabetes also have carpal tunnel syndrome (Wilbourn, 1999). In a population-based prevalence study of diabetics, generalized

peripheral neuropathy, symptomatic carpal tunnel syndrome, and asymptomatic slowing of median nerve conduction across the carpal tunnel were all common (Table 5-3) (Dyck, Kratz, Karnes, Litchy, Klein, Pach, Wilson, O'Brien & Melton, 1993). By the time they develop symptoms of carpal tunnel syndrome, diabetics usually have some evidence of a generalized peripheral neuropathy by examination or by nerve conduction studies (Leffert, 1969). Diabetic carpal tunnel syndrome is very rare in diabetic children (Rosenbloom, 1984). Carpal tunnel syndrome becomes more prevalent with increasing duration of diabetes.

Nerve conduction studies in diabetics without symptoms of carpal tunnel syndrome often show focal abnormalities of motor and sensory conduction across the carpal tunnel in excess of the abnormalities noted in the ipsilateral ulnar nerve (Ozaki, Baba, Matsunaga & Takebe, 1988). More than 20% of diabetics have asymptomatic abnormalities of median nerve conduction across the carpal tunnel (Dyck et al., 1993; Albers, Brown, Sima & Greene, 1996). In diabetics, abnormal conduction across the carpal tunnel increases in frequency with increasing age and duration of diabetes; in patients with non–insulin-dependent diabetes, abnormal median nerve conduction is more common in women and people with higher body mass index (Albers et al., 1996). Conduction is sometimes abnormal across the carpal tunnel when other nerve conduction studies do not give evidence of a more diffuse neuropathy (Comi, Lozza, Galardi, Ghilardi, Medaglini & Canal, 1985; Albers et al., 1996).

The mechanism of the increased incidence of carpal tunnel syndrome in diabetics is unproven but is probably multifactorial. In diabetics, nerve conduction studies often show evidence of peripheral neuropathy before any signs or symptoms of neuropathy are present; electrophysiologic research techniques, such as determination of conduction velocity distribution, can show nerve abnormalities when standard nerve conduction studies are normal (Bertora, Valla, Dezuanni, Osio, Mantica, Bevilacqua, Norbiato, Caccia & Mangoni, 1998). The neuropathic median nerve might be more vulnerable to compression than a healthy nerve would be. Additionally, diabetics have increased hand joint and tendon abnormalities, such as trigger finger, Dupuytren's contracture, and limited joint mobility syndrome (Gamstedt, Holm-Glad, Ohlson & Sundström, 1993; Renard et al., 1994; Chammas, Bousquet, Renard, Poirier, Jaffiol & Allieu, 1995; Rosenbloom & Silverstein, 1996). Thus, they can develop tendinopathies that contribute to median nerve compression within the carpal tunnel.

In patients who present with carpal tunnel syndrome and who are not known to be diabetic, the chance of detecting diabetes by routine screening is very low. Pal and colleagues (1986) screened 42 patients with idiopathic carpal tunnel syndrome and found only one patient with an abnormal glucose tolerance test. Chaplin and Kasdan (1985) found that 2 of 100 carpal tunnel syndrome patients had high fasting blood sugars; both of these patients had absent Achilles tendon reflexes. Isselin and Gariot (1989) found a fasting plasma glucose greater than 140 mg/dl in 3% of patients with carpal tunnel syndrome or other nerve entrapment in the arm.

There is an interesting case report linking the symptoms of carpal tunnel syndrome to the site of insulin injection (Bell & Clements, 1983):

> A 27-year-old woman with a 14-year history of insulin-dependent diabetes presented with bilateral hand pain, thenar atrophy, median distribution sensory loss, and abnormal median nerve conduction. She switched her insulin injection sites from her arms to elsewhere on her body with resultant improvement in hand symptoms and in median sensory finger-to-wrist nerve conduction studies. Arm symptoms recurred temporarily when insulin injection in the arms was briefly resumed.

Unfortunately, treatment of diabetic carpal tunnel syndrome is rarely this simple. There are preliminary reports that treatment of diabetics who have carpal tunnel syndrome with an aldose-reductase inhibitor sometimes improves hand and wrist pain and paresthesias and median transcarpal nerve conduction (Monge, De Mattei, Dani, Sciarretta & Carta, 1995). The scant available data on surgery for diabetic carpal tunnel syndrome are reviewed in Chapter 15.

Thyroid Disease

Both hypothyroidism and hyperthyroidism can cause carpal tunnel syndrome. In a combined series of 2,705 carpal tunnel syndrome patients,

there were 94 cases of thyroid disease. Hypothyroidism was more frequent than hyperthyroidism. However, after performing thyroid function tests in 100 patients with carpal tunnel syndrome, Chaplin and Kasdan (1985) found only one thyroid abnormality, which was not confirmed on repeat testing.

In hypothyroid patients, swelling of the contents of the carpal tunnel can cause median nerve compression with typical carpal tunnel syndrome symptoms. At times, in addition to synovial swelling, hypothyroid patients have a more generalized arthropathy that can affect multiple joints and cause arthralgia, joint swelling, and stiffness (Frymoyer & Bland, 1973). Carpal tunnel syndrome can be the initial clinical manifestation of hypothyroidism (Golding, 1970; Olive & Hennessey, 1988). A mild elevation of thyroid-stimulating hormone is sometimes the earliest laboratory confirmation of the thyroid deficiency.

Estimates of the incidence of carpal tunnel syndrome in hypothyroid patients vary. Murray and Simpson (1958) reported that 26 of 35 myxedematous patients had acroparesthesias. In one series of 51 hypothyroid patients, only one was found to have carpal tunnel syndrome, but focal abnormality of median motor nerve conduction was the only diagnostic criterion (Scarpalezos, Lygidakis, Papageorgiou, Maliara, Koukoulommati & Koutras, 1973). Among another 20 patients with hypothyroidism, three patients had clinical symptoms of carpal tunnel syndrome, and six patients had asymptomatic prolongation of median distal sensory latency (Rao, Katiyar, Nair & Misra, 1980). Among 24 patients with central nervous system effects of hypothyroidism, six had carpal tunnel syndrome, and four others had evidence of peripheral neuropathy (Cremer, Goldstein & Paris, 1969). In a prospective study with careful clinical and electrodiagnostic evaluation, 29% of patients had clinical evidence of carpal tunnel syndrome at the time hypothyroidism was newly diagnosed (Duyff, Van den Bosch, Laman, van Loon & Linssen, 2000). Hypothyroidism infrequently causes a diffuse peripheral neuropathy (Fincham & Cape, 1968; Duyff et al., 2000). Most hypothyroid patients with carpal tunnel syndrome do not have clinical or electrical evidence of more diffuse neuropathy; however, they can have concomitant tarsal tunnel syndrome (Schwartz, Mackworth-Young & McKeran, 1983). Thyroid replacement therapy can lead to complete relief of carpal tunnel syndrome symptoms, but many patients have persistent symptoms of carpal tunnel syndrome even after they are chemically euthyroid (Frymoyer & Bland, 1973; Palumbo, Szabo & Olmsted, 2000).

Carpal tunnel syndrome has been reported in patients receiving lithium for manic-depressive illness (Wood & Jacoby, 1986; Deahl, 1988). In these cases the mechanism appeared to be lithium-induced hypothyroidism, and symptoms of carpal tunnel syndrome resolved with thyroid replacement therapy despite continuation of lithium treatment.

Carpal tunnel syndrome and other mononeuropathies can accompany hyperthyroidism. In prospective surveys of 81 patients with untreated hyperthyroidism, there were eight cases of definite carpal tunnel syndrome (classic symptoms plus abnormal median nerve conduction), three cases of hand paresthesias with normal nerve conduction studies, and seven instances of asymptomatic slowing of median transcarpal nerve conduction studies (Roquer & Cano, 1993; Duyff et al., 2000). Tinel's sign over the median nerve at the wrist is more likely to be present in patients with hyperthyroidism than in control subjects (Ijichi, Niina, Tara, Nakamura, Ijichi, Izumo & Osame, 1992). Both the symptoms and electrical abnormalities of carpal tunnel syndrome usually improve after treatment of hyperthyroidism; however, when treatment of hyperthyroidism leads to hypothyroidism, carpal tunnel syndrome can develop (Beard, Kumar & Estep, 1985; Roquer & Cano, 1993).

Estrogens, Progesterone, Gonadotrophins

Carpal tunnel syndrome is a frequent complication of pregnancy (Tobin, 1967). Symptoms begin in any trimester but typically increase in frequency and severity in the third trimester and usually resolve rapidly postpartum or even toward the end of the pregnancy (Gould & Wissinger, 1978; Massey, 1978; Wand, 1990; Stolp-Smith, Pascoe & Ogburn, 1998). More than 20% of pregnant women have symptoms of carpal tunnel syndrome; symptoms are bilateral in approximately one-half of the women. However, the incidence of physical signs of carpal tunnel syndrome (positive Phalen's test, abnormal sensory signs or opponens weak-

ness) is much lower, 2% in one series (Ekman-Ordeberg, Salgeback & Ordeberg, 1987). In a retrospective review of 14,579 pregnancies in 10,873 women, the diagnosis of carpal tunnel syndrome was recorded in the chart of only 90 women (Stolp-Smith et al., 1998).

Gestational carpal tunnel syndrome is usually uncomplicated by other arm conditions, but cases have been reported of carpal tunnel syndrome with eosinophilic fasciitis, with de Quervain's tenosynovitis, and with "reflex sympathetic dystrophy" in pregnancy (Schumacher Jr, Dorwart & Korzeniowski, 1985; Simon, Mokriski, Malinow & Martz, 1988; Amdur & Levin, 1989).

Gestational carpal tunnel syndrome is probably more common in primiparas (Ekman-Ordeberg et al., 1987). Recurrence with subsequent pregnancies is not inevitable (Tobin, 1967). Among women who undergo carpal tunnel surgery, initiation of symptoms of carpal tunnel syndrome during pregnancy is unusual (al Qattan, Manktelow & Bowen, 1994).

Nerve conduction findings in women with gestational carpal tunnel syndrome vary, as expected, based on techniques used and patient referral patterns. A survey of Thai woman in the third trimester of pregnancy found that 28% had abnormal nerve conduction across the carpal tunnel in at least one hand (i.e., median distal motor latency greater than 4.0 msec, distal sensory latency greater than 3.5 msec, or median nerve minus the radial nerve latency between wrist and thumb greater than 0.48 msec); 23% with abnormal median conduction compared to only 4% of women with normal median conduction had symptoms of carpal tunnel syndrome (Atisook, Benjapibal, Sunsaneevithayakul & Roongpisuthipong, 1995). However, other series report that median nerve conduction studies are normal more often than not in gestational carpal tunnel syndrome (Melvin, Burnett & Johnson, 1969; Nicholas, Noone & Graham, 1971). Among women with findings severe enough to warrant referral for electrodiagnostic testing, sensitive techniques will usually show abnormal median nerve conduction (Seror, 1998). When the latencies are abnormal, they typically improve postpartum and rarely remain mildly abnormal after symptoms have resolved (Gould & Wissinger, 1978).

Symptoms usually can be controlled during pregnancy with use of nocturnal wrist splints

(Ekman-Ordeberg et al., 1987; Courts, 1995). Local steroid injection in the carpal canal can relieve symptoms (Godfrey, 1983; Seror, 1998). Vitamin B_6 therapy, 100 to 200 mg daily, has also been proposed (Ellis, 1987). (The controversy surrounding vitamin B_6 therapy for carpal tunnel syndrome is discussed in Chapter 14.) An occasional patient with gestational carpal tunnel syndrome requires surgical release of the flexor retinaculum (Seror, Albert & Saraby, 1993; Assmus & Hashemi, 2000). Women who develop carpal tunnel symptoms before the last trimester or have abnormal two-point discrimination at the median-innervated fingertips are more likely to need carpal tunnel surgery (Stahl, Blumenfeld & Yarnitsky, 1996).

The high incidence of carpal tunnel syndrome during pregnancy is commonly attributed to fluid retention with an increase in carpal canal pressure secondary to edema. A dog model gives some evidence of an additional mechanism: that peripheral nerves might be more vulnerable to compression during pregnancy (Takayama, 1990). One study suggests that the median nerves of pregnant women have an increased susceptibility to local anesthetics (Butterworth, Walker & Lysak, 1990). Whether this susceptibility is evidence of median nerve compression in the carpal tunnel or of hormonally induced changes in nerve physiology is unknown.

Occurrence of symptoms of carpal tunnel syndrome during breast-feeding is rarer than occurrence of symptoms during pregnancy (Snell, Coysh & Snell, 1980; Yagnik, 1987). Wand (1989, 1990) described 24 women who developed symptoms of carpal tunnel syndrome during lactation. They typically became symptomatic a few weeks postpartum, had persistent symptoms during the months of lactation, and improved within a few weeks of weaning. Compared to women with gestational carpal tunnel syndrome, women with lactational carpal tunnel syndrome are older, more likely to be primiparous, and less likely to have peripheral edema. It is unclear whether carpal tunnel syndrome with lactation has a hormonal cause or whether it is related to wrist positioning during breast-feeding.

Kotowicz and colleagues (1988) reported an unusual case of carpal tunnel syndrome accompanying galactorrhea and amenorrhea secondary to a prolactin-secreting pituitary adenoma. This case, lactation-associated carpal tunnel syndrome, and the observation that prolactin levels are sometimes increased in acromegaly and hypothyroidism have led to speculation about the role of prolactin in the pathogenesis of carpal tunnel syndrome. Rossi and colleagues (1984) measured prolactin levels in patients with idiopathic carpal tunnel syndrome and did not find evidence for an association.

Use of oral contraceptives can be followed by development of carpal tunnel syndrome. Sabour and Fadel (1970) reported 62 women who developed carpal tunnel syndrome symptoms while on oral contraceptives and who had resolution of symptoms within 1 month of stopping the medication. They suggest that the risk is higher when the estrogen content of the oral contraceptive is higher. Another study of premenopausal women found that those who had been on oral contraceptives for 10 years were nearly twice as likely to have carpal tunnel syndrome as those who had never taken these hormones (Vessey, Villard-MacIntosh & Yeates, 1990). This relationship between oral contraceptive use and risk of carpal tunnel syndrome has not been proven in other epidemiologic surveys (Cannon, Bernacki & Walter, 1981; De Krom, Kester, Knipschild & Spaans, 1990; Ferry et al., 2000).

Two case-control studies have suggested that postmenopausal estrogen use might be a risk factor for carpal tunnel syndrome with an odds ratio in both studies of 2.4 (Cannon et al., 1981; Dieck & Kelsey, 1985). In one of these, the results fell slightly short of statistical significance, and neither study controlled for patient age as a confounding variable. Another case-control study did not confirm hormone replacement therapy as a risk factor for development of carpal tunnel syndrome (Ferry et al., 2000).

In contrast to these instances of carpal tunnel syndrome occurring during times of high ovarian hormone levels, there is an increased incidence of carpal tunnel syndrome after oophorectomy. Furthermore, case reports suggest that in some postmenopausal women, hormone replacement therapy leads to improvement in symptoms of carpal tunnel syndrome (Confino-Cohen, Lishner, Savin, Lang & Ravid, 1991). Bjorkqvist and colleagues (1977) studied 20 women before and after oophorectomy. Three of the 20 developed symptoms consistent with carpal tunnel syndrome within 4 months of surgery. Two of these women, who had normal median distal latencies documented before oophorectomy, developed prolonged median distal latencies when they were symptomatic. In a case-control study, hysterectomy with bilateral oophorectomy was a risk factor for developing carpal tunnel syndrome (Cannon et al., 1981). In another case-control study, women aged 36 to 44 years who had undergone oophorectomy 1 to 4 years previously and who were not on hormone replacement therapy were compared to age-matched premenopausal controls; 32% of the oophorectomized women had clinical evidence of carpal tunnel syndrome compared to 10% of controls (Pascual, Giner, Aróstegui, Conill, Ruiz & Picó, 1991). Commonly, the symptoms of carpal tunnel syndrome develop within the first year after oophorectomy. Further complicating the interpretation of any relationship between oophorectomy and risk of carpal tunnel syndrome, one study found an increased risk of carpal tunnel syndrome in women who had undergone hysterectomy without oophorectomy (De Krom et al., 1990).

A 31-year-old woman developed symptoms of carpal tunnel syndrome after taking danazol for treatment of endometriosis (Gray, 1978). She also developed a knee effusion. Carpal tunnel syndrome symptoms and the knee effusion resolved 1 week after stopping danazol.

Somatotropin (Growth Hormone)

Carpal tunnel syndrome is a common complication of acromegaly. In 1891 Sternberg identified nocturnal hand paresthesias as an early manifestation of acromegaly (Pickett, Layzer, Levin, Scheider, Campbell & Sumner, 1975). Woltman (1941) reported that 10 of 213 acromegalic patients complained of periodic hand pain and documented that, in at least some cases, the pain was associated with an isolated median neuropathy. In series of acromegalic patients, the incidence of carpal tunnel syndrome ranges from 35% to 64% (Bluestone, Bywaters, Hartog, Holt & Hyde, 1971; Pickett et al., 1975; Baum, Ludecke & Herrmann, 1986; Podgorski, Robinson, Weissberger, Stiel, Wang & Brooks, 1988). Furthermore, most patients with acromegaly have at least

mild slowing of median transcarpal nerve conduction, even if they do not have symptoms of carpal tunnel syndrome (Kameyama, Tanaka, Hasegawa, Tamura & Kuroki, 1993; Verma & Mahapatra, 1994). Carpal tunnel syndrome symptoms can fluctuate with somatotropin levels and activity of acromegaly: 34 of the 63 patients whose acromegaly was active had carpal tunnel syndrome symptoms; only one patient without active acromegalic findings had carpal tunnel syndrome symptoms (O'Duffy, Randall & MacCarty, 1973).

Symptoms of carpal tunnel syndrome can be one of the earliest clinical indications of acromegaly. However, acromegalics can also have a polyarthropathy that complicates the interpretation of their extremity symptoms (Bluestone et al., 1971; Podgorski et al., 1988). The development of carpal tunnel syndrome is independent of glucose intolerance, abnormalities of thyroid function, or development of more diffuse peripheral neuropathy (Jamal, Kerr, McLellan, Weir & Davies, 1987).

The pathogenic import of raised somatotropin levels is further supported by the development of carpal tunnel syndrome in patients receiving somatotropin as experimental treatment for osteoporosis or in an athlete taking it as part of a body-building program (Aloia, Zanzi, Ellis, Jowsey, Roginsky, Wallach & Cohn, 1976; Dickerman, Douglas & East, 2000). Elderly men who receive somatotropin for treatment of low levels of insulin-like growth factor I often develop symptoms of carpal tunnel syndrome, especially if their plasma insulin-like growth factor-I level is raised to more than 1.0 unit/ml (Cohn, Feller, Draper, Rudman & Rudman, 1993). However, children receiving somatotropin for treatment of renal insufficiency, growth hormone deficiency, or short stature and men receiving high–dose growth hormone for treatment of acquired immunodeficiency syndrome–associated wasting have a low risk of developing carpal tunnel syndrome (Blethen, Allen, Graves, August, Moshang & Rosenfeld, 1996; Van Loon, 1998).

MRI studies of the carpal tunnel in patients with acromegaly suggest that acromegalics who have carpal tunnel syndrome have enlarged median nerves that appear brighter than normal on T2-weighted images (Jenkins, Sohaib, Akker, Phillips, Spillane, Wass, Monson, Grossman, Besser & Reznek, 2000). Other contents of the canal do not appear enlarged. The imaging abnormalities of the median nerve improve after treating the acromegaly.

In unselected patients with carpal tunnel syndrome, the incidence of acromegaly is very low. The cost-effectiveness of screening for acromegaly in carpal tunnel syndrome patients is unknown. A reasonable approach is to be clinically alert for acromegaly but not to undertake laboratory screening for it unless prompted by clinical clues.

In most acromegalic patients treatment of the acromegaly relieves the symptoms of carpal tunnel syndrome (Nabarro, 1987). The symptoms of carpal tunnel syndrome can regress within 2 weeks after the fall of somatotropin levels (O'Duffy et al., 1973). Carpal tunnel syndrome can also improve after suppression of somatotropin secretion with bromocriptine or lergotrile (Kleinberg, Schaaf & Frantz, 1978; Luboshitzky & Barzilai, 1980). The median distal motor latency can improve within 1 week of surgical removal of a pituitary adenoma (Baum et al., 1986). Other median conduction abnormalities usually improve after pituitary adenomectomy, but mild conduction slowing persists in some patients (Kameyama et al., 1993; Verma & Mahapatra, 1994).

Calcium Abnormalities

Carpal tunnel syndrome is rarely associated with disorders of calcium metabolism. Some case reports deserve mention:

A 78-year-old man had had symptoms of carpal tunnel syndrome for years. After carpal tunnel surgery, pseudogout was diagnosed based on finding pyrophosphate crystals in the carpal canal. The pseudogout was caused by hypercalcemia secondary to hyperparathyroidism (Weinstein, Dick & Grantham, 1968).

A patient with carpal tunnel syndrome had hypocalcemia, chronic renal failure, and secondary hyperparathyroidism. Wrist x-rays revealed ectopic calcification in the carpal canal (Firooznia, Golimbu & Rafii, 1981).

A 57-year-old woman presented with bilateral nocturnal hand paresthesias and pain. Serum calcium was elevated to 11.8 mg/dl, and serum parathormone levels were over twice

the upper limit of normal. Bilateral median distal motor latencies were markedly prolonged (6.5 and 7.2 msecs). Two weeks after surgical removal of a parathyroid adenoma, the hand symptoms were absent and median distal motor latencies had improved to 3.8 and 3.7 msecs (Palma, 1983).

A 55-year-old woman acutely developed symptoms of carpal tunnel syndrome after carpopedal spasm caused by hypocalcemic tetany (Massey, O'Brian & Georges, 1978). Symptoms slowly resolved after episodes of spasm were stopped by correction of serum calcium.

References

Abbott LC, Saunders JBdeCM. Injuries of the median nerve in fractures of the lower end of the radius. Surg. Gynecol. Obstet. 1933;57:507–16.

Ahmed T, Braun AI. Carpal tunnel syndrome with polymyalgia rheumatica. Arthritis Rheum. 1978;21:221–23.

Akizuki S, Matsui T. Entrapment neuropathy caused by tophaceous gout. J. Hand Surg. 1984;9B:331–2.

Albers JW, Brown MB, Sima AA, Greene DA. Frequency of median mononeuropathy in patients with mild diabetic neuropathy in the early diabetes intervention trial (EDIT). Tolrestat Study Group For Edit (Early Diabetes Intervention Trial). Muscle Nerve 1996;19:140–46.

Ali T, Hofford R, Mohammed F, Maharaj D, Sookhoo S, van Velzen D. Tophaceous gout: a case of bilateral carpal tunnel syndrome. West Indian Med. J. 1999;48:160–62.

Aloia JF, Zanzi I, Ellis K, Jowsey J, Roginsky M, Wallach S, Cohn SH. Effects of growth hormone in osteoporosis. J. Clin. Endocrinol. Metab. 1976;43:992–99.

Alonso-Ruiz A, Zea-Mendoza AC, Salazar-Vallinas JM, Rocamora-Ripoll A, Beltrán-Gutierrez J. Toxic oil syndrome: a syndrome with features overlapping those of various forms of scleroderma. Semin. Arthritis Rheum. 1986;15:200–212.

al Qattan MM, Manktelow RT, Bowen CVA. Pregnancy-induced carpal tunnel syndrome requiring surgical release longer than 2 years after delivery. Obstet. Gynecol. 1994;84:249–51.

Amdur HS, Levin RE. Eosinophilic fasciitis during pregnancy. Obstet. Gynecol. 1989;73:843–47.

Andonopoulos AP, Lagos G, Drosos AA, Moutsopoulos HM. The spectrum of neurological involvement in Sjögren's syndrome. Br. J. Rheumatol. 1990;29:21–23.

Assmus H, Hashemi B. Surgical treatment of carpal tunnel syndrome in pregnancy: results from 314 cases. Nervenarzt 2000;71:470–73.

Atisook R, Benjapibal M, Sunsaneevithayakul P, Roongpisuthipong A. Carpal tunnel syndrome during pregnancy: prevalence and blood level of pyridoxine. Med. Assoc. Thai. 1995;78:410–14.

Barnes CG, Currey HL. Carpal tunnel syndrome in rheumatoid arthritis. A clinical and electrodiagnostic survey. Ann. Rheum. Dis. 1967;26:226–33.

Barnes L, Rodnan GP, Medsger TA, Short D. Eosinophilic fasciitis. A pathologic study of twenty cases. Am. J. Pathol. 1979;96:493–517.

Barr WG, Blair SJ. Carpal tunnel syndrome as the initial manifestation of scleroderma. J. Hand Surg. 1988;13A:366–68.

Baum H, Ludecke DK, Herrmann HD. Carpal tunnel syndrome and acromegaly. Acta. Neurochir. (Wien). 1986;83:54–55.

Beard L, Kumar A, Estep HL. Bilateral carpal tunnel syndrome caused by Graves' disease. Arch. Intern. Med. 1985;145:345–46.

Belcher HJ, Varma S, Schonauer F. Endoscopic carpal tunnel release in selected rheumatoid patients. J. Hand Surg. 2000;25B:451–52.

Bell DS, Clements RS Jr. Reversal of the carpal tunnel syndrome after change of insulin injection sites. Diabetes Care 1983;6:211–12.

Berth-Jones J, Coates PA, Graham-Brown RA, Burns DA. Neurological complications of systemic sclerosis—a report of three cases and review of the literature. Clin. Exp. Dermatol. 1990;15:91–94.

Bertora P, Valla P, Dezuanni E, Osio M, Mantica D, Bevilacqua M, Norbiato G, Caccia MR, Mangoni A. Prevalence of subclinical neuropathy in diabetic patients: assessment by study of conduction velocity distribution within motor and sensory nerve fibres. J. Neurol. 1998;245:81–86.

Binder AI, Sheppard MN, Paice E. Extensor tendon rupture related to calcium pyrophosphate crystal deposition disease. Br. J. Rheumatol. 1989;28:251–53.

Binder A, Snaith ML, Isenberg D. Sjogren's syndrome: a study of its neurological complications. Br. J. Rheumatol. 1988;27:275–80.

Bjorkqvist SE, Lang AH, Punnonen R, Rauramo L. Carpal tunnel syndrome in ovariectomized women. Acta. Obstet. Gynecol. Scand. 1977;56:127–30.

Bleecker ML, Bohlman M, Moreland R, Tipton A. Carpal tunnel syndrome: role of carpal canal size. Neurology 1985;35:1599–1604.

Blethen SL, Allen DB, Graves D, August G, Moshang T, Rosenfeld R. Safety of recombinant deoxyribonucleic acid-derived growth hormone: the National Cooperative Growth Study experience. J. Clin. Endocrinol. Metab. 1996;81:1704–10.

Bluestone R, Bywaters EG, Hartog M, Holt PJ, Hyde S. Acromegalic arthropathy. Ann. Rheum. Dis. 1971;30:243–58.

Bohr T. Problems with myofascial pain syndrome and fibromyalgia syndrome. Neurology 1996;46:593–97.

Butterworth JF 4th, Walker FO, Lysak SZ. Pregnancy increases median nerve susceptibility to lidocaine. Anesthesiology 1990;72:962–5.

Cannon BW, Love JG. Tardy median palsy; median neuritis; median thenar neuritis amenable to surgery. Surgery 1946;20:210–16.

Cannon LJ, Bernacki EJ, Walter SD. Personal and occupational factors associated with carpal tunnel syndrome. J. Occ. Med. 1981;23:255–58.

Caselli RJ, Daube JR, Hunder GG, Whisnant JP. Peripheral neuropathic syndromes in giant cell (temporal) arteritis. Neurology 1988;38:685–89.

Chamberlain MA, Corbett M. Carpal tunnel syndrome in early rheumatoid arthritis. Ann. Rheum. Dis. 1970;29:149–52.

Chammas M, Bousquet P, Renard E, Poirier JL, Jaffiol C, Allieu Y. Dupuytren's disease, carpal tunnel syndrome, trigger finger, and diabetes mellitus. J. Hand Surg. 1995;20A:109–14.

Champion D. Gouty tenosynovitis and the carpal tunnel syndrome. Med. J. Aust. 1969;1:1030–32.

Chan MK, Kaye RL. Carpal tunnel syndrome as a precursor of polymyalgia rheumatica. Ariz. Med. 1982;39:517–19.

Chaplin E, Kasdan ML. Carpal tunnel syndrome and routine blood chemistries. Plast. Reconstr. Surg. 1985;75:722–24.

Chen CK, Chung CB, Yeh L, Pan HB, Yang CF, Lai PH, Liang HL, Resnick D. Carpal tunnel syndrome caused by tophaceous gout: CT and MR imaging features in 20 patients. AJR. Am. J. Roentgenol. 2000;175:655–59.

Chiu KY, Wong WB, Choi CH, Chow SP. Acute carpal tunnel syndrome caused by pseudogout. J. Hand Surg. 1992;17A:299–302.

Cimmino MA, Parisi M, Moggiana G, Accardo S. The association between fibromyalgia and carpal tunnel syndrome in the general population. Ann. Rheum. Dis. 1996;55:780.

Cobb TK, Bond JR, Cooney WP, Metcalf BJ. Assessment of the ratio of carpal contents to carpal tunnel volume in patients with carpal tunnel syndrome: a preliminary report. J. Hand Surg. 1997;22A:635–39.

Cohn L, Feller AG, Draper MW, Rudman IW, Rudman D. Carpal tunnel syndrome and gynaecomastia during growth hormone treatment of elderly men with low circulating IGF-I concentrations. Clin. Endocrinol. 1993;39:417–25.

Comi G, Lozza L, Galardi G, Ghilardi MF, Medaglini S, Canal N. Presence of carpal tunnel syndrome in diabetics: effect of age, sex, diabetes duration and polyneuropathy. Acta. Diabetol. Lat. 1985;22:259–62.

Confino-Cohen R, Lishner M, Savin H, Lang R, Ravid M. Response of carpal tunnel syndrome to hormone replacement therapy. BMJ. 1991;303:1514.

Courts RB. Splinting for symptoms of carpal tunnel syndrome during pregnancy. J. Hand Ther. 1995;8:31–34.

Craig EV, House JH. Dorsal carpal dislocation and flexor tendon rupture in rheumatoid arthritis: a case report. J. Hand Surg. 1984;9A:261–64.

Cremer GM, Goldstein NP, Paris J. Myxedema and ataxia. Neurology 1969;19:37–46.

Crow RS. Treatment of the carpal-tunnel syndrome. BMJ. 1960;1:1611–15.

Deahl MP. Lithium-induced carpal tunnel syndrome. Br. J. Psychiatry. 1988;153:250–51.

Dekel S, Papaioannou T, Rushworth G, Coates R. Idiopathic carpal tunnel syndrome caused by carpal stenosis. BMJ. 1980;280:1297–99.

De Krom MCT, Kester ADM, Knipschild PG, Spaans F. Risk factors for carpal tunnel syndrome. Am. J. Epidemiol. 1990;132:1102–10.

Dennis RH 2nd, Ransome JR. Giant cell arteritis presenting as a carpal tunnel syndrome. J. Nat. Med. Assoc. 1996;88:524–25.

Dickerman RD, Douglas JA, East JW. Bilateral median neuropathy and growth hormone use: a case report. Arch. Phys. Med. Rehabil. 2000;81:1594–95.

Dieck GS, Kelsey JL. An epidemiologic study of the carpal tunnel syndrome in an adult female population. Prev. Med. 1985;14:63–69.

Duyff RF, Van den Bosch J, Laman DM, van Loon BJ, Linssen WH. Neuromuscular findings in thyroid dysfunction: a prospective clinical and electrodiagnostic study. J. Neurol. Neurosurg. Psychiatry 2000;68:750–55.

Dyck PJ, Kratz KM, Karnes JL, Litchy WJ, Klein R, Pach JM, Wilson DM, O'Brien PC, Melton LJ. The prevalence by staged severity of various types of diabetic neuropathy, retinopathy, and nephropathy in a population-based cohort: the Rochester Diabetic Neuropathy Study. Neurology 1993;43:817.

Dyck PJ, Thomas PK (eds). Diabetic Neuropathy. Philadelphia: Saunders, 1999.

Ekman-Ordeberg G, Salgeback S, Ordeberg G. Carpal tunnel syndrome in pregnancy. A prospective study. Acta Obstet. Gynecol. Scand. 1987;66:233–35.

Ellis JM. Treatment of carpal tunnel syndrome with vitamin B_6. South. Med. J. 1987;80:882–84.

Engel J, Zinneman H, Tsur H, Farin I. Carpal tunnel syndrome due to carpal osteophyte. Hand 1978;10:283–84.

Fassler PR, Stern PJ, Kiefhaber TR. Asymptomatic SLAC wrist: does it exist? J. Hand Surg. 1993;18A:682–86.

Ferlic DC. Rheumatoid flexor tenosynovitis and rupture. Hand Clin. 1996;12:561–72.

Ferry S, Hannaford P, Warskyj M, Lewis M, Croft P. Carpal tunnel syndrome: a nested case-control study of risk factors in women. Am. J. Epidemiol. 2000;151:566–74.

Fincham RW, Cape CA. Neuropathy in myxedema. A study of sensory nerve conduction in the upper extremities. Arch. Neurol. 1968;19:464–66.

Firooznia H, Golimbu C, Rafii M. Carpal tunnel syndrome as a manifestation of secondary hyperparathyroidism. Arch. Intern. Med. 1981;141:959.

Flam M, Ryan SC, Mah-Poy GL, Jacobs KF, Neldner KH. Multicentric reticulohistiocytosis. Report of a case, with atypical features and electron microscopic study of skin lesions. Am. J. Med. 1972;52:841–48.

Fleming A, Dodman S, Crown JM, Corbett M. Extra-articular features in early rheumatoid disease. BMJ. 1976;1:1241–43.

Florack TM, Miller RJ, Pellegrini VD, Burton RI, Dunn MG. The prevalence of carpal tunnel syndrome in patients with basal joint arthritis of the thumb. J. Hand Surg. 1992;17A:624–30.

Frymoyer JW, Bland J. Carpal-tunnel syndrome in patients with myxedematous arthropathy. J. Bone Joint Surg. 1973;55:78–82.

Gainer JV Jr., Nugent GR. Carpal tunnel syndrome: report of 430 operations. South. Med. J. 1977;70:325–28.

Gama C, Meira JBB. Occupational acro-osteolysis. J. Bone Joint Surg. 1978;60A:86–90.

Gamstedt A, Holm-Glad J, Ohlson C-G, Sundström M. Hand abnormalities are strongly associated with the duration of diabetes mellitus. J. Intern. Med. 1993;234:189–93.

Gelmers HJ. Primary carpal tunnel stenosis as a cause of entrapment of the median nerve. Acta Neurochir. (Wien.) 1981;55:317–20.

Gerster JC, Lagier R, Boivin G, Schneider C. Carpal tunnel syndrome in chondrocalcinosis of the wrist. Clinical and histologic study. Arthritis Rheum. 1980;23:926–31.

Godfrey CM. Carpal tunnel syndrome in pregnancy. Can. Med. Assoc. J. 1983;129:928.

Golding DN. Hypothyroidism presenting with musculoskeletal symptoms. Ann. Rheum. Dis. 1970;29:10–14.

Goodwin DR, Arbel R. Pseudogout of the wrist presenting as acute median nerve compression. J. Hand Surg. 1985;10B:261–62.

Gould JS, Wissinger HA. Carpal tunnel syndrome in pregnancy. South. Med. J. 1978;71:144–45,154.

Gray RG. Bilateral carpal tunnel syndrome and arthritis associated with Danazol administration. Arthritis Rheum. 1978;21:493–94.

Gray RG, Gottlieb NL. Hand flexor tenosynovitis in rheumatoid arthritis. Prevalence, distribution, and associated rheumatic features. Arthritis Rheum. 1977;20:1003–8.

Green EJ, Dilworth JH, Levitin PM. Tophaceous gout. An unusual cause of bilateral carpal tunnel syndrome. JAMA. 1977;237:2747–48.

Herbison GJ, Teng C, Martin JH, Ditunno JF Jr. Carpal tunnel syndrome in rheumatoid arthritis. Am. J. Phys. Med. 1973;52:68–74.

Herrera B, Sanmarti R, Ponce A, Lopez-Soto A, Munoz-Gomez J. Carpal tunnel syndrome heralding polymyalgia rheumatica. Scand. J. Rheumatol. 1997;26:222–24.

Hooper J. The surgery of the wrist in rheumatoid arthritis. Aust. N. Z. J. Surg. 1972;42:135–40.

Hoyt RE. Carpal tunnel syndrome and gout: case report. Va. Med. 1986;113:407–9.

Hybbinette CH, Mannerfelt L. The carpal tunnel syndrome. A retrospective study of 400 operated patients. Acta. Orthop. Scand. 1975;46:610–20.

Ijichi S, Niina K, Tara M, Nakamura F, Ijichi N, Izumo S, Osame M. Mononeuropathy associated with hyperthyroidism. J. Neurol. Neurosurg. Psychiatry 1992;53:1109–10.

Isselin J, Gariot P. Tunnel syndromes and blood glucose anomalies. Ann. Chir. Main. 1989;8:344–46.

Izhar-ul-Haque. Carpal tunnel syndrome due to an anomalous distal end of the radius. A case report. J. Bone Joint Surg. 1982;64A:943–44.

Jacoulet P. Double tunnel syndrome of the upper limb in tophaceous gout. Apropos of a case. Ann. Chir. Main Memb. Super. 1994;13:42–45.

Jamal GA, Kerr DJ, McLellan AR, Weir AI, Davies DL. Generalised peripheral nerve dysfunction in acromegaly: a study by conventional and novel neurophysiological techniques. J. Neurol. Neurosurg. Psychiatry 1987;50:886–94.

Janssen T, Rayan GM. Gouty tenosynovitis and compression neuropathy of the median nerve. Clin. Orthop. 1987;216:203–6.

Jenkins PJ, Sohaib SA, Akker S, Phillips RR, Spillane K, Wass JA, Monson JP, Grossman AB, Besser GM, Reznek RH. The pathology of median neuropathy in acromegaly. Ann. Intern. Med. 2000;133:197–201.

Jones HR Jr, Beetham WP Jr., Silverman ML, Margles SW. Eosinophilic fasciitis and the carpal tunnel syndrome. J. Neurol. Neurosurg. Psychiatry 1986;49:324–27.

Kameyama S, Tanaka R, Hasegawa A, Tamura T, Kuroki M. Subclinical carpal tunnel syndrome in acromegaly. Neurol. Med. Chir. (Tokyo) 1993;33:547–51.

Kersting-Sommerhoff B, Hof N, Golder W, Becker K, Werber KD. MRI of the wrist joint: "granulomatous tenovaginitis of the sarcoidosis type"—a rare cause of carpal tunnel syndrome. Rontgenpraxis 1995;48:206–8.

Kleinberg DL, Schaaf M, Frantz AG. Studies with lergotrile mesylate in acromegaly. Fed. Proc. 1978;37:2198–2201.

Ko CY, Jones NF, Steen VD. Compression of the median nerve proximal to the carpal tunnel in scleroderma. J. Hand Surg. 1996;21A:363–65.

Kotowicz MA, Turtle JR, Crouch R. Bilateral carpal tunnel syndrome and galactorrhoea. Med. J. Aust. 1988;148: 252–55.

Lagier R, Boivin G, Gerster JC. Carpal tunnel syndrome associated with mixed calcium pyrophosphate dihydrate and apatite crystal deposition in tendon synovial sheath. Arthritis Rheum. 1984;27:1190–95.

Lakhanpal S, Ginsburg WW, Michet CJ, Doyle JA, Moore SB. Eosinophilic fasciitis: clinical spectrum and therapeutic response in 52 cases. Semin. Arthritis Rheum. 1988;17: 221–31.

Lamberta FJ, Ferlic DC, Clayton ML. Volz total wrist arthroplasty in rheumatoid arthritis: a preliminary report. J. Hand Surg. 1980;5:245–52.

Lanzillo B, Pappone N, Crisci C, di Girolamo C, Massini R, Caruso G. Subclinical peripheral nerve involvement in patients with rheumatoid arthritis. Arthritis Rheum. 1998; 41:1196–1202.

Lee P, Bruni J, Sukenik S. Neurological manifestations in systemic sclerosis (scleroderma). J. Rheumatol. 1984;11:480–83.

Leffert RD. Diabetes mellitus initially presenting as peripheral neuropathy in the upper limb. J. Bone Joint Surg. 1969; 51A:1004–10.

Lewis D, Miller EM. Peripheral nerve injuries associated with fractures. Trans. Am. Surg. Assoc. 1922;40:489–580.

Lewis SL, Fiddian NJ. Acute carpal tunnel syndrome a rare complication of chondrocalcinosis. Hand 1982;14:164–67.

Lianga J, Waslen GD, Penney CJ. Tophaceous gout presenting with bilateral hand contractures and carpal tunnel syndrome. J. Rheumatol. 1986;13:230–31.

Loong SC. The carpal tunnel syndrome: a clinical and electrophysiological study of 250 patients. Proc. Aust. Assoc. Neurol. 1977;14:51–65.

Lori S, Matucci-Cerinic M, Casale R, Generini S, Lombardi A, Pignone A, Scaletti C, Gangemi PF, Cagnoni M. Peripheral nervous system involvement in systemic sclerosis: the median nerve as target structure. Clin. Exp. Rheumatol. 1996;14:601–5.

Luboshitzky R, Barzilai D. Bromocriptine for an acromegalic patient. Improvement in cardiac function and carpal tunnel syndrome. JAMA 1980;244:1825–7.

Luchetti R, Mingione A, Monteleone M, Cristiani G. Carpal tunnel syndrome in Madelung's deformity. J. Hand Surg. 1988;13B:19–22.

Machet L, Vaillant L, Machet MC, Esteve E, Muller C, Khallouf R, Lorette G. Carpal tunnel syndrome and systemic sclerosis. Dermatol. 1992;185:101–3.

March LM, Francis H, Webb J. Benign joint hypermobility with neuropathies: documentation and mechanism of median, sciatic, and common peroneal nerve compression. Clin. Rheumatol. 1988;7:35–40.

Massey EW. Carpal tunnel syndrome in pregnancy. Obstet. Gynecol. Surv. 1978;33:145–48.

Massey EW, O'Brian JT, Georges LP. Carpal tunnel syndrome secondary to carpopedal spasm. Ann. Intern. Med. 1978;88:804–5.

Maxwell JA, Clough CA, Reckling FW, Kelly CR. Carpal tunnel syndrome. A review of cases treated surgically. J. Kans. Med. Soc. 1973;74:190–93.

McGrory BJ, Schmidt IU, Wold LE, Amadio PC. Carpal tunnel syndrome associated with eosinophilic fasciitis. Orthopedics 1998;21:368–70.

Medsger TA, Dixon JA, Garwood VF. Palmar fasciitis and polyarthritis associated with ovarian carcinoma. Ann. Intern. Med. 1982;96:424–31.

Melvin JL, Burnett CN, Johnson EW. Median nerve conduction in pregnancy. Arch. Phys. Med. Rehabil. 1969;50:75–80.

Merianos P, Smyrnis P, Tsomy K, Hager J. Giant cell arteritis of the median nerve simulating carpal tunnel syndrome. Hand 1983;15:249–51.

Miller DG. The association of immune disease and malignant lymphoma. Ann. Intern. Med. 1967;66:507–21.

Miller LD, Stevens MB. Skeletal manifestations of polymyalgia rheumatica. JAMA 1978;240:27–29.

Molina R, Provost TT, Alexander EL. Peripheral inflammatory vascular disease in Sjögren's syndrome. Association with nervous system complications. Arthritis Rheum. 1985; 28:1341–47.

Monge L, De Mattei M, Dani F, Sciarretta A, Carta Q. Effect of treatment with an aldose-reductase inhibitor on symptomatic carpal tunnel syndrome in type 2 diabetes. Diabetic Med. 1995;12:1097–1101.

Moore JR, Weiland AJ. Gouty tenosynovitis in the hand. J. Hand Surg. 1985;10A:291–95.

Moran H, Chen SL, Muirden KD, Jiang SJ, Gu YY, Hopper J, Jiang PL, Lawler G, Chen RB. A comparison of rheumatoid arthritis in Australia and China. Ann. Rheum. Dis. 1986; 45:572–78.

Murray IPC, Simpson JA. Acroparaesthesia in myxoedema—a clinical and electromyographic study. Lancet 1958;1: 1360–63.

Nabarro JD. Acromegaly. Clin. Endocrinol. (Oxf). 1987;26: 481–512.

Nicholas GG, Noone RB, Graham WP. Carpal tunnel syndrome in pregnancy. Hand 1971;3:80–83.

O'Duffy JD, Hunder GG, Wahner HW. A follow-up study of polymyalgia rheumatica: evidence of chronic axial synovitis. J. Rheumatol. 1980;7:685–93.

O'Duffy JD, Randall RV, MacCarty CS. Median neuropathy (carpal-tunnel syndrome) in acromegaly. A sign of endocrine overactivity. Ann. Intern. Med. 1973;78:379–83.

Olive KE, Hennessey JV. Marked hyperprolactinemia in subclinical hypothyroidism. Arch. Intern. Med. 1988;148: 2278–79.

Olmedo-Garzon FJ, Leiva-Santana C, Alonso-Ruiz A, Riva-Meana C. The toxic-oil syndrome: a new cause of the carpal-tunnel syndrome. N. Engl. J. Med. 1983;309:1455.

Omdal R, Mellgren SI, Husby G. Clinical neuropsychiatric and neuromuscular manifestations in systemic lupus erythematosus. Scand. J. Rheumatol. 1988;17:113–17.

Ostroumova IV. Carpal tunnel syndrome. Sov. Med. 1969; 32:62–65.

Ozaki I, Baba M, Matsunaga M, Takebe K. Deleterious effect of the carpal tunnel on nerve conduction in diabetic polyneuropathy. Electromyogr. Clin. Neurophysiol. 1988;28:301–6.

Pai CH, Tseng CH. Acute carpal tunnel syndrome caused by tophaceous gout. J. Hand Surg. 1993;18A:667–69.

Pal B, Mangion P, Hossain MA. An assessment of glucose tolerance in patients with idiopathic carpal tunnel syndrome. Br. J. Rheumatol. 1986;25:412–13.

Palma G. Carpal tunnel syndrome and hyperparathyroidism. Ann. Neurol. 1983;14:592.

Palumbo CF, Szabo RM, Olmsted SL. The effects of hypothyroidism and thyroid replacement on the development of carpal tunnel syndrome. J. Hand Surg. 2000;25A:734–39.

Pascual E, Giner V, Aróstegui A, Conill J, Ruiz MT, Picó A. Higher incidence of carpal tunnel syndrome in oophorectomized women. Br. J. Rheumatol. 1991;30:60–62.

Perez-Ruiz F, Calabozo M, Alonso-Ruiz A, Herrero A, Ruiz-Lucea E, Otermin I. High prevalence of undetected carpal tunnel syndrome in patients with fibromyalgia syndrome. J. Rheumatol. 1995;22:501–4.

Perez-Ruiz F, Calabozo M, Alonso-Ruiz A, Ruiz-Lucea E. Fibromyalgia and carpal tunnel syndrome. Ann. Rheum. Dis. 1997;56:438–39.

Phalen GS. The carpal-tunnel syndrome. Seventeen years' experience in diagnosis and treatment of six hundred fifty-four hands. J. Bone Joint Surg. 1966;48A:211–28.

Phillips RS. Carpal tunnel syndrome as a manifestation of systemic disease. Ann. Rheum. Dis. 1967;26:59–63.

Pickett JB, Layzer RB, Levin SR, Scheider V, Campbell MJ, Sumner AJ. Neuromuscular complications of acromegaly. Neurology 1975;25:638–45.

Pledger SR, Hirsch B, Freiberg RA. Bilateral carpal tunnel syndrome secondary to gouty tenosynovitis: a case report. Clin. Orthop. 1976;118:188–89.

Podgorski M, Robinson B, Weissberger A, Stiel J, Wang S, Brooks PM. Articular manifestations of acromegaly. Aust. N. Z. J. Med. 1988;18:28–35.

Poskitt BL, Duffill MB. Acrokeratosis paraneoplastica of Bazex presenting with carpal tunnel syndrome. Br. J. Dermatol. 1992;127:544–45.

Quinones CA, Perry HO, Rushton JG. Carpal tunnel syndrome in dermatomyositis and scleroderma. Arch. Dermatol. 1966;94:20–25.

Radford PJ, Matthewson MH. Hypoplastic scaphoid—an unusual cause of carpal tunnel syndrome. J. Hand Surg. 1987;12B:236–38.

Rakic M, Elhosseiny A, Ramadan F, Iyer R, Howard RG, Gross L. Adult-type osteopetrosis presenting as carpal tunnel syndrome. Arthritis Rheum. 1986;29:926–28.

Ranawat C, Straub LR. Volar tenosynovitis of wrist in rheumatoid arthritis. Arthritis Rheum. 1970;13:112–17.

Rao SN, Katiyar BC, Nair KR, Misra S. Neuromuscular status in hypothyroidism. Acta Neurol. Scand. 1980;61:167–77.

Rate AJ, Parkinson RW, Meadows TH, Freemont AJ. Acute carpal tunnel syndrome due to pseudogout. J. Hand Surg. 1992;17B:217–18.

Renard E, Jacques D, Chammas M, Poirier JL, Bonifacj C, Jaffiol C, Simon L, Allieu Y. Increased prevalence of soft tissue hand lesions in type 1 and type 2 diabetes mellitus: various entities and associated significance. Diabetes Metab. 1994;20:513–21.

Richards AJ. Carpal tunnel syndrome in polymyalgia rheumatica. Rheumatol. Rehabil. 1980;19:100–102.

Richards AJ. Chondrocalcinosis and polymyalgia rheumatica in carpal tunnel syndrome. Arthritis Rheum. 1981;24:640.

Roquer J, Cano JF. Carpal tunnel syndrome and hyperthyroidism. A prospective study. Acta. Neurol. Scand. 1993;88: 149–52.

Rosenbloom AL. Skeletal and joint manifestations of childhood diabetes. Pediatr. Clin. North Am. 1984;31:569–89.

Rosenbloom AL, Silverstein JH. Connective tissue and joint disease in diabetes mellitus. Endocrinol. & Metab. Clin. North Am. 1996;25:473–83.

Rossi E, Sighinolfi E, Bortolotti P, De-Santis G, Schoenhuber R, Grandi M, Landi A. Nocturnal prolactin secretion in carpal tunnel syndrome. Ital. J. Neurol. Sci. 1984;5:405–8.

Sabour MS, Fadel HE. The carpal tunnel syndrome—a new complication ascribed to the "pill." Am. J. Obstet. Gynecol. 1970;107:1265–67.

Salvarani C, Cantini F, Macchioni P, Olivieri I, Niccoli L, Padula A, Boiardi L. Distal musculoskeletal manifestations in polymyalgia rheumatica: a prospective follow-up study. Arthritis Rheum. 1998;41:1221–26.

Salvarani C, Hunder GG. Musculoskeletal manifestations in a population-based cohort of patients with giant cell arteritis. Arthritis Rheum. 1999;42:1259–66.

Scarpalezos S, Lygidakis C, Papageorgiou C, Maliara S, Koukoulommati AS, Koutras DA. Neural and muscular manifestations of hypothyroidism. Arch. Neurol. 1973;29:140–44.

Schumacher Jr., HR, Dorwart BB, Korzeniowski OM. Occurrence of de Quervain's tendinitis during pregnancy. Arch. Intern. Med. 1985;145:2083–84.

Schwartz MS, Mackworth-Young CG, McKeran RO. The tarsal tunnel syndrome in hypothyroidism. J. Neurol. Neurosurg. Psychiatry 1983;46:440–42.

Selwa JF, Feldman EL, Blaivas M. Mononeuropathy multiplex in tryptophan-associated eosinophilia-myalgia syndrome. Neurology 1990;40:1632–33.

Seror P. Pregnancy-related carpal tunnel syndrome. J. Hand Surg. 1998;23B:98–101.

Seror P, Albert C, Saraby G. Severe carpal tunnel syndrome during pregnancy. Presse Med. 1993;22:687.

Shulman LE. The eosinophilia-myalgia syndrome associated with ingestion of L-tryptophan. Arthritis Rheum. 1990;33: 913–17.

Sidiq M, Kirsner AB, Sheon RP. Carpal tunnel syndrome. First manifestation of systemic lupus erythematosus. JAMA. 1972;222:1416–17.

Simon JN, Mokriski BK, Malinow AM, Martz DG Jr. Reflex sympathetic dystrophy syndrome in pregnancy. Anesthesiology 1988;69:100–102.

Sivri A, Guler-Uysal F. The electroneurophysiological findings in rheumatoid arthritis patients. Electromyogr. Clin. Neurophysiol. 1999;39:387–91.

Smukler NM, Patterson JR, Lorenz H, Weiner L. The incidence of the carpal tunnel syndrome in patients with rheumatoid arthritis. Arthritis Rheum. 1963;6:298–99.

Snell NJ, Coysh HL, Snell BJ. Carpal tunnel syndrome presenting in the puerperium. Practitioner 1980;224:191–93.

Spiegel PG, Ginsberg M, Skosey JL, Kwong P. Acute carpal tunnel syndrome secondary to pseudogout: case report. Clin. Orthop. 1976;00:185–87.

Stahl S, Blumenfeld Z, Yarnitsky D. Carpal tunnel syndrome in pregnancy: indications for early surgery. J. Neurol. Sci. 1996;136:182–84.

Stephens CJ, Ross JS, Charles-Holmes R, McKee PH, Black MM. An unusual case of transient papular mucinosis associated with carpal tunnel syndrome. Br. J. Dermatol. 1993; 129:89–91.

Stolp-Smith KA, Pascoe MK, Ogburn PL Jr. Carpal tunnel syndrome in pregnancy: frequency, severity, and prognosis. Arch. Phys. Med. Rehabil. 1998;79:1285–87.

Sukenik S, Abarbanel JM, Buskila D, Potashnik G, Horowitz J. Impotence, carpal tunnel syndrome and peripheral neuropathy as presenting symptoms in progressive systemic sclerosis. J. Rheumatol. 1987;14:641–43.

Takayama S. An experimental study on compression neuropathy—the vulnerability of the peripheral nerve associated with pregnancy. Nippon Seikkeigeka Gakkai Zasshi 1990; 64:485–99.

Tobin SM. Carpal tunnel syndrome in pregnancy. Am. J. Obstet. Gynecol. 1967;97:493–98.

Tsai CY, Yu CL, Tsai ST. Bilateral carpal tunnel syndrome secondary to tophaceous compression of the median nerves. Scand. J. Rheumatol. 1996;25:107–8.

Van Loon K. Safety of high doses of recombinant human growth hormone. Horm. Res. 1998;49(suppl 2):78–81.

Veltman G, Lange C-E, Jühe S, Stein G, Bachner U. Clinical manifestations and course of vinyl chloride disease. Ann. N. Y. Acad. Sci. 1975;246:6–17.

Vemireddi NK, Redford JB, PombeJara CN. Serial nerve conduction studies in carpal tunnel syndrome secondary to rheumatoid arthritis: preliminary study. Arch. Phys. Med. Rehabil. 1979;60:393–96.

Verma AK, Mahapatra AK. Pre and postoperative median nerve conduction in patients with pituitary tumour. J. Indian Med. Assoc. 1994 Jul;92(7):225–28.

Vessey MP, Villard-MacIntosh L, Yeates D. Epidemiology of carpal tunnel syndrome in women of childbearing age: findings in a large cohort study. Int. J. Epidemiol. 1990; 19:655.

Vincent FM, Van Houzen RN. Trigeminal sensory neuropathy and bilateral carpal tunnel syndrome: the initial manifestation of mixed connective tissue disease. J. Neurol. Neurosurg. Psychiatry 1980;43:458–60.

Wand JS. The natural history of carpal tunnel syndrome in lactation. J. R. Soc. Med. 1989;82:349–50.

Wand JS. Carpal tunnel syndrome in pregnancy and lactation. J. Hand Surg. 1990;15B:93–95.

Weinstein JD, Dick HM, Grantham SA. Pseudogout, hyperparathyroidism, and carpal-tunnel syndrome. A case report. J. Bone Joint Surg. 1968;50:1669–74.

Weinzweig J, Fletcher JW, Linburg RM. Flexor tendinitis and median nerve compression caused by gout in a patient with rheumatoid arthritis. Plast. Reconstr. Surg. 2000;106: 1570–72.

Wells RM, Johnson EW. Study of conduction delay in median nerve of patients with rheumatoid arthritis. Arch. Phys. Med. Rehabil. 1962;43:244–48.

Wilbourn AJ. Diabetic entrapment and compression neuropathies. In PJ Dyck, PK Thomas (eds), Diabetic Neuropathy (2nd ed). Philadelphia: Saunders, 1999;480–508.

Winkelmann RK, Connolly SM, Doyle JA. Carpal tunnel syndrome in cutaneous connective tissue disease: generalized morphea, lichen sclerosus, fasciitis, discoid lupus erythematosus, and lupus panniculitis. J. Am. Acad. Dermatol. 1982;7:94–99.

Winkelmann RK, Stevens JC. Successful treatment response of granuloma annulare and carpal tunnel syndrome to chlorambucil. Mayo Clin. Proc. 1994;69:1163–65.

Winn FJ Jr, Habes DJ. Carpal tunnel area as a risk factor for carpal tunnel syndrome. Muscle Nerve 1990;13:254–58.

Woltman HW. Neuritis associated with acromegaly. Arch. Neurol. Psychiat. (Chicago) 1941;45:680–82.

Wood KA, Jacoby RJ. Lithium induced hypothyroidism presenting with carpal tunnel syndrome. Br. J. Psychiatry. 1986;149:386–87.

Yagnik PM. Carpal tunnel syndrome in nursing mothers. South. Med. J. 1987;80:1468.

Yamaguchi D, Lipscomb P, Soule E. Carpal tunnel syndrome. Minn. Med. 1965;48:22–31.

Chapter 6

Carpal Tunnel Syndrome with Other Medical Conditions: Part II

Amyloidosis

The amyloids are a group of proteins that have specific staining properties and birefringence when viewed with polarized light after staining with Congo red. Amyloid deposition in the tissues of the carpal tunnel is an uncommon cause of carpal tunnel syndrome. Amyloidosis is not evident by gross inspection of canal contents at surgery; its reported incidence increases if the surgeon and pathologist search explicitly for it. Many surgeons do not submit tissue from carpal surgery for histologic evaluation. In one report of 345 carpal tunnel releases, only 87 pathologic specimens were available for review (Bastian, 1974). Two of the 87 stained positive for amyloid. In the Mayo Clinic series of 2,784 patients operated on for carpal tunnel syndrome, 1,500 specimens were reviewed for amyloid deposits (Kyle, Eilers, Linscheid & Gaffey, 1989). Fifty-seven of these specimens were initially reported positive for amyloid, but re-examination of the specimens with Congo red staining and careful searching for amyloid yielded 95 additional cases of carpal tunnel amyloidosis. The 10% prevalence of carpal tunnel amyloid in these patients has been matched in other series (Mohr, 1976; Breda, Richter & Schachenmayr, 1993; Nakamichi & Tachibana, 1996a). In a group of patients who had an even higher prevalence (19%) of amyloid found at the time of carpal tunnel surgery, some amyloid deposits were limited to minute specks of questionable import to the pathogenesis of the carpal tunnel syndrome (Stein, Storkel, Linke & Goebel, 1987).

Carpal tunnel amyloidosis can be subdivided: immunoglobulin light chain amyloidosis including primary systemic amyloidosis, secondary amyloidosis, localized carpal tunnel amyloidosis, familial amyloidosis, and beta-2 microglobulin amyloidosis associated with hemodialysis and renal failure. In the Mayo Clinic series, which did not include hemodialysis cases, the distribution is shown in Figure 6-1. Regardless of the type or cause of amyloid in the carpal tunnel, carpal tunnel surgery is usually successful in relieving the symptoms of carpal tunnel syndrome.

Primary Systemic Amyloidosis

Amyloid can form from immunoglobulin light chains. When this occurs in patients who do not have an underlying malignancy or lymphoproliferative disorder, the diagnosis is primary systemic amyloidosis, also known as *light chain amyloidosis*. Carpal tunnel syndrome is a prominent or initial manifestation of primary systemic amyloidosis in one-fourth of the cases (Kyle & Greipp, 1983). Systemic manifestations may result from infiltration of other organs, especially heart, kidney, tongue, and gastrointestinal tract. If serum and urine of these patients are screened with immunoprotein electrophoresis, nearly 90% have abnormalities, most commonly a monoclonal para-protein (Kelly, Kyle, O'Brien & Dyck, 1979).

Patients who present with a peripheral neuropathy and serum evidence of a monoclonal gammopathy introduce a differential diagnosis that includes primary systemic amyloidosis, multiple myeloma,

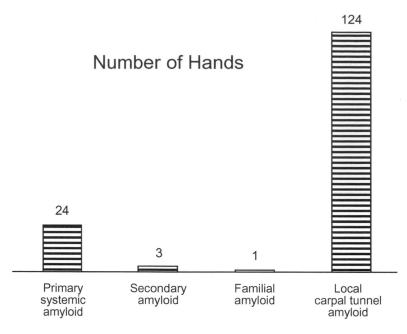

Figure 6-1. Types of amyloid found at the time of carpal tunnel surgery on careful review of 1,500 biopsies. None of the patients with amyloid were on hemodialysis. (Data from RA Kyle, SG Eilers, RL Linscheid, TA Gaffey. Amyloid localized to tenosynovium at carpal tunnel release. Natural history of 124 cases. Am. J. Clin. Pathol. 1989;91:393–97.)

osteoclastic myeloma, Waldenström's macroglobulinemia, non-Hodgkin's lymphoma, or "monoclonal gammopathy of undetermined significance" (Kelly, 1983). In these patients, nerve conduction evidence of focal slowing across the carpal tunnel should prompt a search for primary systemic amyloidosis or multiple myeloma with amyloidosis (Kelly et al., 1979; Kelly, Kyle, Miles, O'Brien & Dyck, 1981). In a series of 19 patients with peripheral neuropathy and monoclonal gammopathy of undetermined significance, only one had evidence of carpal tunnel syndrome (Krol-v-Straaten, Ackerstaff & De-Maat, 1985).

Secondary amyloidosis can accompany chronic inflammatory or infectious diseases. In secondary amyloidosis, the amyloid is usually not deposited in the carpal tunnel (Benson, Cohen, Brandt & Cathcart, 1975). When carpal tunnel syndrome accompanies secondary amyloidosis, the underlying disease, such as rheumatoid arthritis or leprosy, is more likely than amyloidosis to be the cause of the median neuropathy.

Foci of amyloid deposition can be located by scintigraphy with iodine 123–labeled serum amyloid P protein. In a small series of patients, scanning showed amyloid in the carpal region in primary, but not in secondary, amyloidosis patients (Hawkins, Lavender & Pepys, 1990).

Local Carpal Tunnel Amyloid Deposits

Many patients who present with carpal tunnel syndrome and local deposition of amyloid in the carpal tunnel have no evidence of systemic disease or of amyloid elsewhere in their bodies. One hundred twenty-four such patients were followed in the Mayo Clinic series (Kyle et al., 1989). Only four of these patients had systemic manifestations of amyloidosis at follow-up. In these four patients the systemic amyloidosis became apparent 4 to 15 years after the carpal tunnel syndrome was first symptomatic and 4 to 10 years after the amyloid was demonstrated in the carpal tunnel. Nine of the patients had serum evidence of monoclonal gammopathy but did not develop known systemic amyloidosis or multiple myeloma.

Hereditary Neuropathic Amyloidosis

There are a number of different inherited, autosomal dominant amyloid syndromes, some of which, especially those due to mutations in the gene for transthyretin, affect the peripheral nervous system (Hund, Linke, Willig & Grau, 2001). Numerous point mutations in the transthyretin gene are described (Saraiva, 2001). The most common mutation causes substitution of methionine for valine at amino acid position 30, which is one of the mutations that usually present as familial amyloid polyneuropathy I (*Portuguese-Swedish-Japanese type*), a progressive distal symmetric sensorimotor and autonomic neuropathy beginning in the legs in young adults. Familial amyloid polyneuropathy I has a progressive course that can lead to death within 10 to 15 years of onset of symptoms but can be treated with orthotopic liver transplantation. Carpal tunnel syndrome can develop as a later manifestation of familial amyloid polyneuropathy I.

Familial amyloid polyneuropathy II (*Indiana or Rukavina type*) is distinctive for its presentation with carpal tunnel syndrome as the initial symptom (Mahloudji, Teasdall, Adamkiewicz, Hartmann, Lambird & McKusick, 1969). Various transthyretin mutations can cause this presentation (Murakami, Tachibana, Endo, Kawai, Hara, Tanase & Ando, 1994; Saraiva, 1996; Munar-Ques, Saraiva, Ordeig-Calonge, Moreira, Perez-Vidal, Puig-Pujol, Monells-Abel & Badal-Alter, 2000). The carpal tunnel syndrome matches idiopathic carpal tunnel syndrome in its symptoms, distribution of age of onset, varied clinical manifestations, and findings on nerve conduction studies. Amyloid infiltration of the flexor retinaculum can be demonstrated at surgery or by biopsy elsewhere (Lambird & Hartmann, 1969). The illness can slowly progress to a more generalized peripheral neuropathy. Occasionally, cardiac infiltration becomes symptomatic late in the illness. The patients can have vitreous amyloid opacities. Abnormalities of the autonomic nervous system are absent or appear late. Typically, patients survive for many years after onset of symptoms. Inheritance is autosomal dominant. In the United States, large kindreds have been reported from Maryland and Indiana (Rukavina, Block, Jackson, Falls, Carey & Curtis, 1956).

Familial amyloid polyneuropathy type IV, also known as *Finnish type of familial amyloidosis*, is due to a mutation in the gene for a protein called *gesolin*. The prominent clinical manifestations are facial palsy and corneal lattice dystrophy. On nerve conduction studies a slight majority of patients with this condition have focal slowing of nerve conduction across the carpal tunnel, but fewer have clinical symptoms of carpal tunnel syndrome (Kiuru & Seppalainen, 1994).

Beta-2 Microglobulin Amyloid and Renal Disease

Renal dialysis patients, particularly hemodialysis patients, have an increased incidence of carpal tunnel syndrome. Symptoms often worsen after a dialysis session, then improve until the next session (Jain, Cestero & Baum, 1979). The carpal tunnel syndrome occasionally becomes symptomatic within months of institution of dialysis (Mancusi-Ungaro, Corres & Di-Spaltro, 1976). The typical pattern, however, is for carpal tunnel syndrome symptoms to appear after years of dialysis. In some series more than one-half of patients who have been on dialysis for 5 years develop carpal tunnel syndrome (Scardapane, Halter, DeLisa & Sherrard, 1979; Halter, DeLisa, Stolov, Scardapane & Sherrard, 1981).

Early papers noted that symptoms of carpal tunnel syndrome were more common in the arm that had a functioning arteriovenous access fistula (Kumar, Trivedi & Smith, 1975; Warren & Otieno, 1975). The shunt, in some patients, steals radial arterial blood flow from the hand (Gilbert, Robinson, Baez, Gupta, Glabman & Haimov, 1988). However, the carpal tunnel syndrome is often bilateral or may affect an arm that has never been used for a shunt (Jain et al., 1979; Halter et al., 1981; Bicknell, Lim, Raroque & Tzamaloukas, 1991).

Dialysis-associated amyloid is composed primarily of beta-2 microglobulin (Gejyo, Yamada, Odani, Nakagawa, Arakawa, Kunitomo, Kataoka, Suzuki, Hirasawa et al., 1985; Gorevic, Casey, Stone, DiRaimondo, Prelli & Frangione, 1985). The clinical manifestations of beta-2 microglobulin amyloidosis are now known to include carpal tunnel syndrome, juxta-articular radiolucent bone lesions, arthropathy with a predilection for large joints, and destructive spondyloarthropathy, especially in the neck (Bardin, Zingraff, Shirahama, Noel, Droz, Voisin, Drueke, Dryll, Skinner et al., 1987; Kleinman & Coburn, 1989; Sargent, Fleming, Chattopadhyay, Ackrill & Sambrook, 1989; Stone & Hakim, 1989; Ullian, Hammond, Alfrey, Schultz & Molitoris, 1989). Shoulder pain is a common feature (Chattopadhyay, Ackrill & Clague, 1987). Rarely, the spondyloarthropathy can cause clinical radiculomyelopathy (Deforges-Lasseur, Combe, Cernier, Vital & Aparicio, 1993; Sanchez, Praga, Rivas Salas, Araque, Mazuecos, Andres & Rodicio, 1993). Amyloid in flexor tendon synovium can cause trigger digits or other limitations of finger flexion (Le Viet & Gandon, 1992; Lanteri, Ptasznik, Constable & Dawborn, 1997).

Among patients with dialysis-associated carpal tunnel syndrome, biopsy done at the time of carpal tunnel surgery shows amyloid in the tenosynovium in about two-thirds of cases, including one-third of cases that also have amyloid in the transverse carpal ligament (Shiota, Yamaoka, Kawano, Tasaka, Nakamoto & Goya, 1998). Amyloid deposits can be found in joints, bone, tongue, peritoneal fat, or a variety of other organs (Campistol, Cases, Torras, Soler, Muñoz-Gomez, Montoliu, Lopez-Pedret & Revert, 1987; Fuchs, Jagirdar & Schwartz, 1987; Muñoz-Gomez, Gomez-Perez, Llopart-Buisan & Sole-Arques, 1987). However, a negative amyloid stain on a peritoneal fat aspiration does not exclude amyloid deposition in the carpal tunnel or elsewhere (Orfila, Goffinet, Goudable, Eche, Ton-That, Manuel & Suc, 1988).

Nerve conduction studies in hemodialysis patients with carpal tunnel syndrome often give bilateral evidence of median nerve conduction slowing across the carpal tunnel and show electrical evidence of a more diffuse neuropathy (Halter et al., 1981; Hirasawa & Ogura, 2000). The nerve conduction results of 46 patients on chronic dialysis are summarized in Figure 6-2 (Bicknell et al., 1991). Abnormal median nerve conduction and carpal tunnel syndrome were found in both hemodialysis and peritoneal dialysis patients. All patients who had been on dialysis for 7 or more years had abnormal median nerve conduction across the carpal tunnel.

Imaging evidence of beta-2 microglobulin amyloid includes cystic lesions in any of the hand and wrist bones, most commonly in the lunate or middle phalanx (Ueno, Beppu, Shimizu & Komurai, 1999). The lesions can be detected by plain radiography, computed tomography, magnetic resonance imaging (MRI), or ultrasound. Patients on chronic hemodialysis also commonly have radiographic evidence of bone resorption. These abnormalities become more prevalent the longer the patient has been on dialysis and are common in patients with dialysis-associated carpal tunnel syndrome. Beta-2 microglobulin amyloid deposition in the carpal tunnel can also cause changes visible by ultrasound or MRI, including thickening of the palmar radiocarpal ligament, which forms the dorsal border of the canal, widening or deepening of the carpal tunnel, or fluid collections or echogenic masses in the carpal tunnel (Ikegaya, Hishida, Sawada, Furuhashi, Maruyama, Kumagai, Kobayashi & Yamamoto, 1995; Lanteri et al., 1997).

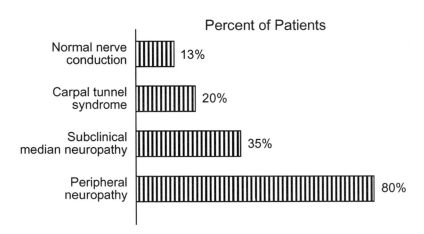

Figure 6-2. Nerve conduction results of 46 patients on chronic dialysis. Peripheral neuropathy and subclinical median neuropathy were diagnosed on the basis of nerve conduction studies. Carpal tunnel syndrome was diagnosed on the basis of typical symptoms and signs and was always accompanied by abnormal median nerve conduction. (Data from JM Bicknell, AC Lim, HG Raroque, AH Tzamaloukas. Carpal tunnel syndrome, subclinical median mononeuropathy, and peripheral polyneuropathy: common early chronic complications of chronic peritoneal dialysis and hemodialysis. Arch. Phys. Med. Rehabil. 1991;72:378–81.)

Hemodialysis patients with carpal tunnel syndrome usually report symptomatic relief from carpal tunnel surgery (Teitz, DeLisa & Halter, 1985; Shiota et al., 1998). Some surgeons routinely perform tenosynovectomy at the time of carpal tunnel surgery because of the high prevalence of amyloid-induced tendonopathy (Le Viet & Gandon, 1992).

Beta-2 microglobulin amyloid is most common with hemodialysis using cuprophan membranes but also occurs with other dialysis techniques including continuous ambulatory peritoneal dialysis (Vandenbroucke, Jadoul, Maldague, Huaux, Noel & van-Ypersele-de-Strihou, 1986; Gagnon, Lough & Bourgouin, 1988). Varied approaches to improving dialysis clearance of beta-2 microglobulin include use of an adsorbent column that removes the beta-2 microglobulin, hemodiafiltration, and use of dialysis membranes that are more permeable to amyloid (Gejyo, Homma, Hasegawa & Arakawa, 1993; Lornoy, Becaus, Billiouw, Sierens, Van Malderen, & D'Haenens, 2000; Schiffl, Fischer, Lang & Mangel, 2000). Case reports suggest that carpal tunnel syndrome symptoms and transcarpal median nerve conduction can improve after switching to dialysis techniques that remove beta-2 microglobulin (Gejyo, Teramura, Ei, Arakawa, Nakazawa, Azuma, Suzuki, Furuyoshi, Nankou & Takata, 1995; Shiota & Fujinaga, 2000). The carpal tunnel syndrome in patients on hemodialysis usually, but not invariably, improves after renal transplantation (Nelson, Sharpstone & Kingswood, 1993).

Even with a careful search, amyloid is not found in all hemodialysis patients with carpal tunnel syndrome (Cornelis, Bardin, Faller, Verger, Allouache, Raymond, Rottembourg, Tourliere et al., 1989). In individual cases, contributory mechanisms of median nerve compression include local edema, deposition of other substances such as iron in synovial tissue, co-existent peripheral neuropathy, vascular effects of the dialysis shunt, or other co-existing disease (Cary, Sethi, Brown, Erhardt, Woodrow & Gower, 1986).

Disorders of Peripheral Nerve

Generalized Peripheral Neuropathy

Common clinical lore is that patients with peripheral neuropathies are susceptible to carpal tunnel syndrome and other forms of local nerve entrapment (Potts, Shahani & Young, 1980). This susceptibility varies depending on the pathophysiology of the neuropathy. For example, diabetic peripheral neuropathy, as discussed previously, has a clear association with carpal tunnel syndrome, but for peripheral neuropathy of other causes, the association is less well documented. The problem of interpreting nerve conduction data in patients with peripheral neuropathy and suspected carpal tunnel syndrome is discussed in Chapter 8.

Patients with demyelinating neuropathies seem particularly susceptible to developing abnormalities at sites of focal nerve compression. Symptoms of carpal tunnel syndrome are usually not a clinical feature of Guillain-Barré syndrome; nonetheless, in some patients with Guillain-Barré syndrome, there is preferential slowing of nerve conduction at common sites of nerve compression (Lambert & Mulder, 1964). This preferential slowing is most evident on sensory nerve conduction studies. Albers and colleagues (1985) found that in 42% of their patients with Guillain-Barré syndrome, median sensory conduction was abnormal, but sural nerve conduction was normal.

Diphtheritic neuropathy provides an experimental model of an acute demyelinating neuropathy. Guinea pigs with experimentally induced diphtheritic neuropathy are more vulnerable than guinea pigs without neuropathy to developing focal conduction delay in the plantar nerve (Hopkins & Morgan-Hughes, 1969). This local pressure effect is prevented if the guinea pigs are not allowed to put pressure on their hind legs.

Hereditary neuropathy with liability to pressure palsies is another example of a neuropathy that affects myelin and predisposes to development of acute or chronic pathology from focal nerve compression. The condition is autosomal dominant, due to a chromosome 17p11.2 deletion. Patients with this condition develop recurrent mononeuropathies at common nerve compression sites, including at the carpal tunnel (Earl, Fullerton, Wakefield & Schutta, 1964; Roos & Thygesen, 1972; Cruz Martinez, Perez Conde, Ramón y Cajal & Martinez, 1977; Debruyne, Dehaene & Martin, 1980). For example, Cruz Martinez and colleagues (1977) found six cases of clinical median neuropathy among 25 patients with this syndrome. The median neuropathy may be accompanied by radial or ulnar neuropathies. The mononeuropathies can develop suddenly following relatively minor trauma or without obvious cause. Symptoms usually begin before age 20 years, and childhood onset of carpal tunnel syndrome is a known but uncommon presentation of hereditary neuropathy with liability to pressure palsies (Cruz Martinez & Arpa, 1998). Patients with the syndrome usually have evidence on nerve conduction studies of diffuse peripheral neuropathy or of additional mononeuropathies that are not clinically evident (Andersson, Yuen, Parko & So, 2000). Only 2 of the 25 patients reported by Cruz Martinez and colleagues and none of the 28 studied by Gouider and colleagues had completely normal median nerve conduction studies. Additional evidence that these patients have a generalized underlying diathesis of peripheral nerve is that they often eventually develop a more symmetric diffuse peripheral neuropathy, and that their sural nerve biopsies often show structural abnormalities, even if no symptoms of neuropathy are present in the biopsied limb (Figure 6-3) (Behse, Buchthal, Carlsen & Knappeis, 1972).

Patients with hereditary sensory motor neuropathy (Charcot-Marie-Tooth disease) commonly develop hand and arm symptoms a few years after developing leg symptoms. Rarely, investigation of an adult, whose only neuropathic symptoms are those of carpal tunnel syndrome, shows diffuse severe slowing of motor nerve conduction due to a hereditary motor and sensory neuropathy (Isaacs, 1972). A small surgical series, with incomplete electrodiagnostic detail, suggests that when patients with hereditary sensory neuropathy have hand pain, the pain may be relieved by carpal tunnel surgery if provocative tests and nerve conduction studies favor median nerve compression at the wrist (Brown, Zamboni, Zook & Russell, 1992). Of course, the generalized neuropathy, including hand intrinsic muscle weakness and atrophy, continues to worsen despite the nerve decompression, and hand function can sometimes improve after tendon transfers or other surgical hand reconstruction.

Despite the high prevalence of alcoholic peripheral neuropathy, there is little literature on carpal tunnel syndrome in alcoholics. Is this because diabetics are studied more closely than alcoholics for variations in their peripheral neuropathy? Or is the predominantly axonal neuropathy of alcoholics less vulnerable than diabetic neuropathy to focal nerve compression? Alcoholic peripheral neuropathy regularly involves the feet before it affects the hands, and when it affects the hands, the sensory loss follows a "glove" distribution rather than a median cutaneous pattern (Victor, 1984). Patients with alcoholic neuropathy are more likely to show abnormal nerve conduction in sural or peroneal nerves than in the median nerve (Behse & Buchthal, 1977).

Casey and Le Quesne (1972b) studied median sensory nerve conduction in 16 alcoholics. They compared digital conduction from the tip to the base of the middle finger with more proximal conduction from the tip of the finger to the wrist. The characteristic abnormality in these alcoholic subjects was loss of amplitude of the digital nerve action potential. None of the alcoholics had slowed sensory conduction across the carpal tunnel; in contrast, sensory conduction velocity across the carpal tunnel was reduced in patients with carpal tunnel syndrome and in some patients with diabetic neuropathy (Casey & Le Quesne, 1972a).

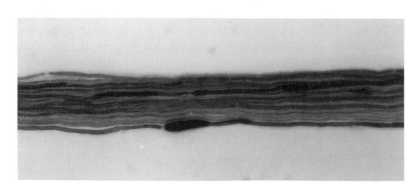

Figure 6-3. Nerve pathology in hereditary liability to pressure palsies. This microdissected bundle of nerve fibers shows several myelin tomaculae ("sausages").

A survey of patients with advanced liver disease found electrodiagnostic or quantitative sensory testing evidence of distal sensorimotor neuropathy in 71% (Chaudhry, Corse, O'Brian, Cornblath, Klein & Thuluvath, 1999). The incidence of neuropathy was high even if alcohol was not the cause of the liver disease. Among the liver disease patients, one-third had focal transcarpal slowing of median nerve conduction.

Double Crush Syndrome

Upton and McComas (1973) offered the hypothesis that many patients with carpal tunnel syndrome presented atypical features because nerve fibers were being compressed both at the carpal tunnel and more proximally, often at the level of the cervical nerve roots. They proposed that constriction of axonal flow at a proximal site along the axon made the median nerve unusually sensitive to compression in the carpal canal. This hypothesis is intuitively appealing; and the catch phrase, "double crush," has often been used in discussions of occurrence of radiculopathies, brachial plexopathies, and proximal median neuropathies in patients with carpal tunnel syndrome. However, the double crush hypothesis has been cogently criticized (Wilbourn & Gilliatt, 1997). In regard to the role of double crush in the combination of carpal tunnel syndrome and cervical radiculopathy, neither theoretical analysis nor empiric data support the hypothesis (Morgan & Wilbourn, 1998; Richardson, Forman & Riley, 1999).

Upton and McComas estimated that over three-fourths of their patients with carpal tunnel syndrome had evidence of cervical pathology. In some of their patients, there was dermatomal sensory loss beyond the territory of the median nerve, or there was electromyographic evidence of denervation in a myotomal pattern in arm muscles not supplied by the median nerve; however, in many instances, their evidence of cervical radiculopathy was as unreliable as radiologic demonstration of cervical spondylosis, complaints of neck pain or stiffness, or remote history of "whiplash" injury. The significance of these coincidences is in doubt because Upton and McComas offered no control data on the incidence of these common neck abnormalities in the general population. Other authors have presented similarly problematic observations linking carpal tunnel syndrome to cervical radiculopathy (Crymble, 1968; Yu, Bendler & Mentari, 1979; Massey, Riley & Pleet, 1981; Frith & Litchy, 1985; Hurst, Weissberg & Carroll, 1985; Cassvan, Rosenberg & Rivera, 1986; Osterman, 1988; Golovchinsky, 2000). In contrast, in a large series in which carpal tunnel syndrome and cervical radiculopathy were carefully defined, only about 5% of patients with carpal tunnel syndrome had an ipsilateral cervical radiculopathy, and in less than 1% of the cases, the level of the radiculopathy corresponded to the origin of the nerve fibers injured in the carpal tunnel (Morgan & Wilbourn, 1998).

The anatomy and physiology of the brachial plexus and median nerve are inconsistent with a double crush effect as an explanation of cases of coincident carpal tunnel syndrome and cervical radiculopathy. As the median nerve arises from nerve roots C6, C7, C8, and T1, abnormality of one or two of these roots cannot explain combined motor and sensory dysfunction of the median nerve. In milder cases of carpal tunnel syndrome with only sensory manifestations, the distribution of sensory findings at times overlaps those of C6 or C7 radiculopathy. However, in patients with cervical radiculopathy sensory roots are compressed proximal to the dorsal root ganglions, a site of compression that does not affect nerve conduction or function in the sensory axons distal to the dorsal root ganglians that run in the median nerve.

Observations in patients support this theoretical analysis. An analysis of a possible role of radiculopathy in causing carpal tunnel syndrome must compare sensory and motor aspects of carpal tunnel syndrome with specific nerve roots involved. When this is done carefully, there is no electrophysiologic support for the double crush hypothesis as an explanation for carpal tunnel syndrome and cervical radiculopathy occurring in the same patient (Richardson et al., 1999).

Occasional cases suggest that cases of carpal tunnel syndrome can occur co-incident with more proximal median compression or with brachial plexus compression (Zamora, Rose, Rosario & Noon, 1986). These random observations of coincident pathology neither prove nor disprove the double crush hypothesis.

In summary, a small percentage of patients with carpal tunnel syndrome have another neuropathic condition contributing to arm symptoms. In these patients thorough neurologic examination and careful electrodiagnostic studies usually yield the correct diagnoses. The concept of double crush syndrome rarely needs to be invoked to explain the clinical profile of these patients.

Infectious Diseases

Rubella Arthritis

Carpal tunnel syndrome sometimes complicates the polyarthritis that is an occasional sequel of rubella infection or of live rubella immunization (Blennow, Bekassy, Eriksson & Rosendahl, 1982; Tingle, Chantler, Pot, Paty & Ford, 1985). Adults are more commonly affected than children (Lefebvre, de-Seze, Lerique, Hamonet, Chaumont, Bigot & Dreyfus, 1969). The syndrome is usually self-limited or improves with anti-inflammatory medication (Hale & Ruderman, 1973). In one postrubella case that came to carpal tunnel surgery, synovial pathology showed infiltration with polymorphonuclear leukocytes (Ellis, 1973).

Out of 23,000 children immunized, nine developed symptoms suggestive of carpal tunnel syndrome (Kilroy, Schaffner, Fleet, Lefkowitz, Karzon & Fenichel, 1970). In another series, the incidence of postimmunization arthralgia was 3%. When a sample of the arthralgic population was questioned closely, over three-fourths of those with arthralgias had symptoms, other than joint pains, that might reflect carpal tunnel syndrome (Thompson, Ferreyra & Brackett, 1971). Symptoms appear 10 days to 2 months after immunization and resolve in 1 month or less. Median nerve conduction studies are usually normal or show transient mild abnormalities.

Lyme Borreliosis

Of 76 patients with symptoms of Lyme disease of greater than 4 weeks' duration and of sufficient severity to require referral to a Lyme disease clinic, over one-fourth had symptoms of carpal tunnel syndrome (Halperin, Volkman, Luft & Dattwyler, 1989). Carpal tunnel syndrome also occurs in patients with chronic manifestations of Lyme disease, such as acrodermatitis chronica atrophica (Kindstrand, 1992).

Only two of the 76 patients studied by Halperin and colleagues had clinical evidence of active wrist tenosynovitis. Median nerve conduction studies were abnormal in nearly three-fourths of the patients with carpal tunnel symptoms. In addition, 3 of 68 patients studied had asymptomatic median nerve conduction abnormalities. The patients often had clinical improvement in carpal tunnel symptoms, and sometimes had median nerve conduction improvement, following antibiotic treatment of the Lyme disease. Patients with carpal tunnel syndrome sometimes have other peripheral nervous system manifestations of Lyme disease. In areas of Sweden where Lyme disease is endemic, most patients with carpal tunnel syndrome do not have positive Lyme serology, and the diagnosis of carpal tunnel syndrome is not an indication for serologic screening for Lyme disease (Kindstrand, 1992).

Granulomatous Infections of the Hand

Carpal tunnel syndrome can complicate varied granulomatous infections in the carpal canal; Table 6-1 gives examples.

These patients often present with insidious onset of carpal tunnel syndrome symptoms, and the syndrome typically evolves gradually over months or years. Local wrist swelling and other signs of focal inflammation are sometimes present (Klofkorn & Steigerwald, 1976; Bush & Schneider, 1984). Histoplasmosis can infect the carpal tunnel with or without radiographic evidence of infection of the carpal bones (Perlman, Jubelirer & Schwarz, 1972; Care & Lacey, 1998). In patients with sporotrichosis, the classic cutaneous nodules on the hand or in a lymphangitic pattern on the arm are not always present (Hagemann, 1968).

Some cases have been treated with local steroid injections before coming to carpal tunnel surgery; however, the effect of the steroids on the natural history of the infection is unknown (Langa, Posner, Hoffman & Steiner, 1986). In a patient with bilateral tuberculous infection of the carpal canal, one side had previously been treated with steroid injec-

Table 6-1. Granulomatous Infection of the Carpal Tunnel

Organism	References
Histoplasma capsulatum	Omer, Lockwood & Travis, 1963; Vanek & Schwarz, 1971; Perlman, Jubelirer & Schwarz, 1972; Strayer, Gutwein, Herbold & Bresalier, 1981; Randall, Smith, Korbitz & Owen, 1982; Mascola & Rickland, 1991; Eglseder, 1992; Care & Lacey, 1998
Leishmania infantum	Chagnon, Carli, Paris, Cameli & Carloz, 1993
Mycobacterium avium-intracellulare	Kelly, Karlson, Weed & Lipscomb, 1967; Cheatum, Hudman & Jones, 1976; Kozin & Bishop, 1994; Regnard, Barry & Isselin, 1996
Mycobacterium bovis Bacille Calmette-Guérin	Janier, Gheorghiu, Cohen, Mazas & Duroux, 1982
Mycobacterium chelonei	Zachary, Clark, Kleinert & O'Donovan, 1988
Mycobacterium fortuitum	Randall, Smith, Korbitz & Owen, 1982
Mycobacterium kansasii	Kelly, Karlson, Weed & Lipscomb, 1967; Kaplan & Clayton, 1969; Gunther & Elliot, 1976; Dorff, Frerichs, Zabransky, Jacobs & Spankus, 1978; Wada, Nomura & Ihara, 2000
Mycobacterium malmoense	Prince, Ispahani & Baker, 1988
Mycobacterium marinum	Williams & Riordan, 1973; Chow, Ip, Lau, Collins, Luk, So & Pun, 1987
Mycobacterium szulgai	Horusitzky, Puechal, Dumont, Begue, Robineau & Boissier, 2000; Stratton, Phelps & Reller, 1978; Merlet, Aberrane, Chilot & Laroche, 2000
Mycobacterium terrae	Deenstra, 1988; Kozin & Bishop, 1994
Mycobacterium tuberculosis	Klofkorn & Steigerwald, 1976; Bush & Schneider, 1984; Gouet, Castets, Touchard, Payen & Alcalay, 1984; Lee, 1985; Langa, Posner, Hoffman & Steiner, 1986; Suso, Peidro & Ramón, 1988; Regnard, Barry & Isselin, 1996; Andersson & Willcox, 1999
Sporothrix schenckii	Hagemann, 1968; Stratton, Lichtenstein, Lowenstein, Phelps & Reller, 1981

tion without evidence that this retarded or promoted the course of the infection (Gouet, Castets, Touchard, Payen & Alcalay, 1984).

Carpal tunnel syndrome is sometimes the first evidence of a systemic granulomatous infection. The classical gross surgical finding of granulomatous infection is "rice bodies" (Stratton, Phelps & Reller, 1978). These are fibrinous masses, shaped like rice grains, 2 to 20 mm long, visible in the carpal canal. They can also develop in noninfectious inflammatory diseases. At times the granulomatous tenosynovitis is not recognized until a second or third exploration of the carpal tunnel is undertaken, after the initial surgery has given no more than transient relief of symptoms (Kelly, Karlson, Weed & Lipscomb, 1967; Langa et al., 1986).

Treatment requires antibiotics for the offending organism, release of the transverse carpal ligament, and debridement of the granulomatous tissue within the carpal tunnel. Even with treatment, an infection can remain asymptomatic for many years, and then cause recurrent carpal tunnel syndrome in the same wrist (Care & Lacey, 1998).

Leprosy

Leprosy is the one granulomatous infection that specifically affects nerves. Patients often have cutaneous sensory neuropathies from disease of intradermal nerve branches (Callaway, Fite & Riordan, 1965). In addition, patients with leprosy can develop a progressive median neuropathy, or more commonly ulnar neuropathy (Baccaredda-Boy, Mastropaoli, Pastorino, Sacco & Farris, 1963; Callaway, Fite & Riordan, 1965; Brown, Kovindha, Wathanadilokkol, Piefer, Smith & Kraft, 1996). Initially, intermittent symptoms can mimic those of carpal tunnel syndrome. Later in the disease, motor and sensory loss becomes irreversible. Brand (1956) examined over 2,000 affected hands and found the following patterns:

Isolated ulnar neuropathy	46%
Median and ulnar neuropathy	52%
Median, ulnar, and radial neuropathy	1.5%
Isolated median neuropathy	0.5%

Table 6-2. Anomalous Carpal Canal Contents in 2,705 Patients with Carpal Tunnel Syndrome

Canal Abnormailty	Number of Cases
Ganglion	12
Tumor	3
Anomalous muscle belly	7
Thrombosed median artery	2

The median nerve infection is usually in the forearm (Antia, Pandya & Dastur, 1970). Leprosy limitcd to the carpal tunnel is quite unusual. When it occurs, the median neuropathy can be due both to compression and to nerve infection (Koss, Reardon & Groves, 1993). The median nerve at the wrist is sometimes visibly or palpably swollen (Husain, Mishra, Prakash & Malaviya, 1997). At carpal tunnel surgery, the median nerve can be thickened, edematous, and show necrosis, giant cells, and occasionally acid fast organisms on biopsy (Callaway et al., 1965; Selby, 1974). In patients with leprous median neuropathy at the wrist, division of the flexor retinaculum, epineurotomy, and combined steroid and antileprous drug therapy can lead to neurologic improvement in some patients and at least cessation of disease progression in most (Bernardin & Thomas, 1997; Husain et al., 1997; Sugumaran, 1997).

Miscellaneous Infections

Carpal tunnel syndrome occasionally accompanies toxic shock syndrome (Sahs, Helms & DuBois, 1983). In some patients with the toxic shock syndrome, the carpal tunnel syndrome develops acutely secondary to hand swelling.

A case report details carpal tunnel syndrome in a 47-year-old woman whose symptoms started 3 weeks after receiving the swine flu/Victoria A influenza vaccine (Hasselbacher, 1977).

References to cases of acute median nerve compression by gonococcal, parvovirus B19, granulomatous, or pyogenic infections of the wrist are discussed later in this chapter (see Acute Carpal Tunnel Syndrome).

Anomalous Canal Contents or Masses

Anomalous contents of the canal are rare in patients with carpal tunnel syndrome. Examples include ganglians, ectopic or accessory muscles, bony anomalies, a persistent median artery, or a variety of tumors. Table 6-2 lists the anomalous canal contents reported in the combined series of 2,705 patients. Anomalies are often present for years before the patient develops symptoms of carpal tunnel syndrome; in some patients, symptoms of carpal tunnel syndrome develop after a change in the anomaly, such as thrombosis of a persistent median artery or hypertrophy of an ectopic muscle.

On occasion physical examination findings such as a palpable palmar mass or swelling, triggering of a flexor tendon, or clicking with wrist movement are clues to these structures (Neviaser, 1974; Aghasi, Rzetelny & Axer, 1980; Asai, Wong, Matsunaga & Akahoshi, 1986; Desai, Pearlman & Patel, 1986). The palmar mass might be present for years before development of symptoms of carpal tunnel syndrome (Hayes, 1974).

Carpal tunnel radiographs at times reveal a deformity or unexpected calcification (Sutro, 1969; Louis & Dick, 1973; Pritsch, Engel & Horowitz, 1980; Firooznia, Golimbu & Rafii, 1981; Edwards, Sill & Macfarlane, 1984; Weiber & Linell, 1987). Soft tissue anomalies or tumors may be detected preoperatively by computed tomography, MRI scanning, or ultrasonography (Mesgarzadeh, Schneck, Bonakdarpour, Mitra & Conaway, 1989; Feyerabend, Schmitt, Lanz & Warmuth-Metz, 1990; Reicher & Kellerhouse, 1990; Nakamichi & Tachibana, 1993a, 1993b; Zeiss & Jakab, 1995; Pierre-Jerome, Bekkelund, Husby, Mellgren, Osteaux & Nordstrom, 1996). These anomalies are rare, and awareness of their existence preoperatively is rarely important for patient management. Some surgeons routinely take radiographs of the wrist before carpal tunnel surgery; but radiographs infrequently (0.4% of the time in one series) show findings of therapeutic significance (Bindra, Evanoff, Chough, Cole, Chow & Gelberman, 1997). Extensive preoperative imaging to study canal contents is seldom needed.

The most common presentation of an anomaly is as an unexpected finding at the time of carpal tunnel syndrome surgery. Phalen (1966) qualified his estimation of the incidence of anomalies, stating that he might have overlooked some because of his operative approach through a transverse incision without careful exploration of the contents of the canal.

Table 6-3. Anomalous Muscles in Carpal Tunnel Syndrome

Anomalous Muscle	References
Palmaris longus	Backhouse & Churchill-Davidson, 1975; Brones & Wilgis, 1978; Crandall & Hamel, 1979; Meyer & Pflaum, 1987; Schlafly & Lister, 1987; Bang, Kojima & Tsuchida, 1988; Sgouros & Ali, 1992
Ectopic lumbrical	Touborg-Jensen, 1970; Butler & Bigley, 1971; Eriksen, 1973; Schultz, Endler & Huddleston, 1973; Jabaley, 1978; Nather & Pho, 1981; Asai, Wong, Matsunaga & Akahoshi, 1986; Desai, Pearlman & Patel, 1986; Robinson, Aghasi & Halperin, 1989
Flexor digitorum profundus	Winkelman, 1983
Flexor digitorum superficialis	Smith, 1971; Hayes, 1974; Neviaser, 1974; Probst & Hunter, 1975; Aghasi, Rzetelny & Axer, 1980; Hutton, Kernohan & Birch, 1981; Gleason & Abraham, 1982; Ametewee, Harris & Samuel, 1985; Elias & Schuler-Ellis, 1985; Schon, Kraus, Boller & Kampe, 1992; Kraus, Schon, Boller & Nabavi, 1993
Abductor digiti quinti	Jackson & Harkins, 1972
Palmaris profundus	Walton & Cutler, 1971; Dyreby & Engber, 1982; Carstam, 1984; Fatah, 1984; Floyd, Burger & Sciaroni, 1990; Bauer & Trusell, 1992

Congenital Muscular Anomalies

Table 6-3 lists anomalous muscles that can compress the median nerve in the carpal tunnel or distal forearm. These case reports of anomalies derive from findings in patients operated on for carpal tunnel syndrome. However, partial movement of lumbricals or finger flexor muscles into the canal can be a physiologic event. A cadaver study of arms dissected with the wrists and fingers in the neutral position found some intrusion of the flexor digitorum sublimis muscle belly into the carpal tunnel in 46% of women and 8% of men (Holtzhausen, Constant & de Jager, 1998). The muscles are even more likely to intrude into the canal during wrist extension (Keir & Bach, 2000). In many individuals, the lumbricals routinely move into the carpal tunnel during finger flexion (Cobb, An, Cooney & Berger, 1994; Ham, Kolkman, Heeres, den Boer & Vierhout, 1996). These incursions might contribute to increases of pressure within the canal, and perhaps individuals with greater muscular incursion or with hypertrophic muscles are more likely to develop carpal tunnel syndrome (Cobb, An & Cooney, 1995; Siegel, Kuzma & Eakins, 1995).

The presence of an anomalous muscle within the carpal tunnel does not prove that the anomaly is pathogenic. Occasionally, children with anomalous muscles have symptoms of carpal tunnel syndrome, but most patients with anomalous muscles do not develop carpal tunnel syndrome until adulthood. At times anomalous muscles become symptomatic following or in association with other pathology within the canal; an example is accessory lumbricals discovered in conjunction with a fibroma or with a degenerative synovial cyst (Butler & Bigley, 1971; Nather & Pho, 1981; Asai et al., 1986; Desai et al., 1986). The anomalous muscle within the canal might not cause nerve compression until it hypertrophies with use (Jabaley, 1978). The anomaly can be present unilaterally in patients with bilateral carpal tunnel syndrome (Gleason & Abraham, 1982). In many instances, the muscle anomaly is an incidental finding at surgery and seems no more important in the pathogenesis of the nerve compression than any of the standard contents of the canal.

The palmaris profundus originates deep in the forearm, becomes superficial above the wrist, and passes through the carpal canal to insert in the deep palmar fascia. It was found only once in 1,600 hand dissections (Reimann, Daseler, Anson & Beaton, 1944). The muscle sometimes is attached to the median nerve with connective tissue (Walton & Cutler, 1971; Floyd, Burger & Sciaroni, 1990). It can be an incidental finding at carpal tunnel surgery; it has been noted in patients presenting with carpal tunnel syndrome at ages 62, 72, and 85 years (Carstam, 1984; Fatah, 1984).

The palmaris longus typically originates in the forearm. Its tendon usually passes volar to the flexor retinaculum to insert on the palmar fascia or thenar muscles. The muscle is subject to numerous variations (Reimann et al., 1944). The tendon of palmaris longus has been found under the flexor retinaculum or between the ligament and the median nerve in cases of carpal tunnel syndrome (Brones & Wilgis, 1978; Mobbs & Chandran, 2000).

In another variant, the body of the palmaris longus compresses the median nerve just proximal to the carpal canal (Backhouse & Churchill-Davidson, 1975; Dorin & Mann, 1984; Meyer & Pflaum, 1987; Schlafly & Lister, 1987; Dent & Hadden, 1992; Sgouros & Ali, 1992; Giunta, Brunner & Wilhelm, 1993; Depuydt, Schuurman & Kon, 1998). This is sometimes termed a *reversed palmaris longus* because the usual sequence of proximal muscle belly and distal tendon is inverted. In patients with a reversed palmaris longus muscle, the muscle belly is sometimes visible as a bluish subcutaneous mass in the distal forearm. The paresthetic symptoms are characteristically induced by effort rather than occurring at rest. The anomaly can be visualized by MRI (Schuurman & van Gils, 2000). Resection of the anomalous muscle without division of the flexor retinaculum can relieve the paresthetic symptoms.

Arterial Abnormalities

A persistent median artery accompanies the median nerve in the carpal canal in 1% to 16% of arms (Coleman & Anson, 1961; Pecket, Gloobe & Nathan, 1973). It is more common in neonatal than in adult hands (Kopuz, Gulman & Baris, 1995). The median nerve at times is bifid with branches on either side of the artery. The anomalous artery can be unilateral or bilateral. At times the pulse of the median artery is palpable in the proximal palm.

The pathogenic import of a patent median artery is not always clear. Individuals can have palpable median arteries without evidence of carpal tunnel syndrome or bilateral carpal tunnel syndrome with a unilateral median artery (Chalmers, 1978; Barfred, Hjlund & Bertheussen, 1985). Chalmers found a persistent median artery in 6% of his patients with carpal tunnel syndrome, and Barfred and colleagues found a persistent median artery in 2% of their patients, not clearly more than would be found in an asymptomatic population. However, both Chalmers and Barfred and colleagues argue that carpal tunnel syndrome patients with persistent median arteries are more likely than other carpal tunnel syndrome patients to have symptoms occurring during hand use and less likely to experience nocturnal hand paresthesias. There was a lower mean age and a higher percentage of male subjects among the patients with patent median arteries.

Barfred and colleagues recommend median artery resection at the time of carpal tunnel surgery if normal digital blood supply can be proven while the median artery is clamped. In contrast, Chalmers recommends flexor retinaculum release without resection of the artery.

The median artery can thrombose, spontaneously or posttraumatically, causing subacute presentation of symptoms of carpal tunnel syndrome, sudden onset of hand pain and paresthesias, or sudden deterioration of chronic carpal tunnel syndrome (Jackson & Campbell, 1970; Maxwell, Kepes & Ketchum, 1973; Levy & Pauker, 1978). The median artery can have an aneurysmal dilation and present as a mass proximal to the carpal tunnel, causing chronic symptoms of median nerve compression (Wright & MacFarlane, 1994). Treatment includes carpal tunnel exploration and resection of the thrombosed artery.

A patient on hemodialysis developed carpal tunnel syndrome secondary to an enlarged median artery with ectopic calcification (Dickinson & Kleinert, 1991). A patient had an arteriovenous malformation in the palm that caused chronic symptoms of carpal tunnel syndrome (Chopra, Khanna & Murthy, 1979). On physical examination, the hand was warm and swollen. Symptoms were relieved after release of the flexor retinaculum. A 12-year-old boy had swelling of the palm and forearm and mild symptoms of carpal tunnel syndrome due to an arteriovenous malformation of the median artery (Gutowski, Olivier, Mehrara & Friedman, 2000). Other rare anomalies found in patients who had carpal tunnel syndrome had been aneurysms of the superficial palmar arch or of the ulnar artery in the hand (Fricker & Troeger, 1994; Iossifidis, As'ad & Sutaria, 1995).

Median Nerve Anomalies

Brachial hypertrophy is a rare condition characterized by progressive unilateral limb hypertrophy with onset in childhood (Figure 6-4). When patients with brachial hypertrophy develop carpal tunnel syndrome, the nerve may be thickened with

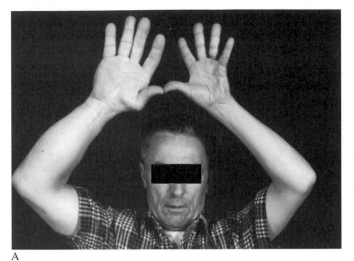

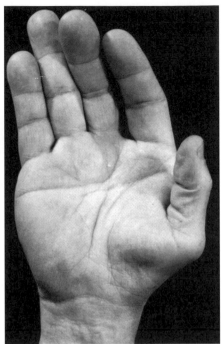

Figure 6-4. (A) Right brachial hemihypertrophy. This patient had severe carpal tunnel syndrome in the hypertrophic right upper limb. Note striking thenar wasting, highlighted in **B**.

B

proliferation of perineural collagen (Shenoy, Saha & Ravindran, 1980). Carpal tunnel syndrome is an infrequent complication of the angio-osteohypertrophy syndrome (Klippel-Trenaunay-Weber syndrome), which is characterized by congenital large vascular nevus, limb hypertrophy, and varied other anomalies (Owens, Garcia, Pierce & Castrow, 1973; Poilvache, Carlier, Rombouts, Partoune & Lejeune, 1989; McGrory & Amadio, 1993; Swinn & Hargreaves, 1996). The association of carpal tunnel syndrome with macrodactyly is discussed in Chapter 19.

A bifid median nerve is a rare variation that is usually not associated with nerve pathology (Lanz, 1977). However, Schweitzer and Miller (1973) described a bifid median nerve with unexplained thickening of epineurium and perineurium in a patient with carpal tunnel syndrome. In another patient with bilateral carpal tunnel syndrome and bilateral bifid median nerves, the radial portion of the nerve ran in an accessory ligamentous tunnel within the carpal tunnel, so that release of compression of this branch required additional dissection after division of the flexor retinaculum (Szabo & Pettey, 1994). In other patients with carpal tunnel syndrome and a bifid median nerve, the anoma-lous nerve division is not necessarily the cause of the carpal tunnel syndrome (Baruch & Hass, 1977; Moneim, 1982; Amadio, 1987; Artico, Cervoni, Stevanato, D'Andrea & Nucci, 1995).

Space-Occupying Lesions

Masses of varied histology are discovered, in rare instances, at the time of carpal tunnel surgery. The most common are ganglions (Trevaskis, Tilly, Marcks & Heffernan, 1967; Hvid-Hansen, 1970; Harvey & Bosanquet, 1981; McMinn, 1985; Lewis, Jr., Nordyke & Foreman, 1986; Kerrigan, Bertoni & Jaeger, 1988). Table 6-4 lists other hand tumors and masses that have been found in the carpal canal. A lipoma can develop in the deep palmar space, distal to the carpal tunnel, and cause median nerve compression (Oster, Blair & Steyers, 1989).

Other Unusual Canal Contents

The ulnar nerve has been found beside the median nerve in the carpal canal (Eskesen, Rosenrn &

Table 6-4. Tumors and Masses in the Carpal Tunnel

Tumor or Mass	References
Calcified mass	Sutro, 1969; Tegner, Leven & Lysholm, 1983; Nakamichi, Tachibana & Tamai, 1994; Takada, Fujioka & Mizuno, 2000
Carpal osteophyte	Engel, Zinneman, Tsur & Farin, 1978
Cavernous hemangioma	Johnson, Kilgore & Newmeyer, 1985
Chondroma, osteo-chondroma	Tompkins, 1967; Gahhos & Cuono, 1984; Nather & Chong, 1986
Degenerative or detritus cyst	Pritsch, Engel & Horowitz, 1980
Distended ulnar bursa	Linscheid, 1979
Epithelioid sarcoma	Patel, Desai & Gordon, 1986
Lipoma	Paarlberg, Linscheid & Soule, 1972; DeLuca & Cowen, 1975; Brand & Gelberman, 1988; Kremchek & Kremchek, 1988; Oster, Blair & Steyers, 1989; Babins & Lubahn, 1994; De Smet, Bande & Fabry, 1994
Median nerve tumors	See Chapter 19
Mesodermal tumor	Ernst & Konermann, 1982
Osteoid osteoma	Herndon, Eaton & Littler, 1974
Pigmented villonodular synovitis	Chidgey, Szabo & Wiese, 1988
Squamous cell carcinoma	Dandy & Munro, 1973; Mackay & Barua, 1990
Synovial nodule	Nakamichi & Tachibana, 1996b
Synovial sarcoma	Weiss & Steichen, 1992
Tendon fibrous histiocytoma	Iqbal, 1982
Tendon fibroma	Brown & Coulson, 1974; Chung & Enzinger, 1979; Sarma, Weilbaecher & Rodriguez, 1986; Evangelisti & Reale, 1992

Osgaard, 1981; Galzio, Magliani, Lucantoni & D'Arrigo, 1987). Both nerves may be compressed so that the patient presents with evidence of both median and ulnar neuropathy at the wrist.

Iatrogenic objects that may be found in the canal and compress the median nerve include a tendon graft prosthesis, a piece of Kirschner's wire, or a prosthetic carpal bone (DeLuca & Cowen, 1975; Lichtman, Alexander, Mack & Gunther, 1982; Bjornsson, Gestsson, Ekelund & Haffajee, 1984; Jou & Lai, 1998). In one patient the broken tip of an acupuncture needle was found imbedded in the median nerve at the time of surgery (Southworth & Hartwig, 1990).

Obesity

Obesity is a definite risk factor for development of carpal tunnel syndrome. Obesity is conveniently assessed by calculating body mass index (BMI), which is the body weight (in kilograms) divided by the square of the body height (in meters). The BMI is called the *Quetelet index* in some papers (De Krom, Kester, Knipschild & Spaans, 1990). Typical operational definitions are as follows: slender, BMI <20 kg/m^2; overweight, BMI >25 kg/m^2; and obese, BMI >29 kg/m^2. The relation between BMI and development of carpal tunnel syndrome has been demonstrated in various settings and using various definitions of carpal tunnel syndrome (De Krom et al., 1990; Vessey, Villard-MacIntosh & Yeates, 1990; Nathan, Keniston, Myers & Meadows, 1992; Radecki, 1996; Stallings, Kasdan, Soergel & Corwin, 1997; Werner, Franzblau, Albers & Armstrong, 1997; Lam & Thurston, 1998; Kouyoumdjian, Morita, Rocha, Miranda & Gouveia, 2000). For example, in a population-based case-control study in which carpal tunnel syndrome was diagnosed clinically, there was in linear relationship between BMI and risk of developing carpal tunnel syndrome; each additional 1 kg/m^2 was associated with an additional 8% risk (Nordstrom, Vierkant, DeStefano & Layde, 1997). Among patients referred to an electrodiagnostic laboratory to evaluate right arm symptoms, the risk of having carpal tunnel syndrome was 2.5 times higher among obese patients than among slender patients (Werner et al., 1994). The mean BMI of patients with bilateral carpal tunnel syndrome is higher than the mean BMI of patients with unilateral carpal tunnel syndrome (Sungpet, Suphachatwong & Kawinwonggowit, 1999). BMI only accounts for part of the risk of developing carpal tunnel syndrome; for example, among the patients in one study, 20% of slender or normal individuals had carpal tunnel syndrome, whereas 65% of obese individuals did not (Werner et al., 1994). Speculation on the mechanism for the association between BMI and carpal tunnel syndrome has considered distribution of adipose tissue and body fluid and variations in hand use affecting carpal canal pressure, but the pathophysiology of this association is unknown.

A study comparing women undergoing reduction mammoplasty to women with smaller breasts suggested that large breast size is a risk factor for development of carpal tunnel syndrome beyond any effect of BMI (Pernia, Ronel, Leeper & Miller, 2000). Women with breasts in the upper quartile of size had a relative risk for development of carpal tunnel syndrome of 8.43 compared with women with breast sizes in the lower two quartiles.

Other Personal Factors

Other personal factors have been mentioned in a few studies as risk factors for development of carpal tunnel syndrome (Table 6-5). The evidence on these risk factors is often contradictory. For example, other studies have not confirmed cigarette smoking as a risk factor for development of carpal tunnel syndrome (Dieck & Kelsey, 1985; Ferry, Hannaford, Warskyj, Lewis & Croft, 2000). If these factors truly contribute to the risk of developing carpal tunnel syndrome, their contribution is relatively small, and the pathophysiology of any effect is unknown.

Hand Edema

Hand swelling of diverse causes can trigger carpal tunnel syndrome. Reported cases are as varied as congestive heart failure, hand edema after large volume intravenous fluid administration during liposuction, hand swelling after an insect sting, vibration-induced angioedema, or postmastectomy lymphedema (Lazaro, 1972; Arnold, 1977; Ganel, Engel, Sela & Brooks, 1979; Wener, Metzger & Simon, 1983; Mandawat, 1985; Barker, Bloch, Vakili & Waller, 1986; Lombardi, Quirke & Rauscher, 1998; Seror, Alliot, Cluzan & Pascot, 1999; Soldado-Carrera, Vilar-Coromina & Rodriguez-Baeza, 2000). Of course, in patients who

Table 6-5. Reported Possible Minor Risk Factors for Development of Carpal Tunnel Syndrome

Factor	References
Cigarette smoking	Vessey, Villard-MacIntosh & Yeates, 1990; Tanaka, Wild, Seligman, Halperin, Behrens & Putz-Anderson, 1995; Nathan, Keniston, Lockwood & Meadows, 1996
Coffee consumption	Nathan, Keniston, Lockwood & Meadows, 1996
Alcohol abuse	Nathan, Keniston, Lockwood & Meadows, 1996
Lack of avocational exercise	Nathan, Keniston, Myers & Meadows, 1992

have hand edema and neurologic symptoms after mastectomy for breast cancer, neoplastic, or radiation-induced brachial plexopathies are often important considerations in the differential diagnosis (Seror et al., 1999).

Wrist Deformities

Patients who develop dystonic wrist flexion deformities after traumatic brain injury or other central nervous system insult can develop carpal tunnel syndrome, apparently as a result of median nerve compression due to chronic wrist flexion (Orcutt, Kramer, Howard, Keenan, Stone, Waters & Gellman, 1990).

Acute Carpal Tunnel Syndrome

Carpal tunnel syndrome can develop suddenly in rare circumstances. Recognition and treatment of these instances is important because emergent nerve decompression is sometimes needed to prevent permanent nerve injury. Trauma is the most common cause of acute median neuropathy at any point along the nerve. A major management issue is whether the median neuropathy is due to direct nerve injury or due to increased pressure within the carpal tunnel (i.e., acute carpal tunnel syndrome). With open injuries, acute nerve laceration or contusion is sometimes evident. With closed injuries, onset of symptoms of median neuropathy at the time of injury can be due to direct nerve injury or acute nerve compression; onset of neuropathic symptoms hours after the injury favors evolving compression rather than direct nerve injury.

Colles' fracture of the distal radius is the prototypic injury. While most patients do not develop median neuropathy after Colles' fracture, some do report mild paresthesias in the median cutaneous distribution that resolve spontaneously as focal swelling recedes. The reported incidence of median neuropathy after distal radius fracture ranges from less than 1% in some series to over 20% in others (Schlesinger & Liss, 1959; Cooney, Dobyns & Linscheid, 1980; Knirk & Jupiter, 1986; Stark, 1987). Development of carpal tunnel syndrome after wrist fracture is unusual in children (Krum-Moller, Jensen & Hansen, 1999). The risk of median nerve compression increases with volar displacement of a fragment of the distal radius (Paley & McMurtry, 1987). Sometimes median nerve function improves after readjusting the patient's splint to neutral rather than wrist-flexed or wrist-extended posture, because neutral splinting minimizes pressure within the carpal tunnel (Gelberman, Szabo & Mortensen, 1984). Even with neutral splinting, some patients have mild symptoms of median neuropathy but do not have objective neurologic deficit; these patients can be observed, but some eventually need carpal tunnel surgery (Sponsel & Palm, 1965). In those patients who have objective median nerve deficits, measuring carpal tunnel pressures with a wick catheter can be helpful in distinguishing between median nerve contusion and ongoing median nerve compression (Mack, McPherson & Lutz, 1994); patients who have canal pressures over 40 mm Hg usually need urgent carpal tunnel surgery. Patients who have total absence of median nerve function also need exploration, regardless of canal pressure, to exclude a rare complication of Colles' fracture, transection of the median nerve (Lusthaus, Matan, Finsterbush, Chaimsky, Mosheiff & Ashur, 1993). Patients who have some preserved median nerve function and lower canal pressures presumably have median nerve contusions, and can be observed without surgery if the canal pressure measurement is reliable and if clinical and imaging studies have excluded direct bony laceration of the median nerve or nerve compression by hematoma or bone displacement in the forearm (Lewis, 1978; Goldie & Powell, 1991).

Acute carpal tunnel syndrome can also complicate other wrist and hand fractures, such as fractures of the scaphoid, capitate, or metacarpals, or with carpal-metacarpal fracture dislocations (McClain & Wissinger, 1976; Weiland, Lister & Villarreal-Rios, 1976; Olerud & Lonnquist, 1984; Allen, Gibbon & Evans, 1994). Acute carpal tunnel syndrome or median nerve contusion (see Figure 12-4) can also follow blunt palm trauma without fracture (Ametewee, 1983).

When hand trauma is severe, for example, after wringer or roller hand-crushing injuries, acute median nerve compression is common, and many surgeons prophylactically section the flexor retinaculum (Primiano & Reef, 1974; Askins, Finley, Parenti, Bush & Brotman, 1986). In the most severe cases a forearm fasciotomy is required to prevent development of a forearm compartment syndrome.

Carpal tunnel syndrome can develop after hand or forearm surgery. For example, a case developed following placement of a compression plate for nonunion of an ulnar fracture, and another occurred after tendon graft prosthesis placement (DeLuca & Cowen, 1975; Bauman, Gelberman, Mubarak & Garfin, 1981).

Foreign bodies that penetrate the wrist can cause acute median nerve injury either directly or by increasing pressure in the carpal tunnel. Examples include thorns; a broken tip of an acupuncture needle; Kirschner's wires placed to fix carpal fractures; or glass, wood, or metal fragments (El-Adwar, 1972; Sterling, Eshraghi, Anderson & Habermann, 1972; Goldberg & Levy, 1977; Browett & Fiddian, 1985; Southworth & Hartwig, 1990; Faithfull & Petchell, 1995; Jou & Lai, 1998). Whether due to carpal tunnel syndrome or to direct nerve penetration, the median neuropathy might first become symptomatic many years, even decades, after the initial, apparently mild, penetrating injury.

Hemorrhage in the carpal canal can cause acute nerve compression. Potential causes of hemorrhage include anticoagulation, acute or chronic leukemia, hemorrhagic diathesis such as hemophilia or von Willebrand's disease, or minor trauma in a patient with pigmented villonodular synovitis of the flexor synovium; rarely, hemorrhage is unexplained (Hartwell & Kurtay, 1966; Case, 1967; Kohn, Bush & Kessler, 1976; McClain & Wissinger, 1976;

Khunadorn, Schlagenhauff, Tourbaf & Papademetriou, 1977; Howie & Buxton, 1984; Moneim & Gribble, 1984; Kilpatrick, Leyden, Sullivan, Lawler & Grossman, 1985; Nkele, 1986; Chidgey, Szabo & Wiese, 1988; Copeland, Wells & Puckett, 1989; Bonatz & Seabol, 1993; Dumontier, Sautet, Man, Bennani & Apoil, 1994; Bindiger, Zelnik, Kuschner & Gellman, 1995; Black, Flowers & Saleh, 1997; Chaudhuri & Madhok, 1998; Parthenis, Karagkevrekis & Waldram, 1998). The acutely compressed nerve often requires surgical decompression, but successful decompression can occasionally be achieved by imaging-guided aspiration of the hematoma (Chaudhuri & Madhok, 1998).

Table 6-6 lists some other uncommon causes of acute carpal tunnel syndrome. Often the patient gives a history of chronic mild acroparesthesias preceding a sudden symptomatic crescendo (Weiber & Linell, 1987). Sometimes investigation of a patient with acute carpal tunnel syndrome reveals a long-standing carpal anomaly or mass, but the cause of the sudden deterioration is not evident (Ametewee, Harris & Samuel, 1985).

Delayed Effects of Trauma

Chronic carpal tunnel syndrome may persist as a residual symptom after Colles' fracture and other wrist or hand injuries (Cooney, Dobyns & Linscheid, 1980; Chapman, Bennett, Bryan & Tullos, 1982). Paget's (1865) original cases of distal median

Table 6-6. Unusual Causes of Acute Carpal Tunnel Syndrome

Cause	References
Acute calcification in the carpal tunnel	Boström & Svartengren, 1993; Knight & Gibson, 1993; Verfaillie, De Smet, Leemans, Van Damme & Fabry, 1996; el Maghraoui, Lecoules, Lechevalier, Magnin & Eulry, 2001
Diving decompression illness	Isakov, Broome & Dutka, 1996
Hand burns	Adamson, Srouji, Horton & Mladick, 1971
Gonococcal tenosynovitis	Balcomb, 1982; Barrick, 1983; DeHertogh, Ritland & Green, 1988
Gout	Morgan, 1985; Ogilvie & Kay, 1988; Pai & Tseng, 1993
Insect sting	Lazaro, 1972; Barker, Bloch, Vakili & Waller, 1986
Intense wrist use	Jones & Scheker, 1988
Leprosy	Gaur, Kulshreshtha & Swarup, 1994
Liposuction using tumescent fluid administration	Lombardi, Quirke & Rauscher, 1998
Median artery thrombosis	Jackson & Campbell, 1970; Maxwell, Kepes & Ketchum, 1973; Levy & Pauker, 1978; de-Graad & Rodseth, 1989
Partially ruptured flexor digitorum profundus tendons secondary to chronic palmar subluxation of the distal ulna	Seiler, Havig & Carpenter, 1996
Parvovirus B19 infection	Samii, Cassinotti, de Freudenreich, Gallopin, Le Fort & Stalder, 1996
Pregnancy	Adamson, Srouji, Horton & Mladick, 1971
Prolonged wrist flexion	Belsole & Greeley, 1988
Pseudogout	Spiegel, Ginsberg, Skosey & Kwong, 1976; Lewis & Fiddian, 1982; Goodwin & Arbel, 1985; Chiu, Wong, Choi & Chow, 1992; Rate, Parkinson, Meadows & Freemont, 1992
Pyogenic hand infection	Bailey & Carter, 1955; Oates, 1960; Gerardi, Mack & Lutz, 1989; Flynn, Bischoff & Gelberman, 1995
Pyogenic forearm infection	Williams Jr. & Geer, 1963
Radial artery cannulation	Martin, Sharrock, Mineo, Sobel & Weiland, 1993
Ruptured palmaris longus tendon	Lourie, Levin, Toby & Urbaniak, 1990
Snake bite	Schweitzer & Lewis, 1981
Tight handcuffs (usually accompanied by superficial radial neuropathy)	Dorfman & Jayaram, 1978; Levin & Felsenthal, 1984; Stone & Laureno, 1991

nerve compression were post-traumatic. The incidence of chronic carpal tunnel syndrome was 31% in one group of patients followed after Colles' fractures (Mundt, Kallwellis & Roder, 1986). In some patients the symptoms resolve slowly in the months after the fracture: In a group of patients with displaced fractures, 17% had symptoms of median neuropathy 3 months after injury, but only 12% had symptoms 6 months after injury (Stewart, Innes & Burke, 1985). In patients who have persistent carpal tunnel syndrome after Colles' fracture, sagittal MRI of the wrist and distal forearm can clarify the pathologic anatomy of compression, showing changes such as angular deviations of the distal radial epiphysis, volar dislocation of the structures in the canal in relation to the distal radial epiphysis, or variations in the course of the median nerve in relation to the flexor tendons (Soccetti, Carloni, Giovagnoni & Misericordia, 1993).

Carpal tunnel syndrome is reported as a delayed effect of arm crush injuries, hook of the hamate fractures, or post-traumatic ulna-minus (Manske, 1978; Murray, Meuller, Rosenthal & Jauernek, 1979; Askins et al., 1986; Nathan & Meadows, 1987). When an episode of heavy lifting causes wrist trauma and synovial edema, carpal tunnel syndrome is a potential delayed complication (Elliott & Elliott, 1979).

The median nerve can be compressed in or just proximal to the carpal tunnel by dislocations or subluxations of the carpal bones, such as the scaphoid or lunate (Monsivais & Scully, 1992; Chen, 1995; Cooney, Linscheid & Dobyns, 1996; Cara, Narvaez, de la Varga & Guerado, 1998; Garcia-Elias, 1999). Patients can present years after an initial wrist injury with findings of carpal tunnel syndrome combined with wrist deformity or impaired wrist motion. Carpal tunnel syndrome can occur as a postoperative complication of wrist arthrodesis (Hastings II, Weiss, Quenzer, Wiedeman, Hanington & Strickland, 1996).

Hand burns, even if superficial, predispose to delayed appearance of carpal tunnel syndrome (Fissette, Onkelinx & Fandi, 1981). Electrical burns of the hand, in particular, can cause distal median nerve injury (DiVincenti, Moncrief & Pruitt Jr., 1969; Solem, Fischer & Strate, 1977; Rosenberg, 1989). The mechanism of injury can include tenosynovial edema, nerve compression in the forearm by damaged tissue such as necrotic muscle, or direct electrical injury to the nerve.

Carpal tunnel syndrome complicates some distal hand tendon injuries (Browne & Snyder, 1975). The injuries need not be severe enough to disrupt the tendons. In an extreme case, a 23-year-old man had resection in the distal palm of an injured flexor digitorum superficialis tendon. Four weeks later he developed median distribution hypesthesia. Surgical exploration of the carpal tunnel revealed that the proximal portion of the divided tendon and adherent scar tissue were compressing the median nerve (Sturim & Edmond, 1980). A similar sequence of events can follow digital avulsion injuries (Milroy, Aldred & Vickers, 1984).

The tendon of flexor digitorum profundus can rupture without evident trauma. Hypertrophic synovial reaction can develop around the ruptured tendon in the carpal tunnel and contribute to median nerve compression (Jackson, 1990).

Symptoms of median neuropathy are a potential late effect of partial median nerve laceration in the forearm. Surgical exploration might reveal a neuroma in continuity in the forearm with the nerve distal to the neuroma swollen and compressed as it enters the carpal tunnel. Symptoms can resolve after section of the flexor retinaculum, while the neuroma is left undisturbed (McGrath & Polayes, 1979; Martinelli, Poppi, Gaist, Padovani & Pozzati, 1985).

Distal median neuropathy can occur after motor vehicle accidents (Guyon & Honet, 1977). Typically, the driver is gripping the steering wheel tightly at the time of impact. Symptoms of median neuropathy develop immediately or within 2 weeks of the accident (Haas, Nord & Bome, 1981). Others arbitrarily accept an interval of up to 2 months between the accident and onset of symptoms as evidence that the accident caused the carpal tunnel syndrome (Ames, 1996). Among 21 patients with carpal tunnel syndrome resulting from steering wheel impact, Label (1991) found that 71% recovered within 5 months when treated with splinting; the remaining 29% underwent carpal tunnel surgery.

The relationship between chronic avocational or occupational hand use and development of carpal tunnel syndrome is discussed in Chapter 13.

Genetic Considerations

A survey of 421 patients who had carpal tunnel syndrome confirmed by abnormal median nerve conduction studies or by need for carpal tunnel surgery found that more than 27% of patients reported at least one family member with carpal tunnel syndrome (Radecki, 1994). The family history was considered positive if any relative (degree not specified) had previously been diagnosed as having carpal tunnel syndrome or had hand paresthesias. Mechanisms underlying familial aggregation of carpal tunnel syndrome are varied and include nongenetic factors, such as random coincidence of a common condition, increased attentiveness to hand symptoms among family members once one member is diagnosed with the condition, and familial tendency to pursue similar vocations. A small fraction of patients with familial carpal tunnel syndrome have currently recognized genetic predispositions to carpal tunnel syndrome. Undoubtedly, other mechanisms of genetic predisposition will be recognized in the future.

Familial Autosomal Dominant Carpal Tunnel Syndrome

Familial autosomal dominant carpal tunnel syndrome (McKusick number MIM 115430) is distinguished from sporadic carpal tunnel syndrome not only by family history but also by consistently bilateral involvement, relatively early age of onset, and equal involvement of men and women (Hess & Baumann, 1969; Danta, 1975; Mochizuki, Ohkubo & Motomura, 1981; Braddom, 1985; Serratrice, Roger, Guastalla & Saint-Jean, 1985; McDonnell, Makley & Horwitz, 1987; Golik, Modai, Pervin, Marcus & Fried, 1988). One reported family had both autosomal dominant carpal tunnel syndrome and autosomal dominant congenital myopathy with central cores and nemaline rods, but the two traits segregated independently (Casado, Arenas, Segura, Chinchón, Gonzalez & Bautista, 1995). Symptoms begin in childhood or adulthood; in some families, there appears to be genetic anticipation manifest by onset of the syndrome in childhood only in later generations (Vadasz, Chance, Epstein & Lou, 1997; Stoll & Maitrot, 1998). The flexor retinaculum is abnormally thickened in some patients (Michaud, Hays, Dudgeon & Kropp, 1990; Leifer, Cros, Halperin, Gallico 3rd & Pierce, 1992). In some families, subjects with carpal tunnel syndrome have an increased incidence of trigger finger or of susceptibility to mallet finger (Gray, Poppo & Gottlieb, 1979; Jones & Peterson, 1988). The condition is not due to hereditary liability to pressure palsies or hereditary sensory motor neuropathy abnormalities on chromosome 17 (Vadasz et al., 1997; Gossett & Chance, 1998). At least one attempt to find a genetic linkage has failed to do so (Braddom, 1985).

Autosomal dominant familial carpal tunnel syndrome sometimes becomes symptomatic in childhood, but onset in infancy is distinctly unusual. A 7-month-old boy who had mutilating hand syndrome, apparent congenital insensitivity to pain, and electrical evidence of carpal tunnel syndrome stopped hand mutilation after carpal tunnel surgery (Swoboda, Engle, Scheindlin, Anthony & Jones, 1998). His parents were consanguineous, and the parents, a paternal uncle and aunt, and both paternal grandparents had carpal tunnel syndrome. His physicians speculated that he might be homozygous for a dominant familial carpal tunnel syndrome gene.

Hereditary Neuropathy

In some families, entrapment neuropathies are evidence of more widespread familial disease (Fowler, Harrison & Snaith, 1986). On occasion, carpal tunnel syndrome is the first symptomatic manifestation of hereditary motor sensory neuropathy or of hereditary liability to pressure palsies, which are discussed previously with other peripheral neuropathies. Some types of familial amyloidosis, also discussed previously, can cause carpal tunnel syndrome, but in many familial aggregations of carpal tunnel syndrome, amyloid stains have been negative.

Mucopolysaccharidoses and Other Inherited Connective Tissue Disorders

Watson-Jones (1949) gave one of the earliest descriptions of carpal tunnel syndrome in an inherited connective tissue disorder, describing bilateral

Table 6-7. Carpal Tunnel Syndrome in Mucopoly-saccharidoses (MPSs) and Mucolipidoses (MLs)

Syndrome	References
Hurler (MPS-IH)	MacDougal, Weeks & Wray, 1977; Giuseffi, Wall, Siegel & Rojas, 1991; Gschwind & Tonkin, 1992
Scheie (MPS-IS)	McKusick, 1972; Fisher, Horner & Wood, 1974; Miner & Schimke, 1975; Vinals-Torras, Garcia, Barreiro-Tella, Diez-Tejedor, Cruz Martinez & Arpa-Gutierrez, 1985
Hunter (MPS-II)	Miner & Schimke, 1975; Bona, Vial, Brunet, Couturier, Girard-Madoux, Bady & Guibaud, 1994; Norman-Taylor, Fixsen & Sharrard, 1995
Maroteaux-Lamy (MPS-VI)	McKusick, 1972; Peterson, Bacchus, Seaich & Kelly, 1975
Pseudo-Hurler (ML-III)	Starreveld & Ashenhurst, 1975; Gellis, Feingold & Kelly, 1975; MacDougal, Weeks & Wray, 1977; Umehara, Matsumoto, Kuriyama, Sukegawa, Gasa & Osame, 1997; Haddad, Hill & Vellodi, 2000
I-cell disease (ML-II)	MacDougal, Weeks & Wray, 1977; Gschwind & Tonkin, 1992
Unknown metabolic defect	Karpati, Carpenter, Eisen & Feindel, 1973; Bundey, Ashenhurst & Dorst, 1974

Table 6-8. Carpal Tunnel Syndrome in Other Inherited Disorders

Disorder	References
Acrodysostosis	Steiner & Pagon, 1992
Adult polyglucosan body disease	Gil-Neciga, Pareja, Chincon, Jarrin & Chaparro, 1995
Lipoid proteinosis	Gordon, Gordon, Botha & Edelstein, 1971
Osteochondritis dissecans	Auld & Chesney, 1979
Progressive laryngotracheal stenosis with short stature and arthropathy	Hopkin, Cotton, Langer & Saal, 1998
Schwartz-Jampel syndrome	Cruz Martinez, Arpa, Perez-Conde & Ferrer, 1984
Weill-Marchesani syndrome	Dellon, Trojak & Rochman, 1984

carpal tunnel syndrome in a 20-year-old man with Léri pleonosteosis, an autosomal dominant condition manifested by short stature and a number of musculoskeletal changes including short spadelike hands, broad thumbs in valgus position, thickened palmar fascia, and limited joint mobility. Yeoman (1961) reported a similar case.

Mucopolysaccharidoses or mucolipidoses are the inherited connective tissue diseases that are most commonly complicated by carpal tunnel syndrome. These storage diseases present in childhood with coarse features, stiff joints, dwarfism, and other anomalies. Inheritance is usually recessive. Carpal tunnel syndrome develops after 2 years of age and is typically manifest by thenar atrophy, hand clumsiness, or decreased median-distribution sweating rather than by sensory symptoms (Wraith & Alani, 1990; Haddad, Jones, Vellodi, Kane & Pitt, 1997; Van Heest, House, Krivit & Walker, 1998). Patients sometimes have

trigger finger and other evidence of flexor tenosynovitis. At surgery the flexor retinaculum is often thickened, and the flexor tenosynovium can be white and exuberant. Despite the severity of the nerve compression, many patients improve following carpal tunnel surgery, but tendon release and postoperative hand therapy may be necessary (Pronicka, Tylki-Szymanska, Kwast, Chmielik, Maciejko & Cedro, 1988). Bone marrow transplant improves survival of some children with these conditions, but, in limited experience, does not appear to improve the carpal tunnel syndrome (Wraith & Alani, 1990; Haddad et al., 1997; Guffon, Souillet, Maire, Straczek & Guibaud, 1998).

Table 6-7 gives additional references linking carpal tunnel syndrome to these disorders, and Table 6-8 lists examples of carpal tunnel syndrome occurring in other inherited disorders. In patients with Sanfilippo syndrome (mucopolysaccharidosis III) or Morquio-Brailsford syndrome (mucopolysaccharidosis IV), carpal tunnel syndrome has been sought and not found (Haddad et al., 1997; Van Heest et al., 1998).

Carpal Tunnel Syndrome in Children

Carpal tunnel syndrome is rare in children. At the Boston Children's Hospital, less than 3% of children referred for electromyography had carpal

Table 6-9. Causes of Childhood Carpal Tunnel Syndrome

Cause	References
Aberrant lumbricals with cystic degeneration of the synovium	Asai, Wong, Matsunaga & Akahoshi, 1986
Angio-osteohypertrophy (Klippel-Trenaunay-Weber syndrome)	Poilvache, Carlier, Rombouts, Partoune & Lejeune, 1989
Anomalous flexor digitorum sublimis	al-Qattan, Thomson & Clarke, 1996
Bleeding diathesis (e.g., hemophilia)	Case, 1967; Khunadorn, Schlagenhauff, Tourbaf & Papademetriou, 1977
Brachial hypertrophy	Shenoy, Saha & Ravindran, 1980
Hypoplastic scaphoid	Radford & Matthewson, 1987
Lipoblastomatosis	Paarlberg, Linscheid & Soule, 1972
Lipofibromatous hamartoma of the median nerve	al-Qattan, Thomson & Clarke, 1996
Lipofibromatous hamartoma of the median nerve in child with Proteus syndrome	Choi, Wey & Borah, 1998
Median nerve tumors	See Chapter 19
Melorheostosis	Barfred & Ipsen, 1985; Bostman & Bakalim, 1985
Poland's syndrome (congenital pectoral muscular defect with hand anomalies)	Harpf, Schwabegger & Hussl, 1999
Rubella infection or immunization	Cooper, Ziring, Weiss, Matters & Krugman, 1969; Kilroy, Schaffner, Fleet, Lefkowitz, Karzon & Fenichel, 1970; Thompson, Ferreyra & Brackett, 1971; Blennow, Bckassy, Eriksson & Rosendahl, 1982

tunnel syndrome; less than 0.1% of patients studies at the Mayo Clinic for carpal tunnel syndrome were younger than 14 years (Stevens, Sun, Beard, O'Fallon & Kurland, 1988; Deymeer & Jones, 1994). In other series of patients who have carpal tunnel syndrome, 1% to 2% are younger than 20 years (Tropet, Brientini, Monnier & Vichard, 1990). For most cases of childhood carpal tunnel syndrome, an underlying cause can be found, but a few cases remain idiopathic (Lettin, 1965; Feingold, Hidvegi & Horwitz, 1980; Sainio, Merikanto & Larsen, 1987; Wilson & Buehler, 1994; Sanchez-Andrada, Martinez-Salcedo, de Mingo-Casado, Domingo-Jimenez & Puche-Mira, 1998). The more common causes, trauma, first, and mucopolysaccharidoses, a distant second, are discussed previously. In some teenagers symptoms are temporally related to increasing arm use in athletics (Loyau, 1987; Tropet et al., 1990). In a 5-year-old boy, symptoms improved after steroid injection in the wrist and after he stopped the habit of sleeping with his wrists flexed (Lagos, 1971). A 9-year-old boy developed carpal tunnel syndrome from a hypertrophic flexor retinaculum, 7 years after partial laceration of the ligament (Poilvache et al., 1989). Some children have a combination of carpal tunnel syndrome and trig-

ger finger (McArthur, Hayles, Gomez & Bianco, 1969; Maurer, Fenske & Samii, 1980; Poilvache et al., 1989; Cruz Martinez & Arpa, 1998). In addition to the familial and metabolic causes mentioned in the preceding sections, some additional causes are listed in Table 6-9.

Two newborns had long median distal motor latencies on nerve conduction studies, one after a wrist hematoma developed following radial artery puncture for blood gas sampling and the other after a radial artery cutdown (Koenigsberger & Moessinger, 1977).

Medication Side Effects

Carpal tunnel syndrome has been reported as a side effect of some drugs (Table 6-10). These are all rare occurrences, documented only with case reports.

Screening

If no clues to the cause of the carpal tunnel syndrome are evident on a general history and physical examination, laboratory screening for causes of carpal tunnel syndrome is rarely worthwhile. In

Table 6-10. Carpal Tunnel Syndrome as a Drug Side Effect

Drug	Notes
Danazol (Sikka, Kemmann, Vrablik & Grossman, 1983)	See Estrogens in Chapter 5.
Diazepam (Hines & Hughes, 1974)	Wrist phlebitis at site of intravenous injection.
Disulfiram (Howard, 1982)	Associated with wrist arthritis.
Fluoxetine (Barnhart, 1991)	Associated with allergic rash.
Lithium (Wood & Jacoby, 1986; Deahl, 1988)	Secondary to hypothyroidism.
Interferon alfa-2b (*Physicians' Desk Reference*, 2002)	Occurs in <5% of patients taking this drug.
Interleukin-2 (Heys, Mills & Eremin, 1992; Puduvalli, Sella, Austin & Forman, 1996)	—
Megestrol acetate (*Physicians' Desk Reference*, 2002)	See Estrogens in Chapter 5.
Nonsteroidal anti-inflammatories	Occasional patients report worsening when these are used to treat carpal tunnel syndrome.
Oral contraceptives	See Estrogens in Chapter 5.
Propanolol, metoprolol (Emara & Saadah, 1988; Lipponi, Lucantoni, Antonicelli Gaetti, 1992; Anand, Mittal & Singh, 1993)	—
Protease inhibitors for treatment of human immunodeficiency virus-1 infection (Sclar, 2000)	—
Quinidine (Sukenik et al., 1987)	Might also occur with drug-induced lupus from other drugs.
Somatropin (*Physicians' Desk Reference*, 1999)	Occurred in <2% of adult patients being treated for somatotropin deficiency.
Thalidomide (Clemmensen, Olsen & Andersen, 1984)	Three patients reported.
Tranylcypromine (Harrison, Stewart, Lovelace & Quitkin, 1983)	Debatable role of B_6 deficiency.
Warfarin (Hartwell & Kurtay, 1966; Nkele, 1986; Copeland, Wells & Puckett, 1989; Bonatz & Seabol, 1993; Bindiger, Zelnik, Kuschner & Gellman, 1995; Black, Flowers & Saleh, 1997)	Hemorrhage in carpal tunnel.

100 patients with carpal tunnel syndrome who underwent laboratory screening, the abnormalities found were two high fasting blood sugars, one abnormal thyroid function test, and two high sedimentation rates (Chaplin & Kasdan, 1985). The thyroid function was normal when rechecked. Both patients with high blood sugars had absent Achilles' tendon reflexes.

Summary

Most cases of carpal tunnel syndrome are idiopathic or occupational, but carpal tunnel syndrome is also a manifestation of a wide variety of medical conditions. At times, it is the first clinical evidence of a systemic disease. Every patient with carpal tunnel syndrome deserves a general history and physical examination to avoid overlooking one of these medical conditions.

References

Adamson JE, Srouji SJ, Horton CE, Mladick RA. The acute carpal tunnel syndrome. Plast. Reconstr. Surg. 1971;47:332–36.

Aghasi MK, Rzetelny V, Axer A. The flexor digitorum superficialis as a cause of bilateral carpal-tunnel syndrome and trigger wrist. A case report. J. Bone Joint Surg. 1980;62:134–35.

Albers JW, Donofrio PD, McGonagle TK. Sequential electrodiagnostic abnormalities in acute inflammatory demyelinating polyradiculoneuropathy. Muscle Nerve 1985;8:528–39.

Allen H, Gibbon WW, Evans RJ. Stress fracture of the capitate. J. Accid. Emerg. Med. 1994;11:59–60.

al-Qattan MM, Thomson HG, Clarke HM. Carpal tunnel syndrome in children and adolescents with no history of trauma. J. Hand Surg. 1996;21B:108–11.

Amadio PC. Bifid median nerve with a double compartment within the transverse carpal canal. J. Hand Surg. 1987;12A:366–68.

Ames EL. Carpal tunnel syndrome and motor vehicle accidents. J. Am. Osteopath. Assoc. 1996;96:223–26.

Ametewee K. Carpal tunnel syndrome produced by a post-traumatic calcific mass. Hand 1983;15:212–15.

Ametewee K, Harris A, Samuel M. Acute carpal tunnel syndrome produced by anomalous flexor digitorum superficialis indicis muscle. J. Hand Surg. 1985;10B:83–84.

Anand KS, Mittal S, Singh NP. Carpal tunnel syndrome with propranolol. J. Assoc. Physicians India 1993;41:313.

Andersson MI, Willcox PA. Tuberculous tenosynovitis and carpal tunnel syndrome as a presentation of HIV disease. J. Infect. 1999;39:240–41.

Andersson PB, Yuen E, Parko K, So YT. Electrodiagnostic features of hereditary neuropathy with liability to pressure palsies. Neurology 2000;54:40–44.

Antia NH, Pandya SS, Dastur DK. Nerves in the arm in leprosy I. Clinical, electrodiagnostic and operative aspects. Int. J. Leprosy 1970;38:12–29.

Arnold AG. The carpal tunnel syndrome in congestive cardiac failure. Postgrad. Med. J. 1977;53:623–24.

Artico M, Cervoni L, Stevanato G, D'Andrea V, Nucci F. Bifid median nerve: report of two cases. Acta Neurochir. (Wien.) 1995;136:160–62.

Asai M, Wong AC, Matsunaga T, Akahoshi Y. Carpal tunnel syndrome caused by aberrant lumbrical muscles associated with cystic degeneration of the tenosynovium: a case report. J. Hand Surg. 1986;11A:218–21.

Askins G, Finley R, Parenti J, Bush D, Brotman S. High-energy roller injuries to the upper extremity. J. Trauma 1986;26:1127–31.

Auld CD, Chesney RB. Familial osteochondritis dissecans and carpal tunnel syndrome. Acta Orthop. Scand. 1979;50:727–30.

Babins DM, Lubahn JD. Palmar lipomas associated with compression of the median nerve. J. Bone Joint Surg. 1994;76A:1360–62.

Baccaredda-Boy A, Mastropaoli C, Pastorino P, Sacco G, Farris G. Electromyographic findings in leprosy. Int. J. Leprosy 1963;31:531–32.

Backhouse KM, Churchill-Davidson D. Anomalous palmaris longus muscle producing carpal tunnel-like compression. Hand 1975;7:22–24.

Bailey D, Carter JFB. Median nerve palsy associated with acute infection of the hand. Lancet 1955;1:530–32.

Balcomb TV. Acute gonococcal flexor tenosynovitis in a woman with asymptomatic gonorrhea—case report and literature review. J. Hand Surg. 1982;7A:521–22.

Bang H, Kojima T, Tsuchida Y. A case of carpal tunnel syndrome caused by accessory palmaris longus muscle. Handchir. Mikrochir. Plast. Chir. 1988;20:141–43.

Bardin T, Zingraff J, Shirahama T, Noel LH, Droz D, Voisin MC, Drueke T, Dryll A, Skinner M, Cohen AS, et al. Hemodialysis-associated amyloidosis and beta-2 microglobulin. Clinical and immunohistochemical study. Am. J. Med. 1987;83:419–24.

Barfred T, Hjlund AP, Bertheussen K. Median artery in carpal tunnel syndrome. J. Hand Surg. 1985;10A:864–67.

Barfred T, Ipsen T. Congenital carpal tunnel syndrome. J. Hand Surg. 1985;10A:246–48.

Barker B, Bloch T, Vakili ST, Waller BF. One pathologist went to mow, went to mow a meadow. JAMA 1986;255:200.

Barnhart ER, ed. Physicians' Desk Reference (45th ed). Oradell, NJ: Medical Economics Data, 1991.

Barrick EF. Acute gonococcal flexor tenosynovitis in a woman with asymptomatic gonorrhea. J. Hand Surg. 1983;8A:224–25.

Baruch A, Hass A. Anomaly of the median nerve. J. Hand Surg. 1977;2:331–32.

Bastian FO. Amyloidosis and the carpal tunnel syndrome. Am. J. Clin. Pathol. 1974;61:711–17.

Bauer JM, Trusell JJ. Palmaris profundus causing carpal tunnel syndrome. Orthopedics 1992;15:1348–50.

Bauman TD, Gelberman RH, Mubarak SJ, Garfin SR. The acute carpal tunnel syndrome. Clin. Orthop. 1981;151–56.

Behse F, Buchthal F. Alcoholic neuropathy: clinical, electrophysiological, and biopsy findings. Ann. Neurol. 1977;2:95–110.

Behse F, Buchthal F, Carlsen F, Knappeis GG. Hereditary neuropathy with liability to pressure palsies. Brain 1972;95:777–94.

Belsole RJ, Greeley JM. Surgeon's acute carpal tunnel syndrome: an occupational hazard? J. Fla. Med. Assoc. 1988;75:369–70.

Benson MD, Cohen AS, Brandt KD, Cathcart ES. Neuropathy, M components, and amyloid. Lancet 1975;1:10–12.

Bernardin R, Thomas B. Surgery for neuritis in leprosy: indications for and results of different types of procedures. Lep. Rev. 1997;68:147–54.

Bicknell JM, Lim AC, Raroque HG, Tzamaloukas AH. Carpal tunnel syndrome, subclinical median mononeuropathy, and peripheral polyneuropathy: common early chronic complications of chronic peritoneal dialysis and hemodialysis. Arch. Phys. Med. Rehabil. 1991;72:378–81.

Bindiger A, Zelnik J, Kuschner S, Gellman H. Spontaneous acute carpal tunnel syndrome in an anticoagulated patient. Bull. Hosp. Joint Dis. 1995;54:52–53.

Bindra RR, Evanoff BA, Chough LY, Cole RJ, Chow JC, Gelberman RH. The use of routine wrist radiography in the evaluation of patients with carpal tunnel syndrome. J. Hand Surg. 1997;22A:115–19.

Bjornsson HA, Gestsson J, Ekelund L, Haffajee D. Silastic scaphoid implants in osteoarthritis of the radioscaphoid joint. J. Hand Surg. 1984;9B:177–80.

Black PR, Flowers MJ, Saleh M. Acute carpal tunnel syndrome as a complication of oral anticoagulant therapy. J. Hand Surg. 1997;22B:50–51.

Blennow G, Bekassy AN, Eriksson M, Rosendahl R. Transient carpal tunnel syndrome accompanying rubella infection. Acta Paediatr. Scand. 1982;71:1025–28.

Bona I, Vial C, Brunet P, Couturier JC, Girard-Madoux M, Bady B, Guibaud P. Carpal tunnel syndrome in mucopolysaccharidoses. A report of four cases in child. Electromyogr. Clin. Neurophysiol. 1994;34:471–75.

Bonatz E, Seabol KE. Acute carpal tunnel syndrome in a patient taking Coumadin: case report. J. Trauma 1993;35:143–44.

Bostman OM, Bakalim GE. Carpal tunnel syndrome in a melorheostotic limb. J. Hand Surg. 1985;10B:101–2.

Boström L, Svartengren G. Acute carpal tunnel syndrome caused by peritendinitis calcarea. Case report. Scand. J. Plast. Reconstr. Surg. Hand Surg. 1993;27:157–59.

Braddom RL. Familial carpal tunnel syndrome in three generations of a black family. Am. J. Phys. Med. 1985;64:227–34.

Brand MG, Gelberman RH. Lipoma of the flexor digitorum superficialis causing triggering at the carpal canal and median nerve compression. J. Hand Surg. 1988;13A:342–44.

Brand PW. Treatment of leprosy II. The role of surgery. N. Engl. J. Med. 1956;254:64–67.

Breda S, Richter HP, Schachenmayr W. Incidence of biopsy-detectable amyloid deposits in the retinaculum flexorum and in the tenosynovial tissue in carpal tunnel syndrome. Zentralbl. Neurochir. 1993;54:72–76.

Brones MF, Wilgis EF. Anatomical variations of the palmaris longus, causing carpal tunnel syndrome: case reports. Plast. Reconstr. Surg. 1978;62:798–800.

Browett JP, Fiddian NJ. Delayed median nerve injury due to retained glass fragments. A report of two cases. J. Bone Joint Surg. 1985;67B:382–84.

Brown LP, Coulson DB. Triggering at the carpal tunnel with incipient carpal-tunnel syndrome. Report of an unusual case. J. Bone Joint Surg. 1974;56-A:623–24.

Brown RE, Zamboni WA, Zook EG, Russell RC. Evaluation and management of upper extremity neuropathies in Charcot-Marie-Tooth disease. J. Hand Surg. 1992;17A:523–30.

Brown TR, Kovindha A, Wathanadilokkol U, Piefer A, Smith T, Kraft GH. Leprosy neuropathy: correlation of clinical and electrophysiological tests. Indian J. Lepr. 1996;68:1–14.

Browne EZ Jr, Snyder CC. Carpal tunnel syndrome caused by hand injuries. Plast. Reconstr. Surg. 1975;56:41–43.

Bundey SE, Ashenhurst EM, Dorst JP. Mucolipidosis, probably a new variant with joint deformity and peripheral nerve dysfunction. Birth Defects 1974;10:484–90.

Bush DC, Schneider LH. Tuberculosis of the hand and wrist. J. Hand Surg. 1984;9A:391–98.

Butler B Jr, Bigley EC Jr. Aberrant index (first) lumbrical tendinous origin associated with carpal-tunnel syndrome. A case report. J. Bone Joint Surg. 1971;53:160–62.

Callaway JC, Fite GL, Riordan DC. Ulnar and median neuritis due to leprosy. Int. J. Leprosy 1965;32:285–91.

Campistol JM, Cases A, Torras A, Soler M, Muñoz-Gomez J, Montoliu J, Lopez-Pedret J, Revert L. Visceral involvement of dialysis amyloidosis. Am. J. Nephrol. 1987;7: 390–93.

Cara J, Narvaez A, de la Varga V, Guerado E. Median nerve neuropathy from an old lunate dislocation. Acta Orthop. Belg. 1998;64:100–103.

Care SB, Lacey SH. Recurrent histoplasmosis of the wrist: a case report. J. Hand Surg. 1998;23A:1112–14.

Carstam N. A rare anomalous muscle, palmaris profundus, found when operating at the wrist for neurological symptoms. A report of two cases. Bull. Hosp. Joint Dis. 1984;44:163–67.

Cary NR, Sethi D, Brown EA, Erhardt CC, Woodrow DF, Gower PE. Dialysis arthropathy: amyloid or iron? BMJ. 1986;293:1392–94.

Casado JL, Arenas C, Segura D, Chinchón I, Gonzalez R, Bautista J. Congenital myopathy with cores and nemaline rods in one family. Neurologia 1995;10:145–48.

Case DB. An acute carpal tunnel syndrome in a haemophiliac. Br. J. Clin. Pract. 1967;21:254–55.

Casey EB, Le Quesne PM. Digital nerve action potentials in healthy subjects, and in carpal tunnel and diabetic patients. J. Neurol. Neurosurg. Psychiatry 1972a;35:612–23.

Casey EB, Le Quesne PM. Electrophysiological evidence for a distal lesion in alcoholic neuropathy. J. Neurol. Neurosurg. Psychiatry 1972b;35:624–30.

Cassvan A, Rosenberg A, Rivera LF. Ulnar nerve involvement in carpal tunnel syndrome. Arch. Phys. Med. Rehabil. 1986;67:290–92.

Chagnon A, Carli P, Paris JF, Cameli M, Carloz E. Carpian tunnel syndrome: a most unusual presentation of leishmaniasis. Eur. J. Med. 1993;2:314.

Chalmers J. Unusual causes of peripheral nerve compression. Hand 1978;10:168–75.

Chaplin E, Kasdan ML. Carpal tunnel syndrome and routine blood chemistries. Plast. Reconstr. Surg. 1985;75:722–24.

Chapman DR, Bennett JB, Bryan WJ, Tullos HS. Complications of distal radial fractures: pins and plaster treatment. J. Hand Surg. 1982;7:509–12.

Chattopadhyay C, Ackrill P, Clague RB. The shoulder pain syndrome and soft-tissue abnormalities in patients on long-term haemodialysis. Br. J. Rheumatol. 1987;26:181–87.

Chaudhry V, Corse AM, O'Brian R, Cornblath DR, Klein AS, Thuluvath PJ. Autonomic and peripheral (sensorimotor) neuropathy in chronic liver disease: a clinical and electrophysiologic study. Hepatology 1999;29:1698–1703.

Chaudhuri K, Madhok R. An unusual case of carpal tunnel syndrome. Br. J. Rheumatol. 1998;37:912–14.

Cheatum DE, Hudman V, Jones SR. Chronic arthritis due to Mycobacterium intracellulare. Sacroiliac, knee, and carpal tunnel involvement in a young man and response to chemotherapy. Arthritis Rheum. 1976;19:777–81.

Chen WS. Median-nerve neuropathy associated with chronic anterior dislocation of the lunate. J. Bone Joint Surg. 1995;77A:1853–57.

Chidgey LK, Szabo RM, Wiese DA. Acute carpal tunnel syndrome caused by pigmented villonodular synovitis of the wrist. Clin. Orthop. 1988;254–57.

Chiu KY, Wong WB, Choi CH, Chow SP. Acute carpal tunnel syndrome caused by pseudogout. J. Hand Surg. 1992; 17A:299–302.

Choi ML, Wey PD, Borah GL. Pediatric peripheral neuropathy in proteus syndrome. Ann. Plast. Surg. 1998;40:528–32.

Chopra JS, Khanna SK, Murthy JM. Congenital arteriovenous fistula producing carpal tunnel syndrome. J. Neurol. Neurosurg. Psychiatry 1979;42:815–17.

Chow SP, Ip F, Lau JH, Collins RJ, Luk KD, So YC, Pun WK. Mycobacterium marinum infections of the hand and wrist. Results of conservative treatment in twenty-four cases. J. Bone Joint Surg. 1987;69A:1161–68.

Chung EB, Enzinger FM. Fibroma of tendon sheath. Cancer 1979;44:1945–54.

Clemmensen OJ, Olsen PZ, Andersen KE. Thalidomide neurotoxicity. Arch. Dermatol. 1984;120:338–41.

Cobb TK, An KN, Cooney WP. Effect of lumbrical muscle incursion within the carpal tunnel on carpal tunnel pressure: a cadaveric study. J. Hand Surg. 1995;20A:186–92.

Cobb TK, An KN, Cooney WP, Berger RA. Lumbrical muscle incursion into the carpal tunnel during finger flexion. J. Hand Surg. 1994;19B:434–38.

Coleman SS, Anson BJ. Arterial patterns in the hand based upon a study of 650 specimens. Surg. Gynecol. Obstet. 1961;113:409–24.

Cooney WP III, Dobyns JH, Linscheid RL. Complications of Colles' fractures. J. Bone Joint Surg. 1980;62A:613–19.

Cooney WP III, Linscheid RL, Dobyns JH. Fractures and dislocations of the wrist. In: Rockwood CA JR, Green DP, Bucholz RW, eds. Rockwood and Green's Fractures in Adults (4th ed). Philadelphia: Lippincott, 1996:745–867.

Cooper LZ, Ziring PR, Weiss HJ, Matters BA, Krugman S. Transient arthritis after rubella vaccination. Am. J. Dis. Child. 1969;118:218–25.

Copeland J, Wells HG Jr, Puckett CL. Acute carpal tunnel syndrome in a patient taking coumarin. J. Trauma 1989; 29:131–32.

Cornelis F, Bardin T, Faller B, Verger C, Allouache M, Raymond P, Rottembourg J, Tourliere D, Benhamou C, Noel LH, et al. Rheumatic syndromes and beta 2-microglobulin amyloidosis in patients receiving long-term peritoneal dialysis. Arthritis Rheum. 1989;32:785–88.

Crandall RC, Hamel AL. Bipartite median nerve at the wrist. Report of a case. J. Bone Joint Surg. 1979;61:311.

Cruz Martinez A, Arpa J. Carpal tunnel syndrome in childhood: study of 6 cases. Electroencephalogr. Clin. Neurophysiol. 1998;109:304–8.

Cruz Martinez A, Arpa J, Perez-Conde MC, Ferrer MT. Bilateral carpal tunnel in childhood associated with Schwartz-Jampel syndrome. Muscle Nerve 1984;7:66–72.

Cruz Martinez A, Perez Conde MC, Ramón y Cajal S, Martinez A. Recurrent familiar polyneuropathy with liability to pressure palsies. Electromyogr. Clin. Neurophysiol. 1977;17: 101–24.

Crymble B. Brachial neuralgia and the carpal tunnel syndrome. BMJ. 1968;3:470–71.

Dandy DJ, Munro DD. Squamous cell carcinoma of skin involving the median nerve. Br. J. Dermatol. 1973; 89:527–31.

Danta G. Familial carpal tunnel syndrome with onset in childhood. J. Neurol. Neurosurg. Psychiatry 1975;38:350–55.

Deahl MP. Lithium-induced carpal tunnel syndrome. Br. J. Psychiatry 1988;153:250–51.

Debruyne J, Dehaene I, Martin JJ. Hereditary pressure-sensitive neuropathy. J. Neurol. Sci. 1980;47:385–94.

Deenstra W. Synovial hand infections from *Mycobacterium terrae*. J. Hand Surg. 1988;13B:335–36.

Deforges-Lasseur C, Combe C, Cernier A, Vital JM, Aparicio M. Destructive spondyloarthropathy presenting with progressive paraplegia in a dialysis patient. Recovery after surgical spinal cord decompression and parathyroidectomy. Nephrol. Dial. Transplant. 1993; 8:180–84.

DeHertogh D, Ritland D, Green R. Carpal tunnel syndrome due to gonococcal tenosynovitis. Orthopedics 1988;11:199–200.

De Krom MCTFM, Kester ADM, Knipschild PG, Spaans F. Risk factors for carpal tunnel syndrome. Am. J. Epidemiol. 1990;132:1102–10.

Dellon AL, Trojak JE, Rochman GM. Median nerve compression in Weill-Marchesani syndrome. Plast. Reconstr. Surg. 1984;74:127–30.

DeLuca FN, Cowen NJ. Median-nerve compression complicating a tendon graft prosthesis. J. Bone Joint Surg. 1975; 57:553.

Dent JA, Hadden WA. Not a routine case of carpal tunnel syndrome. J. R. Coll. Surg. Edinb. 1992;37:346–47.

Depuydt KH, Schuurman AH, Kon M. Reversed palmaris longus muscle causing effort-related median nerve compression. J. Hand Surg. 1998;23B:117–19.

Desai SS, Pearlman HS, Patel MR. Clicking at the wrist due to fibroma in an anomalous lumbrical muscle: a case report and review of literature. J. Hand Surg. 1986; 11A:512–14.

De Smet L, Bande S, Fabry G. Giant lipoma of the deep palmar space, mimicking persistent carpal tunnel syndrome. Acta Orthop. Belg. 1994;60:334–35.

Deymeer F, Jones HR Jr. Pediatric median mononeuropathies: a clinical and electromyographic study. Muscle Nerve 1994; 17:755–62.

Dickinson JC, Kleinert JM. Acute carpal-tunnel syndrome caused by a calcified median artery. J. Bone Joint Surg. 1991;73A:610–11.

Dieck GS, Kelsey JL. An epidemiologic study of the carpal tunnel syndrome in an adult female population. Prev. Med. 1985;14:63–69.

DiVincenti FC, Moncrief JA, Pruitt Jr. BA. Electrical injuries: a review of 65 cases. J. Trauma 1969;9:497–507.

Dorff GJ, Frerichs L, Zabransky RJ, Jacobs P, Spankus JD. Musculoskeletal infections due to *Mycobacterium kansasii*. Clin. Orthop. 1978;136:244–46.

Dorfman LJ, Jayaram AR. Handcuff neuropathy. JAMA. 1978;239:957.

Dorin D, Mann RJ. Carpal tunnel syndrome associated with abnormal palmaris longus muscle. South. Med. J. 1984; 77:1210–11.

Dumontier C, Sautet A, Man M, Bennani M, Apoil A. Entrapment and compartment syndromes of the upper limb in haemophilia. J. Hand Surg. 1994;19B:427–29.

Dyreby JR, Engber WD. Palmaris profundus—rare anomalous muscle. J. Hand Surg. 1982;7:513–14.

Earl CJ, Fullerton PM, Wakefield GS, Schutta HS. Hereditary neuropathy, with liability to pressure palsies. QJM. 1964;33:481–98.

Edwards AJ, Sill BJ, Macfarlane I. Carpal tunnel syndrome due to dystrophic calcification. Aust. N. Z. J. Surg. 1984;54: 491–92.

Eglseder WA. Carpal tunnel syndrome associated with histoplasmosis: a case report and literature review. Mil. Med. 1992;157:557–59.

El-Adwar LI. A rare case of wrist injury. A case report. Injury 1972;3:183–84.

Elias LS, Schuler-Ellis FP. Anomalous flexor superficialis indicis: two case reports and literature review. J. Hand Surg. 1985;10A:296–99.

Elliott GB, Elliott KA. The torture or stretch arthritis syndrome (a modern counterpart of the medieval 'manacles' and 'rack'). Clin. Radiol. 1979;30:313–15.

Ellis W. Rubella arthritis. BMJ 1973;4:549.

el Maghraoui A, Lecoules S, Lechevalier D, Magnin J, Eulry F. Acute carpal tunnel syndrome caused by calcific periarthritis of the wrist. Clin. Exp. Rheumatol. 2001;19:107.

Emara MK, Saadah AM. The carpal tunnel syndrome in hypertensive patients treated with beta-blockers. Postgrad. Med. J. 1988;64:191–92.

Engel J, Zinneman H, Tsur H, Farin I. Carpal tunnel syndrome due to carpal osteophyte. Hand 1978;10:283–84.

Eriksen J. A case of carpal tunnel syndrome on the basis of an abnormally long lumbrical muscle. Acta Orthop. Scand. 1973;44:275–77.

Ernst HU, Konermann H. Mesodermal tumor as a cause of carpal tunnel syndrome. Handchir. Mikrochir. Plast. Chir. 1982;14:220–22.

Eskesen V, Rosenrn J, Osgaard O. Atypical carpal tunnel syndrome with compression of the ulnar and median nerves. Case report. J. Neurosurg. 1981;54:668–69.

Evangelisti S, Reale VF. Fibroma of tendon sheath as a cause of carpal tunnel syndrome. J. Hand Surg. 1992;17A:1026–27.

Faithfull DK, Petchell JF. Occult injury of the median nerve. J. Hand Surg. 1995;20B:210–11.

Fatah MF. Palmaris profundus of Frohse and Frankel in association with carpal tunnel syndrome. J. Hand Surg. 1984;9B: 142–44.

Feingold MH, Hidvegi E, Horwitz SJ. Bilateral carpal tunnel syndrome in an adolescent. Am. J. Dis. Child. 1980;134: 394–95.

Ferry S, Hannaford P, Warskyj M, Lewis M, Croft P. Carpal tunnel syndrome: a nested case-control study of risk factors in women. Am. J. Epidemiol. 2000;151:566–74.

Feyerabend T, Schmitt R, Lanz U, Warmuth-Metz M. CT morphology of benign median nerve tumors. Report of three cases and a review. Acta. Radiol. 1990;31:23–25.

Firooznia H, Golimbu C, Rafii M. Carpal tunnel syndrome as a manifestation of secondary hyperparathyroidism. Arch. Intern. Med. 1981;141:959.

Fisher RC, Horner RL, Wood VE. The hand in mucopolysaccharide disorders. Clin. Orthop. 1974;104:191–99.

Fissette J, Onkelinx A, Fandi N. Carpal and Guyon tunnel syndrome in burns at the wrist. J. Hand Surg. 1981;6:13–15.

Floyd T, Burger RS, Sciaroni CA. Bilateral palmaris profundus causing bilateral carpal tunnel syndrome. J. Hand Surg. 1990;15A:364–66.

Flynn JM, Bischoff R, Gelberman RH. Median nerve compression at the wrist due to intracarpal canal sepsis. J. Hand Surg. 1995;20A:864–67.

Fowler CP, Harrison MJ, Snaith ML. Familial carpal and tarsal tunnel syndrome. J. Neurol. Neurosurg. Psychiatry 1986;49: 717–18.

Fricker R, Troeger H. Aneurysm of the ulnar artery as etiology of carpal tunnel syndrome: case report and first description. Handchir. Mikrochir. Plast. Chir. 1994;26:268–69.

Frith RW, Litchy WJ. Electrophysiologic abnormalities of peripheral nerves in patients with cervical radiculopathy. Muscle Nerve 1985;8:613.

Fuchs A, Jagirdar J, Schwartz IS. Beta 2-microglobulin amyloidosis (AB2M) in patients undergoing long-term hemodialysis. A new type of amyloid. Am. J. Clin. Pathol. 1987; 88:302–7.

Gagnon RF, Lough JO, Bourgouin PA. Carpal tunnel syndrome and amyloidosis associated with continuous ambulatory peritoneal dialysis. Can. Med. Assoc. J. 1988;139:753–55.

Gahhos F, Cuono CB. Periosteal chondroma: another cause of carpal tunnel syndrome. Ann. Plast. Surg. 1984;12:275–78.

Galzio RJ, Magliani V, Lucantoni D, D'Arrigo C. Bilateral anomalous course of the ulnar nerve at the wrist causing ulnar and median nerve compression syndromes. J. Neurosurg. 1987;67:754–56.

Ganel A, Engel J, Sela M, Brooks M. Nerve entrapments associated with postmastectomy lymphedema. Cancer 1979; 44:2254–59.

Garcia-Elias M. Carpal instabilities and dislocations. In: Green DP, Hotchkiss RN, Pederson WC, eds. Green's Operative Hand Surgery (4th ed). New York: Churchill Livingstone, 1999:865–928.

Gaur SC, Kulshreshtha K, Swarup S. Acute carpal tunnel syndrome in Hansen's disease. J. Hand Surg. 1994;19B:286–87.

Gejyo F, Homma N, Hasegawa S, Arakawa M. A new therapeutic approach to dialysis amyloidosis: intensive removal of beta 2-microglobulin with adsorbent column. Artif. Organs 1993;17:240–43.

Gejyo F, Teramura T, Ei I, Arakawa M, Nakazawa R, Azuma N, Suzuki M, Furuyoshi S, Nankou T, Takata S, Yasuda A. Long-term clinical evaluation of an adsorbent column (BM-01) of direct hemoperfusion type for beta 2-microglobulin on the treatment of dialysis-related amyloidosis. Artif. Organs 1995;19:1222–6.

Gejyo F, Yamada T, Odani S, Nakagawa Y, Arakawa M, Kunitomo T, Kataoka H, Suzuki M, Hirasawa Y, Shirahama T, et al. A new form of amyloid protein associated with chronic hemodialysis was identified as beta 2-microglobulin. Biochem. Biophys. Res. Commun. 1985;129:701–6.

Gelberman RH, Szabo RM, Mortensen WW. Carpal tunnel pressures and wrist position in patients with Colles' fractures. J. Trauma 1984;24:747–49.

Gellis SS, Feingold M, Kelly TE. Picture of the month. Am. J. Dis. Child. 1975;129:1059–60.

Gerardi JA, Mack GR, Lutz RB. Acute carpal tunnel syndrome secondary to septic arthritis of the wrist. J. Am. Osteopath. Assoc. 1989;89:933–34.

Gilbert MS, Robinson A, Baez A, Gupta S, Glabman S, Haimov M. Carpal tunnel syndrome in patients who are receiving long-term renal hemodialysis. J. Bone Joint Surg. 1988; 70:1145–53.

Gil-Neciga E, Pareja JA, Chincon I, Jarrin S, Chaparro P. Multiple entrapments neuropathy in adult polyglucosan body disease. Neurologia 1995;10:167–70.

Giunta R, Brunner U, Wilhelm K. Bilateral reversed palmaris longus muscle—a rare cause of peripheral median nerve compression syndrome. Case report. [German] Unfallchirurg. 1993;96:538–40.

Giuseffi V, Wall M, Siegel PZ, Rojas PB. Symptoms and disease associations in idiopathic intracranial hypertension (pseudotumor cerebri): a case-control study. Neurology 1991;41: 239–44.

Gleason TF, Abraham E. Bilateral carpal tunnel syndrome associated with unilateral duplication of the flexor digitorum superficialis muscle: a case report. Hand 1982;14:48–50.

Goldberg A, Levy M. Carpal tunnel syndrome and artificial tenodesis of index tendon due to "nailing" of the tendon by a palm tree thorn. Harefuah. 1977;92:514.

Goldie BS, Powell JM. Bony transfixation of the median nerve following Colles' fracture: a case report. Clin. Orthop. 1991;273:275–77.

Golik A, Modai D, Pervin R, Marcus EL, Fried K. Autosomal dominant carpal tunnel syndrome in a Karaite family. Isr. J. Med. Sci. 1988;24:295–97.

Golovchinsky V. Double-Crush Syndrome. Boston: Kluwer Academic Publishers, 2000.

Goodwin DR, Arbel R. Pseudogout of the wrist presenting as acute median nerve compression. J. Hand Surg. 1985;10B: 261–62.

Gordon H, Gordon W, Botha V, Edelstein I. Lipoid proteinosis. Birth Defects 1971;7:164–77.

Gorevic PD, Casey TT, Stone WJ, DiRaimondo CR, Prelli FC, Frangione B. Beta-2 microglobulin is an amyloidogenic protein in man. J. Clin. Invest. 1985;76:2425–29.

Gossett JG, Chance PF. Is there a familial carpal tunnel syndrome? An evaluation and literature review. Muscle Nerve 1998;21:1533–36.

Gouet P, Castets M, Touchard G, Payen J, Alcalay M. Bilateral carpal tunnel syndrome due to tuberculosis tenosynovitis: a case report. J. Rheumatol. 1984;11:721–22.

de-Graad M, Rodseth DJ. Median artery thrombosis as a cause of carpal tunnel syndrome. S. Afr. Med. J. 1989;76:78–79.

Gray RG, Poppo MJ, Gottlieb NL. Primary familial bilateral carpal tunnel syndrome. Ann. Intern. Med. 1979;91:37–40.

Gschwind C, Tonkin MA. Carpal tunnel syndrome in children with mucopolysaccharidosis and related disorders. J. Hand Surg. 1992;17A:44–47.

Guffon N, Souillet G, Maire I, Straczek J, Guibaud P. Follow-up of nine patients with Hurler syndrome after bone marrow transplantation. J. Pediatr. 1998;133:119–25.

Gunther SF, Elliot RC. Mycobacterium kansasii infection in the deep structures of the hand. Report of two cases. J. Bone Joint Surg. 1976;58A:140–42.

Gutowski KA, Olivier WA, Mehrara BJ, Friedman DW. Arteriovenous malformation of a persistent median artery with a bifurcated median nerve. Plast. Reconstr. Surg. 2000;106:1336–39.

Guyon MA, Honet JC. Carpal tunnel syndrome or trigger finger associated with neck injury in automobile accidents. Arch. Phys. Med. Rehabil. 1977;58:325–27.

Haas DC, Nord SG, Bome MP. Carpal tunnel syndrome following automobile collisions. Arch. Phys. Med. Rehabil. 1981;62:204–6.

Haddad FS, Hill RA, Vellodi A. Orthopaedic manifestations of mucolipidosis III: an illustrative case. J. Pediatr. Orthop. B. 2000;9:58–61.

Haddad FS, Jones DH, Vellodi A, Kane N, Pitt MC. Carpal tunnel syndrome in the mucopolysaccharidoses and mucolipidoses. J. Bone Joint Surg. 1997;79B:576–82.

Hagemann PO. Sporotrichosis tendonitis and tenosynovitis. Trans. Am. Clin. Climatol. Assoc. 1968;79:193–98.

Hale MS, Ruderman JE. Carpal tunnel syndrome associated with rubella immunization. Am. J. Phys. Med. 1973; 52:189–94.

Halperin JJ, Volkman DJ, Luft BJ, Dattwyler RJ. Carpal tunnel syndrome in Lyme borreliosis. Muscle Nerve 1989;12:397–400.

Halter SK, DeLisa JA, Stolov WC, Scardapane D, Sherrard DJ. Carpal tunnel syndrome in chronic renal dialysis patients. Arch. Phys. Med. Rehabil. 1981;62:197–201.

Ham SJ, Kolkman WFA, Heeres J, den Boer JA, Vierhout PAM. Changes in the carpal tunnel due to action of the flexor tendons: visualization with magnetic resonance imaging. J. Hand Surg. 1996;21A:997–1003.

Harpf C, Schwabegger A, Hussl H. Carpal median nerve entrapment in a child associated with Poland's syndrome. Ann. Plast. Surg. 1999;42:458–59.

Harrison W, Stewart J, Lovelace R, Quitkin F. Case report of carpal tunnel syndrome associated with tranylcypromine. Am. J. Psychiatry 1983;140:1229–30.

Hartwell SW Jr, Kurtay M. Carpal tunnel compression caused by hematoma associated with anticoagulant therapy. Report of a case. Cleve. Clin. Q. 1966;33:127–29.

Harvey FJ, Bosanquet JS. Carpal tunnel syndrome caused by a simple ganglion. Hand 1981;13:164–66.

Hasselbacher P. Neuropathy after influenza vaccination. Lancet 1977;1:551–52.

Hastings II H, Weiss A-PC, Quenzer D, Wiedeman GP, Hanington KR, Strickland JW. Arthrodesis of the wrist for post-traumatic disorders. J. Bone Joint Surg. 1996;78A: 897–902.

Hawkins PN, Lavender JP, Pepys MB. Evaluation of systemic amyloidosis by scintigraphy with I123-labeled serum amyloid P component. N. Engl. J. Med. 1990;323:508–13.

Hayes CW Jr. Anomalous flexor sublimis muscle with incipient carpal tunnel syndrome. Case report. Plast. Reconstr. Surg. 1974;53:479–83.

Herndon JH, Eaton RG, Littler JW. Carpal-tunnel syndrome. An unusual presentation of osteoid-osteoma of the capitate. J. Bone Joint Surg. 1974;56A:1715–18.

Hess H, Baumann F. Über das familiäre Vorkommen eines Karpaltunnelsyndroms. Ztschr. Orthop. Grenzgebiete 1969;106: 565–69.

Heys SD, Mills KL, Eremin O. Bilateral carpal tunnel syndrome associated with interleukin 2 therapy. Postgrad. Med. J. 1992;68:587–88.

Hines RA, Hughes CV. Carpal tunnel syndrome and diazepam (intravenously). JAMA. 1974;228:697.

Hirasawa Y, Ogura T. Carpal tunnel syndrome in patients on long-term haemodialysis. Scand. J. Plast. Reconstr. Surg. Hand Surg. 2000;34:373–81.

Holtzhausen LM, Constant D, de Jager W. The prevalence of flexor digitorum superficialis and profundus muscle bellies beyond the proximal limit of the carpal tunnel: a cadaveric study. J. Hand Surg. 1998;23A:32–37.

Hopkin RJ, Cotton R, Langer LO, Saal HM. Progressive laryngotracheal stenosis with short stature and arthropathy. Am. J. Med. Genet. 1998;80:241–46.

Hopkins AP, Morgan-Hughes JA. The effect of local pressure in diphtheritic neuropathy. J. Neurol. Neurosurg. Psychiatry 1969;32:614–23.

Horusitzky A, Puechal X, Dumont D, Begue T, Robineau M, Boissier MC. Carpal tunnel syndrome caused by *Mycobacterium szulgai*. J. Rheumatol. 2000;27:1299–1302.

Howard JF. Arthritis and carpal tunnel syndrome associated with disulfiram (Antabuse) therapy. Arthritis Rheum. 1982; 25:1494–96.

Howie CR, Buxton R. Acute carpal tunnel syndrome due to spontaneous haemorrhage. J. Hand Surg. 1984;9B:137–38.

Hund E, Linke RP, Willig F, Grau A. Transthyretin-associated neuropathic amyloidosis. Pathogenesis and treatment. Neurology 2001;56:431–35.

Hurst LC, Weissberg D, Carroll RE. The relationship of the double-crush to carpal tunnel syndrome (an analysis of

1,000 cases of carpal tunnel syndrome). J. Hand Surg. 1985;10B:202–4.

Husain S, Mishra B, Prakash V, Malaviya GN. Evaluation of results of surgical decompression of median nerve in leprosy in relation to sensory–motor functions. Acta Leprologica 1997;10:199–201.

Hutton P, Kernohan J, Birch R. An anomalous flexor digitorum superficialis indicis muscle presenting as carpal tunnel syndrome. Hand 1981;13:85–86.

Hvid-Hansen O. On the treatment of ganglia. Acta Chir. Scand. 1970;136:471–76.

Ikegaya N, Hishida A, Sawada K, Furuhashi M, Maruyama Y, Kumagai H, Kobayashi S, Yamamoto T, Yamazaki K. Ultrasonographic evaluation of the carpal tunnel syndrome in hemodialysis patients. Clin. Nephrol. 1995;44:231–37.

Iossifidis A, As'ad S, Sutaria PD. Aneurysm of the superficial palmar arch. A case report. Int. Orthop. 1995;19:403–4.

Iqbal QM. Triggering of the finger at the flexor retinaculum. Hand 1982;14:53–55.

Isaacs H. An unusual form of carpal tunnel compression. S. Afr. Med. J. 1972;46:637–39.

Isakov AP, Broome JR, Dutka AJ. Acute carpal tunnel syndrome in a diver: evidence of peripheral nervous system involvement in decompression illness. Ann. Emerg. Med. 1996;28:90–93.

Jabaley ME. Personal observations on the role of the lumbrical muscles in carpal tunnel syndrome. J. Hand Surg. 1978;3:82–84.

Jackson DW, Harkins PD. An aberrant muscle belly of the abductor digiti quinti associated with median nerve paresthesias. Bull. Hosp. Joint. Dis. 1972;33:111–15.

Jackson IT, Campbell JC. An unusual cause of carpal tunnel syndrome. A case of thrombosis of the median artery. J. Bone Joint Surg. 1970;52:330–33.

Jackson SH. Profundus tendon disruption resulting in carpal tunnel syndrome. Orthopedics 1990;13:887–89.

Jain VK, Cestero RV, Baum J. Carpal tunnel syndrome in patients undergoing maintenance hemodialysis. JAMA. 1979;242:2868–69.

Janier M, Gheorghiu M, Cohen P, Mazas F, Duroux P. Syndrome du canal carpien a *mycobacterium bovis BCG*. Sem. Hôp. Paris 1982;58:977–79.

Johnson J, Kilgore E, Newmeyer W. Tumorous lesions of the hand. J. Hand Surg. 1985;10A:284–86.

Jones NF, Peterson J. Epidemiologic study of the mallet finger deformity. J. Hand Surg. 1988;13A:334–38.

Jones WA, Scheker LR. Acute carpal tunnel syndrome: a case report. J. Hand Surg. 1988;13B:400–01.

Jou IM, Lai KA. Acute median nerve injury due to migration of a Kirschner wire. J. Hand Surg. 1998;23B:112–13.

Kaplan H, Clayton M. Carpal tunnel syndrome secondary to *Mycobacterium kansasii* infection. JAMA. 1969;208: 1186–88.

Karpati G, Carpenter S, Eisen AA, Feindel W. Familial multiple peripheral nerve entrapments—an unusual manifestation of a peripheral neuropathy. Trans. Am. Neurol. Assoc. 1973;98:267–69.

Keir PJ, Bach JM. Flexor muscle incursion into the carpal tunnel: a mechanism for increased carpal tunnel pressure? Clin. Biomech. (Bristol, Avon). 2000;15:301–5.

Kelly JJ, Kyle RA, O'Brien PC, Dyck PJ. The natural history of peripheral neuropathy in primary systemic amyloidosis. Ann. Neurol. 1979;6:1–7.

Kelly JJ Jr. The electrodiagnostic findings in peripheral neuropathy associated with monoclonal gammopathy. Muscle Nerve 1983;6:504–9.

Kelly JJ Jr, Kyle RA, Miles JM, O'Brien PC, Dyck PJ. The spectrum of peripheral neuropathy in myeloma. Neurology 1981;31:24–31.

Kelly PJ, Karlson AG, Weed LA, Lipscomb PR. Infection of synovial tissues by mycobacteria other than *mycobacterium tuberculosis*. J. Bone Joint Surg. 1967;49A: 1521–30.

Kerrigan JJ, Bertoni JM, Jaeger SH. Ganglion cysts and carpal tunnel syndrome. J. Hand Surg. 1988;13A:763–65.

Khunadorn N, Schlagenhauff RE, Tourbaf K, Papademetriou T. Carpal tunnel syndrome in hemophilia. N. Y. State J. Med. 1977;77:1314–15.

Kilpatrick T, Leyden M, Sullivan J, Lawler G, Grossman H. Acute median nerve compression by haemorrhage from acute myelomonocytic leukaemia. Med. J. Aust. 1985; 142:51–52.

Kilroy AW, Schaffner W, Fleet WF Jr, Lefkowitz LB Jr, Karzon DT, Fenichel GM. Two syndromes following rubella immunization. Clinical observations and epidemiological studies. JAMA 1970;214:2287–92.

Kindstrand E. Antibodies to *Borrelia burgdorferi* in patients with carpal tunnel syndrome. Acta Neurol. Scand. 1992;86: 73–75.

Kiuru S, Seppalainen AM. Neuropathy in familial amyloidosis, Finnish type (FAF): electrophysiological studies. Muscle Nerve 1994;17:299–304.

Kleinman KS, Coburn JW. Amyloid syndromes associated with hemodialysis. Kidney. Int. 1989;35:567–75.

Klofkorn RW, Steigerwald JC. Carpal tunnel syndrome as the initial manifestation of tuberculosis. Am. J. Med. 1976; 60:583–86.

Knight DJ, Gibson PH. Acute calcification and carpal tunnel syndrome. J. Hand Surg. 1993;18B:335–36.

Knirk JL, Jupiter JB. Intra-articular fractures of the distal end of the radius in young adults. J. Bone Joint Surg. 1986; 68A:647–59.

Koenigsberger MR, Moessinger AC. Iatrogenic carpal tunnel syndrome in the newborn infant. J. Pediatr. 1977;91:443–45.

Kohn D, Bush A, Kessler I. Risk of venepuncture. BMJ. 1976;2:1133.

Kopuz C, Gulman B, Baris S. Persistent median artery: an anatomical study in neonatal and adult cadavers. Acta Anat. Nippon 1995;70:577–80.

Koss SD, Reardon TF, Groves RJ. Recurrent carpal tunnel syndrome due to tuberculoid leprosy in an Asian immigrant. J. Hand Surg. 1993;18A:740–42.

Kouyoumdjian JA, Morita MD, Rocha PR, Miranda RC, Gouveia GM. Body mass index and carpal tunnel syndrome. Arq. Neuropsiquiatr. 2000;58:252–56.

Kozin SH, Bishop AT. Atypical Mycobacterium infections of the upper extremity. J. Hand Surg. 1994;19A:480–87.

Kraus E, Schon R, Boller O, Nabavi A. Muscle anomalies of the upper extremity as an atavistic cause of peripheral nerve disorder. Zentralbl. Neurochir. 1993;54:84–89.

Kremchek TE, Kremchek EJ. Carpal tunnel syndrome caused by flexor tendon sheath lipoma. Orthop. Rev. 1988;17: 1083–85.

Krol-v-Straaten MJ, Ackerstaff RG, De-Maat CE. Peripheral polyneuropathy and monoclonal gammopathy of undetermined significance. J. Neurol. Neurosurg. Psychiatry 1985;48:706–8.

Krum-Moller D, Jensen MK, Hansen TB. Carpal tunnel syndrome after epiphysiolysis of the distal radius in a 5-year-old child. Case report. Scand. J. Plast. Reconstr. Surg. Hand Surg. 1999;33:123–24.

Kumar S, Trivedi HL, Smith EK. Carpal tunnel syndrome: a complication of arteriovenous fistula in hemodialysis patients. Can. Med. Assoc. J. 1975;113:1070–72.

Kyle RA, Eilers SG, Linscheid RL, Gaffey TA. Amyloid localized to tenosynovium at carpal tunnel release. Natural history of 124 cases. Am. J. Clin. Pathol. 1989;91: 393–97.

Kyle RA, Greipp PR. Amyloidosis (AL). Clinical and laboratory features in 229 cases. Mayo Clin. Proc. 1983;58:665–83.

Label LS. Carpal tunnel syndrome resulting from steering wheel impact. Muscle Nerve 1991;14:904.

Lagos JC. Compression neuropathy in childhood. Dev. Med. Child. Neurol. 1971;13:531–32.

Lam N, Thurston A. Association of obesity, gender, age and occupation with carpal tunnel syndrome. Aust. N. Z. J. Surg. 1998;68:190–93.

Lambert EH, Mulder DW. Nerve conduction in the Guillain-Barré syndrome. Electroencephalogr. Clin. Neurophysiol. 1964;17:86P.

Lambird PA, Hartmann WH. Hereditary amyloidosis, the flexor retinaculum, and the carpal tunnel syndrome. Am. J. Clin. Pathol. 1969;52:714–19.

Langa V, Posner MA, Hoffman S, Steiner GC. Carpal tunnel syndrome secondary to tuberculous tenosynovitis. Bull. Hosp. Joint. Dis. 1986;46:137–42.

Lanteri M, Ptasznik R, Constable L, Dawborn JK. Ultrasound changes in the wrist and hand in hemodialysis patients. Clin. Nephrol. 1997;48:375–80.

Lanz U. Anatomical variations of the median nerve in the carpal tunnel. J. Hand Surg. 1977;2:44–53.

Lazaro L 3d. Carpal-tunnel syndrome from an insect sting. A case report. J. Bone Joint Surg. 1972;54:1095–96.

Lee KE. Tuberculosis presenting as carpal tunnel syndrome. J. Hand Surg. 1985;10A:242–45.

Lefebvre J, de-Seze S, Lerique JL, Hamonet C, Chaumont P, Bigot B, Dreyfus P. Aetiology of the carpal tunnel syndrome. Electroencephalogr. Clin. Neurophysiol. 1969; 27:107–8.

Leifer D, Cros D, Halperin JJ, Gallico 3rd GG, Pierce DS. Familial bilateral carpal tunnel syndrome: report of two families. Arch. Phys. Med. Rehabil. 1992;73:393–97.

Lettin AWF. Carpal tunnel syndrome in a girl aged 11. Proc. R. Soc. Med. 1965;58:183.

Le Viet D, Gandon F. Carpal tunnel syndrome in hemodialysed patients. Analysis of 110 surgically-treated cases. Chirurgie 1992; 118:546–50.

Levin RA, Felsenthal G. Handcuff neuropathy: two unusual cases. Arch. Phys. Med. Rehabil. 1984;65:41–43.

Levy M, Pauker M. Carpal tunnel syndrome due to thrombosed persisting median artery. A case report. Hand 1978;10:65–68.

Lewis MH. Median nerve decompression after Colles's fracture. J. Bone Joint Surg. 1978;60–B:195–96.

Lewis RC Jr, Nordyke MD, Foreman KA. Median nerve compression caused by a synovial cyst. Bull. Hosp. Joint Dis. 1986;46:68–71.

Lewis SL, Fiddian NJ. Acute carpal tunnel syndrome a rare complication of chondrocalcinosis. Hand 1982;14:164–67.

Lichtman DM, Alexander AH, Mack GR, Gunther SF. Kienbock's disease—update on silicone replacement arthroplasty. J. Hand Surg. 1982;7:343–47.

Linscheid RL. Carpal tunnel syndrome secondary to ulnar bursa distension from the intercarpal joint: report of a case. J. Hand Surg. 1979;4:191–92.

Lipponi G, Lucantoni C, Antonicelli R, Gaetti R. Clinical and electromyographic evidence of carpal tunnel syndrome in a hypertensive patient with chronic beta-blocker treatment. Ital. J. Neurol. Sci. 1992;13:157–59.

Lombardi AS, Quirke TE, Rauscher G. Acute median nerve compression associated with tumescent fluid administration. Plast. Reconstr. Surg. 1998;102:235–37.

Lornoy W, Becaus I, Billiouw JM, Sierens L, Van Malderen P, D'Haenens P. On-line haemodiafiltration. Remarkable removal of beta2-microglobulin. Long-term clinical observations. Nephrol. Dial. Transplant. 2000;15[Suppl 1]:49–54.

Louis DS, Dick HM. Ossifying lipofibroma of the median nerve. J. Bone Joint Surg. 1973;55:1082–84.

Lourie GM, Levin LS, Toby B, Urbaniak J. Distal rupture of the palmaris longus tendon and fascia as a cause of acute carpal tunnel syndrome. J. Hand Surg. 1990;15A:367–69.

Loyau G. The carpal tunnel syndrome. Diagnosis and treatment. Phlebologie. 1987;40:495–501.

Lusthaus S, Matan Y, Finsterbush A, Chaimsky G, Mosheiff R, Ashur H. Traumatic section of the median nerve: an unusual complication of Colles' fracture. Injury; Br. J. Accid. Surg. 1993;24:339–40.

MacDougal B, Weeks PM, Wray RC Jr. Median nerve compression and trigger finger in the mucopolysaccharidoses and related diseases. Plast. Reconstr. Surg. 1977; 59:260–63.

Mack GR, McPherson SA, Lutz RB. Acute median neuropathy after wrist trauma. The role of emergent carpal tunnel release. Clin. Orthop. 1994;300:141–46.

Mackay IR, Barua JM. Perineural tumour spread: an unusual cause of carpal tunnel syndrome. J. Hand Surg. 1990; 15B:104–5.

Mahloudji M, Teasdall RD, Adamkiewicz JJ, Hartmann WH, Lambird PA, McKusick VA. The genetic amyloidoses with particular reference to hereditary neuropathic amyloidosis, type II (Indiana or Rukavina type). Medicine 1969;48:1–37.

Mancusi-Ungaro A, Corres JJ, Di-Spaltro F. Median carpal tunnel syndrome following a vascular shunt procedure in the forearm. Case report. Plast. Reconstr. Surg. 1976;57:96–97.

Mandawat MK. Congestive heart failure and carpal tunnel syndrome: a rare association. J. Indian Med. Assoc. 1985; 83:287.

Manske PR. Fracture of the hook of the hamate presenting as carpal tunnel syndrome. Hand 1978;10:181–83.

Martin SD, Sharrock NE, Mineo R, Sobel M, Weiland AJ. Acute exacerbation of carpal tunnel syndrome after radial artery cannulation. J. Hand Surg. 1993;18A:455–58.

Martinelli P, Poppi M, Gaist G, Padovani R, Pozzati E. Posttraumatic neuroma of the median nerve: a cause of carpal tunnel syndrome. Eur. Neurol. 1985;24:13–15.

Mascola JR, Rickland LS. Infectious causes of carpal tunnel syndrome. Rev. Infect. Dis. 1991;13:911–17.

Massey EW, Riley TL, Pleet AB. Coexistent carpal tunnel syndrome and cervical radiculopathy (double-crush syndrome). South. Med. J. 1981;74:957–59.

Maurer K, Fenske A, Samii M. Carpal tunnel syndrome combined with trigger finger in early childhood. J. Neurol. Neurosurg. Psychiatry 1980;43:1148.

Maxwell JA, Kepes JJ, Ketchum LD. Acute carpal tunnel syndrome secondary to thrombosis of a persistent median artery. Case report. J. Neurosurg. 1973;38:774–77.

McArthur RG, Hayles AB, Gomez MR, Bianco AJ Jr. Carpal tunnel syndrome and trigger finger in childhood. Am. J. Dis. Child. 1969;117:463–69.

McClain EJ, Wissinger HA. The acute carpal tunnel syndrome: nine case reports. J. Trauma 1976;16:75–78.

McDonnell JM, Makley JT, Horwitz SJ. Familial carpal-tunnel syndrome presenting in childhood. Report of two cases. J. Bone Joint Surg. 1987;69:928–30.

McGrath MH, Polayes IM. Posttraumatic median neuroma: a cause of carpal tunnel syndrome. Ann. Plast. Surg. 1979;3:227–30.

McGrory BJ, Amadio PC. Klippel-Trenaunay syndrome: orthopaedic considerations. Orthop. Rev. 1993;22:41–50.

McKusick VA. Heritable Disorders of Connective Tissue (4th ed). St. Louis: Mosby, 1972.

McMinn DJ. Carpal tunnel syndrome caused by a simple ganglion. J. R. Coll. Surg. Edinb. 1985;30:325–26.

Merlet C, Aberrane S, Chilot F, Laroche JM. Carpal tunnel syndrome complicating hand flexor tenosynovitis due to *Mycobacterium szulgai*. Joint Bone Spine 2000;67:247–48.

Mesgarzadeh M, Schneck CD, Bonakdarpour A, Mitra A, Conaway D. Carpal tunnel: MR imaging. Part II. Carpal tunnel syndrome. Radiology 1989;171:749–54.

Meyer FN, Pflaum BC. Median nerve compression at the wrist caused by a reversed palmaris longus muscle. J. Hand Surg. 1987;12A:369–71.

Michaud LJ, Hays RM, Dudgeon BJ, Kropp RJ. Congenital carpal tunnel syndrome: case report of autosomal dominant inheritance and review of the literature. Arch. Phys. Med. Rehabil. 1990;71:430–32.

Milroy BC, Aldred RJ, Vickers D. Digital avulsion injuries: the shish kebab effect of the fibrous flexor sheath. Aust. N. Z. J. Surg. 1984;54:67–71.

Miner ME, Schimke RN. Carpal tunnel syndrome in pediatric mucopolysaccharidoses. Report of four cases. J. Neurosurg. 1975;43:102–3.

Mobbs RJ, Chandran KN. Variation of palmaris longus tendon. Aust. N. Z. J. Surg. 2000;70:538.

Mochizuki Y, Ohkubo H, Motomura T. Familial bilateral carpal tunnel syndrome. J. Neurol. Neurosurg. Psychiatry 1981;44:367–69.

Mohr W. Amyloid deposits in the periarticular tissue. Z. Rheumatol. 1976;35:412–17.

Moneim MS. Unusually high division of the median nerve. J. Hand Surg. 1982;7:13–14.

Moneim MS, Gribble TJ. Carpal tunnel syndrome in hemophilia. J. Hand Surg. 1984;9A:580–83.

Monsivais JJ, Scully S. Rotary subluxation of the scaphoid resulting in persistent carpal tunnel syndrome. J. Hand Surg. 1992;17A:642–44.

Morgan LM. Acute median nerve compression. Med. J. Aust. 1985;142:620.

Morgan G, Wilbourn AJ. Cervical radiculopathy and coexisting distal entrapment neuropathies: double-crush syndromes? Neurology 1998;50:78–83.

Munar-Ques M, Saraiva MJ, Ordeig-Calonge J, Moreira P, Perez-Vidal R, Puig-Pujol X, Monells-Abel J, Badal-Alter JM. Familial amyloid polyneuropathy in a Spanish family with a transthyretin deletion (deltaVal 122) presenting with carpal tunnel syndrome. Clin. Genet. 2000; 58:411–12.

Mundt B, Kallwellis G, Roder H. [Thermographic studies with fluid crystals in peripheral nerve damage]. Psychiatr. Neurol. Med. Psychol. (Leipz.) 1986;38:9–15.

Muñoz-Gomez J, Gomez-Perez R, Llopart-Buisan E, Sole-Arques M. Clinical picture of the amyloid arthropathy in patients with chronic renal failure maintained on haemodialysis using cellulose membranes. Ann. Rheum. Dis. 1987;46:573–79.

Murakami T, Tachibana S, Endo Y, Kawai R, Hara M, Tanase S, Ando M. Familial carpal tunnel syndrome due to amyloidogenic transthyretin His 114 variant. Neurology 1994;44:315–18.

Murray WT, Meuller PR, Rosenthal DI, Jauernek RR. Fracture of the hook of the hamate. AJR. Am. J. Roentgenol. 1979; 133:899–903.

Nakamichi K, Tachibana S. Ultrasonography in the diagnosis of carpal tunnel syndrome caused by an occult ganglion. J. Hand Surg. 1993a;18B:174–75.

Nakamichi K, Tachibana S. Unilateral carpal tunnel syndrome and space-occupying lesions. J. Hand Surg. 1993b;18B: 748–49.

Nakamichi K-I, Tachibana S. Amyloid deposition in the synovium and ligament in idiopathic carpal tunnel syndrome. Muscle Nerve 1996a;19:1349–51.

Nakamichi K, Tachibana S. Carpal tunnel syndrome caused by a synovial nodule of the flexor digitorum profundus tendon of the index finger. J. Hand Surg. 1996b; 21A:282–84.

Nakamichi K, Tachibana S, Tamai K. Carpal tunnel syndrome caused by a mass of calcium phosphate. J. Hand Surg. 1994;19A:111–13.

Nathan PA, Keniston RC, Lockwood RS, Meadows KD. Tobacco, caffeine, alcohol, and carpal tunnel syndrome in American industry. A cross-sectional study of 1464 workers. J. Occup. Environ. Med. 1996;38:290–98.

Nathan PA, Keniston RC, Myers LD, Meadows KD. Obesity as a risk factor for slowing of sensory conduction of the median nerve in industry. J. Occup. Med. 1992;34:379–83.

Nathan PA, Meadows KD. Ulna-minus variance and Kienbock's disease. J. Hand Surg. 1987;12A:777–78.

Nather A, Chong PY. A rare case of carpal tunnel syndrome due to tenosynovial osteochondroma. J. Hand Surg. 1986;11B: 478–80.

Nather A, Pho RW. Carpal tunnel syndrome produced by an organising haematoma within the anomalous second lumbrical muscle. Hand 1981;13:87–91.

Nelson SR, Sharpstone P, Kingswood JC. Does dialysis-associated amyloidosis resolve after transplantation? Nephrol. Dial. Transplant. 1993;8:369–70.

Neviaser RJ. Flexor digitorum superficialis indicis and carpal tunnel syndrome. Hand 1974;6:155–56.

Nkele C. Acute carpal tunnel syndrome resulting from haemorrhage into the carpal tunnel in a patient on warfarin. J. Hand Surg. 1986;11B:455–56.

Nordstrom DL, Vierkant RA, DeStefano F, Layde PM. Risk factors for carpal tunnel syndrome in a general population. Occup. Environ. Med. 1997;54:734–40.

Norman-Taylor F, Fixsen JA, Sharrard WJ. Hunter's syndrome as a cause of childhood carpal tunnel syndrome: a report of three cases. J. Pediatr. Orthop. 1995;4B:106–9.

Oates GD. Median-nerve palsy as a complication of acute pyogenic infections of the hand. BMJ. 1960;1:1618–20.

Ogilvie C, Kay NRM. Fulminating carpal tunnel syndrome due to gout. J. Hand Surg. 1988;13B:42–43.

Olerud C, Lonnquist L. Acute carpal tunnel syndrome caused by fracture of the scaphoid and the 5th metacarpal bones. Injury 1984;16:198–99.

Omer GEJ, Lockwood RS, Travis LO. Histoplasmosis involving the carpal joint. J. Bone Joint Surg. 1963;45A:1699–1703.

Orcutt SA, Kramer WG 3rd, Howard MW, Keenan MA, Stone LR, Waters RL, Gellman H. Carpal tunnel syndrome secondary to wrist and finger flexor spasticity. J. Hand Surg. 1990;15A:940–44.

Orfila C, Goffinet F, Goudable C, Eche JP, Ton-That H, Manuel Y, Suc JM. Unsuitable value of abdominal fat tissue aspirate examination for the diagnosis of amyloidosis in long-term hemodialysis patients. Am. J. Nephrol. 1988;8:454–56.

Oster LH, Blair WF, Steyers CM. Large lipomas in the deep palmar space. J. Hand Surg. 1989;14A:700–704.

Osterman AL. The double-crush syndrome. Orthop. Clin. North Am. 1988;19:147–55.

Owens DW, Garcia E, Pierce RR, Castrow FF 2d. Klippel-Trenaunay-Weber syndrome with pulmonary vein varicosity. Arch. Dermatol. 1973;108:111–13.

Paarlberg D, Linscheid RL, Soule EH. Lipomas of the hand. Including a case of lipoblastomatosis in a child. Mayo Clin. Proc. 1972;47:121–24.

Paget J. Lectures on Surgical Pathology. Philadelphia: Lindsay & Blakiston, 1865. Third American.

Pai CH, Tseng CH. Acute carpal tunnel syndrome caused by tophaceous gout. J. Hand Surg. 1993;18A:667–69.

Paley D, McMurtry RY. Median nerve compression by volarly displaced fragments of the distal radius. Clin. Orthop. 1987;7:139–47.

Parthenis DG, Karagkevrekis CB, Waldram MA. von Willebrand's disease presenting as acute carpal tunnel syndrome. J. Hand Surg. 1998;23B:114.

Patel MR, Desai SS, Gordon SL. Functional limb salvage with multimodality treatment in epithelioid sarcoma of the hand: a report of two cases. J. Hand Surg. 1986;11A:265–69.

Pecket P, Gloobe H, Nathan H. Variations in the arteries of the median nerve. With special considerations on the ischemic factor in the carpal tunnel syndrome (CTS). Clin. Orthop. 1973;97:144–47.

Perlman R, Jubelirer RA, Schwarz J. Histoplasmosis of the common palmar tendon sheath. J. Bone Joint Surg. 1972;54A:676–87.

Pernia LR, Ronel DN, Leeper JD, Miller HL. Carpal tunnel syndrome in women undergoing reduction mammaplasty. Plast. Reconstr. Surg. 2000;105:1314–19.

Peterson DI, Bacchus H, Seaich L, Kelly TE. Myelopathy associated with Maroteaux-Lamy syndrome. Arch. Neurol. 1975;32:127–29.

Phalen GS. The carpal-tunnel syndrome. Seventeen years' experience in diagnosis and treatment of six hundred fifty-four hands. J. Bone Joint Surg. 1966;48A:211–28.

Physician's Desk Reference. Montvale, NJ: Medical Economics Company, 2002.

Pierre-Jerome C, Bekkelund SI, Husby G, Mellgren SI, Osteaux M, Nordstrom R. MRI of anatomical variants of the wrist in women. Surg. Radiol. Anat. 1996;18:37–41.

Poilvache P, Carlier A, Rombouts JJ, Partoune E, Lejeune G. Carpal tunnel syndrome in childhood: report of five new cases. J. Pediatr. Orthop. 1989;9:687–90.

Potts F, Shahani BT, Young RR. A study of the coincidence of carpal tunnel syndrome and generalized peripheral neuropathy. Muscle Nerve 1980;3:440.

Primiano GA, Reef TC. Disruption of the proximal carpal arch of the hand. J. Bone Joint Surg. 1974;56A:328–32.

Prince H, Ispahani P, Baker M. A *Mycobacterium malmoense* infection of the hand presenting as carpal tunnel syndrome. J. Hand Surg. 1988;13B:328–30.

Pritsch M, Engel J, Horowitz A. Cystic change in the wrist, causing carpal tunnel syndrome. Plast. Reconstr. Surg. 1980;65:494–95.

Probst CE, Hunter JM. A digastric flexor digitorum superficialis. Bull. Hosp. Joint Dis. 1975;36:52–57.

Pronicka E, Tylki-Szymanska A, Kwast O, Chmielik J, Maciejko D, Cedro A. Carpal tunnel syndrome in children with mucopolysaccharidoses: needs for surgical tendons and median nerve release. J. Ment. Defic. Res. 1988;32:79–82.

Puduvalli VK, Sella A, Austin SG, Forman AD. Carpal tunnel syndrome associated with interleukin-2 therapy. Cancer 1996;77:1189–92.

Radecki P. The familial occurrence of carpal tunnel syndrome. Muscle Nerve 1994;17:325–30.

Radecki P. Variability in the median and ulnar nerve latencies: implications for diagnosing entrapment. J. Occup. Environ. Med. 1996;37:1293–99.

Radford PJ, Matthewson MH. Hypoplastic scaphoid—an unusual cause of carpal tunnel syndrome. J. Hand Surg. 1987;12B:236–38.

Randall G, Smith PW, Korbitz B, Owen DR. Carpal tunnel syndrome caused by *Mycobacterium fortuitum* and *Histoplasma capsulatum*. Report of two cases. J. Neurosurg. 1982;56:299–301.

Rate AJ, Parkinson RW, Meadows TH, Freemont AJ. Acute carpal tunnel syndrome due to pseudogout. J. Hand Surg. 1992;17B:217–18.

Regnard P-J, Barry P, Isselin J. Mycobacterial tenosynovitis of the flexor tendons of the hand. A report of five cases. J. Hand Surg. 1996;21B:351–54.

Reicher MA, Kellerhouse LE. Carpal tunnel disease, flexor and extensor tendon disorders. In: Reicher MA, Kellerhouse LE, eds. MRI of the Wrist and Hand. New York: Raven Press, 1990:49–68.

Reimann AF, Daseler EH, Anson BJ, Beaton LE. The palmaris longus muscle and tendon. A study of 1600 extremities. Anat. Rec. 1944;89:495–505.

Richardson JK, Forman GM, Riley B. An electrophysiological exploration of the double-crush hypothesis. Muscle Nerve 1999;22:71–77.

Robinson D, Aghasi M, Halperin N. The treatment of carpal tunnel syndrome caused by hypertrophied lumbrical muscles. Case reports. Scand. J. Plast. Reconstr. Surg. Hand Surg. 1989;23:149–51.

Roos D, Thygesen P. Familial recurrent polyneuropathy. Brain 1972;95:235–48.

Rosenberg DB. Neurologic sequelae of minor electric burns. Arch. Phys. Med. Rehabil. 1989;70:914–15.

Rukavina JG, Block WD, Jackson CE, Falls HF, Carey JH, Curtis AC. Primary systemic amyloidosis: an experimental, genetic, and clinical study of 29 cases with particular emphasis on the familial form. Medicine 1956;35:239–334.

Sahs AL, Helms CM, DuBois C. Carpal tunnel syndrome. Complication of toxic shock syndrome. Arch. Neurol. 1983;40:414–15.

Sainio K, Merikanto J, Larsen TA. Carpal tunnel syndrome in childhood. Dev. Med. Child. Neurol. 1987;29:794–97.

Samii K, Cassinotti P, de Freudenreich J, Gallopin Y, Le Fort D, Stalder H. Acute bilateral carpal tunnel syndrome associated with human parvovirus B19 infection. Clin. Infect. Dis. 1996;22:162–64.

Sanchez R, Praga M, Rivas Salas JJ, Araque A, Mazuecos A, Andres A, Rodicio JL. Compressive myelopathy due to dialysis-associated amyloidosis. Nephron 1993;65:463–65.

Sanchez-Andrada RM, Martinez-Salcedo E, de Mingo-Casado P, Domingo-Jimenez R, Puche-Mira A, Casas-Fernandez C. Carpal tunnel syndrome in childhood. A case of early onset. Revista de Neurologia 1998;27:988–91.

Saraiva MJ. Molecular genetics of familial amyloidotic polyneuropathy. J. Peripher. Nerv. Syst. 1996;1:179–88.

Saraiva MJ. Transthyretin mutations in hyperthyroxinemia and amyloid diseases. Hum. Mutat. 2001;17:493–503.

Sargent MA, Fleming SJ, Chattopadhyay C, Ackrill P, Sambrook P. Bone cysts and haemodialysis-related amyloidosis. Clin. Radiol. 1989;40:277–81.

Sarma DP, Weilbaecher TG, Rodriguez FH Jr. Fibroma of tendon sheath. J. Surg. Oncol. 1986;32:230–32.

Scardapane D, Halter S, DeLisa JA, Sherrard DJ. Hand dysfunction due to carpal tunnel syndrome: a common sequela of dialysis. Proc. Clin. Dial. Transplant. Forum 1979;9:15–16.

Schiffl H, Fischer R, Lang SM, Mangel E. Clinical manifestations of AB-amyloidosis: effects of biocompatibility and flux. Nephrol. Dial. Transplant. 2000;15:840–45.

Schlafly B, Lister G. Median nerve compression secondary to bifid reversed palmaris longus. J. Hand Surg. 1987;12A:371–73.

Schlesinger EB, Liss HR. Fundamentals, fads and fallacies in the carpal tunnel syndrome. Am. J. Surg. 1959;97:466.

Schon R, Kraus E, Boller O, Kampe A. Anomalous muscle belly of the flexor digitorum superficialis associated with carpal tunnel syndrome: case report. Neurosurgery 1992;31:969–70.

Schultz RJ, Endler PM, Huddleston HD. Anomalous median nerve and an anomalous muscle belly of the first lumbrical associated with carpal-tunnel syndrome. J. Bone Joint Surg. 1973;55:1744–46.

Schuurman AH, van Gils AP. Reversed palmaris longus muscle on MRI: report of four cases. Eur. Radiol. 2000;10:1242–44.

Schweitzer G, Lewis JS. Puff adder bite—an unusual cause of bilateral carpal tunnel syndrome. A case report. S. Afr. Med. J. 1981;60:714–15.

Schweitzer G, Miller RD. Carpal tunnel syndrome due to median nerve enlargement. S. Afr. Med. J. 1973;47:2222–24.

Sclar G. Carpal tunnel syndrome in HIV-1 patients: a metabolic consequence of protease inhibitor use? AIDS 2000;14:336–38.

Seiler JG 3rd, Havig M, Carpenter W. Acute carpal tunnel syndrome complicating chronic palmar subluxation of the distal ulna. J. South. Orthop. Assoc. 1996;5:108–10.

Selby RC. Neurosurgical aspects of leprosy. Surg. Neurol. 1974;2:165–77.

Seror P, Alliot F, Cluzan RV, Pascot M. Results of a neurophysiologic consultation in patients with secondary lymphedema of the arm after breast cancer associated with neurological symptoms. J. Mal. Vasc. 1999;24: 294–99.

Serratrice G, Roger J, Guastalla B, Saint-Jean JC. Amyotrophies thenariennes familiales d'origine carpienne. Rev. Neurol. (Paris) 1985;141:746–749.

Sgouros S, Ali MS. An unusual cause of carpal tunnel syndrome. Case report. Scand. J. Plast. Reconstr. Surg. Hand Surg. 1992;26:335–37.

Shenoy KT, Saha PK, Ravindran M. Carpal tunnel syndrome: an unusual presentation of brachial hypertrophy. J. Neurol. Neurosurg. Psychiatry 1980;43:82–84.

Shiota E, Fujinaga M. Remission of a recurrent carpal tunnel syndrome by a new device of the hemodialysis method in a long-term hemodialysis patient. Clin. Nephrol. 2000; 53:230–34.

Shiota E, Yamaoka K, Kawano O, Tasaka Y, Nakamoto M, Goya T. Surgical treatments for orthopaedic complications in long-term haemodialysis patients—a review of 546 cases over the last 8 years. Fukuoka Igaku Zasshi 1998;89:261–76.

Siegel DB, Kuzma G, Eakins D. Anatomic investigation of the role of the lumbrical muscles in carpal tunnel syndrome. J. Hand Surg. 1995;20A:860–63.

Sikka A, Kemmann E, Vrablik RM, Grossman L. Carpal tunnel syndrome associated with danazol therapy. Am. J. Obstet. Gynecol. 1983;147:102–3.

Smith RJ. Anomalous muscle belly of the flexor digitorum superficialis causing carpal-tunnel syndrome. Report of a case. J. Bone Joint Surg. 1971;53:1215–16.

Soccetti A, Carloni S, Giovagnoni M, Misericordia M. MR findings in post-traumatic carpal tunnel syndrome. Chir. Organi Mov. 1993;78:233–39.

Soldado-Carrera F, Vilar-Coromina N, Rodriguez-Baeza A. An accessory belly of the abductor digiti minimi muscle: a case report and embryologic aspects. Surg. Radiol. Anat. 2000;22:51–54.

Solem L, Fischer RP, Strate RG. The natural history of electrical injury. J. Trauma 1977;17:487–92.

Southworth SR, Hartwig RH. Foreign body in the median nerve: a complication of acupuncture. J. Hand Surg. 1990;15B:111–12.

Spiegel PG, Ginsberg M, Skosey JL, Kwong P. Acute carpal tunnel syndrome secondary to pseudogout: case report. Clin. Orthop. 1976;00:185–87.

Sponsel KH, Palm ET. Carpal tunnel syndrome following Colles' fracture. Surg. Gynecol. Obstet. 1965;121:1252–56.

Stallings SP, Kasdan ML, Soergel TM, Corwin HM. A case-control study of obesity as a risk factor for carpal tunnel syndrome in a population of 600 patients presenting for independent medical examination. J. Hand Surg. 1997; 22A:211–15.

Stark WA. Neural involvement in fractures of the distal radius. Orthopedics 1987;10:333.

Starreveld E, Ashenhurst EM. Bilateral carpal tunnel syndrome in childhood. A report of two sisters with mucolipidosis III (pseudo-Hurler polydystrophy). Neurology 1975;25: 234–38.

Stein K, Storkel S, Linke RP, Goebel HH. Chemical heterogeneity of amyloid in the carpal tunnel syndrome. Virchows Arch. A Pathol. Anat. Histpathol. 1987;412:37–45.

Steiner RD, Pagon RA. Autosomal dominant transmission of acrodysostosis. Clin. Dysmorph. 1992;1:201–6.

Sterling AP, Eshraghi A, Anderson WJ, Habermann ET. Acute carpal tunnel syndrome secondary to a foreign body within the median nerve. Bull. Hosp. Joint Dis. 1972;33: 130–34.

Stevens JC, Sun S, Beard CM, O'Fallon WM, Kurland LT. Carpal tunnel syndrome in Rochester, Minnesota, 1961 to 1980. Neurology 1988;38:134–38.

Stewart HD, Innes AR, Burke FD. The hand complications of Colles' fractures. J. Hand Surg. 1985;10B:103–6.

Stoll C, Maitrot D. Autosomal dominant carpal tunnel syndrome. Clin. Genet. 1998;54:345–48.

Stone DA, Laureno R. Handcuff neuropathies. Neurology 1991;41:145–47.

Stone WJ, Hakim RM. Beta-2-microglobulin amyloidosis in long-term dialysis patients. Am. J. Nephrol. 1989;9:177–83.

Stratton CW, Lichtenstein KA, Lowenstein SR, Phelps DB, Reller LB. Granulomatous tenosynovitis and carpal tunnel syndrome caused by *Sporothrix schenckii*. Am. J. Med. 1981;71:161–64.

Stratton CW, Phelps DB, Reller LB. Tuberculoid tenosynovitis and carpal tunnel syndrome caused by *Mycobacterium szulgai*. Am. J. Med. 1978;65:349–51.

Strayer DS, Gutwein MB, Herbold D, Bresalier R. Histoplasmosis presenting as the carpal tunnel syndrome. Am. J. Surg. 1981;141:286–88.

Sturim HS, Edmond JA. Carpal tunnel compression syndrome secondary to a retracted flexor digitorum sublimis tendon. Plast. Reconstr. Surg. 1980;66:846–48.

Sugumaran DS. Steroid therapy for paralytic deformities in leprosy. Int. J. Lepr. Other Mycobact. Dis. 1997;65:337–44.

Sukenik S, Horowitz J, Katz A, Henkin J, Buskila D. Quinidine-induced lupus erythematosus-like syndrome: three case reports and a review of the literature. Isr. J. Med. Sci. 1987;23:1232–34.

Sungpet A, Suphachatwong C, Kawinwonggowit V. The relationship between body mass index and the number of sides of carpal tunnel syndrome. J. Med. Assoc. Thailand 1999;82:182–85.

Suso S, Peidro L, Ramón R. Tuberculous synovitis with "rice bodies" presenting as carpal tunnel syndrome. J. Hand Surg. 1988;13A:574–76.

Sutro CJ. Carpal tunnel syndrome caused by calcification in the deep or volar radio-carpal ligament. Bull. Hosp. Joint Dis. 1969;30:23–27.

Swinn MJ, Hargreaves DG. Consequences of lymphatic malformations in the Klippel-Trenaunay syndrome. J. R. Soc. Med. 1996;89:106P–7P.

Swoboda KJ, Engle EC, Scheindlin B, Anthony DC, Jones HR. Mutilating hand syndrome in an infant with familial carpal tunnel syndrome. Muscle Nerve 1998;21:104–11.

Szabo RM, Pettey J. Bilateral median nerve bifurcation with an accessory compartment within the carpal tunnel. J. Hand Surg. 1994;19B:22–23.

Takada T, Fujioka H, Mizuno K. Carpal tunnel syndrome caused by an idiopathic calcified mass. Arch. Orthop. Trauma Surg. 2000;120:226–27.

Tanaka S, Wild DK, Seligman PJ, Halperin WE, Behrens VJ, Putz-Anderson V. Prevalence and work-relatedness of self-reported carpal tunnel syndrome among U.S. workers: analysis of the Occupational Health Supplement data of 1988 National Health Interview Survey. Am. J. Ind. Med. 1995;27:451–70.

Tegner Y, Leven P, Lysholm J. Acute surgery of carpal tunnel syndrome. Lakartidningen 1983;80:3189.

Teitz CC, DeLisa JA, Halter SK. Results of carpal tunnel release in renal hemodialysis patients. Clin. Orthop. 1985;5:197–200.

Thompson GR, Ferreyra A, Brackett RG. Acute arthritis complicating rubella vaccination. Arthritis Rheum. 1971;14: 19–26.

Tingle AJ, Chantler JK, Pot KH, Paty DW, Ford DK. Postpartum rubella immunization: association with development of prolonged arthritis, neurological sequelae, and chronic rubella viremia. J. Infect. Dis. 1985;152:606–12.

Tompkins DG. Median neuropathy in the carpal tunnel caused by tumor-like conditions. Report of two cases. J. Bone Joint Surg. 1967;49A:737–40.

Touborg-Jensen A. Carpal-tunnel syndrome caused by an abnormal distribution of the lumbrical muscles. Case report. Scand. J. Plast. Reconstr. Surg. 1970;4:72–74.

Trevaskis AE, Tilly D, Marcks KM, Heffernan AH. Loss of nerve function in the hand caused by ganglions. Plast. Reconstr. Surg. 1967;39:97–100.

Tropet Y, Brientini JM, Monnier G, Vichard P. Carpal tunnel syndrome before 20 years of age. A report of 7 cases. Ann. Chir. Main. 1990;9:29–31.

Ueno E, Beppu M, Shimizu H, Komurai M. Bone lesions of the hand and wrist in patients undergoing hemodialysis for ten years. Hand Surg. 1999;4:159–65.

Ullian ME, Hammond WS, Alfrey AC, Schultz A, Molitoris BA. Beta-2-microglobulin-associated amyloidosis in chronic hemodialysis patients with carpal tunnel syndrome. Medicine 1989;68:107–15.

Umehara F, Matsumoto W, Kuriyama M, Sukegawa K, Gasa S, Osame M. Mucolipidosis III (pseudo-Hurler polydystrophy); clinical studies in aged patients in one family. J. Neurol. Sci. 1997;146:167–72.

Upton AR, McComas AJ. The double crush in nerve entrapment syndromes. Lancet 1973;2:359–62.

Vadasz AG, Chance PF, Epstein LG, Lou JS. Familial autosomal-dominant carpal tunnel syndrome presenting in a 5-year old case report and review of the literature. Muscle Nerve 1997;20:376–78.

Vandenbroucke JM, Jadoul M, Maldague B, Huaux JP, Noel H, van-Ypersele-de-Strihou C. Possible role of dialysis membrane characteristics in amyloid osteoarthropathy. Lancet 1986;1:1210–11.

Vanek J, Schwarz J. The gamut of histoplasmosis. Am. J. Med. 1971;50:89–104.

Van Heest AE, House J, Krivit W, Walker K. Surgical treatment of carpal tunnel syndrome and trigger digits in children with mucopolysaccharide storage disorders. J. Hand Surg. 1998;23A:236–43.

Verfaillie S, De Smet L, Leemans A, Van Damme B, Fabry G. Acute carpal tunnel syndrome caused by hydroxyapatite crystals: a case report. J. Hand Surg. 1996;21A:360–62.

Vessey MP, Villard-MacIntosh L, Yeates D. Epidemiology of carpal tunnel syndrome in women of childbearing age: findings in a large cohort study. Int. J. Epidemiol. 1990;19:655.

Victor M. Polyneuropathy due to nutritional deficiency and alcoholism. In: Dyck PJ, Thomas PK, Lambert EH, Bunge R, eds. Peripheral Neuropathy (2nd ed). Philadelphia: Saunders, 1984:1899–940.

Vinals-Torras M, Garcia AF, Barreiro-Tella P, Diez-Tejedor E, Cruz Martinez A, Arpa-Gutierrez J. Manifestation of Scheie mucopolysaccharidosis I: carpal tunnel syndrome in childhood. Case report. Arch. Neurobiol. (Madr) 1985;48:113–23.

Wada A, Nomura S, Ihara F. Mycobacterium kansasii flexor tenosynovitis presenting as carpal tunnel syndrome. J. Hand Surg. 2000;25B:308–10.

Walton S, Cutler CR. Carpal tunnel syndrome. Case report of unusual etiology. Clin. Orthop. 1971;74:138–40.

Warren DJ, Otieno LS. Carpal tunnel syndrome in patients on intermittent haemodialysis. Postgrad. Med. J. 1975;51:450–52.

Watson-Jones R. Leri's pleonosteosis, carpal tunnel compression of the median nerves and Morton's metatarsalgia. J. Bone Joint Surg. 1949;31B:560–71.

Weiber H, Linell F. Tumoral calcinosis causing acute carpal tunnel syndrome. Case report. Scand. J. Plast. Reconstr. Surg. Hand Surg. 1987;21:229–30.

Weiland AJ, Lister GD, Villarreal-Rios A. Volar fracture dislocations of the second and third carpometacarpal joints associated with acute carpal tunnel syndrome. J. Trauma 1976;16:672–75.

Weiss AP, Steichen JB. Synovial sarcoma causing carpal tunnel syndrome. J. Hand Surg. 1992;17A:1024–25.

Wener MH, Metzger WJ, Simon RA. Occupationally acquired vibratory angioedema with secondary carpal tunnel syndrome. Ann. Intern. Med. 1983;98:44–46.

Werner RA, Albers JW, Franzblau A, Armstrong TJ. The relationship between body mass index and the diagnosis of carpal tunnel syndrome. Muscle Nerve 1994;17:632–36.

Werner RA, Franzblau A, Albers JW, Armstrong TJ. Influence of body mass index and work activity on the prevalence of median mononeuropathy at the wrist. Occup. Environ. Med. 1997;54:268–71.

Wilbourn AJ, Gilliatt RW. Double-crush syndrome: a critical analysis. Neurology 1997;49:21–29.

Williams CS, Riordan DC. Mycobacterium marinum (atypical acid-fast bacillus) infections of the hand: a report of six cases. J. Bone Joint Surg. 1973;55A:1042–50.

Williams Jr. LF, Geer T. Acute carpal tunnel syndrome secondary to pyogenic infection of the forearm. JAMA. 1963; 185:409–10.

Wilson KM, Buehler MJ. Bilateral carpal tunnel syndrome in a normal child. J. Hand Surg. 1994;19A:913–14.

Winkelman NZ. An accessory flexor digitorum profundus indicis. J. Hand Surg. 1983;8:70–71.

Wood KA, Jacoby RJ. Lithium induced hypothyroidism presenting with carpal tunnel syndrome. Br. J. Psychiatry 1986;149:386–87.

Wraith JE, Alani SM. Carpal tunnel syndrome in the mucopolysaccharidoses. Arch. Dis. Childhood 1990;65:962.

Wright C, MacFarlane I. Aneurysm of the median artery causing carpal tunnel syndrome. Aust. N. Z. J. Surg. 1994; 64:66–67.

Yeoman PM. Leri's pleonosteosis. Proc. R. Soc. Med. 1961; 54:275.

Yu J, Bendler EM, Mentari A. Neurological disorders associated with carpal tunnel syndrome. Electromyogr. Clin. Neurophysiol. 1979;19:27–32.

Zachary LS, Clark GL Jr, Kleinert JM, O'Donovan C 3d. Mycobacterium chelonei tenosynovitis. Ann. Plast. Surg. 1988; 20:360–62.

Zamora JL, Rose JE, Rosario V, Noon GP. Double entrapment of the median nerve in association with PTFE hemodialysis loop grafts. South. Med. J. 1986;79:638–40.

Zeiss J, Jakab E. MR demonstration of an anomalous muscle in a patient with coexistent carpal and ulnar tunnel syndrome. Case report and literature summary. Clin. Imaging 1995;19: 102–5.

Chapter 7
Electrodiagnostic Methods for Evaluation of Carpal Tunnel Syndrome

Electrodiagnostic tests are invaluable aids to the diagnosis of carpal tunnel syndrome. In addition to assisting in the diagnosis, they are helpful in characterizing the severity of the median mononeuropathy, investigating the patient for alternative or co-existing forms of neurologic pathology, and providing a baseline for evaluating the results of therapy. However, carpal tunnel syndrome remains a clinical diagnosis, so that electrodiagnostic results cannot make or exclude the diagnosis of carpal tunnel syndrome; the electrodiagnostic results must always be interpreted in clinical context.

Table 7-2 lists some of the more important electrodiagnostic methods and parameters, which are discussed in greater detail in this chapter. Chapter 8 reviews the interpretation of electrodiagnostic results in patients being investigated for possible carpal tunnel syndrome.

History of Electrodiagnosis of Carpal Tunnel Syndrome

Dawson and Scott (1949) pioneered surface stimulation and recording of nerve action potentials. Simpson (1958) stimulated the median nerve at the wrist and recorded a compound muscle action potential (CMAP) over the thenar eminence. He reported prolonged distal motor latency (DML) of the median nerve in 11 of 15 patients with carpal tunnel syndrome. Thomas (1960) found a similar diagnostic sensitivity in 95 patients. Gilliatt and Sears (1958) described the use of sensory nerve conduction studies in the diagnosis of carpal tunnel syndrome. Subsequent authors have

described a number of approaches to improving diagnostic sensitivity of nerve conduction tests. The American Association of Electrodiagnostic Medicine, the American Academy of Neurology, and the American Academy of Physical Medicine and Rehabilitation (1993, 2002) have jointly issued practice guidelines for nerve conduction testing in patients with suspected carpal tunnel syndrome. Stevens (1997) has written a useful brief review of nerve conduction tests for carpal tunnel syndrome.

Electrodiagnostic Methods

Motor Nerve Conduction Studies

Technique

The most commonly used median motor nerve conduction test measures conduction of the nerve impulse to muscles of the thenar eminence (Liveson & Ma, 1992). Surface recording electrodes should be on the thenar eminence with the active electrode over the motor point of the abductor pollicis brevis, two-thirds of the way along a line running from the metacarpal-phalangeal joint to the carpal-metacarpal joint of the thumb (Figure 7-1). In this position the electrode detects potentials from multiple thenar muscles including abductor pollicis brevis, opponens pollicis, and flexor pollicis brevis, as well as from neighboring muscles such as adductor pollicis and first dorsal interosseous. The reference electrode should be at the metacar-

Table 7-1. Electrodiagnostic Abbreviations

Abbreviation	Definition
CMAP	Compound muscle action potential
CSI	Combined sensory index
CSP	Cutaneous silent period
DML	Distal motor latency
DSL	Distal sensory latency
EMG	Needle electromyography
MLD	Maximum serial sensory latency difference
MNCV	Motor nerve conduction velocity
RF	Repeater F-wave
%RF	Percent repeater F-waves
RML	Residual motor latency
SNAP	Sensory nerve action potential
SNCV	Sensory nerve conduction velocity
SSEP	Somatosensory evoked potential
SSR	Sympathetic skin response
TLI	Terminal latency index

Table 7-2. Electrodiagnostic Methods and Parameters for Evaluation of Carpal Tunnel Syndrome

Motor nerve conduction studies
   Distal motor latency to the thenar muscles
   Residual motor latency
   Terminal latency index
   Compound muscle action potential amplitude and duration
   Distal motor latency to the second lumbrical muscle
   Palmar stimulation
   Palmar serial motor stimulation
   Forearm motor conduction velocity
   Anterior interosseus comparison
   Martin-Gruber anastomosis
   Threshold distal motor latency
   F-wave studies
Sensory nerve conduction studies
   Digit-to-wrist conduction
   Palm-to-wrist conduction
   Variability of digital nerves
   Ultradistal sensory conduction
   Palmar serial sensory stimulation
   Ipsilateral comparison methods
      Median-ulnar
      Median-radial
      Sensory nerve action potential amplitude comparisons
      Hand-forearm
      Palm-wrist versus digit-palm
      Median thumb-wrist versus median palmar cutaneous
      Combined sensory index
Electromyography
   Evidence of axonal interruption
   Repetitive neuronal firing
   Cutaneous silent period
Somatosensory evoked potentials
Transcranial magnetic stimulation
Autonomic tests
   Sympathetic skin response

pal-phalangeal joint of the thumb. The ground electrode may be on the dorsum of the hand. The stimulation sites are typically at the wrist, just medial to the tendon of flexor carpi radialis, and in the antecubital space just medial to the biceps tendon. The examiner records the amplitude of the CMAP in millivolts and the latency in milliseconds between the time of stimulation and the onset of the CMAP.

The distance from the wrist stimulation site to the active electrode should be measured and kept constant from study to study. Because the recurrent motor branch of the median nerve reaches the thenar muscles along a curved path, the measurement is only an approximation of nerve length. Some examiners measure directly between the stimulating and recording electrodes, while others bend the measuring tape, guessing at the course of the nerve. The measuring technique must be consistent from study to study.

The stimulus intensity is increased until the maximum amplitude CMAP is obtained to ensure that all motor nerve fibers in the median nerve are stimulated. When stimulating the median nerve at the wrist, the examiner must be careful to obtain supramaximal stimulation without stimulating the ulnar nerve (Carpay, Schimsheimer & de Weerd,

1997). A thenar CMAP to median nerve stimulation at the wrist that is initially positive suggests volume-conducted contributions from ulnar-innervated muscles. A thenar CMAP to median stimulation at the wrist that is much larger than the CMAP to median stimulation in the antecubital space may be caused by volume-conducted ulnar stimulation at the wrist, by abnormal median nerve conduction in the forearm, or by inadequate proximal stimula-

Figure 7-1. Electrode placement for studying median nerve motor conduction to the thenar muscles. The compound muscle action potentials (CMAPs) obtained over the thenar muscles from stimulation at the wrist and at the antecubital space are shown. The wave-forms shown in this chapter are artist's renditions rather than pictures of actual recordings.

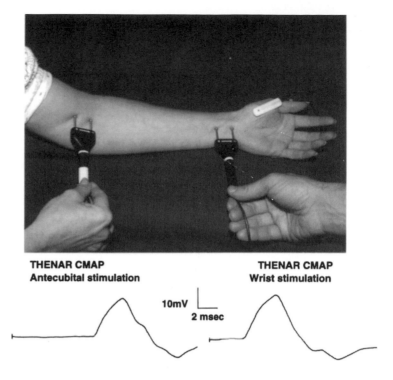

THENAR CMAP
Antecubital stimulation

THENAR CMAP
Wrist stimulation

10mV

2 msec

tion. To avoid inadvertent ulnar stimulation during median stimulation at the wrist, the stimulus can be decreased or the stimulator moved slightly radially. Sometimes use of a needle recording electrode in abductor pollicis brevis is necessary to measure the median motor latencies accurately.

The thenar CMAP evoked by median nerve stimulation is often preceded by a bifid low amplitude (10 to 50 μV) negative wave, which may not be noted at gains such as 1 mV/division commonly used for clinical recording of thenar motor conduction. The origin of these so-called premotor potentials has been debated (Dumitru & King, 1995; Park & Del Toro, 1995; Mandel, 1998); they are not of clinical diagnostic value.

Normal Values

Liveson and Ma (1992) summarize the normal values from a number of different clinics. Typical values, shown in Table 7-3, are those from the Mayo Clinic, based on a 7-cm distance between the recording electrode and wrist stimulation site (Stevens, 1987).

Median DML is also considered abnormal by the Mayo Clinic criteria if it is 1.0 msec longer than the contralateral median DML or 1.8 msec longer than the ipsilateral ulnar DML. By the methods used in some other laboratories, the upper limit of normal for DML is less than 4.6 msec.

Table 7-3. Median Motor Conduction: Normal Values

Distal Motor Latency (msec)		Compound Muscle Action Potential Amplitude (mV)		Forearm Motor Nerve Conduction Velocity (m/sec)	
Mean	Upper normal	Mean	Lower normal	Mean	Lower normal
3.2	4.6	10.7	3.7	59	49

Data from JC Stevens. AAEE minimonograph 26: the electrodiagnosis of carpal tunnel syndrome. Muscle Nerve 1987;10:99–113.

Findings in Carpal Tunnel Syndrome

Distal Motor Latency to Thenar Muscles. In early published series of patients with carpal tunnel syndrome, two-thirds to over four-fifths of symptomatic hands had a prolonged median DML (Thomas, PK, 1960; Thomas, Lambert & Cseuz, 1967; Kopell & Goodgold, 1968; Buchthal et al., 1974). The diagnostic sensitivity of median DML is lower in contemporary laboratories where it is common to test patients who have relatively milder carpal tunnel syndrome. For example, in the series of Buchthal, Rosenfalck, and Trojaborg (1974), 82% of the patients had abnormal median DML; in this series one-half the patients had clinical thenar weakness or atrophy, an incidence of clinical motor abnormality that would be quite high in contemporary clinics. In contrast, at the Mayo Clinic from 1961 to 1980, 51% of patients who had clinical evidence of carpal tunnel syndrome and underwent electrodiagnostic studies had an abnormal median DML (Stevens, 1987).

Residual Motor Latency. The median DML is too long to be explained solely by the conduction velocity of median myelinated fibers (Hodes, Larrabee & German, 1948). The median DML varies with (1) the length of nerve between sites of stimulation and recording, (2) the overall conduction velocity of the median nerve, (3) any delay in conduction attributable to focal nerve compression or disease, (4) any delay between arrival of the nerve action potential at the terminal unmyelinated axonal branches and activation of the muscle across the neuromuscular junction, and (5) systematic slowing of distal relative to proximal conduction (e.g., due to decrease in axon diameter distally or to distal temperature being less than proximal temperature). In healthy subjects there is a relatively wide standard deviation and range of the median DML. Kraft and Halvorson (1983) corrected for the portion of this variation attributed to differences in distance between the stimulating and recording electrodes and to diffuse variations in conduction in the median nerve by calculating a *residual motor latency* (RML) using the following definition:

$$RML = DML - \left(10 \times \frac{D}{MNCV} \right)$$

where RML = residual motor latency (milliseconds), DML = distal motor latency (milliseconds), D = distance from recording electrode to distal stimulating electrode (centimeters), and

MNCV = motor nerve conduction velocity in the forearm (meters per second). The factor 10 in the formula corrects the dimensions so that although D is in centimeters and MNCV is in meters per second, the result is in milliseconds.

The recurrent median motor branch follows a curved and variable course in the palm, but D is measured on the surface; therefore, D is only an approximation of actual nerve length.

Kraft and Halvorson (1983) found an upper limit of normal median RML of 2.6 msec and gave examples of patients with clinical diagnoses of carpal tunnel syndrome who had normal median DML but prolonged median RML. One advantage of the RML over the DML is that the RML is less dependent on patient age.

Terminal Latency Index. Calculation of a *terminal latency index* (TLI) is another approach to correcting the DML for variations in the median forearm MNCV (Shahani, Young, Potts & Maccabee, 1979). The TLI is defined by the following formula:

$$TLI = \frac{D}{(MNCV \times DML)}$$

In healthy subjects, the range of the TLI in one series was 0.36 to 0.55 (Shahani et al., 1979). Like the RML, the TLI may be abnormal in patients with carpal tunnel syndrome, even though the median DML and palm to wrist conductions are normal (Simovic & Weinberg, 1997). Among 52 patients who had a clinical diagnosis of carpal tunnel syndrome, 82% had an abnormal TLI (<0.34), and the TLI was a more sensitive indicator of carpal tunnel syndrome than palm-wrist latency, ring finger median to ulnar comparison, wrist to index finger distal sensory latencies (DSL), or DML (Simovic & Weinberg, 1999).

Compound Muscle Action Potential Amplitude and Duration. The normal amplitude and duration of the thenar CMAP to supramaximal stimulation have a large range and standard deviation (Hodes et al., 1948; Chan, Yang, Penn & Chuang, 1998). Table 7-4 gives sample values.

The amplitude is influenced by technical factors such as electrode placement or amount of electrode paste used and by patient idiosyncrasies such as local swelling, sweating, or callosity (Felsenthal, 1978b). Slight variations in recording electrode placement or thumb position can change the measured amplitude (Lateva, McGill & Burgar, 1996; van Dijk, van Benten, Kramer & Stegeman, 1999). In a healthy individual, the thenar CMAP amplitude of one hand may be as low as 40% of the CMAP amplitude of the contralateral hand (Felsenthal, 1978b).

In a population of patients with carpal tunnel syndrome, the mean thenar CMAP amplitude was 60% of the normal mean, but few individuals with carpal tunnel syndrome had CMAP amplitudes below the normal range (Thomas et al., 1967). There is a correlation between CMAP amplitude and slowing of forearm median MNCV (Thomas et al., 1967).

Rarely, patients who have carpal tunnel syndrome have decrement of the thenar CMAP to repetitive median nerve stimulation at 2 to 3 Hz (Singer & Lin, 1982). The reported patients had electromyographic (EMG) evidence of denervation in abductor pollicis brevis and normal response to repetitive stimulation in other nerves.

Distal Motor Latency to the Second Lumbrical Muscle. Median motor nerve conduction can also be measured to the second lumbrical muscle. The active surface recording electrode can be placed

Table 7-4. Compound Muscle Action Potential Amplitude and Duration: Normal Values

	Mean	Standard Deviation	Range
Thenar compound muscle action potential amplitude (mV)	15.6	5.8	3.6–29.0
Thenar compound muscle action potential duration (msec)	12.23	1.64	9.0–16.0

Data from G Felsenthal. Median and ulnar muscle and sensory evoked potentials. Am. J. Phys. Med. 1978b;57:167–82.

on the palm on the radial side of the third metacarpal, over the motor point of the lumbrical, approximately at the midpoint of the metacarpal (Figure 7-2). Alternatively, a needle-recording electrode can be inserted into the lumbrical. The reference electrode is placed 3 cm distal to the active electrode (Logigian, Busis, Berger, Bruyninckx, Khalil, Shahani & Young, 1987). In control subjects, the median DML from the wrist is similar whether measured to the abductor pollicis brevis or to the second lumbrical. In some patients

Figure 7-2. To study median nerve motor conduction to the lumbricals, the active surface electrode can be placed on the radial side of the third metacarpal, over the motor point of the lumbrical, approximately at the midpoint of the metacarpal. (CMAP = compound muscle action potential.)

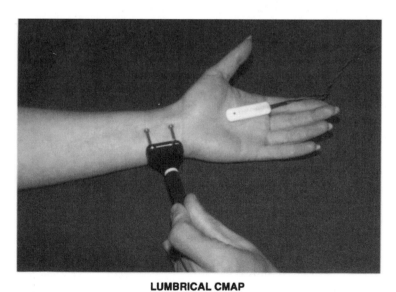

LUMBRICAL CMAP
Wrist stimulation

10mV

2 msec

who have carpal tunnel syndrome, the DML to the abductor pollicis brevis is significantly longer than the DML to the second lumbrical. Logigian and colleagues (1987) classified patients who had carpal tunnel syndrome as having "lumbrical sparing" if the DML to abductor pollicis brevis was greater than or equal to 0.4 msec more than the DML to the ipsilateral second lumbrical. They found that four-fifths of their carpal tunnel syndrome patients had lumbrical sparing. In 60 hands affected by carpal tunnel syndrome, the thenar DML was normal in 17. Of the 17 patients who had normal thenar DML, 14 were classified as abnormal by demonstration of lumbrical sparing. Lumbrical sparing was noted in five patients who had normal palm-to-wrist mixed nerve conduction velocity.

Lumbrical sparing is sometimes demonstrable in patients who have severe carpal tunnel syndrome. When the thenar CMAP has an initial positive deflection to both wrist and antecubital stimulation, the source can be a volume-conducted CMAP from the median-innervated lumbricals (Yates, Yaworski & Brown, 1981). The median lumbrical CMAP sometimes is preserved when the thenar muscles are severely atrophic (Yates, Yaworski & Brown, 1981).

In the carpal tunnel, the median nerve fascicles that form the recurrent thenar motor branch are usually located on the anterior surface of the nerve, whereas the fascicles that form terminal branches to the lumbricals are farther from the surface of the nerve. Lumbrical sparing might reflect greater vulnerability to compression of the more superficial nerve fascicles.

Lumbrical sparing is not specific to carpal tunnel syndrome. It can also occur in patients who have injuries to the recurrent median motor nerve, true neurogenic thoracic outlet syndrome, partial median nerve transection, or median nerve injury in the axilla (Yates et al., 1981; Logigian et al., 1987).

Using the same recording electrode placement and stimulating the ulnar nerve at the wrist, the ulnar nerve motor latency to the interossei can be measured (Preston & Logigian, 1992). Using identical stimulation-to-recording distances of 10 cm, the ulnar-to-interossei and median-to-lumbrical latencies should differ by no more than 0.4 msec. The median-lumbrical latency is abnormal compared with the ulnar-interossei latency in many patients with carpal tunnel syndrome, with approximately the same sensitivity as median palm-to-wrist versus ulnar palm-to-wrist comparisons (Sheean, Houser & Murray, 1995; Loscher, Auer-Grumbach, Trinka, Ladurner & Hartung, 2000; Resende, Adamo, Bononi, Castro, Kimaid, Fortinguerra & Schelp, 2000). Other investigators have found higher upper limits of normal for the median-lumbrical versus ulnar-interossei difference and, hence, found this test to have a lower sensitivity for the diagnosis of carpal tunnel syndrome (Uncini, Di Muzio, Awad, Manente, Tafuro & Gambi, 1993; Seror, 1995).

Palmar Stimulation. Although the median DML is commonly obtained by stimulating the nerve at the wrist and recording over the thenar muscles, the median nerve can be stimulated more distally, in the palm (Figure 7-3). The site for palmar stimulation is approximated by asking the patient to flex the ring finger; the flexed finger points to the point in the palm that is chosen for stimulation. A more exact site of stimulation can be determined by starting slightly distal to this point in the palm and slowly moving the stimulating cathode proximally until stimulation elicits a twitch of the median thenar muscles. The anode is distal to the cathode (Pease, Cunningham, Walsh & Johnson, 1988). Co-activation of the deep ulnar nerve during palmar stimulation can lead to erroneous values for median CMAP amplitude (Di Guglielmo, Torrieri, Repaci & Uncini, 1997; Park, Welshofer, Dzwierzynski, Erickson & Del, 2001).

Kimura (1979) measured wrist-to-palm motor conduction in 122 control hands and 172 hands affected by symptomatic carpal tunnel syndrome (Table 7-5). He found that 61% of carpal tunnel syndrome patients had prolonged median DML (wrist to muscle). In an additional 23% of carpal tunnel syndrome patients, the wrist-to-palm motor conduction velocity was greater than two standard deviations below the mean of the normal controls. Others have agreed that wrist-to-palm motor conduction velocity is more sensitive than DML as a test for carpal tunnel syndrome (Di Guglielmo et al., 1997).

In healthy subjects the amplitude of the CMAP from palmar stimulation is slightly larger than the

Figure 7-3. The site of palmar stimulation of the median nerve for motor conduction test is found by asking the patient to flex the ring finger; the flexed finger points to the approximate stimulation site. The stimulating electrode should explore the vicinity to find the optimal site of stimulation.

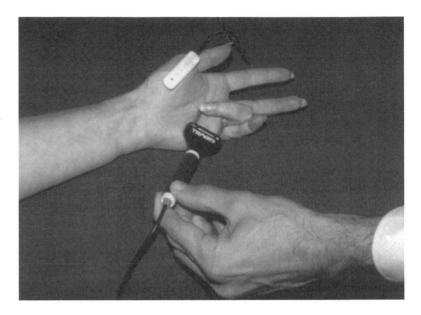

amplitude of the CMAP from wrist stimulation. In many patients who have carpal tunnel syndrome, the loss of amplitude with the more proximal wrist stimulation is greater, suggesting that, in these patients, conduction block ("neurapraxia") is causing at least part of the loss of CMAP amplitude (Kimura, J 1979; Pease et al., 1988; Lesser, Venkatesh, Preston & Logigian, 1995; Di Guglielmo et al., 1997). Table 7-6 gives illustrative data.

Median sensory conduction block across the carpal can be assessed in a similar fashion, recording sensory nerve action potential (SNAP) amplitude in a finger and comparing responses on wrist and palm stimulation. Lesser and colleagues (1995) found that 61% of a group of their patients who had carpal tunnel syndrome had conduction block. The presence of conduction block establishes that the blocked axons are probably intact as they run through the carpal tunnel and that improvement may be relatively rapid after treatment of the nerve compression.

Palmar Serial Motor Stimulation. Median motor conduction in the palm can be further studied by *inching*, that is, serially stimulating the nerve at 1-cm increments in an effort to localize nerve segments with excessive slowing of conduction. The technique is difficult because of the recurrent

course of the motor branch to the thenar muscles, which makes it hard to stimulate only the median nerve in the palm without also stimulating the recurrent motor branch. Kimura (1979) found that motor inching was often impossible to perform accurately.

White and colleagues (1988) took care to stimulate in the palm as far medially as possible in an effort to stimulate the median nerve without also stimulating the recurrent motor branch. They discuss criteria for ensuring the technical accuracy of the stimulation. They found an abnormal 1-cm motor segment in 72% of *asymptomatic* hands in patients who had contralateral unilateral carpal tunnel syndrome. They also describe a technique for performing median nerve palmar inching studies with recording over the second lumbrical.

Table 7-5. Wrist-to-Palm Median Motor Nerve Conduction

	Velocity (m/sec) (Mean ± Standard Deviation)
Controls	49.0 ± 5.7
Carpal tunnel syndrome	28.2 ± 7.5

Data from J Kimura. The carpal tunnel syndrome: localization of conduction abnormalities within the distal segment of the median nerve. Brain 1979;102:619–35.

Table 7-6. Thenar Compound Muscle Action Potential Amplitude: Wrist versus Palmar Stimulation

	Mean Compound Muscle Action Potential Amplitude (mV Mean ± Standard Deviation)		Compound Muscle Action Potential Palm-Wrist Amplitude Ratio (Mean ± Standard Deviation)
	From Palm	From Wrist	
Controls	11.3 ± 2.9	10.9 ± 2.3	1.0 ± 0.1
Carpal tunnel syndrome patients	7.3 ± 3.4	6.2 ± 3.4	1.6 ± 1.3

Data from EA Lesser, S Venkatesh, DC Preston, EL Logigian. Stimulation distal to the lesion in patients with carpal tunnel syndrome. Muscle Nerve 1995;18:503–7.

Median Nerve Conduction in the Forearm. The median forearm MNCV is mildly slowed in some patients who have carpal tunnel syndrome and prolonged median DML (Thomas, 1960). Table 7-7 shows the incidence of this finding in selected series.

Slowed median forearm MNCV is evidence of more severe median nerve compression in the carpal tunnel, but correlations between median forearm MNCV and median DML are imperfect (Uchida & Sugioka, 1993). The series with higher incidences of slowing included more patients with severe carpal tunnel syndrome. Patients with decreased amplitude of the thenar CMAP or prolonged median DML are more likely to have slowing of median forearm MNCV (Stoehr, Petruch, Scheglmann & Schilling, 1978; Kimura & Ayyar, 1985; Tzeng, Wu & Chu, 1990).

Median nerve conduction in the forearm can also be assessed by stimulating the median nerve at the wrist and recording a mixed nerve action potential in the antecubital space or more proximally or by stimulating in the antecubital space and recording a mixed nerve action potential at the wrist (Stoehr, Petruch, Scheglmann & Schilling, 1978; Pease, Lee & Johnson, 1990; White, 1997). The median nerve

Table 7-7. Incidence of Forearm Motor Nerve Conduction Velocity Slowing in Carpal Tunnel Syndrome Patients

Study	Incidence (%)
Buchthal & Rosenfalck, 1971	50–65
Thomas, Lambert & Cseuz, 1967	43
Kimura & Ayyar, 1985	23
Stevens, 1987	11
Fox & Bangash, 1996	18
Tzeng, Wu & Chu, 1990	11

between the wrist and the antecubital space includes motor fibers for median-innervated hand intrinsic muscles, sensory fibers for median digital nerves, and sensory fibers for the median palmar cutaneous nerve. In patients who have carpal tunnel syndrome, the forearm mixed nerve conduction velocity is usually not slowed, presumably because the median palmar cutaneous nerve is unaffected by carpal tunnel syndrome (Hansson, 1994; Fox & Bangash, 1996). However, in patients who have more severe carpal tunnel syndrome, the amplitude of the mixed nerve action potential recorded at the antecubital space is decreased (Stoehr et al., 1978; Uchida & Sugioka, 1993; Hansson, 1994). The median forearm sensory conduction velocity is also reduced in some patients who have carpal tunnel syndrome; the reduction is usually less than the reduction in forearm motor conduction velocity (Hansson, 1994).

In patients who have carpal tunnel syndrome and median motor conduction slowing in the forearm, a cause for the slowing other than carpal tunnel syndrome must be considered. In one small sample, over 40% of patients who had carpal tunnel syndrome and forearm median motor conduction velocity that was even slower than 3 m/sec below the lower normal limit had an additional neuropathic diagnosis such as diffuse peripheral neuropathy (Donahue, Raynor & Rutkove, 1998).

Two mechanisms can contribute to slowing of forearm motor conduction in patients with carpal tunnel syndrome. First, the largest, fastest conducting myelinated fibers can be compressed severely enough to develop conduction block across the carpal tunnel, so that forearm motor conduction velocity calculated by stimulation at the wrist and antecubital space does not measure their function. This hypothesis is supported by showing that median forearm mixed nerve conduction velocity, obtained by stimulating the wrist and recording a mixed nerve action potential in the antecubital space, is not slowed in some patients who have carpal tunnel syndrome and slowed forearm motor conduction. However, in other patients forearm mixed nerve conduction is slowed, supporting the second mechanism: More severely compressed nerve fibers can develop retrograde changes, such as distortion of myelin (Anderson, Fullerton, Gilliatt & Hern, 1970; Pease, Lee & Johnson, 1990; Chang, Chiang, Ger, Yang & Lo, 2000).

Anterior Interosseus Nerve Conduction. In some patients who have severe carpal tunnel syndrome and thenar muscle atrophy, a reproducible median thenar CMAP is unobtainable, and median forearm motor conduction to the thenar muscles cannot be assessed. In these patients, one approach to excluding a median neuropathy proximal to the carpal tunnel or a more diffuse neuropathy is to measure the conduction in the anterior interosseus nerve (see Chapter 17 for techniques), which is unaffected by median nerve compression in the carpal tunnel but is often impaired with more proximal median nerve dysfunction (Shafshak & El-Hinawy, 1995). Anterior interosseus nerve conduction studies can also be helpful in deciding whether median forearm motor conduction slowing in patients with carpal tunnel syndrome is attributable to the compression at the carpal tunnel or to some additional neuropathy.

Martin-Gruber Anastomosis. The anatomy of the Martin-Gruber anastomosis is discussed in Chapter 1 (Figure 7-4). The fibers participating in the Martin-Gruber anastomosis are motor components of the median nerve at the level of the antecubital space. These fibers then cross to the ulnar nerve in the forearm, usually via the anterior interosseous nerve. The fibers cross the wrist with the ulnar nerve and may then innervate hypothenar, thenar, or interosseous muscles.

Sun and Streib (1983) searched systematically for the Martin-Gruber anastomosis in 150 arms by comparing the amplitude of the thenar, hypothenar, and first dorsal interosseous CMAPs from median nerve stimulation at the wrist and at the antecubital space. The electrodiagnostic criteria for the anomaly were as follows:

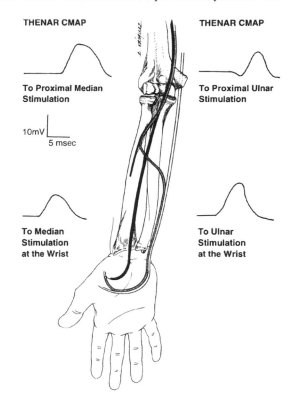

Figure 7-4. Martin-Gruber anastomosis. The compound muscle action potentials (CMAPs) recorded over the thenar eminence to median and to ulnar nerve stimulation are shown. This patient meets Sun and Streib's (1983) criteria 1 and 2 for presence of the anastomosis.

1. A thenar CMAP that was larger with median nerve stimulation at the antecubital space than at the wrist,
2. A thenar CMAP that was at least 25% smaller with ulnar stimulation above the elbow compared by ulnar stimulation at the wrist,
3. A hypothenar CMAP with initial negative deflection obtained by median stimulation at the antecubital space, or
4. A first dorsal interosseous CMAP that was at least 25% larger with median stimulation at the antecubital space than with median stimulation at the wrist.

Note that application of the second criterion assumes that there is no co-existing ulnar conduction block between the two stimulating sites. Figure 7-4 shows typical CMAPs obtained over the

Table 7-8. Incidence of Martin-Gruber Anastomosis

Muscle Innervated by Anastomotic Fibers	Percent
First dorsal interosseus	34
Thenar	12
Hypothenar	16
At least one of the above	34

Data from SF Sun, EW Streib. Martin-Gruber anastomosis: electromyographic studies. Electromyogr. Clin. Neurophysiol. 1983;23:271–85.

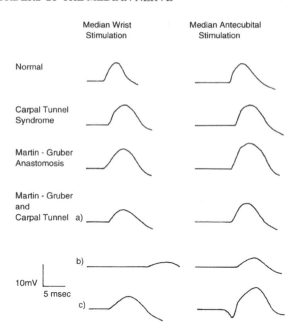

Figure 7-5. Typical waveforms of thenar compound muscle action potential in patients who have both carpal tunnel syndrome and Martin-Gruber anastomosis. The stimulation sites are shown in Figure 7-4.

thenar eminence in a patient with Martin-Gruber anastomosis.

Table 7-8 shows the incidence of detection of Martin-Gruber anastomosis at the different recording sites (Sun & Streib, 1983).

Even in the absence of the Martin-Gruber anastomosis, a volume-conducted response from thenar muscles is routinely recorded over the first dorsal interosseous and the hypothenar eminence after median nerve stimulation. To eliminate the effect of volume-conducted responses, Kimura and colleagues (1976) used a collision technique, stimulating the median nerve at the wrist followed by a paired stimulus in the antecubital space. Using this technique, recording from thenar and hypothenar muscles, but not from the first dorsal interosseous, they found Martin-Gruber anastomosis in 17% of arms.

Patients who have both carpal tunnel syndrome and a Martin-Gruber anastomosis often show distinctive findings on nerve conduction studies. The median latency to thenar muscles after antecubital stimulation can be normal despite prolongation of the DML (Figure 7-5, example a) (Iyer & Fenichel, 1976). This combination can lead to an erroneously high calculated value for forearm MNCV. At the extreme, the median DML may be longer than the latency from antecubital stimulation to the thenar CMAP (see Figure 7-5, example b). Another variation is a bifid or double-humped thenar CMAP to median nerve stimulation in the antecubital area (Lambert, 1962).

When carpal tunnel syndrome and Martin-Gruber anastomosis co-exist, the thenar CMAP from median nerve stimulation at the wrist may have an initial negative deflection, while the thenar CMAP from median nerve stimulation at the antecubital space has an initial positive deflection (see Figure 7-5, example c) (Gutmann, 1977). The positive deflection is explained by volume-conducted potentials from thenar or first dorsal interosseous muscles that are innervated via fibers that are in the median nerve at the antecubital space, then cross with the anastomosis, and enter the hand in the ulnar nerve. Fibers that cross in the anastomosis do not go through the carpal tunnel, and conduction in these fibers is not slowed in carpal tunnel syndrome. This finding may be present even when median DML and transcarpal sensory conduction are normal (Gutmann, Gutierrez & Riggs, 1986).

Individuals who have a Martin-Gruber anastomosis can have unusual nerve conduction responses following injuries to the median or ulnar nerves in the forearm (Kingery, Wu & Date, 1996).

A much more unusual finding is ulnar-to-median motor anastomosis in the forearm (Resende, Adamo, Kimaid, Castro, Canheu & Schelp, 2000). The characteristic is a median antecubital-stimulation CMAP that is lower in amplitude than the median wrist-stimulation

CMAP over the thenar muscles, coupled with a thenar CMAP to ulnar stimulation at the elbow with an initial negative deflection.

Threshold Distal Motor Latency. Preswick (1963) proposed measuring conduction in other than fastest median motor fibers. He recorded in the abductor pollicis brevis with a needle electrode while stimulating the median nerve at the wrist. Rather than use supramaximal nerve stimulation, he gradually increased stimulus intensity until the first motor unit was recorded. He then measured latency to onset of this potential. In 25 control subjects, this latency, the *threshold distal motor latency*, was shorter than or equal to 5.2 msec. Preswick studied 29 hands in which carpal tunnel syndrome was clinically suspected. Of these, 83% had a prolonged threshold DML, but only 38% had a prolonged supramaximal DML.

Loong (1977), using surface recording electrodes, found that 52% of patients who had a clinical diagnosis of carpal tunnel syndrome had a prolonged median threshold DML, while only 35% had a prolonged supramaximal DML.

In vitro the largest myelinated fibers have the lowest threshold to electrical stimulation; in theory, with threshold stimulation, the largest myelinated fibers are stimulated so that threshold conduction velocity is equal to supramaximal conduction velocity. In contrast, in human median nerve motor conduction studies, stimulating at the wrist, the supramaximal DML and threshold DML are unequal (Preswick, 1963). This inequality implies that topographic factors, such as the proximity of fibers to the stimulating electrode, influence the selection of the fibers responding to threshold stimulus.

Some patients who have carpal tunnel syndrome have a larger than normal range between threshold stimulation voltage (i.e., voltage of the stimulus, not CMAP amplitude) and the maximal stimulation voltage (Brismar, 1985). This is not a useful diagnostic test for carpal tunnel syndrome, first because of low sensitivity and second because the effect is also observed in neuropathies such as those caused by diabetes or uremia (Brismar, 1985).

Motor Unit Number Estimates. The number of thenar motor units innervated by the median nerve can be estimated by comparing the CMAP amplitude to supramaximal stimulation to CMAP amplitudes to selected submaximal stimuli (Cuturic & Palliyath, 2000). This parameter is below normal in some patients who have moderate to severe carpal tunnel syndrome.

F-Wave Studies. The F-wave is a late response recorded from muscle following mixed nerve stimulation. It can be recorded from the median-innervated thenar muscles following median nerve stimulation. The nerve stimulation is performed with the cathode proximal to the anode, the reverse of the normal electrode orientation used for routine nerve conduction studies. A nerve stimulus does not always evoke an F-response. At most, the nerve stimulus evokes an F-response in only a fraction of the stimulated motor neurons; therefore, the amplitude of the F-wave is only a fraction of the amplitude of the CMAP from supramaximal stimulation. The configuration and latency of the F-wave varies from stimulus to stimulus. Multiple stimuli are needed to evaluate the range of F-wave responses from an individual nerve. Normal values for F-waves latency vary with height, age, and gender (Buschbacher, 1999). Many of the studies discussed here measure the *minimum* F-wave latency; subsequent analysis of normative median nerve F-waves values suggests that use of the *mean* F-wave latency might be more reliable and slightly more sensitive (Fisher, Hoffen & Hultman, 1994; Fisher & Hoffen, 1997).

In some patients who have carpal tunnel syndrome and prolonged median DML, the minimum F-wave latency from the wrist is proportionately prolonged (Eisen, Schomer & Melmed, 1977). In other patients the DML is prolonged out of proportion to the F-wave latency (Kimura, 1983). Table 7-9 shows representative data.

The prolongation of median nerve F-wave latency in patients who have carpal tunnel syndrome can reflect both delayed conduction across the carpal tunnel, as measured by DML, and delayed median nerve conduction proximal to the carpal tunnel. The effects of conduction proximal to the carpal tunnel can be isolated by calculating an F-wave conduction velocity, using a formula that subtracts the median DML from the minimal median F-wave latency from wrist stimulation. The proximal median nerve conduction velocity to thenar muscles can be compared with the con-

Table 7-9. Median Nerve F-Wave Latency in Patients with Carpal Tunnel Syndrome

	Median Distal Motor Latency (msec; Mean ± Standard Deviation)	Minimum F-Wave Latency (Wrist) (msec; Mean ± Standard Deviation)
Controls	3.4 ± 0.4	26.6 ± 2.2
Patients with carpal tunnel syndrome	5.4 ± 1.2	30.8 ± 3.3

Data from A Eisen, D Schomer, C Melmed. The application of F-wave measurements in the differentiation of proximal and distal upper limb entrapments. Neurology 1977;27:662–68.

duction velocity of the median nerve to a more proximal muscle such as pronator quadratus. In patients with carpal tunnel syndrome the proximal conduction to thenar muscles may be slowed, while the conduction velocity to pronator quadratus should be normal unless the patient has an additional abnormality of the median nerve proximal to the carpal tunnel (Anastasopoulos & Chroni, 1997).

In carpal tunnel syndrome patients who have normal motor and sensory conduction studies, minimum median nerve F-wave latency to thenar muscles is sometimes abnormal by virtue of being prolonged in comparison with the minimum ulnar F-wave latency to abductor digiti minimi (Menkes, Hood & Bush, 1997). A prolonged median F-wave latency with a normal median DML does not distinguish between carpal tunnel syndrome and a proximal median neuropathy or brachial plexopathy. Nerves in addition to the median must be studied since a prolonged F-wave latency can also be seen in peripheral neuropathies.

Another way to use the F-wave to evaluate conduction through the carpal tunnel is to compare the minimum median nerve F-wave latency with palmar stimulation with the minimum median F-wave latency with wrist stimulation. In one series, the difference between these two latencies was abnormal in 64% of patients with carpal tunnel syndrome, including some cases with normal median DML and DSL (Maccabee, Shahani & Young, 1980).

The F-wave chronodispersion is the difference between the minimum F-wave latency and the maximum F-wave latency. Accurate measurement of chronodispersion requires many more than the 10 to 20 stimuli that are used in many clinics for F-wave recordings. In patients who have carpal tunnel syndrome, median nerve F-wave chronodispersion is more likely to be increased if the DML is prolonged (Fisher & Hoffen, 1997).

Macleod (1987) recorded 100 consecutive F-waves in the thenar muscles evoked by stimulation of an individual median nerve. He defined a "repeater F-wave" (RF) as an F-wave that was identical in configuration, amplitude, and latency to the F-wave elicited by the preceding stimulus (Figure 7-6). He calculated the ratio of RF responses to total elicited F-waves to obtain a "% repeater F-wave value" (%RF). In 90% of controls the %RF was less than 37; in 84% of carpal tunnel syndrome patients, the %RF was greater than 37. In patients who have carpal tunnel syndrome, the %RF can be abnormal when the DML and palm-to-wrist sensory latency are normal. The %RF can also be abnormal in other disorders of the alpha motor neuron. If the thenar %RF is 60% or greater in a patient who has carpal tunnel syndrome, the patient often has sustained median nerve axonal injury (Fisher & Hoffen, 1997).

Sensory Nerve Conduction

Technique

Median nerve sensory conduction can be assessed by a number of different techniques (Liveson & Ma, 1992). Figure 7-7 illustrates typical electrode placement. The technical details of papers on sensory conduction must be read carefully. Variations of technique between laboratories often make it difficult to compare results of one study with those of another.

For median sensory antidromic stimulation, the nerve is stimulated at the wrist or palm while recording with ring electrodes on any of the first four digits. For median sensory orthodromic stimulation, the nerve is stimulated on a median-innervated digit or at the palm. The potential recorded at the wrist or proximally to palmar stimulation is actually a mixed nerve action potential. The recording electrodes are placed over the median nerve at the wrist or more proximally along its

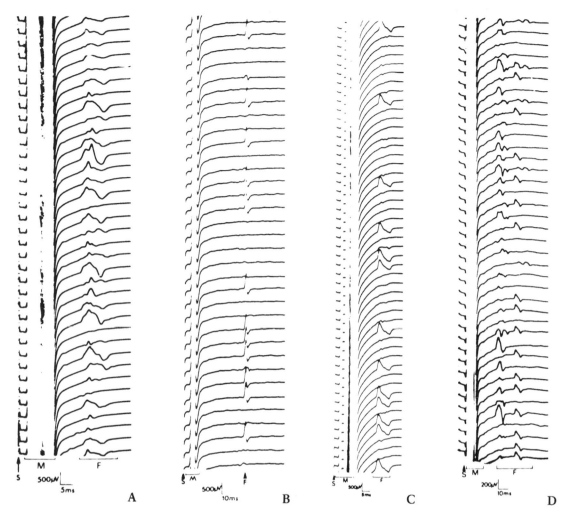

Figure 7-6. (A) F-wave sweeps from a healthy median nerve. Two F-waves recur; % repeater F-wave (RF) value = 12%. **(B–D)** Median nerve F-wave sweeps from patients who have carpal tunnel syndrome. **(B)** RF follows the majority of supramaximal stimuli at a delayed latency. **(C)** Two RFs predominate. **(D)** RFs firing "in series." Two individual RFs repeatedly follow the initial F response. (Reprinted with permission from WN Macleod. Repeater F waves: a comparison of sensitivity with sensory antidromic wrist-to-palm latency and distal motor latency in the diagnosis of carpal tunnel syndrome. Neurology 1987;37:773–78.)

course, such as in the antecubital fossa or in the axilla. Some examiners use needle rather than surface electrodes for stimulation or recording (Johnson & Melvin, 1967; Buchthal & Rosenfalck, 1971). Surface and needle electrodes are equally effective for diagnostic purposes (Smith, 1998).

Latency to negative peak varies with distance between recording electrodes. By changing the positions of the recording electrodes, slight differences can be detected between orthodromic and antidromic latencies (Murai & Sanderson,

1975). Whether orthodromic or antidromic approaches are used has little practical effect on normal or pathologic values (Ludin, Lutschg & Valsangiacomo, 1977; Goddard, Barnes, Berry & Evans, 1983).

To assess conduction velocity in the fastest myelinated sensory fibers, the latency is measured to onset of the SNAP. The SNAP amplitude is measured in microvolts, and an averager is often needed to obtain accurately measurable latencies and amplitudes. Many examiners measure latency

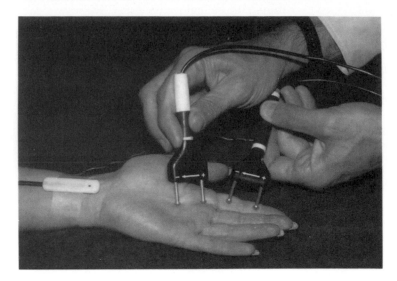

Figure 7-7. Typical electrode placement for measuring sensory nerve conduction between the wrist and index finger. The example shown is an orthodromic study with the stimulating electrodes on the index finger and in the palm and the recording electrode over the wrist.

**MEDIAN SNAP
at Wrist**

Stimulate Index Finger

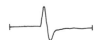

Stimulate Palm

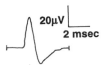

to SNAP initial positive peak or initial negative peak rather than onset; this decreases measurement error, but a conduction velocity calculated based on peak latency does not reflect the velocity of the fastest fibers. Analysis can use latency data obtained with a constant distance between stimulating and recording electrodes; alternatively, conduction velocity can be calculated from distance and latency measurements.

Some examiners measure SNAP amplitude from negative peak to positive peak; others measure from baseline to negative peak. Amplitudes are greater

with antidromic than with orthodromic stimulation and greater with needle than with surface recording electrodes. Amplitude, duration, and configuration depend on the distance between the recording electrodes (Gilliatt, Melville, Velate & Willison, 1965).

The upper limit of normal for median DSL can be decreased, and the diagnostic sensitivity can be increased, with attention to details such as temperature control and careful distance measurement (Di Benedetto, Mitz, Klingbeil & Davidoff, 1986). Table 7-10 shows examples of normal limits for median sensory nerve conduction studies.

Findings in Carpal Tunnel Syndrome

Finger-to-Wrist Conduction. In patients who have carpal tunnel syndrome, median sensory conduction studies are more likely than median DML to be abnormal (Kopell & Goodgold, 1968). Thomas and colleagues (1967) found sensory conduction abnormalities in 85% of their patients who had carpal tunnel syndrome. They did not use an averager, and the most common abnormal-

Table 7-10. Median Sensory Nerve Conduction: Examples of Normal Values

Source	Technique	Normal Limits
Gilliatt & Sears, 1958	Orthodromic digit II	Peak latency ≤4.0 msec; amplitude ≥9 μV
Mayo Clinic (Stevens, 1987)	Antidromic digit II	Peak latency ≤3.5 msec (distance 13 cm); amplitude ≥25 μV

ity was an unobtainable or indiscernible SNAP. Melvin and colleagues (1973) found a prolonged latency from wrist to index finger in 88% of their 17 patients who had carpal tunnel syndrome. In contrast, only 76% of their patients had a prolonged median DML, and only 6% had an abnormally low SNAP amplitude.

Transcarpal Conduction. Sensory conduction time in the segment of the median nerve in the carpal tunnel can be derived by stimulating at the wrist and at the mid-palm while recording the SNAP from a digit. The transcarpal sensory conduction time is the difference of the two measured latencies (Wiederholt, 1970). Transcarpal nerve conduction can also be studied by stimulating the median nerve in the palm and recording over the nerve at the wrist or more proximally (Eklund, 1975; Mills, 1985). In this technique both motor and sensory fibers are stimulated, and a mixed nerve action potential is recorded. Both techniques give similar latency values (Tackmann, Kaeser & Magun, 1981; Monga, Shanks & Poole, 1985). In healthy subjects the median sensory nerve conduction velocity (SNCV) between digit and palm and between palm and wrist is the same (Buchthal & Rosenfalck, 1971). The fascicular contributions of individual common digital nerves to the transcarpal median nerve conduction can be studied by comparing the response at the wrist to distal palmar stimulation between the second and third metacarpal versus stimulation between the third and fourth metacarpal (Rossi, Giannini, Passero, Paradiso, Battistini & Cioni, 1994).

In patients who have carpal tunnel syndrome, conduction in the palm-to-wrist segment of the median nerve is often disproportionately slowed; these patients sometimes have normal digit-to-wrist conduction but abnormally slow palm-to-wrist conduction (Buchthal & Rosenfalck, 1971). However, in other patients who have carpal tunnel syndrome, the SNCV is slowed in both the digit-to-palm and palm-to-wrist segment of the nerve. Patients with diffuse peripheral neuropathies, such as diabetic neuropathy, can also have slowing of both digit-to-palm and palm-to-wrist conduction (Casey & Le-Quesne, 1972).

Median palm-wrist latency is now a standard technique for electrodiagnostic evaluation of carpal tunnel syndrome (Anonymous, 1993; Stevens,

Table 7-11. Variation in Sensory Nerve Conduction Velocity Results by Finger Tested in 30 Patients with Carpal Tunnel Syndrome

	Recording Site			
Result	Thumb	Index	Middle	Ring
Unobtainable	2	1	0	3
Digit-to-wrist slow	18	16	21	21
Palm-to-wrist slow (digit-to-wrist normal)	7	9	8	4
Normal	3	4	1	2

Data from K Toyonaga, CR DeFaria. Electromyographic diagnosis of the carpal tunnel syndrome. Arq. Neuropsiquiatr. 1978;36:127–34.

1997). Typically, a latency to peak of less than or equal to 2.2 msec is normal for a palm-wrist distance of 8 cm.

Variability of Digital Nerves. In most cases of carpal tunnel syndrome, sensory fibers in all median digital nerves are affected. This can be demonstrated by measuring conduction to each digit separately from the wrist or by calculating a transcarpal SNCV for each digit. Table 7-11 shows data from an orthodromic study (Toyonaga & DeFaria, 1978). Note that the index finger is somewhat less likely to show abnormal values, a finding also reported by other laboratories (Cioni, Passero, Paradiso, Giannini, Battistini & Rushworth, 1989; Terzis, Paschalis, Metallinos & Papapetropoulos, 1998). The ring finger-to-wrist median SNAP was the most likely to be absent.

When ring electrodes are used for orthodromic sensory studies, both digital nerves in a digit are stimulated. Macdonell and colleagues (1990) used a pair of stimulating electrodes held against the lateral or medial side of the digit in an effort to stimulate individual digital nerves. They recorded with surface electrodes at the wrist. In hands of women who had a clinical diagnosis of carpal tunnel syndrome, abnormalities varied in frequency from one digital nerve to the next as shown in Figure 7-8. These data are from 29 dominant hands; similar findings were recorded in nondominant hands. Again, the index finger was least likely to yield abnormal results. The SNAP

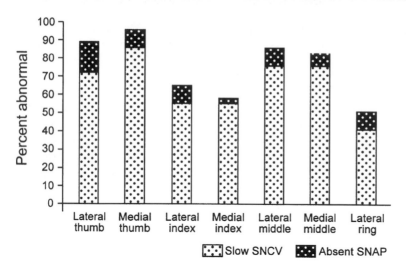

Figure 7-8. The results of digital nerve stimulation in patients who have carpal tunnel syndrome. The site of stimulation is shown at the bottom; recordings were made at the wrist. (SNAP = sensory nerve action potential; SNCV = sensory nerve conduction velocity.) (Data from RA Macdonell, MS Schwartz, M Swash. Carpal tunnel syndrome: which finger should be tested? An analysis of sensory conduction in digital branches of the median nerve. Muscle Nerve 1990;13:601–6.)

from the ring finger was most often absent, perhaps because of ulnar nerve supply of this digital nerve in some patients or perhaps because, in the other digits, volume-conducted stimulation of the adjoining digital nerve was more likely to give a higher-amplitude SNAP.

Ultradistal Sensory Studies. Ultradistal sensory nerve conduction studies are done by stimulating at the tips of each digit of both hands and recording at the ipsilateral wrist (Seror, 1996). Indications of abnormality include low-amplitude SNAP in one or more digits compared with other digits or prolonged latency for some digits but not for others. Some patients who have symptoms of carpal tunnel syndrome have abnormalities on ultradistal sensory studies but not on more conventional median nerve conduction studies. The published data on this technique are limited to a few patients.

Palmar Serial Sensory Studies. Kimura (1979) standardized a technique for studying the sensory conduction in the median nerve centimeter by centimeter. He used ring recording electrodes on the index finger and stimulated the nerve at 1-cm intervals along the distal forearm and palm. Serial studies can also be done orthodromically by stimulating a digit and moving the recording electrodes centimeter by centimeter across the palm and wrist (Seror, 1998, 2000). Kimura measured latency to onset of negative deflection and subtracted successive latencies to obtain a latency

difference for each centimeter of the nerve. In controls the mean latency difference was 0.2 msec/cm. The latency difference for the portions of the nerve under the carpal ligament, 1 to 4 cm distal to the distal wrist crease, were slightly greater than for the adjacent distal and proximal segments of the nerve. For example, mean latency difference was 0.22 msec for the segment 3 to 4 cm past the distal wrist crease and 0.17 msec for the segment 4 to 5 cm past the distal wrist crease.

Approximately one-half of patients who had carpal tunnel syndrome showed slowing of sensory conduction distributed fairly evenly along the palm-to-wrist portion of the nerve; the other one-half of the patients showed localized conduction delay in one segment. Kimura used delay of *greater than* 0.5 msec over 1 cm as abnormal. In 4 of 172 hands with symptoms of carpal tunnel syndrome, he found a delayed conduction latency difference over 1 cm, even though wrist-to-palm latencies were normal.

Other authors have proposed increasing the diagnostic sensitivity of serial palmar sensory studies by using a latency difference over 1 cm of *greater than or equal to* 0.4 msec as abnormal. For example, Seror (1988) found this measure abnormal in each of 45 cases of carpal tunnel syndrome and initially thought this criteria could eliminate false-negative results; later Seror (1990, 1998) found cases with typical carpal tunnel syndrome symptoms but no abnormality on palmar median serial sensory latency studies.

Nathan and colleagues (1988) studied segmental sensory latency values over 1 cm in 70 hands of 38 controls who had no clinical suggestion of carpal tunnel syndrome and in 54 hands affected by carpal tunnel syndrome. Using criteria for carpal tunnel syndrome that relied heavily on classical clinical history, they found that the maximum segmental latency difference was greater than or equal to 0.4 msec in 81% and greater than or equal to 0.5 msec in 54% of hands affected by carpal tunnel syndrome (see Table 8-11).

Imaoka and colleagues (1992) suggested another version of the serial technique: median nerve stimulation at the antecubital space and recording along the nerve between the wrist and fingers using a linear array of electrodes spaced at 15-mm intervals. Bipolar recordings were made from adjacent paired electrodes.

Ipsilateral Comparison Methods. Comparing conduction in the median nerve with conduction in ipsilateral radial or ulnar nerves minimizes confounding personal factors, such as age and temperature, that decrease diagnostic sensitivity by increasing the variation in healthy subjects.

MEDIAN VERSUS ULNAR COMPARISON. When median wrist-to-index finger and ulnar wrist-to-little finger sensory latencies are obtained over identical distances in the same hand, they are normally within 0.4 msec. of each other (Felsenthal, 1977). When median wrist-to-ring finger and ulnar wrist-to-ring finger sensory latencies are compared over 14 cm in the same hand, the difference in latencies is normally 0.3 msec or less (Johnson, Kukla, Wongsam & Piedmont, 1981). In patients who have carpal tunnel syndrome and normal ulnar nerve function, stimulating the ring finger and recording over the median nerve at the wrist may elicit a bifid or double-peak SNAP since the volume-conducted ulnar SNAP may arrive before the delayed median response (Haloua, Soulier & Collin, 1994; Seror, 1994). One disadvantage of using the ring finger for studies is the lower amplitude of the ring finger SNAP for either nerve compared with the amplitudes from other digits. Another disadvantage is the possibility of anomalous sensory patterns: Ring finger innervation can be solely median or solely ulnar (Monga & Laidlow, 1982). If the median nerve ring finger SNAP is absent, either because of carpal tunnel syndrome

or because of anomalous innervation, the SNAP recorded over the median nerve at the wrist after ring finger stimulation can actually be a volume-conducted ulnar nerve SNAP (Capone, Pentore, Lunazzi & Schonhuber, 1998). Felsenthal (1978a) studied 82 hands affected by carpal tunnel syndrome and found that 17 had an increased median minus ulnar latency difference even though the median wrist-to-index finger sensory latency was normal. Others have also found that comparing ulnar and median nerve responses to ring finger stimulation is a sensitive test for carpal tunnel syndrome (Uncini, Lange, Solomon, Soliven, Meer & Lovelace, 1989; Uncini, Di Muzio, Cutarella, Awad & Gambi, 1990; Lauritzen, Liguori & Trojaborg, 1991).

In some series, patients who had carpal tunnel syndrome were more likely than controls to show abnormalities of ulnar nerve conduction. Sedal and colleagues (1973) found low amplitude ulnar SNAPs in 39% and delayed ulnar DSL in 5% of hands that had both clinical and nerve conduction evidence of carpal tunnel syndrome. Patients who have generalized peripheral neuropathy or an illness, such as diabetes, that might predispose to neuropathy were excluded. Harrison (1978) disagreed, finding normal ulnar SNAP amplitude in 60 consecutive patients who had carpal tunnel syndrome. Cassvan and colleagues (1986) found an ulnar DSL greater than or equal to 3.7 msec. in 46% of patients who had carpal tunnel syndrome. Mortier and colleagues (1988) found a prolonged ulnar DML in 18% of patients who had carpal tunnel syndrome. The mechanism underlying these ulnar nerve conduction abnormalities may vary from patient to patient. If ulnar abnormalities are present, they decrease the sensitivity of median-ulnar comparison methods.

Median and ulnar motor conduction can also be used for comparison studies. For example, in healthy subjects the difference between the median DML to the thenar muscles and an ulnar latency from wrist stimulation to a response at the thenar muscles is no more than 0.8 msec; the ulnar and median action potentials are recorded with the same electrode placement, so the ulnar CMAP is initially positive rather than negative (Sander, Quinto, Saadeh & Chokroverty, 1999). Normal values and diagnostic sensitivities have also been proposed for comparing median wrist-

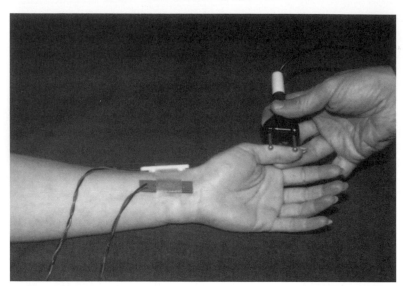

Figure 7-9. Typical electrode placement for comparing orthodromic nerve conduction in the radial and median nerves between the thumb and the wrist.

to-thenar with ulnar wrist-to-hypothenar latencies or for comparing median with ulnar F-wave latencies.

MEDIAN VERSUS RADIAL COMPARISON. With stimulation of the thumb, a SNAP can be recorded over the median nerve at the wrist or over the superficial radial nerve as it crosses the extensor pollicis longus tendon to course along the lateral aspect of the radius (Figure 7-9). For comparison, the distance for the two nerves from the stimulating to the recording electrodes should be the same (Carroll, 1987). When the median latency is prolonged, a double-peak SNAP is sometimes recorded over the median nerve at the wrist from a volume-conducted radial SNAP arriving before the delayed-median SNAP (Padua, LoMonaco, Gregori, Valente & Tonali, 1996). Alternatively, ring recording electrodes can be placed on the thumb at the metacarpal-phalangeal and interphalangeal joints, and the median or radial nerves may be stimulated 10 cm proximally (Johnson, Sipski & Lammertse, 1987). Measured orthodromically or antidromically, the difference between the sensory latencies of the two nerves normally should be less than 0.5 msec (Carroll, 1987; Johnson et al., 1987).

Another approach to median versus radial comparison is to check the median wrist to digit latency against the superficial radial latency for conduction in the forearm, recording over the nerve as it crosses the extensor pollicis longus tendon on the dorsal radial wrist (Ghavanini, Kazemi, Jazayeri & Khosrawi, 1996).

Carroll (1987) found that 49% of 161 patients who had a clinical diagnosis of carpal tunnel syndrome had abnormal thumb-to-wrist median sensory latencies. An additional 21% of patients showed abnormal median nerve conduction demonstrated by a prolonged median-radial sensory latency difference. Others have also noted high sensitivity for median versus radial comparisons (Cassvan, Ralescu, Shapiro, Moshkovski & Weiss, 1988; Pease, Cannell & Johnson, 1989).

SENSORY NERVE ACTION POTENTIAL AMPLITUDE COMPARISONS. The median SNAP amplitude, whether antidromically or orthodromically determined, is normal in most patients who have mild carpal tunnel syndrome. Diagnostic sensitivity can be increased by comparing it with the ulnar SNAP amplitude. For example, Table 7-12 shows the results of Loong and Seah (1971, 1972) using surface electrodes and orthodromic technique.

Of their 23 patients who had carpal tunnel syndrome, only 37% had a subnormal median SNAP amplitude, but 91% had a median to ulnar SNAP amplitude ratio below the normal range. In four of the patients, the digit-to-wrist median sensory latency was normal, but the median to ulnar SNAP amplitude ratio was abnormal.

Felsenthal (1978a) extended this approach to antidromic studies, comparing SNAP amplitudes in the index finger from median wrist stimulation and in the ring finger from ulnar wrist stimulation. He found that the normal range of ratios of median to ulnar SNAP amplitudes was 0.67 to 2.0. A ratio less than 0.67 was more sensitive than median SNAP amplitude alone in identifying carpal tunnel syndrome patients.

HAND VERSUS FOREARM SENSORY NERVE CONDUCTION VELOCITY COMPARISON. Kimura and Ayyar (1985) calculated median sensory conduction velocity from wrist to index finger and from antecubital space to wrist based on latencies to negative peak. They found, in patients who had carpal tunnel syndrome, but never in controls, that the ratio of hand SNCV to forearm SNCV was always less than 0.75. This ratio was abnormal even in carpal tunnel syndrome patients with normal DSL and conduction velocities. Scelsa and colleagues (1998) used a similar concept by subtracting the median palm-to-wrist mixed nerve conduction velocity from the median forearm mixed nerve conduction velocity or the median palm-to-digit sensory conduction velocity and reported a sensitivity of 87% and specificity of 98% for the diagnosis of carpal tunnel syndrome.

PALM-WRIST VERSUS DIGIT-PALM COMPARISON. Padua and colleagues (1996) compared median nerve conduction from the middle finger to the palm versus conduction from palm to wrist. Stimulating the middle finger and recording in the palm and at the wrist, they calculated SNCVs, then calculated the ratio of distal conduction velocity to proximal conduction velocity:

$$\text{Distal-proximal ratio} = \frac{\text{SNCV}_{\text{middle finger-to-palm}}}{\text{SNCV}_{\text{palm-wrist}}}$$

In all control subjects, the distal-proximal ratio was less than 1.0; in 98% of hands with a clinical diagnosis of carpal tunnel syndrome, the distal-proximal ratio was greater than 1.0. The distal-proximal ratio was a more sensitive test for carpal tunnel syndrome than palm-to-wrist conduction, median versus ulnar comparison, or median versus radial comparison.

MEDIAN THUMB-WRIST VERSUS MEDIAN PALMAR CUTANEOUS NERVE COMPARISON.   Chang and Lien (1991) compared orthodromic sensory conduction of median nerve from the thumb to the wrist versus the palmar cutaneous branch of the median

Table 7-12. Ratio of Median to Ulnar Sensory Nerve Action Potential Amplitude in Controls and Patients Who Had Carpal Tunnel Syndrome

	Median Sensory Nerve Action Potential Amplitude (μV)		Ratio of Median to Ulnar Amplitude	
	Mean	Range	Mean	Range
Controls	28.6	9–48	1.5	1.1–2.4
Patients who had carpal tunnel syndrome		0–18		0.4–1.3

Data from SC Loong, CS Seah. Comparison of median and ulnar sensory nerve action potentials in the diagnosis of the carpal tunnel syndrome. J. Neurol. Neurosurg. Psychiatry 1971;34: 750–54; and SC Loong, CS Seah. A sensitive diagnostic test for carpal tunnel syndrome. Singapore Med. J. 1972;13: 249–55.

nerve from the thenar eminence to the wrist. The palmar cutaneous branch leaves the median nerve proximal to the carpal tunnel, so it is spared by median nerve compression in the carpal tunnel. Among patients who had carpal tunnel syndrome, 84% had an abnormal increase of the difference between these two latencies, providing a more sensitive test than median palm-to-wrist latency in this series. Obtaining a reproducible SNAP from median palmar cutaneous nerve stimulation can be technically challenging (Foresti, Quadri, Rasella, Tironi, Viscardi & Ubiali, 1996).

COMBINED SENSORY INDEX. The combined sensory index (CSI) is the sum of three comparative latency differences: (1) median minus ulnar palm-to-wrist (8 cm), (2) median minus ulnar wrist-to-ring finger (14 cm), and (3) median minus radial wrist-to-thumb (10 cm) (Robinson, Micklesen & Wang, 1998). Using the normal values shown in Table 7-13, the CSI has better specificity and sensitivity for the diagnosis of carpal tunnel syndrome than does any one of the individual comparison latencies and has better reliability than a single comparison latency (Bland, 2000). An electrodiagnostic approach that maintains the specificity and sensitivity of the CSI while minimizing the number of tests per patient is to start by measuring the wrist-to-ring finger latency difference (Robinson et al., 2000; Kaul, Pagel & Dryden, 2001). If the median minus ulnar wrist-

Table 7-13. Upper Limits of Normal Used for Combined Sensory Index from Robinson, Micklesen & Wang (1998)

Latency Parameter	Upper Limit of Normal (msec)
Median minus ulnar palm-to-wrist (8 cm)	0.3
Median minus ulnar wrist-to-ring finger (14 cm)	0.4
Median minus radial wrist-to-thumb (10 cm)	0.5
Combined sensory index (sum of three latency differences above)	0.9

to-ring finger latency difference is greater than 0.4 msec, the findings are compatible with carpal tunnel syndrome and no further components of the CSI need to be determined. Similarly, if median minus ulnar wrist-to-ring finger latency difference is 0.0 msec or less, the findings are normal and no further components of the CSI need to be determined. However, if the latency difference is between 0.0 and 0.4 msec, the testing for CSI should be completed.

Provocative Tests. EFFECTS OF COMPRESSION ON NERVE CONDUCTION. Changes in median nerve conduction during and after median nerve compression or ischemia are pathophysiologically interesting but do not provide clinically useful diagnostic tests for carpal tunnel syndrome. Marin and colleagues (1983) tested median DML and DSL with the wrist in neutral position and after 5 and 10 minutes of sustained maximum wrist flexion or extension. In healthy controls, the DML and DSL increased slightly with this procedure; for example, the mean DML increased by 0.13 msec after 10 minutes of wrist extension. Smaller changes in mean DML were noted with wrist flexion or with briefer wrist extension. In patients who had carpal tunnel syndrome, the changes in DML were often greater. Of five patients with normal DML and DSL in the neutral position, three developed prolonged DSL after 5 minutes of sustained wrist flexion or extension.

Two other papers report median DML and DSL after 2 minutes of wrist flexion (Schwartz,

Gordon & Swash, 1980; White et al., 1988). In some patients who have carpal tunnel syndrome, DML increases more than 0.2 msec with this test. On rare occasions median DML after wrist flexion is abnormal when DML and DSL with the wrist in the neutral position are normal. In a larger series of patients and controls tested after 5 minutes of sustained flexion, postflexion median nerve conduction testing was not a useful technique for diagnosing carpal tunnel syndrome (Dunnan & Waylonis, 1991).

Werner and colleagues (1994) measured median distal sensory conduction before and immediately after 1 minute of sustained wrist extension. In controls who had no hand symptoms, the DSL had a mean increase of 0.05 msec after wrist extension; in patients who had carpal tunnel syndrome, the mean increase was 0.13 msec. Although this demonstrated a statistically significant difference between the patient and control groups, it provides no validation of the test in individuals.

A provocative maneuver consisting of 2 minutes of repetitive alternating wrist flexion and extension at 2-second intervals followed by 2 minutes of repetitive alternating finger flexion and extension did elicit paresthesias in some patients who had carpal tunnel syndrome, but did not have a significant effect on median nerve conduction (Clifford & Israels, 1994).

In healthy subjects and in patients who have carpal tunnel syndrome, sustained wrist flexion leads to gradual reduction of the median SNAP amplitude recorded at a finger while stimulating at the wrist. The reduction in amplitude does not occur until flexion has been sustained for many minutes; for example, in healthy subjects the amplitude falls to one-half of its initial value after 25 minutes or more of sustained flexion. In patients who have carpal tunnel syndrome, the amplitude falls more quickly, so that early decrease in the SNAP amplitude during sustained flexion may offer another test for carpal tunnel syndrome (Hansson & Nilsson, 1995). When patients who have carpal tunnel syndrome are compared with healthy controls, the median SNAP amplitude for some patients returns to normal more slowly after flexion is released (Rosecrance, Cook & Bingham, 1997). These preliminary reports suggest that these tests are more time consuming and no more sensitive than other sensitive median conduction tests for carpal tunnel syndrome.

EFFECTS OF ISCHEMIA ON NERVE CONDUCTION. Fullerton (1963) studied median motor conduction before and during ischemia of the forearm and hand, induced by a pneumatic cuff applied to the upper arm. Nerve conduction studies were repeated every 2 to 5 minutes after occlusion of blood flow. In control subjects, the amplitude and area of the thenar CMAP from median stimulation at the wrist remained unchanged for at least 20 minutes but fell as much as 50% by the thirtieth minute of ischemia. The thenar CMAP amplitude from median stimulation in the antecubital space often fell more quickly.

In two-thirds of patients who had carpal tunnel syndrome, the fall in thenar CMAP amplitude occurred more rapidly than in controls. There was a correlation in the patients between the severity of pain and paresthesias and the rate of fall in thenar CMAP amplitude during ischemia.

Sustained occlusion of blood flow by cuff on the upper arm also leads to gradual loss of amplitude of the median nerve SNAP recorded at the wrist to digital stimulation (Cruz Martinez, Perez Conde & Ferrer, 1980). In patients who have carpal tunnel syndrome, SNAP amplitude falls faster than normal. In contrast, in some patients who have metabolic disturbances such as diabetes and chronic renal failure, the SNAP amplitude falls more slowly than normal.

Minimum Sensory Nerve Conduction Velocity. Buchthal and colleagues (1974) used near-nerve needle recording electrodes and averaged the responses to between 500 and 1,000 stimuli. They measured the latencies to the last peak distinguishable from noise to calculate a minimum detectable SNCV. In healthy subjects the mean minimum SNCV was 16 m/sec with lower limits of normal of 12 m/sec. The amplitude of the slowest component was 0.05 to 0.1 μV.

In patients who had carpal tunnel syndrome, the SNAP often showed temporal dispersion over as long as 30 msec. Fibers conducting at 16 m/sec created a potential of 0.2 to 3.0 μV, much higher than the amplitude from the slowest fibers in normal nerve.

Minimum SNCV is less sensitive than maximum SNCV in the diagnosis of carpal tunnel syndrome. Of 11 patients who had carpal tunnel and abnormal median maximum SNCV or SNAP amplitude, only three had reduced median minimum SNCV (Shefner, Buchthal & Krarup, 1991).

The duration of the SNAP is a measure of temporal dispersion between conduction in fastest and slower fibers. The value measured for duration is dependent on technical factors such as filter and gain settings, surface versus needle electrodes, and whether an averager is used. Using surface electrodes for antidromic recording without an averager, Bhala and Thoppil (1981) found a prolonged SNAP duration in 64% of their carpal tunnel patients.

Repetitive Sensory Stimulation. Repetitive sensory stimulation is another technique that increases diagnostic sensitivity in patients with carpal tunnel syndrome. Lehmann and Tackmann (1974) studied the response of median sensory fibers to trains of stimuli. They stimulated the index finger with ring electrodes and recorded from the median nerve at the wrist with needle electrodes. They stimulated the nerve with trains of stimuli at 100 to 500 Hz and compared the latencies and amplitudes of the first and tenth responses. They found differences in the responses of healthy and carpal tunnel syndrome subjects. Table 7-14 gives representative data from 500-Hz stimulation.

They also found an increase in latency of the tenth response, compared with the first. For example, at 200 Hz the mean latency of the tenth response in carpal tunnel syndrome patients was 109% of the latency of the first response, but no prolongation of mean latency was noted in control patients. For both latency and amplitude comparisons, the abnormalities were noted at 100-Hz

Table 7-14. Amplitude Ratio of Tenth to First Sensory Nerve Action Potential in Response to Repetitive Index Finger Stimulation at 500 Hz

	Mean	Range
Controls	0.70	0.50–0.89
Hands with carpal tunnel syndrome	0.31	0.19–0.40

Data from HJ Lehmann, W Tackmann. Neurographic analysis of trains of frequent electric stimuli in the diagnosis of peripheral nerve diseases. Investigations in the carpal tunnel syndrome. Eur. Neurol. 1974;12:293–308.

stimulation, and differences between controls and patients increased as stimulation frequency increased to 500 Hz. All patients with clinical history suggesting carpal tunnel syndrome had abnormal responses to trains of stimuli, even though 5 of the 24 patients with carpal tunnel syndrome had normal routine DML and DSL. Tackmann and Lehmann (1974) also compared responses to paired stimuli spaced 1.0 to 50.0 msec apart and found abnormal "relative refractory periods of median sensory fibers in the carpal tunnel syndrome."

Gilliatt and Meer (1990) studied the refractory period of transmission by stimulating the median nerve at the wrist with paired stimuli at intervals of 0.8 to 1.0 msec. They recorded nerve action potentials over the index or middle fingers and over the median nerve at the antecubital space. Controls always showed transmission of paired responses at both the distal and proximal recording sites. Eleven of 14 patients with carpal tunnel syndrome showed an impaired or absent response to the second stimulus at the distal recording site. Two of these patients had normal transcarpal SNCVs. In contrast, among a group of patients who had mild carpal tunnel syndrome, only 10% had an abnormal refractory period of transmission, a much lower test sensitivity than shown by other parameters, such as median palm-wrist latency or median-ulnar comparisons (Girlanda, Quartarone, Sinicropi, Pronesti, Nicolosi, Macaione, Picciolo & Messina, 1998). Gilliatt and Meer posited that refractory period of transmission might normalize following remyelination even if SNCV remained abnormal.

Electrodiagnostic Screening Devices

Portable automated devices are available to perform some aspects of electrodiagnostic studies. The NervePace electroneurometer (NeuMed, Pennington, NJ) is the best known of these. Early models of this device detected onset latency of the thenar CMAP after stimulation at the wrist and automatically reported the DML. The test correlates well with DML measured with traditional techniques and has good test-retest reliability (Pransky, Long, Hammer, Schulz, Himmelstein & Fowke, 1997; Atroshi, Gummesson, Johnsson,

Ornstein & Rosén, 2000). Another automated device (NC-Stat, NeuroMetrix, Inc., Cambridge, MA) measures DML and F-waves latency by recording a volume-conducted response over the wrist, and results correlate well with standard electrodiagnostic measurements of DML (Leffler, Gozani & Cros, 2000). A number of papers document that automated measurement of DML has limited sensitivity for diagnosis of carpal tunnel syndrome (Grant, Congleton, Koppa, Leonard & Huchingson, 1992; Steinberg, Gelberman, Rydevik & Lundborg, 1992; Beckenbaugh & Simonian, 1995; Atroshi & Johnsson, 1996; Cherniack, Moalli & Viscolli, 1996; Dunne, Thompson, Cole, Dunning, Martyn, Coggon & Cooper, 1996), a finding that is expected given the limited sensitivity of measuring DML in isolation and the technical limitations imposed by automated detection of waveform onset and inability to observe the actual waveform to confirm supramaximal stimulation, lack of ulnar stimulation, or anomalous innervation patterns (Chaudhry, 1997). Some models of the electroneurometer can also be used to measure median DSL (Durnil, Rosecrance, Cook, Birgen, Dostal & McMurray, 1993; Rosecrance, Cook & Bingham, 1993). Newer models of the portable devices display waveforms and permit testing of multiple nerves, including sensory and mixed nerve studies. To the extent that these newer devices are now portable versions of traditional electrodiagnostic equipment, their utility depends on the training and skill of the electrodiagnostician, and adequate studies should follow the American Association of Electrodiagnostic Medicine guidelines given at the end of Chapter 8.

Needle Electromyography

The EMG examination of thenar muscles is normal in most patients with carpal tunnel syndrome. The diagnostic and prognostic value of thenar EMG in patients who have carpal tunnel syndrome is debated (Mazur, 1998). The early Mayo Clinic series found fibrillations in 44% of patients (Thomas et al., 1967). Fasciculations were found in approximately 12% of patients.

Buchthal and colleagues (1974) examined patients whose carpal tunnel syndrome was often

Table 7-15. Electromyographic Abnormalities in Abductor Pollicis Brevis in 585 Hands with Carpal Tunnel Syndrome

	Fibrillations or Sharp Waves (%)	Fasciculations (%)	Decreased Recruitment (%)	Increased Polyphasics (%)
All hands	22	6	31	18
Distal motor latency <4.7 msec	13	3	19	10
Distal motor latency >7.7 msec	46	14	60	43

Data from I Kimura, DR Ayyar. The carpal tunnel syndrome: electrophysiological aspects of 639 symptomatic extremities. Electromyogr. Clin. Neurophysiol. 1985;25:151–64.

clinically severe; one-half of the patients had wasting or severe weakness of abductor pollicis brevis. As expected, these patients had a high incidence of EMG abnormalities in abductor pollicis brevis: Only one-third of the patients had a full interference pattern; the mean motor unit potential duration was prolonged in one-half the patients; and one-half the patients had fibrillations or positive sharp waves. The probability of finding an EMG abnormality increased, as median DML increased.

The later Mayo series covering 1961 to 1980 found fibrillations in only 18% of patients (Stevens, 1987). Decreased recruitment or abnormal motor units were present in 41% of patients. Kimura and Ayyar (1985) found a similar incidence of abnormalities in their series of EMGs in 585 abductor pollicis brevis muscles of patients who had carpal tunnel syndrome (Table 7-15). Patients who have a clinical history suggestive of carpal tunnel syndrome but have normal nerve conductions are unlikely to have abnormal EMG findings in thenar muscles unless they also have another neurologic cause of the abnormal EMG (Balbierz, Cottrell & Cottrell, 1998). The probability of finding an abnormality by thenar EMG increases when the DML is prolonged or the CMAP amplitude is lower (Kimura & Ayyar, 1985; Murga, Moreno, Menendez & Castilla, 1994; Werner & Albers, 1995; Vennix, Hirsh, Chiou-Tan & Rossi, 1998).

Repetitive Nerve Fiber Discharge

Simpson (1958) used a needle electrode in abductor pollicis brevis for his pioneering motor nerve conduction studies. In patients who had carpal tunnel syndrome, he noted occasional repetitive firing of individual motor units, particularly of the unit elicited by threshold stimulation.

In patients who have carpal tunnel syndrome, thenar muscle EMG occasionally shows spontaneous myokymic discharges (Figure 7-10) (Albers,

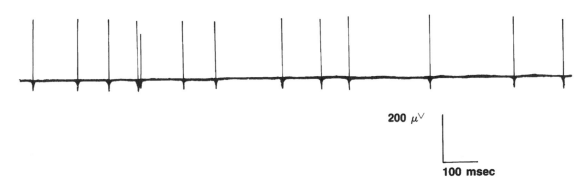

200 μ^V

100 msec

Figure 7-10. In this patient with carpal tunnel syndrome, electromyography done with a needle electrode in the abductor pollicis brevis shows spontaneous rhythmic firing at rest; there were no fibrillations or abnormalities of configuration of voluntary motor units. Median sensory latencies were abnormal. Median distal motor latency was normal. (Courtesy of Dr. Patrick Radecki.)

Allen, Bastron & Daube, 1981). Spaans (1982) found spontaneous rhythmic firing of motor unit potentials in the thenar muscle EMG in 8% of hands affected by carpal tunnel syndrome. Single-fiber EMG supported the hypothesis that these rhythmic discharges originated in the motor axon rather than in muscle fibers. The spontaneously discharging motor units were found in mild or severe cases of carpal tunnel syndrome; in contrast, fibrillations and positive sharp waves were much more common in severe cases. When spontaneously discharging motor units were present, they became more abundant after 1 or 2 minutes of forearm ischemia. They were not abolished by local anesthetic block of the median nerve in the antecubital space. Other authors have not reported a similar incidence of spontaneous motor unit potential firing; for example, Kimura and Ayyar (1985) found myokymia in abductor pollicis brevis only four times out of 585 muscles tested.

Simpson and Thomaides (1988) used a linearly rising current stimulation of the median nerve and found that this would evoke repetitive firing in abductor pollicis brevis more easily in patients who had carpal tunnel syndrome than in controls. The term *motor Tinel sign* has been suggested for the phenomenon of evoking a burst of thenar muscle motor unit firing, detectable by needle EMG, after taping over the median nerve at the wrist; this sign is present in perhaps one-half of patients who have carpal tunnel syndrome, but can also be elicited in some individuals who do not have carpal tunnel syndrome (Montagna & Liguori, 2000).

Electromyography and Differential Diagnosis

The EMG is particularly important in searching for other neuropathic conditions that might mimic or co-exist with carpal tunnel syndrome. When the EMG examination of abductor pollicis brevis is abnormal or when otherwise clinically indicated, the EMG should be extended to more proximal median-innervated muscles, to ulnar-innervated muscles, and to additional muscles as needed to search for mononeuritis multiplex, brachial plexopathy, or cervical radiculopathy.

Cutaneous Silent Period

EMG during sustained voluntary contraction shows brief cessation of motor activity after painful stimulation of an appropriate dermatome. The absence of motor activity, called the *cutaneous silent period* (CSP), typically begins many milliseconds after the stimulus and lasts many milliseconds. The afferent mediators of the CSP are A delta fibers. The CSP can be induced in the thenar muscles by painful electrical stimulation of a finger or by supramaximal stimulation of the median nerve at the wrist. When a group of patients with carpal tunnel syndrome were compared with controls, the mean duration of the CSP was longer in the patients who had carpal tunnel syndrome, and two patients who had severe carpal tunnel syndrome had no CSP after index finger stimulation but normal CSP after little finger stimulation (Aurora, Ahmad & Aurora, 1998). However, CSP is not a sensitive test for carpal tunnel syndrome; CSP abnormalities do not indicate the severity of carpal tunnel syndrome (Resende, Alves, Castro, Kimaid, Fortinguerra & Schelp, 2000).

Somatosensory Evoked Potentials

Somatosensory evoked potentials (SSEPs) recorded over the contralateral cerebral cortex while stimulating the median nerve at the index finger are sometimes abnormal in carpal tunnel syndrome patients (Constantinovici, 1989). In these patients, comparison of latencies measured over the contralateral scalp with stimulation at wrist and at the index finger can demonstrate distal slowing, and the cerebral SSEP can sometimes be obtained when a SNAP is unobtainable (Desmedt, Manil, Borenstein, Debecker, Lambert, Franken & Danis, 1966). For example, in patients who have severe carpal tunnel syndrome and unrecordable thenar CMAP, the median distal sensory conduction time can be measured by subtracting the cortical N60 latency to median stimulation at the wrist from the N60 latency to median stimulation at the middle finger (Kawasaki, Saito & Ogawa, 1995).

In some patients who have carpal tunnel syndrome and abnormal median nerve conduction, the SSEP from the ipsilateral ulnar nerve has increased amplitude (Tinazzi, Zanette, Volpato, Testoni, Bonato, Manganotti, Miniussi & Fiaschi, 1998). Magnetoencephalographic scalp recordings during repetitive pressure stimulation of digits showed that a patient who had long-standing carpal tunnel syndrome had a decreased area of median nerve representation in the contralateral primary somatosensory cortex (Druschky, Kaltenhauser, Humel, Druschky, Huk, Stefan & Neundorfer, 2000). Cortical somatosensory potentials evoked by painful stimuli to the middle finger using argon laser stimulation can also be abnormal in patients who have carpal tunnel syndrome (Arendt-Nielsen, Gregersen, Toft & Bjerring, 1991).

Transcranial Magnetic Stimulation

Transcranial magnetic stimulation can evoke peripheral motor responses. The latency of the CMAP recorded over the thenar eminence after transcranial magnetic stimulation is prolonged in some patients who have carpal tunnel syndrome (Kaneko, Kawai, Taguchi, Fuchigami & Shiraishi, 1997). This is not a particularly sensitive test for carpal tunnel syndrome; however, the technique can be used to calculate a central motor conduction time and to investigate the possibility of cervical spinal cord dysfunction in patients suspected of having both a peripheral nerve entrapment and a cervical myelopathy (Kaneko et al., 1997).

Autonomic Tests

Sympathetic Skin Response

The sympathetic skin response (SSR) is a triphasic potential, with amplitude typically of many hundred microvolts, that can be recorded on a digit 1.3 seconds or longer after stimulation (Shahani, Halperin, Boulu & Cohen, 1984). It can be evoked by deep inspiration or by diverse stimuli. The latency does not differ significantly between controls and patients who have carpal tunnel syndrome (Caccia, Galimberti, Valla, Salvaggio, Dezuanni & Mangoni, 1993; Sener, Tascilar, Balaban & Selcuki, 2000). The ulnar SSR can be compared with the median by simultaneous recording of the response of median-innervated and-ulnar innervated digits. In healthy subjects, the amplitude of the SSR does not differ between the index finger and the little finger. Some patients who have carpal tunnel syndrome have an absent, low amplitude, or low area SSR recorded from the index finger, or the SSR recorded at the index finger is lower in amplitude than the SSR recorded at the little finger (Schoenhuber, Grenzi, Di Donato & Gibertoni, 1988; Kanzato, Komine, Kanaya & Fukiyama, 2000; Reddeppa, Bulusu, Chand, Jacob, Kalappurakkal & Tharakan, 2000). SSR studies have low diagnostic sensitivity; for example, using a lower limit of normal for the median to ulnar SSR amplitude ratio of 0.36, only 10% of patients who had carpal tunnel syndrome had abnormal results of this test (Kuntzer, 1994). The SSR is more likely to be abnormal in patients who have severe carpal tunnel syndrome, especially if the patient has autonomic symptoms (Verghese, Galanopoulou & Herskovitz, 2000). In patients who have carpal tunnel syndrome and abnormal SSR, the SSR sometimes improves after surgery (Kanzato, Komine, Kanaya & Fukiyama, 2000; Mondelli, Vecchiarelli, Reale, Marsili & Giannini, 2001).

To Be Continued

This chapter reviews myriad techniques for electrodiagnostic study of the median nerve. The challenge to the electrodiagnostician of choosing and interpreting electrodiagnostic tests is discussed in Chapter 8.

References

Albers JW, Allen AA 2nd, Bastron JA, Daube JR. Limb myokymia. Muscle Nerve 1981;4:494–504.

American Association of Electrodiagnostic Medicine, American Academy of Neurology, American Academy of Physical Medicine and Rehabilitation. Practice parameter for electrodiagnostic studies in carpal tunnel syndrome: summary statement. Muscle Nerve 1993;16:1390–91

Anastasopoulos D, Chroni E. Effect of carpal tunnel syndrome on median nerve proximal conduction estimated by F-waves. J. Clin. Neurophysiol. 1997;14:63–67.

Anderson MH, Fullerton PM, Gilliatt RW, Hern JEC. Changes in the forearm associated with median nerve compression at the wrist in the guinea pig. J. Neurol. Neurosurg. Psychiatry 1970;33:70–79.

Arendt-Nielsen L, Gregersen H, Toft E, Bjerring P. Involvement of thin afferents in carpal tunnel syndrome: evaluated quantitatively by argon laser stimulation. Muscle Nerve 1991;14:508–14.

Atroshi I, Gummesson C, Johnsson R, Ornstein E, Rosén I. Median nerve latency measurement agreement between portable and conventional methods. J. Hand Surg. 2000;25B:73–77.

Atroshi I, Johnsson R. Evaluation of portable nerve conduction testing in the diagnosis of carpal tunnel syndrome. J. Hand Surg. 1996;21A:651–54.

Aurora SK, Ahmad BK, Aurora TK. Silent period abnormalities in carpal tunnel syndrome. Muscle Nerve 1998;21:1213–15.

Balbierz JM, Cottrell AC, Cottrell WD. Is needle examination always necessary in evaluation of carpal tunnel syndrome? Arch. Phys. Med. Rehabil. 1998;79:514–16.

Beckenbaugh RD, Simonian PT. Clinical efficacy of electroneurometer screening in carpal tunnel syndrome. Orthopedics 1995;18:549–52.

Bhala RP, Thoppil E. Early detection of carpal tunnel syndrome by sensory nerve conduction. Electromyogr. Clin. Neurophysiol. 1981;21:155–64.

Bland JD. The value of the history in the diagnosis of carpal tunnel syndrome. J. Hand Surg. 2000;25B:445–50.

Brismar T. Changes in electrical threshold in human peripheral neuropathy. J. Neurol. Sci. 1985;68:215–23.

Buchthal F, Rosenfalck A. Sensory conduction from digit to palm and from palm to wrist in the carpal tunnel syndrome. J. Neurol. Neurosurg. Psychiatry 1971;34:243–52.

Buchthal F, Rosenfalck A, Trojaborg W. Electrophysiological findings in entrapment of the median nerve at wrist and elbow. J. Neurol. Neurosurg. Psychiatry 1974;37:340–60.

Buschbacher RM. Median nerve F-wave latencies recorded from the abductor pollicis brevis. Am. J. Phys. Med. Rehabil. 1999;78:S32–37.

Caccia MR, Galimberti V, Valla PL, Salvaggio A, Dezuanni E, Mangoni A. Peripheral autonomic involvement in the carpal tunnel syndrome. Acta. Neurol. Scand. 1993;88:47–50.

Capone L, Pentore R, Lunazzi C, Schonhuber R. Pitfalls in using the ring finger test alone for the diagnosis of carpal tunnel syndrome. Ital. J. Neurol. Sci. 1998;19:387–90.

Carpay JA, Schimsheimer RJ, de Weerd AW. Coactivation of the ulnar nerve in motor tests for carpal tunnel syndrome. Neurophysiol. Clin. 1997;27:309–13.

Carroll GJ. Comparison of median and radial nerve sensory latencies in the electrophysiological diagnosis of carpal tunnel syndrome. Electroencephalogr. Clin. Neurophysiol. 1987;68:101–6.

Casey EB, Le-Quesne PM. Digital nerve action potentials in healthy subjects, and in carpal tunnel and diabetic patients. J. Neurol. Neurosurg. Psychiatry 1972;35:612–23.

Cassvan A, Ralescu S, Shapiro E, Moshkovski FG, Weiss J. Median and radial sensory latencies to digit I as compared with other screening tests in carpal tunnel syndrome. Am. J. Phys. Med. Rehabil. 1988;67:221–24.

Cassvan A, Rosenberg A, Rivera LF. Ulnar nerve involvement in carpal tunnel syndrome. Arch. Phys. Med. Rehabil. 1986;67:290–92.

Chan R-C, Yang T-F, Penn I-W, Chuang T-Y. Compound muscle action potential amplitude and area changes in normal subjects and patients with carpal tunnel syndrome. Electromyogr. Clin. Neurophysiol. 1998;38:317–20.

Chang C-W, Lien I-N. Comparison of sensory nerve conduction in the palmar cutaneous branch and first digital branch of the median nerve: a new diagnostic method for carpal tunnel syndrome. Muscle Nerve 1991;14:1173–76.

Chang MH, Chiang HT, Ger LP, Yang DA, Lo YK. The cause of slowed forearm median conduction velocity in carpal tunnel syndrome. Clin. Neurophysiol. 2000;111:1039–44.

Chaudhry V. Technology review: NervePace digital electroneurometer. Muscle Nerve 1997;20:1200–3.

Cherniack MG, Moalli D, Viscolli C. A comparison of traditional electrodiagnostic studies, electroneurometry, and vibrometry in the diagnosis of carpal tunnel syndrome. J. Hand Surg. 1996;21A:122–31.

Cioni R, Passero S, Paradiso C, Giannini F, Battistini N, Rushworth G. Diagnostic specificity of sensory and motor nerve conduction variables in early detection of carpal tunnel syndrome. J. Neurol. 1989;236:208–13.

Clifford JC, Israels H. Provocative exercise maneuver: its effect on nerve conduction studies in patients with carpal tunnel syndrome. Arch. Phys. Med. Rehabil. 1994;75:8–11.

Constantinovici A. The diagnostic value of somatosensory evoked potentials in the diseases of peripheral nervous system. Neurol. Psychiatr. (Bucur) 1989;27:111–25.

Cruz Martinez A, Perez Conde MC, Ferrer MT. Effect of ischaemia on sensory evoked potentials. 2. Study in patients with diabetes mellitus, alcoholism, chronic renal failure, carpal tunnel syndrome and hyperparathyroidism. Electromyogr. Clin. Neurophysiol. 1980;20:193–203.

Cuturic M, Palliyath S. Motor unit number estimate (MUNE) testing in male patients with mild to moderate carpal tunnel syndrome. Electromyogr. Clin. Neurophysiol. 2000;40:67–72.

Dawson GD, Scott JW. The recording of nerve action potentials through the skin in man. J. Neurol. Neurosurg. Psychiatry 1949;12:259–67.

Desmedt JE, Manil J, Borenstein S, Debecker J, Lambert C, Franken L, Danis A. Evaluation of sensory nerve conduction from averaged cerebral evoked potentials in neuropathies. Electromyography 1966;6:263–69.

Di Benedetto M, Mitz M, Klingbeil GE, Davidoff D. New criteria for sensory nerve conduction especially useful in diagnosing carpal tunnel syndrome. Arch. Phys. Med. Rehabil. 1986;67:586–89.

Di Guglielmo G, Torrieri F, Repaci M, Uncini A. Conduction block and segmental velocities in carpal tunnel syndrome. Electroencephalogr. Clin. Neurophysiol. 1997;105:321–27.

Donahue JE, Raynor EM, Rutkove SB. Forearm velocity in carpal tunnel syndrome: when is slow too slow? Arch. Phys. Med. Rehabil. 1998;79:181–83.

Druschky K, Kaltenhauser M, Humel C, Druschky A, Huk WJ, Stefan H, Neundorfer B. Alteration of the somatosensory cortical map in peripheral mononeuropathy due to carpal tunnel syndrome. Neuroreport 2000;27:3925–30.

Dumitru D, King JC. Median/ulnar premotor potential identification and localization. Muscle Nerve 1995;18:518–25.

Dunnan J, Waylonis GW. Wrist flexion as an adjunct to the diagnosis of carpal tunnel syndrome. Arch. Phys. Med. Rehabil. 1991;72:211.

Dunne CA, Thompson PW, Cole J, Dunning J, Martyn CN, Coggon D, Cooper C. Carpal tunnel syndrome: evaluation of a new method of assessing median nerve conduction at the wrist. Ann. Rheum. Dis. 1996;55:396–98.

Durnil WG, Rosecrance JC, Cook TM, Birgen WE, Dostal AJ, McMurray SJ. Reliability of distal sensory latency measures of the median nerve using an electroneurometer. J. Occup. Rehabil. 1993;3:105–12.

Eisen A, Schomer D, Melmed C. The application of F-wave measurements in the differentiation of proximal and distal upper limb entrapments. Neurology 1977;27:662–68.

Eklund G. A new electrodiagnostic procedure for measuring sensory nerve conduction across the carpal tunnel. Ups. J. Med. Sci. 1975;80:63–64.

Felsenthal G. Median and ulnar distal motor and sensory latencies in the same normal subject. Arch. Phys. Med. Rehabil. 1977;58:297–302.

Felsenthal G. Comparison of evoked potentials in the same hand in normal subjects and in patients with carpal tunnel syndrome. Am. J. Phys. Med. 1978a;57:228–32.

Felsenthal G. Median and ulnar muscle and sensory evoked potentials. Am. J. Phys. Med. 1978b;57:167–82.

Fisher MA, Hoffen B. F-wave analysis in patients with carpal tunnel syndrome. Electromyogr. Clin. Neurophysiol. 1997;37:27–31.

Fisher MA, Hoffen B, Hultman C. Normative F wave values and the number of recorded F waves. Muscle Nerve 1994;17:1185–89.

Foresti C, Quadri S, Rasella M, Tironi F, Viscardi M, Ubiali E. Carpal tunnel syndrome: which electrodiagnostic path should we follow? A prospective study of 100 consecutive patients. Electromyogr. Clin. Neurophysiol. 1996;36:377–84.

Fox JE, Bangash IH. Conduction velocity in the forearm segment of the median nerve in patients with impaired conduction through the carpal tunnel. Electroencephalogr. Clin. Neurophysiol. 1996;101:192–96.

Fullerton PM. The effect of ischaemia on nerve conduction in the carpal tunnel. J. Neurol. Neurosurg. Psychiatry 1963; 26:385–97.

Ghavanini MR, Kazemi B, Jazayeri M, Khosrawi S. Median-radial sensory latencies comparison as a new test in carpal tunnel syndrome. Electromyogr. Clin. Neurophysiol. 1996; 36:171–73.

Gilliatt RW, Meer J. The refractory period of transmission in patients with carpal tunnel syndrome. Muscle Nerve 1990;13:445–50.

Gilliatt RW, Melville ID, Velate AS, Willison RG. A study of normal nerve action potentials using an averaging technique (barrier grid storage tube). J. Neurol. Neurosurg. Psychiatry 1965;28:191–200.

Gilliatt RW, Sears TA. Sensory nerve action potentials in patients with peripheral nerve lesions. J. Neurol. Neurosurg. Psychiatry 1958;21:109–18.

Girlanda P, Quartarone A, Sinicropi S, Pronesti C, Nicolosi C, Macaione V, Picciolo G, Messina C. Electrophysiological studies in mild idiopathic carpal tunnel syndrome. Electroencephalogr. Clin. Neurophysiol. 1998;109:44–49.

Goddard DH, Barnes CG, Berry H, Evans S. Measurement of nerve conduction—a comparison of orthodromic and antidromic methods. Clin. Rheumatol. 1983;2:169–74.

Grant KA, Congleton JJ, Koppa RJ, Leonard CS, Huchingson RD. Use of motor nerve conduction testing and vibration sensitivity testing as screening tools for carpal tunnel syndrome in industry. J. Hand Surg. 1992;17A:71–76.

Gutmann L. Median-ulnar nerve communications and carpal tunnel syndrome. J. Neurol. Neurosurg. Psychiatry 1977; 40:982–86.

Gutmann L, Gutierrez A, Riggs JE. The contribution of median-ulnar communications in diagnosis of mild carpal tunnel syndrome. Muscle Nerve 1986;9:319–21.

Haloua JP, Soulier F, Collin JP. The sensory potential of the ring finger. The value of electromyographic diagnosis of carpal tunnel syndrome. Ann. Chir. Main Memb. Super. 1994;13: 64–70.

Hansson S. Does forearm mixed nerve conduction velocity reflect retrograde changes in carpal tunnel syndrome? Muscle Nerve 1994;17:725–29.

Hansson S, Nilsson BY. Median sensory nerve conduction block during wrist flexion in the carpal tunnel syndrome. Electromyogr. Clin. Neurophysiol. 1995;35:99–105.

Harrison MJ. Lack of evidence of generalised sensory neuropathy in patients with carpal tunnel syndrome. J. Neurol. Neurosurg. Psychiatry 1978;41:957–59.

Hodes R, Larrabee MG, German W. The human electromyogram in response to nerve stimulation and the conduction velocity of motor axons. Arch. Neurol. Psychiatry (Chicago) 1948;60:340–65.

Imaoka H, Yorifuji S, Takahashi M, Nakamura Y, Kitaguchi M, Tarui S. Improved inching method for the diagnosis and prognosis of carpal tunnel syndrome. Muscle Nerve 1992;15:318–24.

Iyer V, Fenichel GM. Normal median nerve proximal latency in carpal tunnel syndrome: a clue to coexisting Martin-Gruber anastomosis. J. Neurol. Neurosurg. Psychiatry 1976; 39:449–52.

Johnson EW, Kukla RD, Wongsam PE, Piedmont A. Sensory latencies to the ring finger: normal values and relation to carpal tunnel syndrome. Arch. Phys. Med. Rehabil. 1981;62:206–8.

Johnson EW, Melvin JL. Sensory conduction studies of median and ulnar nerves. Arch. Phys. Med. Rehabil. 1967;48:25–30.

Johnson EW, Sipski M, Lammertse T. Median and radial sensory latencies to digit I: normal values and usefulness in carpal tunnel syndrome [published erratum appears in Arch. Phys. Med. Rehabil. 1987;68:388]. Arch. Phys. Med. Rehabil. 1987;68:140–41.

Kaneko K, Kawai S, Taguchi T, Fuchigami Y, Shiraishi G. Coexisting peripheral nerve and cervical cord compression. Spine 1997;22:636–40.

Kanzato N, Komine Y, Kanaya F, Fukiyama K. Preserved sympathetic skin response at the distal phalanx in patients with carpal tunnel syndrome. Clin. Neurophysiol. 2000;111: 2057–63.

Kaul MP, Pagel KJ, Dryden JD. When to use the combined sensory index. Muscle Nerve 2001;24:1078–82.

Kawasaki M, Saito T, Ogawa R. Somatosensory evoked potentials for the diagnosis of carpal tunnel syndrome. Nippon Seikeigeka Gakkai Zasshi 1995;69:891–98.

Kimura I, Ayyar DR. The carpal tunnel syndrome: electrophysiological aspects of 639 symptomatic extremities. Electromyogr. Clin. Neurophysiol. 1985;25:151–64.

Kimura J. The carpal tunnel syndrome: localization of conduction abnormalities within the distal segment of the median nerve. Brain 1979;102:619–35.

Kimura J. F-wave determination in nerve conduction studies. Adv. Neurol. 1983;39:961–75.

Kimura J, Murphy MJ, Varda DJ. Electrophysiological study of anomalous innervation of intrinsic hand muscles. Arch. Neurol. 1976;33:842–44.

Kingery WS, Wu PB, Date ES. An unusual presentation of a traumatic ulnar mononeuropathy with a Martin-Gruber anastomosis. Muscle Nerve 1996;19:920–22.

Kopell HP, Goodgold J. Clinical and electrodiagnostic features of carpal tunnel syndrome. Arch. Phys. Med. Rehabil. 1968;49:371–75.

Kraft GH, Halvorson GA. Median nerve residual latency: normal value and use in diagnosis of carpal tunnel syndrome. Arch. Phys. Med. Rehabil. 1983;64:221–26.

Kuntzer T. Carpal tunnel syndrome in 100 patients: sensitivity, specificity of multi-neurophysiological procedures and estimation of axonal loss of motor, sensory and sympathetic median nerve fibers. J. Neurol. Sci. 1994;127:221–29.

Lambert EH. Diagnostic value of electrical stimulation of motor nerves. Electroencephalogr. Clin. Neurophysiol. 1962; 22[Suppl]:9–16.

Lateva ZC, McGill KC, Burgar CG. Anatomical and electrophysiological determinants of the human thenar compound muscle action potential. Muscle Nerve 1996; 19:1457–68.

Lauritzen M, Liguori R, Trojaborg W. Orthodromic sensory conduction along the ring finger in normal subjects and in patients with a carpal tunnel syndrome. Electroencephalogr. Clin. Neurophysiol. 1991;81:18–23.

Leffler CT, Gozani SN, Cros D. Median neuropathy at the wrist: diagnostic utility of clinical findings and an automated electrodiagnostic device. J. Occup. Environ. Med. 2000; 42:398–409.

Lehmann HJ, Tackmann W. Neurographic analysis of trains of frequent electric stimuli in the diagnosis of peripheral nerve diseases. Investigations in the carpal tunnel syndrome. Eur. Neurol. 1974;12:293–308.

Lesser EA, Venkatesh S, Preston DC, Logigian EL. Stimulation distal to the lesion in patients with carpal tunnel syndrome. Muscle Nerve 1995;18:503–7.

Liveson JA, Ma DM. Laboratory Reference for Clinical Neurophysiology. Philadelphia: F.A. Davis, 1992.

Logigian EL, Busis NA, Berger AR, Bruyninckx F, Khalil N, Shahani BT, Young RR. Lumbrical sparing in carpal tunnel syndrome: anatomic, physiologic, and diagnostic implications. Neurology 1987;37:1499–1505.

Loong SC. The carpal tunnel syndrome: a clinical and electrophysiological study of 250 patients. Proc. Aust. Assoc. Neurol. 1977;14:51–65.

Loong SC, Seah CS. Comparison of median and ulnar sensory nerve action potentials in the diagnosis of the carpal tunnel syndrome. J. Neurol. Neurosurg. Psychiatry 1971; 34:750–54.

Loong SC, Seah CS. A sensitive diagnostic test for carpal tunnel syndrome. Singapore Med. J. 1972;13:249–55.

Loscher WN, Auer-Grumbach M, Trinka E, Ladurner G, Hartung HP. Comparison of second lumbrical and interosseous latencies with standard measures of median nerve function across the carpal tunnel: a prospective study of 450 hands. J. Neurol. 2000;247:530–34.

Ludin HP, Lutschg J, Valsangiacomo F. Comparison of orthodromic and antidromic sensory nerve conduction. 1. Normals and patients with carpal tunnel syndrome. EEG-EMG 1977;8:173–79.

Maccabee PJ, Shahani BT, Young RR. Usefulness of double simultaneous recording (DSR) and F response studies in the diagnosis of carpal tunnel syndrome (CTS). Electroencephalogr. Clin. Neurophysiol. 1980;49:18P.

Macdonell RA, Schwartz MS, Swash M. Carpal tunnel syndrome: which finger should be tested? An analysis of sensory conduction in digital branches of the median nerve. Muscle Nerve 1990;13:601–6.

Macleod WN. Repeater F waves: a comparison of sensitivity with sensory antidromic wrist-to-palm latency and distal motor latency in the diagnosis of carpal tunnel syndrome. Neurology 1987;37:773–78.

Mandel JD. Premotor potentials. Phys. Med. Rehabil. Clin. North Am. 1998;9:765–6.

Marin EL, Vernick S, Friedmann LW. Carpal tunnel syndrome: median nerve stress test. Arch. Phys. Med. Rehabil. 1983;64:206–8.

Mazur A. Role of thenar electromyography in the evaluation of carpal tunnel syndrome. Phys. Med. Rehabil. Clin. North Am. 1998;9:755–64.

Melvin JL, Schuchmann JA, Lanese RR. Diagnostic specificity of motor and sensory nerve conduction variables in the carpal tunnel syndrome. Arch. Phys. Med. Rehabil. 1973;54:69–74.

Menkes DL, Hood DC, Bush AC. Inversion of the F-waves in median neuropathy at the wrist (carpal tunnel syndrome): an adjunctive diagnostic method. J. Contemp. Neurol, 1997;1:2–8.

Mills KR. Orthodromic sensory action potentials from palmar stimulation in the diagnosis of carpal tunnel syndrome. J. Neurol. Neurosurg. Psychiatry 1985;48:250–55.

Mondelli M, Vecchiarelli B, Reale F, Marsili T, Giannini F. Sympathetic skin response before and after surgical release of carpal tunnel syndrome. Muscle Nerve 2001;24:130–33.

Monga TN, Laidlow DM. Carpal tunnel syndrome. Measurement of sensory potentials using ring and index fingers. Am. J. Phys. Med. 1982;61:123–29.

Monga TN, Shanks GL, Poole BJ. Sensory palmar stimulation in the diagnosis of carpal tunnel syndrome. Arch. Phys. Med. Rehabil. 1985;66:598–600.

Montagna P, Liguori R. The motor Tinel sign: a useful sign in entrapment neuropathy? Muscle Nerve 2000;23:976–78.

Mortier G, Deckers K, Dijs H, Vander Auwera JC. Comparison of the distal motor latency of the ulnar nerve in carpal tunnel syndrome with a control group. Electromyogr. Clin. Neurophysiol. 1988;28:75–77.

Murai Y, Sanderson I. Studies of sensory conduction. J. Neurol. Neurosurg. Psychiatry 1975;38:1187–89.

Murga L, Moreno JM, Menéndez C, Castilla JM. The carpal tunnel syndrome. Relationship between median distal motor latency and graded results of needle electromyography. Electromyogr. Clin. Neurophysiol. 1994;34:377–83.

Nathan PA, Meadows KD, Doyle LS. Sensory segmental latency values of the median nerve for a population of normal individuals. Arch. Phys. Med. Rehabil. 1988; 69:499–501.

Padua L, LoMonaco M, Gregori B, Valente EM, Tonali P. Double-peaked potential in the neurophysiological evaluation of carpal tunnel syndrome. Muscle Nerve 1996;19:679–80.

Padua L, LoMonaco M, Valente EM, Tonali PA. A useful electrophysiologic parameter for diagnosis of carpal tunnel syndrome. Muscle Nerve 1996;19:48–53.

Park TA, Del Toro DR. Generators of the early and late median thenar premotor potentials. Muscle Nerve 1995;18:1000–8.

Park TA, Welshofer JA, Dzwierzynski WW, Erickson SJ, Del TDR. Median "pseudoneurapraxia" at the wrist: reassessment of palmar stimulation of the recurrent median nerve. Arch. Phys. Med. Rehabil. 2001;82:190–97.

Pease WS, Cannell CD, Johnson EW. Median to radial latency difference test in mild carpal tunnel syndrome. Muscle Nerve 1989;12:905–9.

Pease WS, Cunningham ML, Walsh WE, Johnson EW. Determining neurapraxia in carpal tunnel syndrome. Am. J. Phys. Med. Rehabil. 1988;67:117–19.

Pease WS, Lee HH, Johnson EW. Forearm median nerve conduction velocity in carpal tunnel syndrome. Electroencephalogr. Clin. Neurophysiol. 1990;30:299–302.

Pransky G, Long R, Hammer K, Schulz LA, Himmelstein J, Fowke J. Screening for carpal tunnel syndrome in the workplace. An analysis of portable nerve conduction devices. J. Occup. Environ. Med. 1997;39:727–33.

Preston DC, Logigian EL. Lumbrical and interossei recording in carpal tunnel syndrome. Muscle Nerve 1992;15:1253–57.

Preswick G. The effect of stimulus intensity on motor latency in the carpal tunnel syndrome. J. Neurol. Neurosurg. Psychiatry 1963;26:398–401.

Reddeppa S, Bulusu K, Chand PR, Jacob PC, Kalappurakkal J, Tharakan J. The sympathetic skin response in carpal tunnel syndrome. Auton. Neurosci. 2000;84:119–21.

Resende LA, Adamo AS, Bononi AP, Castro HA, Kimaid PA, Fortinguerra CH, Schelp AO. Test of a new technique for the diagnosis of carpal tunnel syndrome. J. Electromyogr. Kinesiol. 2000;10:127–33.

Resende LA, Adamo AS, Kimaid PA, Castro HA, Canheu AC, Schelp AO. Ulnar-to-median nerve anastomosis in the forearm. Review and report of 2 new cases. Electromyogr. Clin. Neurophysiol. 2000;40:253–55.

Resende LA, Alves RP, Castro HA, Kimaid PA, Fortinguerra CR, Schelp AO. Silent period in carpal tunnel syndrome. Electromyogr. Clin. Neurophysiol. 2000;40:31–36.

Robinson LR, Micklesen PJ, Wang L. Strategies for analyzing conduction data: superiority of a summary index over single tests. Muscle Nerve 1998;21:1166–71.

Robinson LR, Micklesen PJ, Wang L. Optimizing the number of tests for carpal tunnel syndrome. Muscle Nerve 2000;23:1880–82.

Rosecrance JC, Cook TM, Bingham RC. Comparison of a digital electroneurometer and formal nerve conduction studies for the measurement of median nerve sensory latency. J. Occup. Rehabil. 1993;3:191–200.

Rosecrance JC, Cook TM, Bingham RC. Sensory nerve recovery following median nerve provocation in carpal tunnel syndrome. Electromyogr. Clin. Neurophysiol. 1997;37:219–29.

Rossi S, Giannini F, Passero S, Paradiso C, Battistini N, Cioni R. Sensory neural conduction of median nerve from digits and palm stimulation in carpal tunnel syndrome. Electroencephalogr. Clin. Neurophysiol. 1994;93:330–34.

Sander HW, Quinto C, Saadeh PB, Chokroverty S. Sensitive median-ulnar motor comparative techniques in carpal tunnel syndrome. Muscle Nerve 1999;22:88–98.

Scelsa SN, Herskovitz S, Bieri P, Berger AR. Median mixed and sensory nerve conduction studies in carpal tunnel syndrome. Electroencephalogr. Clin. Neurophysiol. 1998; 109:268–73.

Schoenhuber R, Grenzi P, Di Donato G, Gibertoni M. Sudomotor nerve fiber impairment in carpal tunnel syndrome. Muscle Nerve 1988;11:974.

Schwartz MS, Gordon JA, Swash M. Slowed nerve conduction with wrist flexion in carpal tunnel syndrome. Ann. Neurol. 1980;8:69–71.

Sedal L, McLeod JG, Walsh JC. Ulnar nerve lesions associated with the carpal tunnel syndrome. J. Neurol. Neurosurg. Psychiatry 1973;36:118–23.

Sener HO, Tascilar NF, Balaban H, Selcuki D. Sympathetic skin response in carpal tunnel syndrome. Clin. Neurophysiol. 2000;111:1395–99.

Seror P. The centrimetric test: a diagnostic test of certainty in carpal tunnel syndrome. Presse Med. 1988;17:588.

Seror P. The centimeter test: diagnostic test for beginning carpal tunnel syndrome. Neurophysiol. Clin. 1990; 20:137–44.

Seror P. Sensitivity of the various tests for the diagnosis of carpal tunnel syndrome. J. Hand Surg. 1994;19B:725–28.

Seror P. The value of special motor and sensory tests for the diagnosis of benign and minor median nerve lesion at the wrist. Am. J. Phys. Med. Rehabil. 1995;74:124–29.

Seror P. The axonal carpal tunnel syndrome. Electroencephalogr. Clin. Neurophysiol. 1996;101:197–200.

Seror P. Orthodromic inching test in mild carpal tunnel syndrome. Muscle Nerve 1998;21:1206–8.

Seror P. Comparative diagnostic sensitivities of orthodromic or antidromic sensory inching test in mild carpal tunnel syndrome. Arch. Phys. Med. Rehabil. 2000;81:442–46.

Shafshak TS, El-Hinawy YM. The anterior interosseous nerve latency in the diagnosis of severe carpal tunnel syndrome with unobtainable median nerve distal conduction. Arch. Phys. Med. Rehabil. 1995;76:471–75.

Shahani BT, Halperin JJ, Boulu P, Cohen J. Sympathetic skin response: a method of assessing unmyelinated axon dysfunction in peripheral neuropathies. J. Neurol. Neurosurg. Psychiatry 1984;47:536–42.

Shahani BT, Young RR, Potts F, Maccabee P. Terminal latency index (TLI) and late response studies in motor neuron disease (MND), peripheral neuropathies and entrapment syndromes. Acta Neurol. Scand. 1979;74:118.

Sheean GL, Houser MK, Murray NM. Lumbrical-interosseous latency comparison in the diagnosis of carpal tunnel syndrome. Electroencephalogr. Clin. Neurophysiol. 1995; 97:285–89.

Shefner JM, Buchthal F, Krarup C. Slowly conducting myelinated fibers in peripheral neuropathy. Muscle Nerve 1991;14:534–42.

Simovic D, Weinberg DH. Terminal latency index in the carpal tunnel syndrome. Muscle Nerve 1997;20:1178–80.

Simovic D, Weinberg DH. The median nerve terminal latency index in carpal tunnel syndrome: a clinical case selection study. Muscle Nerve 1999;22:573–77.

Simpson JA. Electrical signs in the diagnosis of carpal tunnel and related syndromes. J. Neurol. Neurosurg. Psychiatry 1958;19:275–80.

Simpson JA, Thomaides T. Fasciculation and focal loss of nerve accommodation in peripheral neuropathies. Acta Neurol. Scand. 1988;77:133–41.

Singer PA, Lin JTY. Decremental response in carpal tunnel syndrome. Muscle Nerve 1982;5:566.

Smith T. Near-nerve versus surface electrode recordings of sensory nerve conduction in patients with carpal tunnel syndrome. Acta Neurol. Scand. 1998;98:280–82.

Spaans F. Spontaneous rhythmic motor unit potentials in the carpal tunnel syndrome. J. Neurol. Neurosurg. Psychiatry 1982;45:19–28.

Steinberg DR, Gelberman RH, Rydevik B, Lundborg G. The utility of portable nerve conduction testing for patients with carpal tunnel syndrome: a prospective clinical study. J. Hand Surg. 1992;17A:77–81.

Stevens JC. AAEE minimonograph 26: the electrodiagnosis of carpal tunnel syndrome. Muscle Nerve 1987;10:99–113.

Stevens JC. AAEM minimonograph 26: the electrodiagnosis of carpal tunnel syndrome. American Association of Electrodiagnostic Medicine. Muscle Nerve 1997;20:1477–86.

Stoehr M, Petruch F, Scheglmann K, Schilling K. Retrograde changes of nerve fibers with the carpal tunnel syndrome. An electroneurographic investigation. J. Neurol. 1978;218:287–92.

Sun SF, Streib EW. Martin-Gruber anastomosis: electromyographic studies. Electromyogr. Clin. Neurophysiol. 1983;23:271–85.

Tackmann W, Kaeser HE, Magun HG. Comparison of orthodromic and antidromic sensory nerve conduction velocity measurements in the carpal tunnel syndrome. J. Neurol. 1981;224:257–66.

Tackmann W, Lehmann HJ. Relative refractory period of median nerve sensory fibres in the carpal tunnel syndrome. Eur. Neurol. 1974;12:309–16.

Terzis S, Paschalis C, Metallinos IC, Papapetropoulos T. Early diagnosis of carpal tunnel syndrome: comparison of sensory conduction studies of four fingers. Muscle Nerve 1998;21:1543–45.

Thomas JE, Lambert EH, Cseuz KA. Electrodiagnostic aspects of the carpal tunnel syndrome. Arch. Neurol. 1967; 16:635–41.

Thomas PK. Motor nerve conduction in the carpal tunnel syndrome. Neurology 1960;10:1045–50.

Tinazzi M, Zanette G, Volpato D, Testoni R, Bonato C, Manganotti P, Miniussi C, Fiaschi A. Neurophysiological evidence of neuroplasticity at multiple levels of the somatosensory system in patients with carpal tunnel syndrome. Brain 1998;121:1785–94.

Toyonaga K, DeFaria CR. Electromyographic diagnosis of the carpal tunnel syndrome. Arq. Neuropsiquiatr. 1978;36:127–34.

Tzeng SS, Wu ZA, Chu FL. Proximal slowing of nerve conduction velocity in carpal tunnel syndrome. Chin. Med. J. (Taipei) 1990;45:186–90.

Uchida Y, Sugioka Y. Electrodiagnosis of retrograde changes in carpal tunnel syndrome. Electromyogr. Clin. Neurophysiol. 1993;33:55–58.

Uncini A, Di Muzio A, Awad J, Manente G, Tafuro M, Gambi D. Sensitivity of three median-to-ulnar comparative tests in diagnosis of mild carpal tunnel syndrome. Muscle Nerve 1993;16:1366–73.

Uncini A, Di Muzio A, Cutarella R, Awad J, Gambi D. Orthodromic median and ulnar fourth digit sensory conductions in mild carpal tunnel syndrome. Neurophysiol. Clin. 1990;20:53–61.

Uncini A, Lange DJ, Solomon M, Soliven B, Meer J, Lovelace RE. Ring finger testing in carpal tunnel syndrome: a comparative study of diagnostic utility. Muscle Nerve 1989; 12:735–41.

van Dijk JG, van Benten I, Kramer CG, Stegeman DF. CMAP amplitude cartography of muscles innervated by the median, ulnar, peroneal, and tibial nerves. Muscle Nerve 1999;22:378–89.

Vennix MJ, Hirsh DD, Chiou-Tan FY, Rossi CD. Predicting acute denervation in carpal tunnel syndrome. Arch. Phys. Med. Rehabil. 1998;79:306–12.

Verghese J, Galanopoulou AS, Herskovitz S. Autonomic dysfunction in idiopathic carpal tunnel syndrome. Muscle Nerve 2000;23:1209–13.

Werner RA, Albers JW. Relation between needle electromyography and nerve conduction studies in patients with carpal tunnel syndrome. Arch. Phys. Med. Rehabil. 1995;76:246–49.

Werner RA, Bir C, Armstrong TJ. Reverse Phalen's maneuver as an aid in diagnosing carpal tunnel syndrome. Arch. Phys. Med. Rehabil. 1994;75:783–86.

White JC. On the use of upper extremity proximal nerve action potentials in the localization of focal nerve lesions producing axonotmesis. Electromyogr. Clin. Neurophysiol. 1997;37:323–34.

White JC, Hansen SR, Johnson RK. A comparison of EMG procedures in the carpal tunnel syndrome with clinical-EMG correlations. Muscle Nerve 1988;11:1177–82.

Wiederholt WC. Median nerve conduction velocity in sensory fibers through carpal tunnel. Arch. Phys. Med. Rehabil. 1970;51:328–30.

Yates SK, Yaworski R, Brown WF. Relative preservation of lumbrical versus thenar motor fibres in neurogenic disorders. J. Neurol. Neurosurg. Psychiatry 1981;44:768–74.

Zamir D, Amar M, Groisman G, Weiner P. *Toxoplasma* infection in systemic lupus erythematosus mimicking lupus cerebritis. Mayo Clin. Proc. 1999;74:575–78.

Chapter 8
Interpretation of Electrodiagnostic Findings

Importance of Clinical Setting

Despite the abundant variety of available electrodiagnostic tests, carpal tunnel syndrome remains a clinical diagnosis. Test results can support the diagnosis but can never make the diagnosis by themselves. This chapter has a recurring theme: Laboratory evidence of impaired impulse conduction in the median nerve at the wrist does not prove that a patient's clinical signs or symptoms are caused by the conduction abnormality.

Many clinicians diagnose and initiate early treatment of carpal tunnel syndrome based on signs and symptoms before performing electrodiagnostic evaluation. Some hand surgeons operate for carpal tunnel syndrome without obtaining electrodiagnostic tests (Duncan, Lewis, Foreman & Nordyke, 1987; Trojaborg, Kelly-Perez & Sheriff, 1996).

If their limitations are understood, electrodiagnostic tests are very helpful in assessing carpal tunnel syndrome patients, particularly in difficult diagnostic cases. For a number of reasons, we favor electrodiagnostic evaluation of every patient before carpal tunnel surgery. First, electrodiagnosis offers information about the severity of dysfunction of the median nerve. Second, the electrodiagnostician, evaluating the patient with neuropathic arm symptoms, has the opportunity to obtain data on other diagnostic possibilities. Depending on the clinical setting, these possibilities might include other mononeuropathies, mononeuritis multiplex, disease of the median nerve outside the carpal tunnel, brachial plexopathy, cervical radiculopathy, anterior horn cell dis-

ease, or diffuse peripheral neuropathy. Third, preoperative electrodiagnostic studies provide baseline data necessary to evaluate patients who have persistent symptoms after surgery.

Personal Factors Affecting Nerve Conduction

Body Mass Index

The role of obesity in genesis of carpal tunnel syndrome is discussed in Chapter 6. Regardless of presence or absence of symptoms of carpal tunnel syndrome, obese workers are more likely than slender workers to have abnormal conduction across the carpal tunnel (Nathan, Keniston, Myers & Meadows, 1992; Werner, Franzblau, Albers & Armstrong, 1997). In asymptomatic healthy subjects sensory and mixed nerve action potential amplitudes for the median nerve (and for the ulnar, posterior tibial, and peroneal nerves) decrease as body mass index increases; motor amplitudes and motor, sensory, or mixed nerve latencies do not correlate with body mass index (Buschbacher, 1998).

Temperature

Median motor and sensory latencies increase, and sensory nerve action potential (SNAP) amplitudes decrease, as limb temperature increases (Buchthal & Rosenfalck, 1966; Bolton, Sawa & Carter, 1981). For example, in one laboratory median distal sensory latency (DSL) or distal motor latency

(DML) increased approximately 0.2 msec for each degree centigrade decrease in wrist skin temperature; in the forearm, median motor nerve conduction velocity (MNCV) decreased 1.5 m/sec and median sensory nerve conduction velocity (SNCV) decreased 1.4 m/sec for each degree centigrade decrease in temperature (Halar, DeLisa & Soine, 1983). However, correction factors reported from other laboratories range from 1.0 to 2.4 m/sec/degree centigrade (Ashworth, Marshall & Satkunam, 1998). Therefore, whenever possible, the limb should be maintained within a standard temperature range during nerve conduction testing, rather than use a formula or correction factor to attempt to compensate for a limb that is too cool or too warm.

Therapeutic ultrasound can temporarily increase nerve latencies for conduction through treated areas. This effect is explained by ultrasonic heating of subcutaneous tissue (Moore, Gieck, Saliba, Perrin, Ball & McCue, 2000).

In some studies, patients who had carpal tunnel syndrome did not display the same relation of median SNCV to temperature change that had been found in normal median nerves or in ipsilateral ulnar nerves (Fine & Wongjirad, 1985; Ashworth, Marshall & Satkunam, 1998). In contrast, others have found that median DML and DSL responded similarly to changes in temperature whether in patients who had carpal tunnel syndrome or in asymptomatic individuals who had normal median nerve conduction (Baysal, Chang & Oh, 1993; Wang, Raynor, Blum & Rutkove, 1999). There are conflicting data in these studies on the effect of temperature on median SNAP amplitude.

Age

Normally, median nerve conduction velocity decreases with increasing age. The amplitude of the median SNAP decreases, the DML and DSL increase, and MNCV and SNCV decrease with age. For example, in a sample of workers not doing repetitive hand and wrist activity, MNCV decreased 0.8 m/sec per decade of age, and SNCV decreased 1.3 m/sec per decade (Stetson, Albers, Silverstein & Wolfe, 1992). A longitudinal study of industrial workers shows the gradual slowing of DSL over 11 years (Figure 8-1) (Nathan, Keniston, Myers, Meadows & Lockwood, 1998). Table 8-1 shows data obtained using surface electrodes, stimulating at the wrist, and recording at the index finger for sensory studies and at the thenar eminence for motor studies (LaFratta, 1972; LaFratta & Canestrari, 1966). Perhaps, residual motor latency is less sensitive than DML to changes in age (Kraft & Halvorson, 1983).

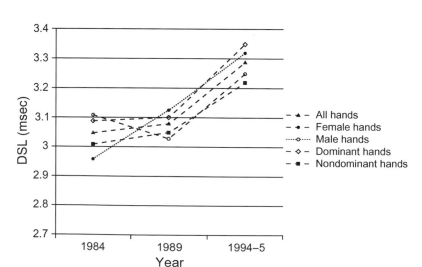

Figure 8-1. Longitudinal changes in median distal sensory latency (DSL) (14-cm distance) for 280 workers followed for 11 years. (Data from PA Nathan, RC Keniston, LD Myers, KD Meadows, RS Lockwood. Natural history of median nerve sensory conduction in industry: relationship to symptoms and carpal tunnel syndrome in 558 hands over 11 years. Muscle Nerve 1998;21:711–21.)

Table 8-1. Effect of Age on Median Nerve Conduction

Decade of age	3rd	4th	5th	6th	7th	8th	9th
Mean sensory nerve action potential amplitude (μV)	55	47	44	36	36	18	23
Mean distal sensory latency (msec)	3.15	3.19	3.43	3.67	3.82	3.96	4.08
Mean distal motor latency (msec)	3.45	3.44	3.71	3.81	3.91	3.77	3.98

Data from CW LaFratta, RE Canestrari. A comparison of sensory and motor nerve conduction velocities as related to age. Arch. Phys. Med. Rehabil. 1972;53:388–89; and CW LaFratta. Relation of age to amplitude of evoked sensory nerve potentials: a supplemental report. Arch. Phys. Med. Rehabil. 1996;47:286–90.

The slowing of nerve conduction with age is more marked in the portion of the median nerve in the carpal tunnel than in the digital nerves or in the palmar portion of the ulnar nerve. Cruz-Martinez and colleagues (1978) measured orthodromic SNCV in median and ulnar nerves in an asymptomatic population. They compared digit-to-palm and palm-to-wrist SNCV in both nerves. In all segments, the mean SNCV was lower in subjects over 50 years old than in younger subjects. The drop in SNCV with age was most marked in the palm-to-wrist segment of the median nerve. Regardless of age, the ulnar palm-to-wrist SNCV remained faster than the ulnar digit-to-palm SNCV. In contrast, in the group older than age 50 years, the median palm-to-wrist SNCV fell slightly below the median digit-to-palm SNCV. The median transcarpal maximum serial sensory latency difference (MLD) also increases with age (Nathan, Meadows & Doyle, 1988a). In older patients, the upper limit of normal for medial-ulnar or median-radial comparison studies is increased (Hennessey, Falco, Braddom & Goldberg, 1994).

The decrease in SNAP amplitude with age, using finger stimulation and recording at the wrist, is greater in median-innervated digits than in ulnar-innervated digits, which can be important if SNAP amplitude ratio is used as a diagnostic test. Table 8-2 shows representative data (Cruz Martinez, Barrio, Perez Conde & Gutierrez, 1978).

The serial sensory MLD increases with age. Table 8-3 shows data for one group of workers randomly chosen without regard to symptoms (Nathan, Meadows & Doyle, 1988a). Is an MLD greater than 0.5 msec abnormal in sexagenarians? The incidence of carpal tunnel syndrome is lower after age 65 years than between the ages of 45 and 64 years (Stevens, Sun, Beard, O'Fallon & Kurland, 1988). If normal limits are not adjusted upward for age, the incidence of false-positive results increases with age.

Finger Circumference

For antidromic ulnar or median sensory studies, SNAP amplitude recorded with surface electrodes

Table 8-2. Effect of Age on Sensory Nerve Action Potential Amplitude

Age (yrs)	Sensory Nerve Action Potential Amplitude (μV)		Ratio
	Middle Finger	Little Finger	
≤30	22.2	11.5	1.93
31–49	18.0	11.0	1.64
≥50	12.0	7.5	1.60

Table 8-3. Variation with Age of Median Serial Sensory Maximum Serial Sensory Latency Difference

	18–29 Yrs (%)	30–39 Yrs (%)	40–49 Yrs (%)	50–69 Yrs (%)
Men with maximum serial sensory latency difference >0.5	8	9	23	32
Women with maximum serial sensory latency difference >0.5	15	20	28	35

Data from PA Nathan, KD Meadows, LS Doyle. Relationship of age and sex to sensory conduction of the median nerve at the carpal tunnel and association of slowed conduction with symptoms. Muscle Nerve 1988a;11:1149–53.

over the digit decreases as finger circumference increases (Bolton & Carter, 1980; Stetson, Albers, Silverstein & Wolfe, 1992). This is probably due to increased distance between the electrodes and the digital nerve caused by subcutaneous tissue of the larger fingers.

Gender

The mean median thenar CMAP amplitude was slightly smaller in a group of normal women (15.0 mV) than of normal men (17.1 mV); the mean antidromic median SNAP amplitude recorded at the index finger with ring electrodes after wrist stimulation was higher in a group of normal women (62.1 μV) than in a group of normal men (45.3 μV) (Felsenthal, 1978). Mean DML to thenar muscles was slightly shorter for normal women than for normal men (Buschbacher, 1999). Others have confirmed the gender effect on SNAP amplitude but not on CMAP amplitude (Hennessey, Falco, Goldberg & Braddom, 1994). These findings are largely explicable by differences in height and finger circumference (Bolton & Carter, 1980; Stetson, Albers, Silverstein & Wolfe, 1992).

Handedness

Mean median DSL and DML do not vary with handedness in groups of healthy subjects (Felsenthal, 1978). The amplitudes of the median thenar CMAP and antidromic SNAP recorded with surface electrodes at the index finger are slightly smaller in the right than in the left hand of asymptomatic right handers (Felsenthal, 1978; Werner & Franzblau, 1996). The amplitude differences might reflect differences in hand callosity; an opposite effect on SNAP amplitude has been noted with orthodromic stimulation (Cruz Martinez, Barrio, Perez Conde & Gutierrez, 1978).

Hand Position

The median nerve slides with wrist motion so that the length of nerve between surface stimulating and recording electrodes varies unless wrist and elbow position are kept constant from test to test (Gordan, 1981; Valls-Solé, Alvarez & Nuñez, 1995). The changes in median nerve latency induced by wrist and elbow movement are reduced in some patients with carpal tunnel syndrome (Valls-Solé, Alvarez & Nuñez, 1995). Changes in thumb position can change thenar CMAP amplitude and morphology (Lateva, McGill & Burgar, 1996).

Height

For practical purposes, height does not significantly affect median nerve conduction parameters. A number of authors have examined this issue with slightly conflicting results (Rivner, Swift, Crout & Rhodes, 1990; Letz & Gerr, 1993; Hennessey, Falco, Goldberg & Braddom, 1994). Results are summarized in Table 8-4.

Table 8-4. Relations between Height and Median Nerve Conduction Parameters

Reference	Effect of Change in Height on Median Nerve Conduction Parameters
Stetson, Albers, Silverstein & Wolfe, 1992	Height negatively associated with sensory nerve action potential amplitude and positively associated with distal sensory latency.
Rivner, Swift, Crout & Rhodes, 1990	Motor nerve conduction velocity not correlated with height, but distal motor latency increase of 0.016 msec/cm of height.
Letz & Gerr, 1993	Motor nerve conduction velocity slows 0.045 m/sec/cm of height; sensory nerve conduction velocity change with height is not significant; sensory nerve action potential amplitude decreases slightly with increasing height.
Hennessey, Falco, Goldberg & Braddom, 1994	Motor nerve conduction velocity is independent of arm length; sensory nerve action potential amplitude decreases slightly with increasing arm length.

Wrist Dimensions

The *wrist ratio* is defined as the wrist anteroposterior diameter divided by the mediolateral diameter based on measurements at the distal wrist crease. The mean wrist ratio in the population is higher for women than for men; it does not correlate with age or body mass index (Radecki, 1994). Both median DML and DSL have a weak, statistically significant, correlation with wrist ratio (Johnson, Gatens, Poindexter & Bowers, 1983; Gordon, Johnson, Gatens & Ashton, 1988; Nathan, Keniston, Myers & Meadows, 1992; Stetson, Albers, Silverstein & Wolfe, 1992; Radecki, 1994, 1995; Nathan, Keniston, Lockwood & Meadows, 1996; Salerno, Franzblau, Werner, Bromberg, Armstrong & Albers, 1998). Ulnar sensory latency may have a weaker correlation with wrist width (Salerno, Franzblau, Werner, Bromberg, Armstrong & Albers, 1998). The pathophysiology of these observations is still unknown.

Among a group of patients referred to an electrodiagnostic laboratory because of symptoms possibly indicative of carpal tunnel syndrome, 69% of those with abnormal median nerve conduction had a wrist ratio greater than or equal to 0.70, while only 27% of those with normal median nerve conduction had this ratio (Kuhlman & Hennessey, 1997). In another group of patients with carpal tunnel syndrome by clinical and electrodiagnostic criteria, those with longer wrist-to-index finger latencies were likely to have higher wrist ratios (Kouyoumdjian, Morita, Rocha, Miranda & Gouveia, 2000). It is unclear whether wrist ratio represents a risk factor for development of carpal tunnel syndrome or affects nerve conduction results without affecting the risk of having carpal tunnel syndrome.

In a study of sensory conduction between wrist and digit in normal hands, both orthodromic and antidromic, median and ulnar, SNAP amplitudes declined as wrist anteroposterior diameter increased (Chira-Adisai, Yan & Turan, 1999).

Test Sensitivity in Carpal Tunnel Syndrome

There is no test that is always abnormal in every patient who has carpal tunnel syndrome; normal tests in patients who have clinical symptoms and signs of carpal tunnel syndrome are *false-negative results*. The *sensitivity* of a test for carpal tunnel syndrome is defined as the ratio of positive tests in patients who have the syndrome (*true-positive results*) to total number of tested patients who have the syndrome (Schulzer, 1994).

$$\text{Test sensitivity} = \frac{(\text{True-positive results})}{\left(\begin{array}{c}\text{True-positive}\\\text{results}\end{array}\right) + \left(\begin{array}{c}\text{False-negative}\\\text{results}\end{array}\right)}$$

Comparing sensitivity of techniques is difficult because different published studies use differing populations of patients and because each laboratory uses an idiosyncratic version of the techniques. Table 8-5 shows the approximate relative sensitivity of different techniques (Evans & Daube, 1984; White et al., 1988; Cruz Martinez, 1991).

A less sensitive test is occasionally abnormal when a more sensitive test is normal. For example, in carpal tunnel syndrome patients, median DML is less likely to be abnormal than median DSL.

Table 8-5. Relative Sensitivity of Electrodiagnostic Tests for Carpal Tunnel Syndrome

More sensitive	Less sensitive
Serial motor studies	Residual motor latency
Serial sensory studies	Terminal latency index
Repetitive sensory stimulation	Distal motor latency
Transcarpal motor conduction	**Insensitive**
Transcarpal sensory conduction	Electromyographic evidence of axonal interruption
Ipsilateral nerve comparisons	**Rare**
Threshold distal motor latency	Electromyographic evidence of spontaneous repetitive
Distal sensory latency	discharges

However, cases with carpal tunnel syndrome in which DML is abnormal, but DSL is normal do rarely occur and raise the question of selective fascicular damage (Stevens, 1987).

There are conflicting data on the relative sensitivity of different parameters. Felsenthal and Spindler (1979) found that median-ulnar sensory latency comparison and median transcarpal sensory conduction values were equally sensitive in diagnosing mild median sensory conduction abnormalities. Median-radial and median-ulnar sensory latency comparisons are approximately equally sensitive in detecting mild median nerve conduction slowing (Pease, Cannell & Johnson, 1989). Pease and colleagues (1989) and Cassvan and colleagues (1988) both found median-radial latency comparisons more sensitive than median palmar conduction values. Monga and colleagues (1985) found median palmar values slightly more sensitive than median-ulnar comparisons. Comparing laboratories is confusing because of differences in techniques, populations, diagnostic criteria for carpal tunnel syndrome, and normal ranges; the variation in reported test sensitivities is illustrated in Table 8-6.

One approach to improving test sensitivity while preserving specificity is to use a summary index of different tests. For example, a *combined sensory index* can be calculated by summing the median-ulnar midpalmar mixed nerve latency difference, the median-ulnar ring finger latency difference, and the median-radial thumb latency difference; the combined sensory index is more sensitive and as specific for the diagnosis of carpal tunnel syndrome as is any of these three differences alone (Robinson, Micklesen & Wang, 1998).

Test Specificity for Carpal Tunnel Syndrome

Any median nerve test result occasionally is abnormal in individuals who have no symptoms of carpal tunnel syndrome; test results can be false positive in asymptomatic individuals or be positive because of median nerve pathology other than the carpal tunnel syndrome. Although abnormal median nerve conduction across the carpal tunnel in an asymptomatic individual is falsely positive as a diagnostic test for symptomatic carpal tunnel syndrome, it can still be truly indicative of abnormal median nerve electrophysiology.

Contralateral Asymptomatic Median Nerve

In patients who have unilateral symptomatic carpal tunnel syndrome, the median nerve in the contralat-

Table 8-6. Sensitivity (Percent Abnormal) of Various Electrodiagnostic Parameters in Groups of Patients Who Have Carpal Tunnel Syndrome

Parameter	References*							
	I	II	III	IV	V	VI	VII	VIII
Median palm-wrist conduction	76		33	93	83		51	76
Palmar median-ulnar comparison		56	61			97		
Digital median-ulnar comparison		77		93	61	91	57	88
Thumb median-radial comparison	74		90					
Digit-palm to palm-wrist sensory nerve conduction velocity ratio	98						81	
Lumbrical-interosseous comparison		13		87		88		
Palmar sensory serial latencies							59	100

*I = Padua, Lo Monaco, Valente & Tonali, 1996; II = Uncini, Di Muzio, Awad, Manente, Tafuro & Gambi, 1993; III = Andary, Fankhauser, Ritson, Spiegel, Hulce, Yosef & Stanton, 1996; IV = Foresti, Quadri, Rasella, Tironi, Viscardi & Ubiali, 1996; V = Kuntzer, 1994; VI = Preston, Ross, Kothari, Plotkin, Venkatesh & Logigian, 1994; VII = Girlanda, Quartarone, Sinicropi, Pronesti, Nicolosi, Macaione, Picciolo & Messina, 1998; VIII = Seror, 1994.

eral asymptomatic hand frequently is abnormal on nerve conduction tests. The frequency of abnormality varies with the test used. Those tests that are more sensitive to abnormalities in the symptomatic hand are the tests that are more likely to be abnormal in the asymptomatic hand. Using repetitive stimulation of sensory fibers at 500 Hz, Lehmann and Tackmann (1974) found abnormalities in seven of eight contralateral asymptomatic hands in patients who had unilateral carpal tunnel syndrome. Table 8-7 gives representative data for asymptomatic hands in patients with unilateral symptoms.

False-Positive Electrodiagnostic Test Results

Electrodiagnostic abnormalities are found in many limbs that do not have symptoms of carpal tunnel syndrome. In the asymptomatic hand that is contralateral to a symptomatic hand, one can argue whether to classify a detected abnormality as *false positive*. Because the hand is asymptomatic, the abnormality is a false-positive indicator of symptomatic carpal tunnel syndrome. However, in many, but probably not all, contralateral asymptomatic hands, the abnormal electrodiagnostic test is a true-positive sign of median nerve microscopic pathology. Another example of the same dichotomy is the persistence of abnormalities of nerve conduction after carpal tunnel surgery that successfully relieves symptoms; the abnormal test signifies persisting neuropathology that is no longer symptomatic.

Abnormal median nerve conduction values can also be present in individuals who have no history of carpal tunnel syndrome. In some, these abnormalities reflect asymptomatic or presymptomatic nerve pathology; it others the abnormalities reflect statistical overlap on the test between the healthy and pathologic populations. The overlap is determined both by biological variability of the normal population and by experimental errors inherent in the nerve conduction techniques. As illustrated by the data from contralateral asymptomatic hands (see Table 8-7), the more sensitive the diagnostic test, the higher the incidence of false-positive test responses.

Despite the inevitability of false-positive responses, there is a dearth of data on the false-positive rate of the various electrodiagnostic tests. Table 8-8 shows false-positive rates in 50 subjects with no history of neurologic disease and no signs or symptoms of carpal tunnel syndrome (Redmond & Rivner, 1988). Table 8-8 also illustrates that doing multiple tests increases the risk that at least one result will be falsely positive. For each test, the incidence of false-positive results could be decreased by using more stringent criteria for abnormality, but such more stringent criteria would decrease the diagnostic sensitivity of the test (Rivner, 1994).

There are few data on the natural history of individuals with asymptomatic abnormalities of median nerve conduction across the carpal tunnel. Among

Table 8-7. Nerve Conduction Abnormalities in Asymptomatic Hand Contralateral to a Hand with Carpal Tunnel Syndrome

	Percent Abnormal
Distal motor latency	9
Distal sensory latency	19
Sensory serial stimulation (maximum serial sensory latency difference ≥0.5 msec)	23
Median-radial sensory latency difference	34
Transcarpal sensory latency	56
Terminal latency index	58
Motor serial stimulation	72

Data from JC White, SR Hansen, RK Johnson. A comparison of EMG procedures in the carpal tunnel syndrome with clinical-EMG correlations. Muscle Nerve 1988;11:1177–82.

Table 8-8. Incidence of Abnormal Nerve Conduction Tests in Healthy Subjects

Distal motor latency >4.5 msec	2%
Median-ulnar palmar sensory latency >0.3 msec	8%
Residual motor latency >2.6 msec	14%
Median/ulnar sensory nerve action potential amplitude ratio <1.1	30%
Abnormality on at least one of previously mentioned tests	46%

Data from MD Redmond, MH Rivner. False positive electrodiagnostic tests in carpal tunnel syndrome. Muscle Nerve 1988; 11:511–18.

asymptomatic workers who had a median wrist-to-index finger minus ulnar wrist-to-little finger sensory latency difference more than or equal to 0.5 msec, 12% had developed symptoms suggestive of carpal tunnel syndrome when questioned a mean of 17 months later; however, 10% of workers with a sensory latency difference less than or equal to 0.2 msec had become symptomatic over the same period of follow-up (Werner, Franzblau, Albers, Buchele & Armstrong, 1997). In a larger group of patients with longer follow-up, Nathan and colleagues (1998) found a correlation between median MLD in asymptomatic hands and the probability of developing carpal tunnel syndrome over the next 11 years (Figure 8-2).

Choice of Normal Control Values

In many electrodiagnostic laboratories, normal values are determined from relatively small samples of easily available volunteers, so-called *convenience* controls. In other laboratories, normal values are adopted from the literature. A large sample of normal values from a cohort of asymptomatic active workers emphasizes the effect of factors such as age, sex, hand temperature, and anthropometric features on normal values; even after correcting for these, the normal (95% confidence limit) median-ulnar sensory latency difference was 0.8 msec, a higher value than that commonly used (Salerno, Franzblau, Werner, Bromberg, Armstrong & Albers, 1998).

Development of a test for carpal tunnel syndrome begins with data from healthy controls and from patients who have carpal tunnel syndrome. Validation of the diagnostic value of the test requires *disease controls*, data from patients with illnesses that might be confused with or co-exist with carpal tunnel syndrome (Nierenberg & Feinstein, 1988). So far, published disease control data are inadequate for most carpal tunnel syndrome electrodiagnostic tests. For example, what are the ranges of median nerve conduction findings for patients with soft tissue abnormalities of the arm such as de Quervain's tenosynovitis. If the range of values for these conditions differs from healthy subjects, do the abnormalities bespeak co-existent symptomatic carpal tunnel syndrome or asymptomatic deterioration of median nerve conduction? The answer requires careful clinical assessment and long-term follow-up. Appropriate data are not yet available in the literature.

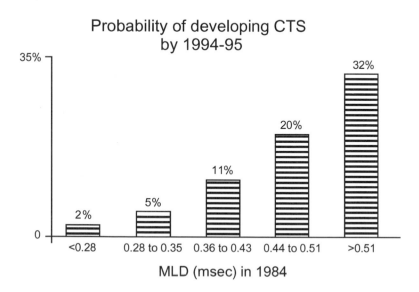

Figure 8-2. Probability of developing carpal tunnel syndrome (CTS) over time as a function of maximum serial sensory latency difference based on 464 asymptomatic hands studied with nerve conduction tests in 1984. (MLD = maximum serial sensory latency difference.) (Data from PA Nathan, RC Keniston, LD Myers, KD Meadows, RS Lockwood. Natural history of median nerve sensory conduction in industry: relationship to symptoms and carpal tunnel syndrome in 558 hands over 11 years. Muscle Nerve 1998;21:711–21.)

Results in Patients with Co-Existent Neuropathy

Normative studies of nerve conduction techniques in patients with carpal tunnel syndrome routinely exclude patients with diffuse polyneuropathy. Interpretation of nerve conduction values across the carpal tunnel in patients with polyneuropathies requires appropriate disease control data. Diabetic peripheral neuropathy is the best-studied example. There is an increased prevalence of symptoms of carpal tunnel syndrome in patients with diabetic peripheral neuropathy (Dieck & Kelsey, 1985). Ozaki and colleagues (1988) compared ulnar and median nerve conduction in insulin-dependent diabetics, most of whom had clinical evidence of peripheral neuropathy. The patients were carefully screened to *exclude* patients with symptoms of carpal tunnel syndrome. As expected, in diabetic polyneuropathy, the median and ulnar nerves of the patient group had abnormal DSL, DML, MNCV, and SNCV compared with controls. In addition, median DSL and DML were often more abnormal than ulnar DSL and DML, suggesting that the median nerve in the carpal tunnel was more vulnerable than the ulnar nerve in the hand to developing conduction abnormality. For example, 14 of 49 asymptomatic diabetic hands (29%) had a median DML at least 2.0 msec more than the ipsilateral ulnar DML. Focal median nerve abnormalities across the carpal tunnel were more common in women than in men.

Some 23% of subjects in the Early Diabetes Intervention Trial who had mild distal symmetric polyneuropathy diagnosed by clinical and electrodiagnostic criteria also had selective slowing of distal median nerve conduction in their nondominant hands (Albers, Brown, Sima & Greene, 1996). Subjects with electrodiagnostic evidence of median mononeuropathy were likely to have had diabetes for longer. Among those with non–insulin-dependent diabetes, risk factors for median mononeuropathy were female gender, shorter height, and higher body mass index.

The Rochester Diabetic Neuropathy Study thoroughly examined a population-based cohort of diabetics (Dyck, Kratz, Karnes, Litchy, Klein, Pach, Wilson, O'Brien & Melton, 1993). As shown in Table 8-9, asymptomatic focal slowing of median nerve conduction in these diabetics was much more common than was symptomatic carpal tunnel syndrome. The prevalence of focal median nerve

Table 8-9. Prevalence of Focal Median Nerve Conduction Slowing or Carpal Tunnel Syndrome in the Rochester Diabetic Neuropathy Study Cohort

	Insulin-Dependent Diabetes Mellitus (%)	Non–Insulin-Dependent Diabetes Mellitus (%)
No clinical or electrodiagnostic evidence of carpal tunnel syndrome	70	65
Electrodiagnostic evidence of focal median slowing, but no symptoms of carpal tunnel syndrome	22	29
Symptoms of carpal tunnel syndrome, regardless of electrodiagnostic findings	9	4
Symptoms and electrodiagnostic findings diagnostic of carpal tunnel syndrome	2	2

Data from PJ Dyck, KM Kratz, JL Karnes, WJ Litchy, R Klein, JM Pach, DM Wilson, PC O'Brien, LJ Melton. The prevalence by staged severity of various types of diabetic neuropathy, retinopathy, and nephropathy in a population-based cohort: the Rochester diabetic neuropathy study. Neurology 1993;43:817.

conduction slowing increased with duration of diabetes but did not correlate with age or gender.

The high incidence of asymptomatic focal slowing of median nerve conduction across the carpal tunnel in patients with diabetic polyneuropathy creates a diagnostic paradox: Symptomatic carpal tunnel syndrome is common in diabetics; nonetheless, the presence of a focal abnormality of median nerve conduction is less helpful in diabetics than in nondiabetics in determining whether hand symptoms are caused by carpal tunnel syndrome.

Guillain-Barré syndrome provides another example of the propensity of the median nerve to show asymptomatic focal abnormalities across the carpal tunnel in patients with polyneuropathies. Patients with Guillain-Barré syndrome often show a prolonged median DSL when sensory conduction is normal in the sural nerve (Albers, Donofrio & McGonagle, 1985).

Vogt and colleagues (1997) compared median and ulnar motor conduction findings in patients with

Table 8-10. Median-to-Lumbrical versus Ulnar-to-Interosseous Motor Latency Difference in Patients with Polyneuropathy with or without Carpal Tunnel Syndrome

	Control	Polyneuropathy Alone	Polyneuropathy and Carpal Tunnel Syndrome
Lumbrical-interosseus latency difference ± standard deviation (msec)	0.45 ± 0.25	1.1 ± 1.2	2.9 ± 2.0
Percent of hands with difference >1.0 msec	0	18	96

Data from T Vogt, A Mika, F Thomke, HC Hopf. Evaluation of carpal tunnel syndrome in patients with polyneuropathy. Muscle Nerve 1997;20:153–57.

polyneuropathy with or without coincident symptoms of carpal tunnel syndrome. The polyneuropathies were of varied causes and were severe enough to cause forearm motor conduction slowing in the median and ulnar nerves. Patients with polyneuropathy and no symptoms of carpal tunnel syndrome often had prolonged median distal motor latencies to the thenar muscles and a median DML to thenar muscles at least 1.6 msec more than the ulnar DML to abductor digiti minimi. The median to lumbrical latency minus the ulnar to interosseous latency was a better but imperfect parameter for separating patients with polyneuropathy alone from patients with polyneuropathy and carpal tunnel syndrome (Table 8-10).

Asymptomatic focal median nerve conduction slowing in patients with polyneuropathy might signify vulnerability of diseased nerve to entrapment; alternatively, nerve fiber demyelination or dropout can unmask pre-existing focal nerve entrapment.

Receiver Operating Characteristic Curves

The continuous measurements of nerve conduction studies (e.g., latencies or nerve conduction velocities) have overlapping distributions of results for patients who have carpal tunnel syndrome and individuals who do not have carpal tunnel syndrome; inevitably, there is an overlap of the values for the two groups (Rivner, 1994; Schulzer, 1994). By changing the cutoff value between normal and abnormal, the specificity and sensitivity of the test can be changed reciprocally: Changing the normal range to increase the specificity decreases the sensitivity (Figure 8-3). In Table 8-11, the relationship between increased diagnostic sensitivity and increased incidence of false-positive results is illustrated for median nerve palmar serial sensory stimulation studies (Nathan, Meadows & Doyle, 1988b).

This relation between sensitivity and specificity for a test can be graphed as a *receiver operator char-*

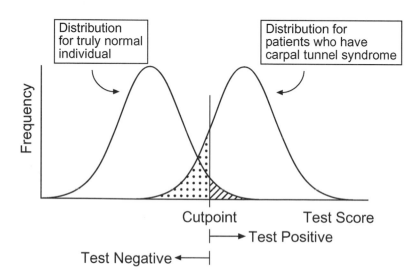

Figure 8-3. For every electrodiagnostic test, values for patients who have carpal tunnel syndrome and values for asymptomatic individuals overlap. Changing the cutpoint leads to reciprocal changes in false-negative (*stippled area*) and false-positive (*cross-hatched area*) rates. (Adapted with permission from Schulzer, 1994.)

Table 8-11. Serial Median Sensory Stimulation: Sensitivity and False-Positive Results Vary with Diagnostic Criteria

Definition of Abnormal	Sensitivity (%)	False-Positive Results (%)
Maximum serial sensory latency difference ≥0.5 msec	54	3
Maximum serial sensory latency difference ≥0.4 msec	81	19

Data from PA Nathan, KD Meadows, LS Doyle. Sensory segmental latency values of the median nerve for a population of normal individuals. Arch. Phys. Med. Rehabil. 1988b;69:499–501.

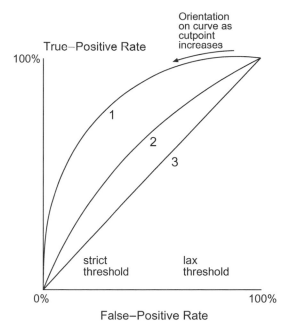

Figure 8-4. Three receiver operating characteristic curves are illustrated. These curves are drawn to show how the true-positive and false-positive rates of three diagnostic tests change with the position of the cutpoint in Figure 8-3. As the cutpoint increases, the corresponding position on the curve moves down and to the left. Curve 1 represents a test with high sensitivity and specificity at all cutpoint values. Curve 2 illustrates a test with lower sensitivity and specificity. Curve 3 corresponds to a totally uninformative test: At any level of the cutpoint, the test has equal chances of labeling a normal and a diseased individual as "positive." (Redrawn with permission from Schulzer, 1994.)

acteristic curve (Figure 8-4) (Schulzer, 1994). Figure 8-5 shows a typical received operator characteristic curve, using DML to distinguish healthy controls from patients who had a clinical diagnosis of carpal tunnel syndrome (Eisen, Schulzer, Pant, MacNeil, Stewart, Trueman, J & Mak, 1993). In this example, the statistical median value for DML in the control group was 3.5 msec, which corresponds to a false-positive rate of 50% on the receiver operator characteristic graph. A larger DML would have a lower probability of being a false-positive result, but also have a lower probability of being abnormal in a patient who had carpal tunnel syndrome. Eisen and colleagues (1993) provide tables illustrating how to estimate the probability that a patient has carpal tunnel syndrome for any given combination of median ulnar palmar latency difference and median DML Tables of this type are dependent on the prevalence of carpal tunnel syndrome in the population being examined, and so cannot be extrapolated from one electrodiagnostic laboratory to another (Grosser, Neuhauser & Katirji, 1994).

Clinical Electrodiagnostic Correlation

In patients with carpal tunnel syndrome, the correlation between symptoms, signs, and electrodiagnostic findings is imperfect. Patients who have pain and paresthesias with normal nerve conduction study results or who have abnormal nerve conduction in an asymptomatic hand are commonplace. In surveys of workers or applicants for work, one-half or more of individuals with mild abnormalities of transcarpal median nerve conduction are asymptomatic (Bingham, Rosecrance & Cook, 1996; Werner, Franzblau, Albers & Armstrong, 1998; Hamann, Werner, Franzblau, Rodgers, Siew & Gruninger, 2001). The presence or absence of pain and paresthesias correlates poorly with routine electrodiagnostic abnormalities (Wilbourn, Hanson, Lederman & Salanga, 1980; Shivde, Dreizin & Fisher, 1981; Ferry, Silman, Pritchard, Keenan & Croft, 1998; Homan, Franzblau, Werner, Albers, Armstrong & Bromberg, 1999). Pain and other symptoms can be prominent when nerve conduction results are normal or minimally abnormal (Padua, Padua, Lo Monaco, Aprile & Tonali, 1999). Nonetheless, there are trends relating the severity of clinical disease and the severity of electrodiagnostic abnormalities (Dhong, Han, Lee & Kim, 2000). Symptoms that correlate best with nerve conduction results include nocturnal

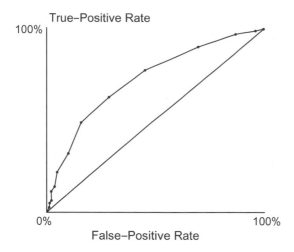

Figure 8-5. This receiver operating characteristic curve shows the use of distal motor latency to distinguish patients who have a clinical diagnosis of carpal tunnel syndrome from healthy controls for the laboratory of A Eisen, M Schulzer, B Pant, M MacNeil, H Stewart, S Trueman, E Mak. Receiver operating characteristic curve analysis in the prediction of carpal tunnel syndrome: a model for reporting electrophysiological data. Muscle Nerve 1993;16:787–96.

awakening, morning symptoms, relief from shaking the hand on awakening, typical median-innervated sensory distribution of paresthesias, and history of benefiting from wrist splinting (You, Simmons, Freivalds, Kothari & Naidu, 1999; Bland, 2000). In contrast, symptoms of hand pain, clumsiness, and weakness correlate less well with nerve conduction results (You, Simmons, Freivalds, Kothari & Naidu, 1999).

Nerve conduction is more likely to be abnormal in patients with longer duration of symptoms. In one series, only one-half of patients with symptoms for less than 3 months had a prolonged median DML; in contrast, three-fourths of patients with symptoms for greater than 1 year had a prolonged median DML (Thomas, Lambert & Cseuz, 1967). Similar differences are noted for median SNAP amplitude or median sensory latencies across the carpal tunnel (Loong, 1977).

Clinical thenar weakness is more likely to be present if there is prolonged median DML, low amplitude thenar CMAP, or neuropathic abnormalities on electromyography (Wilbourn, Hanson, Lederman & Salanga, 1980; Shivde, Dreizin & Fisher, 1981; Pavesi, Olivieri, Misk & Mancia, 1986). Both symptoms of impaired hand function as rated on the Carpal Tunnel Functional Status Scale (see Table 15-10 and findings of median nerve dysfunction by examination are more likely if median sensory responses are unobtainable and DML is prolonged or unobtainable (Padua, Padua, Lo Monaco, Aprile & Tonali, 1999).

The clinical sensory examination is often normal despite mild to moderate abnormalities of sensory conduction. If the clinical sensory examination is abnormal, sensory studies usually show slowed conduction, often with decreased amplitude of the SNAP (Thomas, Lambert & Cseuz, 1967; Pavesi, Olivieri, Misk & Mancia, 1986). Patients with constant rather than intermittent symptoms are more likely to have abnormal nerve conduction findings (White, Hansen & Johnson, 1988). The results depend both on the nerve conduction test used and the clinical sensory test used.

Spindler and Dellon (1982) divided carpal tunnel syndrome patients into those with intermittent and those with constant symptoms. Motor conduction was considered abnormal if the median DML was greater than 4.0 msec or greater than the ulnar DML plus 1.0 msec. Sensory conduction was considered abnormal if the DSL measured at onset was greater than 3.1 msec or greater than the ulnar DSL plus 0.4 msec. Sensory tests were perception of a vibrating tuning fork head or two-point discrimination. Figure 8-6 shows the correlation between sensory symptoms, sensory examination, and nerve conduction results.

Electrodiagnosis and Response to Therapy

Median nerve conduction usually improves following successful treatment of carpal tunnel syndrome, but the time course of improvement in nerve conduction often does not match the pace of symptomatic improvement.

Treatment of carpal tunnel syndrome with splinting or with steroid injection into the carpal tunnel leads to improvement in median DML or DSL in some cases (Goodman & Gilliatt, 1961; Goodwill, 1965; Kruger, Kraft, Deitz, Ameis & Polissar, 1991; Walker, Metzler, Cifu & Swartz, 2000). However, other patients experience relief of symptoms without improvement in DML or have normalization of DML despite persistent symptoms. Patients who

Figure 8-6. Correlating symptoms, signs, and nerve conduction in patients with carpal tunnel syndrome. (DML = distal motor latency; DSL = distal sensory latency.) (Data from HA Spindler, AL Dellon. Nerve conduction studies and sensibility testing in carpal tunnel syndrome. J. Hand Surg. 1982;7:260–63.)

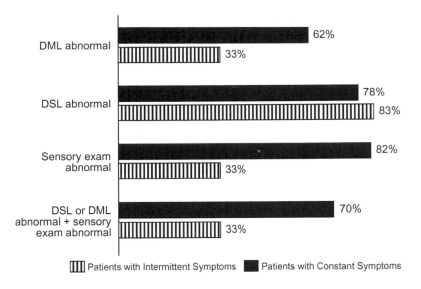

DML abnormal — 62% / 33%

DSL abnormal — 78% / 83%

Sensory exam abnormal — 82% / 33%

DSL or DML abnormal + sensory exam abnormal — 70% / 33%

|||| Patients with Intermittent Symptoms   ■ Patients with Constant Symptoms

have carpal tunnel syndrome and are treated with steroid injection into the carpal tunnel often show some improvement in median nerve sensory transcarpal conduction 1 month after the injection, but the improvement is usually not maintained at later follow-up (Seror, 1992).

After carpal tunnel surgery, changes in median nerve conduction go through a number of phases.

Immediate Postoperative Changes

In many patients with carpal tunnel syndrome some improvement in nerve conduction can be demonstrated intraoperatively within minutes of division of the flexor retinaculum (Hongell & Mattsson, 1971). Whether or not there is intraoperative improvement in nerve conduction, further improvement usually occurs over the ensuing months (Luchetti, Schoenhuber & Landi, 1988).

Eversman and Ritsick (1978) measured median DML in 51 hands before surgery and within 10 minutes of wound closure. DML improved in 44 of the hands. The most dramatic improvement was from 10.8 msec preoperatively to 5.8 msec after surgery. Four patients with high normal DML before surgery showed a drop of DML following surgery. A few patients had a prolongation of DML immediately after surgery; the worst deterioration was an increase from 4.0 to 5.1 msec.

The effect of neurolysis on intraoperative changes in nerve conduction is discussed in Chapter 15.

Long-Term Postoperative Changes

Both sensory and motor conduction across the carpal tunnel improve gradually after successful open or endoscopic surgery (Goodman & Gilliatt, 1961; Hongell & Mattsson, 1971; Schlagenhauff & Glasauer, 1971; Shurr, Blair & Bassett, 1986; Seror, 1992; Genba, Ugawa, Kanazawa, Okutsu & Hamanaka, 1993; Nakamura, Uchiyama, Toriumi, Nakagawa & Miyasaka, 1999). The greatest rate of improvement is in the first few months (Pascoe, Pascoe, Tarrant & Boyle, 1994). If the preoperative DML is less than 4.0 msec, preoperative abnormalities of sensory conduction are usually resolved by the sixth postoperative month (Padua, Lo Monaco, Padua, Tamburrelli, Gregori & Tonali, 1997). However, more sensitive diagnostic parameters, such as median-ulnar palmar latency difference, usually are still abnormal 6 months after successful surgery (Pascoe, Pascoe, Tarrant & Boyle, 1994). Patients with more severe preoperative abnormalities have a greater percentage of improvement (Schlagenhauff & Glasauer, 1971). Goodman and Gilliatt (1961) found that in patients with preoperative median DML greater than 10 msec, DML improved 40% or more within 5 months of surgery; in patients with preoperative DML between 5 and 7 msec, DML improved 20% or more within the same period. Patients who have high normal median DML preoperatively can have postoperative decrease in DML. However, if the preoperative DML is greater than 6 msec, median nerve conduction usually remains at least partially abnormal even 6 months postoperatively (Padua, Lo Monaco, Padua, Tamburrelli, Gregori & Tonali, 1997). Patients often become asymptomatic long before nerve conduction has returned to normal. A few patients with clinically satisfactory responses to surgery have persistent mild abnormalities of nerve conduction even when examined a year or more after surgery (Goodwill, 1965; Melvin, Johnson & Duran, 1968).

Sensory conduction in median digital nerves can be abnormal in patients with carpal tunnel syndrome. This abnormal conduction distal to the site of compression usually remains abnormal if checked 6 to 8 weeks after surgery. By 12 to 18 weeks after surgery, both digital SNCV and SNAP amplitude have often improved (Le-Quesne & Casey, 1974).

Electrodiagnostic Caveats

Various techniques are available to study median nerve conduction. The majority of these measure some aspect of nerve impulse conduction in the fastest conducting myelinated fibers. These large myelinated fibers are the most likely to be damaged in carpal tunnel syndrome, yet the nerve conduction studies are imperfect diagnostic tools in carpal tunnel syndrome for a number of reasons:

1. *Biological variability creates an overlap of normal and abnormal.* Conduction of normal nerves varies with a number of factors. Some personal factors, such as age and temperature are known, and allowances can be made for them. Other factors, such as individual variation in nerve fiber size or anomalous variations in nerve length or course (e.g., the variety of possible courses of the recurrent thenar motor branch), inevitably widen the normal range.

One way to partially correct for biological variability is by comparing conduction across the carpal tunnel against conduction in another nerve segment in the same individual. The residual motor latency and terminal latency index use the proximal median nerve for this purpose. The radial and ulnar comparison tests also decrease the normal range by using the individual as his or her own

control for some factors of individual biological variation. The rationale of these tests is defeated if the nerve segment being used for comparison is also abnormal.

2. *Experimental error increases with increased attention to a short abnormal segment of nerve.* Errors in measuring latencies and conduction distances add to the uncertainty of the results of nerve conduction tests. For example, size of the stimulating electrode, spread of stimulating current through electrode paste, and volume conduction of the stimulus all blur the exact site of nerve stimulation when surface stimulating electrodes are used. Variations in nerve course and sliding of the nerve with changes of hand or arm position increase the error of measurement. The sensory nerve conduction techniques have evolved from examining 13 or 14 cm of nerve between wrist and finger to examining the nerve in 1-cm segments. With longer nerve lengths, sensitivity is lower; biological variability in normal nerve can mask abnormalities in a short segment of compressed nerve. With shorter nerve lengths, a few millimeters of imprecision in localizing site of stimulation can introduce a large relative variation in the measured latency. This imprecision is amplified when using latency differences to compare conduction in adjacent segments. A mismeasured stimulation site results in a longer latency adjacent to a shorter latency.

The ratio of experimental error to conduction velocity increases as both the distance and latency differences decrease, so conduction measured over shorter distances with shorter latency differences has a larger experimental error and hence a larger spread of normal values (Maynard & Stolov, 1972). A large experimental error not only increases the difficulty of separating normal from abnormal, but also decreases the reproducibility of a test repeated in the same subject.

3. *The probability of an abnormal result increases if multiple tests are done on the same patient.* When routine studies such as DML and DSL are normal in a patient suspected of having carpal tunnel syndrome, many examiners proceed to increasingly more sensitive tests and often find abnormalities by doing so. Unfortunately, adding extra tests increases the probability of false-positive results. If each test has a probability of positives in a few percent of the normal population, the probability of a false-positive result increases with

Figure 8-7. This patient developed constant tingling paresthesias projected to the cutaneous territory of the left median nerve after he fell, landing on his wrist. Mild tactile sensory loss was limited to the tips of index and ring fingers. A witness is pointing to the location of Tinel's sign. Conventional median nerve conduction studies were normal, but microneurographic recording through a microelectrode, inserted where he is pointing, revealed abnormal continual spontaneous bursting unitary discharges in a median nerve fascicle that supplied the skin of the index finger.

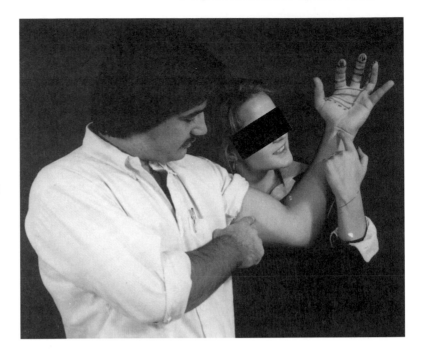

the number of different tests that are performed. An examination algorithm, such as the approach to combined sensory index described in Chapter 7, that plans additional testing in specified contingencies can result in a known specificity and sensitivity for the laboratory. An ad hoc approach, whereby the examiner does more tests if his or her clinical suspicion is high or referring physicians are insistent, invites false-positive errors

4. *Symptoms of carpal tunnel syndrome can occur whether or not nerve conduction is measurably impaired.* The tell-tale early symptoms of carpal tunnel syndrome, intermittent pain and paresthesias, are symptoms not of slowed nerve conduction but rather of *ectopic nerve impulse generation* that is not detected by nerve conduction techniques (see Chapter 12) (Ochoa & Torebjörk, 1980). Figure 8-7 illustrates the pattern of sensory symptoms for a patient in whom abnormal median nerve impulses were recorded by microneurography. Any study for conduction slowing, no matter how refined, is unlikely to correlate perfectly with the phenomena that are causing the patient's symptoms.

Some papers overlook this dissociation between symptoms and nerve conduction findings and demand nerve conduction abnormalities as a criteria for the diagnosis of carpal tunnel syndrome. For

example, as discussed in Chapter 3, systematic reviews that rely on nerve conduction–based criterion standards for carpal tunnel syndrome to evaluate clinical findings necessarily portray a skewed sample of the syndrome.

Patients who have carpal tunnel syndrome occasionally show ectopic impulse generation in motor neurons. Examples include fasciculations or repetitive firing on electromyography and, probably, the repeater F-wave. Unfortunately, these phenomena are observed too infrequently to provide sensitive diagnostic tests. There are no data on how they correlate with symptomatic ectopic impulse generation in sensory neurons.

5. *Nerve conduction slowing or loss of evoked potential amplitude does not actually measure clinical disruption of nerve function.* Examples of asymptomatic slowing of conduction have been given previously. Abnormal signs on sensory examination correlate particularly poorly with nerve conduction studies because only a minority of sensory fibers need to function for the patient to perform normally on common clinical sensory tests. An electrical stimulus is perceptible when it activates only 1 of the approximately 600 median sensory fibers to the normal finger (Johansson & Vallbo, 1979; Ochoa & Torebjörk, 1983). When the median nerve recovers from local anesthesia,

normal sensitivity to two-point discrimination and to von Frey hairs returns when SNAP amplitude is only approximately 20% of normal (Buchthal & Rosenfalck, 1966).

6. *Mild nerve compression is a common finding in the asymptomatic population.* Microscopic evidence of median nerve compression was found in over 40% of cadavers examined in one autopsy series (Neary, Ochoa & Gilliatt, 1975). Approximately 20% of asymptomatic control subjects have serial segmental maximum latency differences of 0.4 msec or greater: Many of these control subjects have asymptomatic focal median nerve pathology; some have normal median nerves but have false-positive results because of measurement error or biological variability. Little is known of the natural history of mild asymptomatic nerve compression or of mild asymptomatic nerve conduction abnormalities. However, given the much lower incidence of symptoms of carpal tunnel syndrome in the population, overattention to asymptomatic electrical abnormalities will usually be misleading (Gilliatt, 1978).

7. *Axonal interruption is a late manifestation of carpal tunnel syndrome.* The best measures of axonal interruption in patients who have carpal tunnel syndrome are electromyography, amplitude of the CMAP and the SNAP, and the forearm MNCV and SNCV. The amplitudes after proximal stimulation can also be reduced as a consequence of conduction block; the differentiation between conduction block and axonal disease requires data on amplitudes from stimulation distal to the carpal tunnel. In patients who have carpal tunnel syndrome, compression and distortion of myelin precedes axonal disruption, so the measures of axonal interruption are rarely abnormal in early or mild cases; conversely, the presence of signs of axonal interruption reflects more severe median nerve injury.

Testing in Suspected Carpal Tunnel Syndrome

The American Association of Electrodiagnostic Medicine, the American Academy of Neurology, and the American Academy of Physical Medicine and Rehabilitation (1993, 2002) have offered a practice recommendation for electrodiagnostic laboratory confirmation in patients with suspected carpal tunnel syndrome:

1. Perform a median sensory nerve conduction study across the wrist with a conduction distance of 13 to 14 cm. If the result is abnormal, comparison of the result of the median sensory nerve conduction study to the result of a sensory nerve conduction study of one other adjacent sensory nerve in the symptomatic limb (Standard).

2. If the initial median sensory nerve conduction study across the wrist has a conduction distance greater than 8 cm and the result is normal, one of the following additional studies is recommended:

   a. Comparison of median sensory nerve conduction across the wrist over a short (7 to 8 cm) conduction distance with ulnar sensory nerve conduction across the wrist over the same short (7 to 8 cm) conduction distance (Standard), or

   b. Comparison of median sensory conduction across the wrist with radial or ulnar sensory conduction across the wrist in the same limb (Standard), or

   c. Comparison of median sensory or mixed nerve conduction through the carpal tunnel to sensory or mixed nerve conduction studies of proximal (forearm) or distal (digit) segments of the medial nerve in the same limb (Standard).

3. Motor conduction study of the median nerve recording from the thenar muscle and of one other nerve in the symptomatic limb to include measurement of distal latency (Guideline).

4. Supplementary nerve conduction study—Comparison of the median motor nerve distal latency (second lumbrical) to the ulnar motor nerve distal latency (second interossei), median motor terminal latency index, median motor nerve conduction between wrist and palm, median motor nerve CMAP wrist to palm amplitude ratio to detect conduction block, median SNAP wrist to palm amplitude ratio to detect conduction block, short segment (1 cm) incremental median sensory nerve conduction across the carpal tunnel (Option).

5. Needle electromyography of a sample of muscles innervated by the C5 to T1 spinal roots,

including a thenar muscle innervated by the median nerve of the symptomatic limb (Option).

We agree with these recommendations and offer the following amendments:

6. Each laboratory should use a selection of the available tests and need not perform every known variation.
7. The motor conduction studies must examine CMAP amplitudes and configurations to avoid overlooking co-existent Martin-Gruber anastomosis or more proximal median neuropathies.
8. If median nerve conduction is normal, the clinical setting will dictate appropriate electrodiagnostic evaluation for alternative diagnoses.
9. If median nerve conduction is abnormal, the ipsilateral ulnar or radial nerve and contralateral median nerve should also be studied. If these nerves are abnormal, the testing must be extensive enough to distinguish between a diffuse peripheral neuropathy and multiple mononeuropathies.
10. If median nerve conduction is abnormal, electromyographic needle examination of at least one median-innervated thenar muscle should be considered. If this muscle is abnormal, other median and C8–T1 muscles will often merit evaluation for radiculopathy, plexopathy, or more proximal median neuropathy.

References

Albers JW, Brown MB, Sima AA, Greene DA. Frequency of median mononeuropathy in patients with mild diabetic neuropathy in the early diabetes intervention trial (EDIT). Tolrestat Study Group For Edit (Early Diabetes Intervention Trial. Muscle Nerve 1996;19:140–46.

Albers JW, Donofrio PD, McGonagle TK. Sequential electrodiagnostic abnormalities in acute inflammatory demyelinating polyradiculoneuropathy. Muscle Nerve 1985;8:528–39.

American Association of Electrodiagnostic Medicine, American Academy of Neurology. Practice parameter for electrodiagnostic studies in carpal tunnel syndrome: summary statement. Muscle Nerve 2002 (in press).

American Association of Electrodiagnostic Medicine, American Academy of Neurology, American Academy of Physical Medicine and Rehabilitation. Practice parameter for electrodiagnostic studies in carpal tunnel syndrome: summary statement. Muscle Nerve 1993;16:1390–91.

Andary MT, Fankhauser MJ, Ritson JL, Spiegel N, Hulce V, Yosef M, Stanton DF. Comparison of sensory mid-palm studies to other techniques in carpal tunnel syndrome. Electromyogr. Clin. Neurophysiol. 1996;36:279–85.

Ashworth NL, Marshall SC, Satkunam LE. The effect of temperature on nerve conduction parameters in carpal tunnel syndrome. Muscle Nerve 1998;21:1089–91.

Baysal AI, Chang CW, Oh SJ. Temperature effects on nerve conduction studies in patients with carpal tunnel syndrome. Acta Neurol. Scand. 1993;88:213–16.

Bingham RC, Rosecrance JC, Cook TM. Prevalence of abnormal median nerve conduction in applicants for industrial jobs. Am. J. Ind. Med. 1996;30:355–61.

Bland JD. A neurophysiological grading scale for carpal tunnel syndrome. Muscle Nerve 2000;23:1280–83.

Bolton CF, Carter KN. Human sensory nerve compound action potential amplitude: variation with sex and finger circumference. J. Neurol. Neurosurg. Psychiatry 1980;43:925–28.

Bolton CF, Sawa GM, Carter K. The effects of temperature on human compound action potentials. J. Neurol. Neurosurg. Psychiatry 1981;44:407–13.

Buchthal F, Rosenfalck A. Evoked action potentials and conduction velocity in human sensory nerves. Brain Res. 1966;3:1–122.

Buschbacher RM. Body mass index effect on common nerve conduction study measurements. Muscle Nerve 1998;21:1398–1404.

Buschbacher RM. Median nerve motor conduction to the abductor pollicis brevis. Am. J. Phys. Med. Rehabil. 1999;78:S1–S8.

Cassvan A, Ralescu S, Shapiro E, Moshkovski FG, Weiss J. Median and radial sensory latencies to digit I as compared with other screening tests in carpal tunnel syndrome. Am. J. Phys. Med. Rehabil. 1988;67:221–24.

Chira-Adisai W, Yan K, Turan B. The influence of wrist thickness on amplitudes of sensory nerve action potentials. Electromyogr. Clin. Neurophysiol. 1999;39:485–88.

Cruz Martinez A, Barrio M, Perez Conde MC, Gutierrez AM. Electrophysiological aspects of sensory conduction velocity in healthy adults. 1. Conduction velocity from digit to palm, from palm to wrist, and across the elbow as a function of age. J. Neurol. Neurosurg. Psychiatry 1978;41:1092–96.

Dhong ES, Han SK, Lee BI, Kim WK. Correlation of electrodiagnostic findings with subjective symptoms in carpal tunnel syndrome. Ann. Plast. Surg. 2000;45:127–31.

Dieck GS, Kelsey JL. An epidemiologic study of the carpal tunnel syndrome in an adult female population. Prev. Med. 1985;14:63–69.

Duncan KH, Lewis RC Jr, Foreman KA, Nordyke MD. Treatment of carpal tunnel syndrome by members of the American Society for Surgery of the Hand: results of a questionnaire. J. Hand Surg. 1987;12A:384–91.

Dyck PJ, Kratz KM, Karnes JL, Litchy WJ, Klein R, Pach JM, Wilson DM, O'Brien PC, Melton LJ. The prevalence by staged severity of various types of diabetic neuropathy, retinopathy, and nephropathy in a population-based cohort: the Rochester diabetic neuropathy study. Neurology 1993;43:817.

Eisen A, Schulzer M, Pant B, MacNeil M, Stewart H, Trueman S, Mak E. Receiver operating characteristic curve analysis in the prediction of carpal tunnel syndrome: a model for reporting electrophysiological data. Muscle Nerve 1993;16:787–96.

Eversmann WW Jr, Ritsick JA. Intraoperative changes in motor nerve conduction latency in carpal tunnel syndrome. J. Hand Surg. 1978;3:77–81.

Felsenthal G. Median and ulnar muscle and sensory evoked potentials. Am. J. Phys. Med. 1978;57:167–82.

Felsenthal G, Spindler H. Palmar conduction time of median and ulnar nerves of normal subjects and patients with carpal tunnel syndrome. Am. J. Phys. Med. 1979;58:131–38.

Ferry S, Silman AJ, Pritchard T, Keenan J, Croft P. The association between different patterns of hand symptoms and objective evidence of median nerve compression: a community-based survey. Arthritis Rheum. 1998;41:720–24.

Fine EJ, Wongjirad C. The fallacy of temperature correction in carpal tunnel syndrome. Muscle Nerve 1985;8:628.

Foresti C, Quadri S, Rasella M, Tironi F, Viscardi M, Ubiali E. Carpal tunnel syndrome: which electrodiagnostic path should we follow? A prospective study of 100 consecutive patients. Electromyogr. Clin. Neurophysiol. 1996;36:377–84.

Genba K, Ugawa Y, Kanazawa I, Okutsu I, Hamanaka I. Physiological assessment of endoscopic surgery for carpal tunnel syndrome. Muscle Nerve 1993;16:567–68.

Gilliatt RW. Sensory conduction studies in the early recognition of nerve disorders. Muscle Nerve 1978;1:352–59.

Girlanda P, Quartarone A, Sinicropi S, Pronesti C, Nicolosi C, Macaione V, Picciolo G, Messina C. Electrophysiological studies in mild idiopathic carpal tunnel syndrome. Electroencephalogr. Clin. Neurophysiol. 1998;109:44–49.

Goodman HV, Gilliatt RW. The effect of treatment on median nerve conduction in patients with the carpal tunnel syndrome. Ann. Phys. Med. 1961;6:137–55.

Goodwill CJ. The carpal tunnel syndrome—long-term follow-up showing relation of latency measurements to response to treatment. Ann. Phys. Med. 1965;8:12–21.

Gordan DS. Nerve sliding and conduction velocity (letter). J. Neurol. Neurosurg. Psychiatry 1981;44:457.

Gordon C, Johnson EW, Gatens PF, Ashton JJ. Wrist ratio correlation with carpal tunnel syndrome in industry. Am. J. Phys. Med. Rehabil. 1988;67:270–72.

Grosser SJ, Neuhauser D, Katirji B. Limitations of receiver operating characteristic curve analysis in the prediction of carpal tunnel syndrome. Muscle Nerve 1994;17:704–5.

Halar EM, DeLisa JA, Soine TL. Nerve conduction studies in upper extremities: skin temperature corrections. Arch. Phys. Med. Rehabil. 1983;64:412–16.

Hamann C, Werner RA, Franzblau A, Rodgers PA, Siew C, Gruninger S. Prevalence of carpal tunnel syndrome and median mononeuropathy among dentists. J. Am. Dent. Assoc. 2001;132:163–70; quiz, 223–24.

Hennessey WJ, Falco FJ, Braddom RL, Goldberg G. The influence of age on distal latency comparisons in carpal tunnel syndrome. Muscle Nerve 1994;17:1215–17.

Hennessey WJ, Falco FJ, Goldberg G, Braddom RL. Gender and arm length: influence on nerve conduction parameters in the upper limb. Arch. Phys. Med. Rehabil. 1994;75:265–69.

Homan MM, Franzblau A, Werner RA, Albers JW, Armstrong TJ, Bromberg MB. Agreement between symptom surveys, physical examination procedures and electrodiagnostic findings for the carpal tunnel syndrome. Scand. J. Work Environ. Health 1999;25:115–24.

Hongell A, Mattsson HS. Neurographic studies before, after, and during operation for median nerve compression in the carpal tunnel. Scand. J. Plast. Reconstr. Surg. 1971; 5:103–9.

Johansson RS, Vallbo ÅB. Detection of tactile stimuli. Thresholds of afferent units related psychophysical thresholds in the human hand. J. Physiol. 1979;297:405–22.

Johnson EW, Gatens T, Poindexter D, Bowers D. Wrist dimensions: correlation with median sensory latencies. Arch. Phys. Med. Rehabil. 1983;64:556–57.

Kouyoumdjian JA, Morita MP, Rocha PR, Miranda RC, Gouveia GM. Wrist and palm indexes in carpal tunnel syndrome. Arq. Neuropsiquiatr. 2000;58:625–29.

Kraft GH, Halvorson GA. Median nerve residual latency: normal value and use in diagnosis of carpal tunnel syndrome. Arch. Phys. Med. Rehabil. 1983;64:221–26.

Kruger VL, Kraft GH, Deitz JC, Ameis A, Polissar L. Carpal tunnel syndrome: objective measures and splint use. Arch Phys Med Rehabil. Arch. Phys. Med. Rehabil. 1991; 72:517–20.

Kuhlman KA, Hennessey WJ. Sensitivity and specificity of carpal tunnel syndrome signs. Am. J. Phys. Med. Rehabil. 1997;76:451–57.

Kuntzer T. Carpal tunnel syndrome in 100 patients: sensitivity, specificity of multi-neurophysiological procedures and estimation of axonal loss of motor, sensory and sympathetic median nerve fibers. J. Neurol. Sci. 1994;127: 221–29.

LaFratta CW. Relation of age to amplitude of evoked antidromic sensory nerve potentials: a supplemental report. Arch. Phys. Med. Rehabil. 1972;53:388–89.

LaFratta CW, Canestrari RE. A comparison of sensory and motor nerve conduction velocities as related to age. Arch. Phys. Med. Rehabil. 1966;47:286–90.

Lateva ZC, McGill KC, Burgar CG. Anatomical and electrophysiological determinants of the human thenar compound muscle action potential. Muscle Nerve 1996;19:1457–68.

Lehmann HJ, Tackmann W. Neurographic analysis of trains of frequent electric stimuli in the diagnosis of peripheral nerve diseases. Investigations in the carpal tunnel syndrome. Eur. Neurol. 1974;12:293–308.

Le-Quesne PM, Casey EB. Recovery of conduction velocity distal to a compressive lesion. J. Neurol. Neurosurg. Psychiatry 1974;37:1346–51.

Letz R, Gerr F. Covariates of human peripheral nerve function: I. nerve conduction velocity and amplitude. Neurotoxicol. Teratol. 1993;16:95–104.

Levine DW, Simmons BP, Koris MJ, Daltroy LH, Hohl GG, Fossel AH, Katz JN. A self-administered questionnaire for the assessment of severity of symptoms and functional status in carpal tunnel syndrome. J. Bone Joint Surg. 1993; 75A:1585–92.

Loong SC. The carpal tunnel syndrome: a clinical and electrophysiological study of 250 patients. Proc. Aust. Assoc. Neurol. 1977;14:51–65.

Luchetti R, Schoenhuber R, Landi A. Assessment of sensory nerve conduction in carpal tunnel syndrome before, during and after operation. J. Hand. Surg. 1988;13B:386–90.

Maynard FM, Stolov WC. Experimental error in determination of nerve conduction velocity. Arch. Phys. Med. Rehabil. 1972;53:362–72.

Melvin JL, Johnson EW, Duran R. Electrodiagnosis after surgery for the carpal tunnel syndrome. Arch. Phys. Med. Rehabil. 1968;49:502–7.

Monga TN, Shanks GL, Poole BJ. Sensory palmar stimulation in the diagnosis of carpal tunnel syndrome. Arch. Phys. Med. Rehabil. 1985;66:598–600.

Moore JH, Gieck JH, Saliba EN, Perrin DH, Ball DW, McCue FC. The biophysical effects of ultrasound on median nerve distal latencies. Electromyogr. Clin. Neurophysiol. 2000; 40:169–80.

Nakamura Y, Uchiyama S, Toriumi H, Nakagawa H, Miyasaka T. Longitudinal median nerve conduction studies after endoscopic carpal tunnel release. Hand Surg. 1999;4:145–49.

Nathan PA, Keniston RC, Lockwood RS, Meadows KD. Tobacco, caffeine, alcohol, and carpal tunnel syndrome in American industry. A cross-sectional study of 1464 workers. J. Occup. Environ. Med. 1996;38:290–98.

Nathan PA, Keniston RC, Myers LD, Meadows KD. Obesity as a risk factor for slowing of sensory conduction of the median nerve in industry. J. Occup. Med. 1992;34:379–83.

Nathan PA, Keniston RC, Myers LD, Meadows KD, Lockwood RS. Natural history of median nerve sensory conduction in industry: relationship to symptoms and carpal tunnel syndrome in 558 hands over 11 years. Muscle Nerve 1998;21:711–21.

Nathan PA, Meadows KD, Doyle LS. Relationship of age and sex to sensory conduction of the median nerve at the carpal tunnel and association of slowed conduction with symptoms. Muscle Nerve 1988a;11:1149–53.

Nathan PA, Meadows KD, Doyle LS. Sensory segmental latency values of the median nerve for a population of normal individuals. Arch. Phys. Med. Rehabil. 1988b;69:499–501.

Neary D, Ochoa J, Gilliatt RW. Sub-clinical entrapment neuropathy in man. J. Neurol. Sci. 1975;24:282–98.

Nierenberg AA, Feinstein AR. How to Evaluate a Diagnostic Marker Test. JAMA. 1988;259:1699–1702.

Ochoa J, Torebjörk E. Sensations evoked by intraneural microstimulation of single mechanoreceptor units innervating the human hand. J. Physiol. 1983;342:633–54.

Ochoa JL, Torebjörk HE. Paraesthesiae from ectopic impulse generation in human sensory nerves. Brain 1980;103:835–53.

Ozaki I, Baba M, Matsunaga M, Takebe K. Deleterious effect of the carpal tunnel on nerve conduction in diabetic polyneuropathy. Electromyogr. Clin. Neurophysiol. 1988;28:301–6.

Padua L, Lo Monaco M, Padua R, Tamburrelli F, Gregori B, Tonali P. Carpal tunnel syndrome: neurophysiological results of surgery based on preoperative electrodiagnostic testing. J. Hand Surg. 1997;22B:599–601.

Padua L, Lo Monaco M, Valente EM, Tonali PA. A useful electrophysiologic parameter for diagnosis of carpal tunnel syndrome. Muscle Nerve 1996;19:48–53.

Padua L, Padua R, Lo Monaco M, Aprile I, Tonali P. Multiperspective assessment of carpal tunnel syndrome: a multicenter study. Italian CTS Study Group. Neurology 1999;53:1654–59.

Parachuri R, Adams EM. Entrapment neuropathies. A guide to avoiding misdiagnoses. Postgrad. Med. 1993;94:39–41,44–6,51.

Pascoe MK, Pascoe RD, Tarrant E, Boyle R. Changes in palmar sensory latencies in response to carpal tunnel release. Muscle Nerve 1994;17:1475–76.

Pavesi G, Olivieri MF, Misk A, Mancia D. Clinical-electrophysiological correlations in the carpal tunnel syndrome. Ital. J. Neurol. Sci. 1986;7:93–96.

Pease WS, Cannell CD, Johnson EW. Median to radial latency difference test in mild carpal tunnel syndrome. Muscle Nerve 1989;12:905–9.

Preston DC, Ross MH, Kothari MJ, Plotkin GM, Venkatesh S, Logigian EL. The median-ulnar latency difference studies are comparable in mild carpal tunnel syndrome. Muscle Nerve 1994;17:1469–71.

Radecki P. A gender specific wrist ratio and the likelihood of a median nerve abnormality at the carpal tunnel. Am. J. Phys. Med. Rehabil. 1994;73:157–62.

Radecki P. Variability in the median and ulnar nerve latencies: implications for diagnosing entrapment. J. Occup. Environ. Med. 1995;37:1293–99.

Redmond MD, Rivner MH. False positive electrodiagnostic tests in carpal tunnel syndrome. Muscle Nerve 1988; 11:511–18.

Rivner MH. Statistical errors and their effect on electrodiagnostic medicine. Muscle Nerve 1994;17:811–14.

Rivner MH, Swift TR, Crout BO, Rhodes KP. Toward more rational nerve conduction interpretations: the effect of height. Muscle Nerve 1990;13:232–39.

Robinson LR, Micklesen PJ, Wang L. Strategies for analyzing conduction data: superiority of a summary index over single tests. Muscle Nerve 1998;21:1166–71.

Salerno DF, Franzblau A, Werner RA, Bromberg MB, Armstrong TJ, Albers JW. Median and ulnar nerve conduction studies among workers: normative values. Muscle Nerve 1998;21:999–1005.

Schlagenhauff RE, Glasauer FE. Pre- and post-operative electromyographic evaluations in the carpal tunnel syndrome. J. Neurosurg. 1971;35:314–19.

Schulzer M. Diagnostic tests: a statistical review. Muscle Nerve 1994;17:815–19.

Seror P. Nerve conduction studies after treatment for carpal tunnel syndrome. J. Hand. Surg. 1992;17B:641–45.

Seror P. Sensitivity of the various tests for the diagnosis of carpal tunnel syndrome. J. Hand Surg. 1994;19B:725–28.

Shivde AJ, Dreizin I, Fisher MA. The carpal tunnel syndrome. A clinical-electrodiagnostic analysis. Electromyogr. Clin. Neurophysiol. 1981;21:143–53.

Shurr DG, Blair WF, Bassett G. Electromyographic changes after carpal tunnel release. J. Hand Surg. 1986;11A:876–80.

Spindler HA, Dellon AL. Nerve conduction studies and sensibility testing in carpal tunnel syndrome. J. Hand. Surg. 1982;7:260–63.

Stetson DS, Albers JW, Silverstein BA, Wolfe RA. Effects of age, sex and anthromorphic features on nerve conduction measurements. Muscle Nerve 1992;15:1095–1104.

Stevens JC. AAEE minimonograph #26: The electrodiagnosis of carpal tunnel syndrome. Muscle Nerve 1987;10:99–113.

Stevens JC, Sun S, Beard CM, O'Fallon WM, Kurland LT. Carpal tunnel syndrome in Rochester, Minnesota, 1961 to 1980. Neurology 1988;38:134–38.

Thomas JE, Lambert EH, Cseuz KA. Electrodiagnostic aspects of the carpal tunnel syndrome. Arch. Neurol. 1967;16:635–41.

Trojaborg W, Kelly-Perez B, Sheriff P. Prolonged latency to 2nd lumbrical signifying an incipient carpal tunnel syndrome: a case report. Muscle Nerve 1996;19:258–60.

Uncini A, Di Muzio A, Awad J, Manente G, Tafuro M, Gambi D. Sensitivity of three median-to-ulnar comparative tests in diagnosis of mild carpal tunnel syndrome. Muscle Nerve 1993;16:1366–73.

Valls-Solé J, Alvarez R, Nuñez M. Limited longitudinal sliding of the median nerve in patients with carpal tunnel syndrome. Muscle Nerve 1995;18:761–67.

Vogt T, Mika A, Thomke F, Hopf HC. Evaluation of carpal tunnel syndrome in patients with polyneuropathy. Muscle Nerve 1997;20:153–57.

Walker WC, Metzler M, Cifu DX, Swartz Z. Neutral wrist splinting in carpal tunnel syndrome: a comparison of night-only versus full-time wear instructions. Arch. Phys. Med. Rehabil. 2000;81:424–29.

Wang AK, Raynor EM, Blum AS, Rutkove SB. Heat sensitivity of sensory fibers in carpal tunnel syndrome. Muscle Nerve 1999;22:37–42.

Werner RA, Franzblau A. Hand dominance effect on median and ulnar sensory evoked amplitude and latency in asymptomatic workers. Arch. Phys. Med. Rehabil. 1996;77:473–76.

Werner RA, Franzblau A, Albers JW, Armstrong TJ. Influence of body mass index and work activity on the prevalence of median mononeuropathy at the wrist. J. Occup. Environ. Med. 1997;54:268–71.

Werner RA, Franzblau A, Albers JW, Armstrong TJ. Median mononeuropathy among active workers: are there differences between symptomatic and asymptomatic workers? Am. J. Ind. Med. 1998;33:374–78.

Werner RA, Franzblau A, Albers JW, Buchele H, Armstrong TJ. Use of screening nerve conduction studies for predicting future carpal tunnel syndrome. J. Occup. Environ. Med. 1997;54:96–100.

White JC, Hansen SR, Johnson RK. A comparison of EMG procedures in the carpal tunnel syndrome with clinical-EMG correlations. Muscle Nerve 1988;11:1177–82.

Wilbourn AJ, Hanson MR, Lederman RJ, Salanga VD. Carpal tunnel syndrome: clinical-electrodiagnostic correlations. Electroencephalogr. Clin. Neurophysiol. 1980;49:18P.

You H, Simmons Z, Freivalds A, Kothari MJ, Naidu SH. Relationships between clinical symptom severity scales and nerve conduction measures in carpal tunnel syndrome. Muscle Nerve 1999;22:497–501.

Chapter 9
Quantitative Sensory Testing

In the evaluation of nerve function, conventional electrophysiologic testing falls short in two major areas: sensory phenomena of positive character and dysfunction of small caliber fiber systems, both afferent and sympathetic efferent (Ochoa, 1987). Supplementary information concerning these two areas of dysfunction may be obtained with quantitative sensory testing and thermography (see Chapter 10).

The bedside sensory examination must be supplemented if a standardized measure of somatosensory function is desired. In quantitative sensory tests, defined amounts of stimulus energy are applied, and the sensory response is measured. Reliable assessment of subjective responses is achieved through standard determination of perception thresholds or through estimation of the psychophysical suprathreshold magnitude function. Precise delivery of stimuli is possible through instruments that generate finite mechanical or thermal energies, noxious or non-noxious, to sensory receptors. Instruments such as the vibrameter, the thermostimulator, and the mechanical algometer have proven to be valuable and sometimes indispensable aids in clinical assessment of certain sensory parameters (Lindblom, 1981; Lindblom & Ochoa, 1992; Triplett & Ochoa, 1990; Verdugo & Ochoa, 1992; Yarnitsky, 1997).

Quantitative Sensory Thermotesting

Quantitative sensory thermotesting is a key method for evaluation of four sensory submodalities served by small-caliber fiber afferent channels (Verdugo & Ochoa, 1992). The method applies measured ramps of ascending or descending temperature to the skin through a thermode based on the Peltier principle. The subjective response is measured by recording detection thresholds; the subject signals onset of a specific sensation (Figure 9-1). The Marstock method (Fruhstorfer, Lindblom & Schmidt, 1976) allows assessment in a noninvasive and yet rigorous fashion of receptor encoding, nerve transmission, and central subjective decoding of cold sensation, warm sensation, pain induced by low temperature, and pain induced by heat. Other methods confine their assessment to cold and warm sensations; measurement of cold and heat pain multiplies the sensitivity of the method so that not only sensory deficits, but also sensory exaggeration, or release, such as heat hyperalgesia or cold hyperalgesia, are detected.

After measuring all four functions, the abnormal patterns may be segregated into three main groups: (1) cold or warm hypoesthesia; (2) heat or cold pain hyperalgesia; and (3) combination of thermal hypoesthesia with thermal hyperalgesia (Figure 9-2). These abnormal thermotest profiles may occur in the absence of hypoesthesia for tactile submodalities served by large-caliber fibers. Moreover, hypoesthesia for low temperature may dissociate from warm hypoesthesia, and thermal hyperalgesia may occur in the absence of deficit of cold or warm sensations. Furthermore, thermal hyperalgesia for heat may dissociate from hyperalgesia for cold. Unfortunately, unlike electrophysiologic methods for testing large-caliber afferent fibers, these psychophysical tests do not specify the level between skin and brain where the abnormality resides. Moreover, abnormal tests may result from pure psychological dysfunction (Verdugo and Ochoa, 1992).

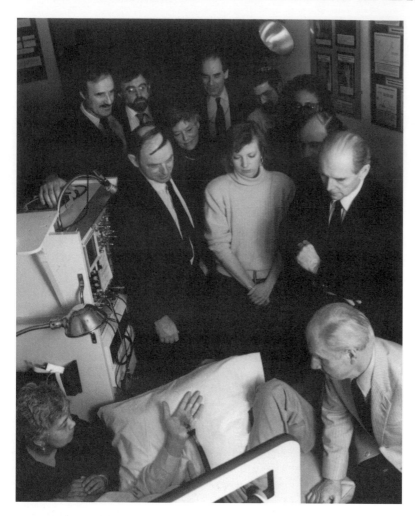

Figure 9-1. Professor U. Lindblom oversees performance of the quantitative thermotest with Marstock apparatus in a patient while a distinguished crowd attends. A Peltier thermoprobe is on the left palm of the subject, who is instructed to signal onset of a specified sensory quality by pressing a switch that reverses the direction of excursion of the temperature record in the plotter. The examiner starts the stimulus ramp by pressing a separate switch, unknown to the subject.

Methodologic Aspects

A contact thermode of standard surface area, based on the Peltier principle, is applied to tested skin. Depending on the direction of electrical current passed through the semiconductor elements within the thermode, a ramp of increasing or decreasing temperature is generated. The slope of the changing temperature generated is determined by the intensity of current applied. Temperature at the surface of the stimulator probe is measured through a thermocouple in the probe. The ramps of applied temperature are displayed by a graphic system connected to the apparatus. The subject is instructed to signal onset of a given sensation by pressing the switch, which automatically reverses the temperature ramp to adapting baseline temperature. The turning point reflects in degrees Celsius the threshold signaled by the individual for a particular sensation.

A typical normal profile of quantitative thermotest for cold, warm, heat pain, and cold pain sensation is shown in Figure 9-2. Examples of profiles of the three major abnormal categories, namely, pure temperature-specific hypoesthesia, pure thermal hyperalgesia, and combinations of hypoesthesia and hyperalgesia, are also shown in Figure 9-2.

Warm Hypoesthesia

In peripheral nerve disease, this abnormal pattern implies dropout of unmyelinated C fibers. Commonly, warm hypoesthesia occurs in the absence of hypoesthesia to pain induced by heat, even though heat pain is also mediated by an afferent system

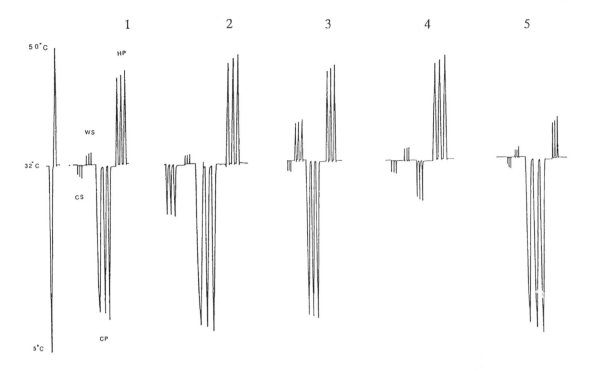

Figure 9-2. Marstock thermotest records of typical pure sensory patterns found in the clinic. Adapting temperature, 32°C. Thermal hypoesthesia, thermal hyperalgesia, and thermal hypoalgesia may combine in various other patterns. (CP = cold pain; CS = cold sensation; HP = heat pain; WS = warm sensation; 1 = normal pattern; 2 = cold hypoesthesia; 3 = warm hypoesthesia; 4 = cold hyperalgesia; 5 = heat hyperalgesia.)

using unmyelinated C fibers. Thus, threshold function remains normal for heat pain but is deficient for warm sensation in the presence of significant depopulation of unmyelinated afferent fibers. This occurs because warm sensation has a marked requirement for spatial summation, whereas heat pain does not. Distal warm hypoesthesia in lower limbs is a "normal" phenomenon in aging.

Cold Hypoesthesia

In peripheral nerve disease, cold hypoesthesia correlates with loss of small-caliber A delta fibers. The distal ends of cold-specific afferents in humans probably are unmyelinated (Campero, Serra, Bostock & Ochoa, 2001). Cold hypoesthesia tends to associate with cold hyperalgesia because deficit of cold-specific input releases pain induced by low temperature (Wahrén, Torcbjörk & Jörum, 1989; Yarnitsky & Ochoa, 1990). Pure cold hypoesthesia is an exceptionally rare finding in organic disease

(Verdugo & Ochoa, 1992). Cold hypoesthesia from experimental block of A delta fibers naturally releases hyperalgesia with a paradoxical burning quality in response to low temperature stimuli (Wahrén, Torebjörk & Jörum, 1989; Yarnitsky & Ochoa, 1990).

Heat and Cold Hyperalgesias

Detection of cold and heat hyperalgesia is an important part of the evaluation of sensory dysfunction of peripheral nerve origin. Fully developed heat hyperalgesia, cold hyperalgesia, or both may occur in the absence of deficit of warm or cold sensations and of tactile modalities of any kind.

Clinical Use

The quantitative sensory thermotest is valuable for evaluation of polyneuropathies involving small-caliber fibers, nerve injuries, and neuropathic pain syndromes. Like thermography, it is of limited value in assessing patients with carpal tunnel syndrome, in whom small-fiber dysfunction is a late and unusual consequence of nerve compression.

Vibration Sense and Vibrametry

Sensibility to vibration is a defined normal skill of the nervous system that has long attracted the interest of neurophysiologists (Lindblom & Lund, 1966; Talbot, Darian-Smith, Kornhuber, & Mountcastle, 1968; Merzenich & Harrington, 1969), clinicians (Goff, Rosner, Detre & Kennard, 1965; Calne & Pallis, 1966; Goldberg & Lindblom, 1979), and psychophysicists (Verrillo, 1980). Vibrating mechanical stimuli excite specifically sensitive receptors encapsulated in Pacinian corpuscles. These connect with somatotopic and modality-specific loci in the somatosensory cortex through large-caliber myelinated fibers in nerves, posterior columns, lemniscal system, and thalamic relays.

The Pacini system is very sensitive in mechanoreception and transmission of high-frequency sustained vibration. This sensitivity derives from the low mechanical thresholds and rapid adaptation of Pacinian corpuscles, which sensitively fire one action potential per mechanical stimulus and adapt instantaneously to become available to respond to further incoming stimuli. The characteristics that make Pacini organs responsive to repetitive mechanical stimuli disable them from responding in a sustained fashion to a slow deformation or to constant pressure.

Intraneural selective microstimulation of identified Pacinian units in humans using repetitive electrical stimuli at various frequencies typically evokes a sensation of vibration with a minimal frequency around 10 Hz for conscious detection. In contrast, slowly adapting units evoke a sustained sensation of pressure in response to intermittent electrical stimuli applied to their nerve fibers in isolation (Ochoa and Torebjörk, 1983). "In everyday tasks of the exploring hand the Pacinian system seems suited to provide an overall idea of very fine textures, without providing the more exact spatio-temporal detail that the rapidly adapting (RA) system probably gives" (Ochoa and Torebjörk, 1983).

Clinical abnormalities of vibration sense correlate with impaired function of afferent pathways served by large-caliber myelinated fibers. Typically, large-caliber axonal polyneuropathies, demyelinating polyneuropathies, and demyelinating disease in posterior columns affect vibration sense early or predominantly. The traditionally acknowledged loss of vibration sense with aging probably relates to cumulative functional impairment along the sensory pathway, between receptor and brain (Pearson, 1928; Critchley, 1956; Steiness, 1957; Verrillo, 1980; Spencer & Ochoa, 1981).

Measurement of vibration sense is an important part of the routine clinical neurologic examination and is usually conducted with a tuning fork delivering mechanical oscillations at 128 Hz. In the clinical evaluation of peripheral nerve injuries, some surgeons view impaired vibration sense as indicative of complete nerve division and therefore of the need for surgical intervention (Dellon, 1980). Although this concept applies to nerve lacerations, it does not apply to acute closed injuries in which nerve block may be due to neurapraxia rather than anatomic interruption of axons.

Quantitative vibrametry through electromagnetic devices introduces precision to assessment of vibration sense both at the level of stimulus delivery and at the level of measurement of sensory response (Goldberg & Lindblom, 1979). Lindblom (1981) rates vibrametry as less reliable for assessment of mononeuropathy than for polyneuropathy because of stimulus spread to areas innervated by neighboring intact nerves. However, when the stimulus can be confined to a specific territory, vibrametry can be quite sensitive. This is the case when specific stimuli are applied to some individual fingers (Borg and Lindblom, 1986). Reference values for vibration sense, as determined through thresholds during vibrametry, are available for carpal, tibial, and tarsal stimulus sites (Goldberg and Lindblom, 1979). In patients with various neurologic disorders, Dyck et al. (1987) and Gerr et al. (1991) found statistically significant correlations between vibrotactile thresholds and electrophysiologic status, particularly sensory nerve action potential (SNAP) parameters.

Gelberman et al. (1983) subjected 12 volunteers to controlled external compression of the median nerve at the carpal tunnel to levels between 40 and

Figure 9-3. Effect of 15 minutes of wrist flexion on vibration perception threshold in patients with carpal tunnel syndrome confirmed by nerve conduction studies, compared with control patients with hand paresthesias and normal nerve conduction studies. (Data from C Borg, U Lindblom. Increase of vibration threshold during wrist flexion in patients with carpal tunnel syndrome. Pain 1986;26:211–19.)

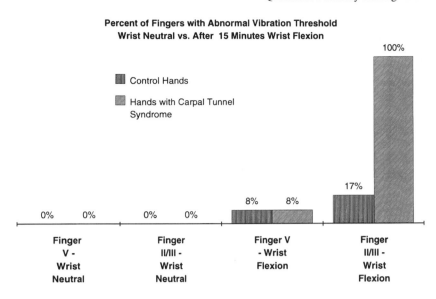

70 mm Hg. Nerve compression was applied externally through a specially designed device, and fluid pressure within the carpal tunnel was registered by a wick catheter. Vibration sense accurately reflected gradual decreases in nerve function as expressed by subjective sensation and by electrodiagnostic testing. Two-point discrimination threshold was insensitive. Median amplitude of the SNAP was 87% of the baseline value at the time when paresthesias in the distribution of the median nerve were first experienced. Median amplitude of the SNAP was 75% of normal when abnormalities in vibration were first noticed. Decreased amplitudes of the SNAP and compound muscle action potential constituted the first objective median nerve impairment in each subject.

Vibration sense has been specifically studied in carpal tunnel syndrome. Dellon (1980) evaluated 36 patients with a history of carpal tunnel syndrome and found abnormal perception of vibratory stimuli in 72%, testing with the head of a tuning fork. Within that subpopulation, electrodiagnostic studies were abnormal in only 63%. The 256-Hz tuning fork appeared to be more specific than a 30-Hz tuning fork for detection of abnormalities in patients with carpal tunnel syndrome. After surgical release for treatment of carpal tunnel syndrome, vibration perception returned to normal in all those patients who were tested. "This study demonstrates that the tuning fork *is* an acceptable, convenient, simple, and quick test instrument for use in emergencies; the patient in pain is not further discomforted, the child views it as a nonthreatening toy, and the intoxicated patient perceives the vibration through his stupor" (Dellon, 1980). Subsequently, Dellon (1983), applying an electromagnetic vibrameter, evaluated 34 patients with carpal tunnel syndrome. He found that threshold, as detected by quantitative electromagnetic vibrametry, was no better than the patient's perception of tuning fork stimulus in diagnosing carpal tunnel syndrome. Increased thresholds were observed in 55% of patients with "moderate" and 85% of patients with "severe" carpal tunnel syndrome in this study.

Using provocation with sustained wrist flexion, Borg and Lindblom (1986) showed that many patients with carpal tunnel syndrome develop an abnormally increased vibration perception threshold in skin of fingers supplied by the median nerve, but not in fingers supplied by the ulnar nerve. The patients flexed their wrists as for Phalen's test but sustained the flexed position for up to 15 minutes. Figure 9-3 compares the results in control patients with hand paresthesias and normal nerve conduction studies and in patients with carpal tunnel syndrome and abnormal median nerve conduction across the carpal tunnel. Borg and Lindblom concluded that provocation increases the sensitivity of quantitative sensory testing in diagnosis of carpal tunnel syndrome.

Over the last decade, there have been a number of focused studies on the use of vibrametry in evaluation of carpal tunnel syndrome and other sensory disorders of the hand. Measurements of test-retest reliability (3- to 5-day interval) of vibration sensibility have been found to be relatively high, even in the workplace (Rosecrance, Cook, Satre, Goode & Schroder, 1994). Gerr et al. (1995) reproduced the results and endorsed the potential usefulness of vibrametry, as reported by Borg and Lindblom, before and after a period of wrist flexion. Lang et al. (1995), from Erlangen, used the vibrameter (Somedic, Stockholm) in 22 patients with carpal tunnel syndrome before, and serially on five follow-up testing sessions up to 18 months postoperatively. At baseline, vibration thresholds in the index finger were significantly increased compared with control subjects. After median nerve decompression, the abnormalities decreased significantly. Another rigorous study ranked vibration threshold of testing as being close to nerve conduction studies in its ability to identify individuals with carpal tunnel syndrome (Winn, Morrissey & Huechtker, 2000). Others have found vibrametry not effective for early carpal tunnel syndrome detection (Werner, Franzblau & Johnston, 1994; Checkosky, Bolanowski & Cohen, 1996).

Current Perception Thresholds in Carpal Tunnel Syndrome

The somatosensory system is certainly capable of detecting and perceiving electric current stimuli and to estimate subjective magnitude of its intensity and frequency, within limits. Like other psychophysical methods, current perception evaluation by examiners relies on cognitive input from the subject. Thus, it lacks the power of objective methods that measure purely physical analogs of function of components of the senses, prominent among which are electrophysiologic methods.

Current perception threshold (CPT) measurement (through a single-blind, forced choice paradigm) has been promoted as a quick and painless method to screen for carpal tunnel syndrome (Katims, Patil, Rendell, Rouvelas, Sadle, Wesely & Bleeker, 1991). Detection sensitivity was assessed as better than clinical sensitivity (75% versus 50% in 20 subjects), which challenges the definition of carpal tunnel syndrome as being a clinical concept. A more robust study (Franzblau, Werner, Johnston & Torrey, 1994) screened 84 workers to estimate prevalence of carpal tunnel syndrome. Clinical, electrophysiologic, and CPT data (Neurometer) were compared. CPT results correlated poorly with electrophysiologic and self-reported symptoms suggestive of carpal tunnel syndrome. Sensitivity, specificity, and predictive value of CPT for carpal tunnel syndrome were low compared with traditional sensory nerve conduction parameters.

The American Association of Electrodiagnostic Medicine (1999) reviewed in the method of CPT, as performed through the Neurometer. After rigorous analysis of multiple issues, the American Association of Electrodiagnostic Medicine Equipment and Computer Committee recommended that further research is necessary to determine sensitivity and specificity of the Neurometer CPT data. Conflicting information and methodologic problems regarding its use were identified, but a potential for the method was recognized.

References

AAEM Practices in electrodiagnostic medicine. American Association of Electrodiagnostic Medicine. Technology review: the Neurometer current perception threshold (CPT). Muscle Nerve 1999;22:523–31.

Borg C, Lindblom U. Increase of vibration threshold during wrist flexion in patients with carpal tunnel syndrome. Pain 1986;26:211–19.

Calne DB, Pallis CA. Vibratory sense: a critical review. Brain 1966;4:723–46.

Campero M, Serra J, Bostock H, Ochoa JL. Slowly conducting afferents activated by innocuous low temperature in human skin. J. Physiol. 2001;535:855–65.

Checkosky CM, Bolanowski SJ, Cohen JC. Assessment of vibrotactile sensitivity in patients with carpal tunnel syndrome. J. Occup. Med. 1996;38:593–601.

Critchley M. Neurological changes in the aged. In: Moore JE, Merritt HH, Masserlink RJ, eds. The Neurologic and Psychiatric Aspects of the Disorders of Aging: Proceedings of the Association for Research in Nervous and Mental Disease, New York, NY, December 9–10, 1955. Baltimore: Williams & Wilkins, 1956;35:198.

Dellon AL. Clinical use of vibratory stimuli to evaluate peripheral nerve injury and compression neuropathy. Plast. Reconstr. Surg. 1980;6S:466–76.

Dellon AL. The vibrameter. Plast. Reconstr. Surg. 1983;71:427–31.

Dyck PJ, Bushek W, Spring EM, Karnes JL, Litchy WJ, O'Brien PC, Service FJ. Vibratory and cooling detection thresholds compared with other tests in diagnosing and staging diabetic neuropathy. Diabetes Care 1987;10:432–40.

Franzblau A, Werner RA, Johnston E, Torrey S. Evaluation of current perception threshold testing as a screening procedure for carpal tunnel syndrome among industrial workers. J. Occup. Med. 1994;36:1015–21.

Fruhstorfer H, Lindblom U, Schmidt WG. Method for quantitative estimation of thermal thresholds in patients. J. Neurol. Neurosurg. Psychiatry 1976;39:1071–75.

Gelberman RH, Szabo RM, Williamson RV, Dimick MP. Sensibility testing in peripheral nerve compression syndromes. An experimental study in humans. J. Bone Joint Surg. 1983;65A:632–38.

Gerr F, Letz R, Hershman D, Farraye J, Simpson D. Comparison of vibrotactile thresholds with physical examination and electrophysiological assessment. Muscle Nerve 1991;14:1059–66.

Gerr F, Letz R, Harris-Abbott D, Hopkins LC. Sensitivity and specificity of vibrometry for detection of carpal tunnel syndrome. J. Occup. Environ. Med. 1995;37(9): 1108–15.

Goff GD, Rosner BS, Detre T, Kennard D. Vibration perception in normal man and medical patients. J. Neurol. Neurosurg. Psychiatry 1965;28:305–509.

Goldberg JM, Lindblom U. Standardized method of determining vibratory perception thresholds of diagnosis and screening in neurological investigation. J. Neurol. Neurosurg. Psychiatry 1979;42:793–803.

Katims JJ, Patil AS, Rendell M, Rouvelas P, Sadler B, Weseley SA, Bleecker ML. Current perception threshold screening for carpal tunnel syndrome. Arch. Environ. Health 1991;37:207–12.

Lang B, Spitzer A, Pfannmüller D, Claus D, Handwerker HO, Neundörfer B. Function of thick and thin nerve fibers in carpal tunnel syndrome before and after surgical treatment. Muscle Nerve 1995;18:207–15.

Lindblom U. Quantitative testing of sensibility including pain. In: Stålberg E, Young RR, eds. Clinical Neurophysiology. London: Butterworth–Heinemann, 1981;168–90.

Lindblom U, Lund L. The discharge from vibration-sensitive receptors in the monkey foot. Exp. Neurol. 1966;15:401–17.

Lindblom U, Ochoa J. Somatosensory function and dysfunction. In: Asbury AK, McKhann GM, McDonald WI, eds. Disease of the Nervous System (2nd ed), Vol 1. Philadelphia: WB Saunders, 1992;213–28.

Merzenich MM, Harrington T. The sense of flutter-vibration evoked by stimulation of the hairy skin of primates: comparison of human sensory capacity with the responses of mechanoreceptive afferents innervating the hairy skin of monkeys. Exp. Brain Res. 1969;9:236–60.

Ochoa JL. Mechanisms of symptoms in neuropathy. The London symposia. EEG Suppl. 1987;39:121–27.

Ochoa JL, Torebjörk HE. Sensations evoked by intraneural microstimulation of single mechanoreceptor units innervating the human hand. J. Physiol. (Lond.) 1983;342: 633–54.

Rosecrance JC, Cook TM, Satre DL, Goode JD, Schroder MJ. Vibration sensibility testing in the work place. Day-to-day reliability. J. Occup. Med, 1994;36:1032–7.

Pearson GHJ. Effect of age on vibratory sensibility. Arch. Neurol. Psychiatry 1928;20:482.

Spencer PS, Ochoa J. The mammalian peripheral nervous system in old age. In: Johnson JE, ed. Aging and Cell Structure. Vol. 1. New York: Plenum Press, 1981;35–103.

Steiness I. Vibratory perception in normal subjects. Acta Med. Scand. 1957;l58:315.

Talbot WH, Darian-Smith I, Kornhuber HH, Mountcastle VB. The sense of flutter-vibration: comparison of the human capacity with response patterns in mechanoreceptive afferents from the monkey hand. J. Neurophysiol. 1968; 31:301–34.

Triplett W, Ochoa JL. Contemporary techniques in assessing peripheral nervous system function. Am. J. EEG. Technol. 1990;30:29–44.

Verdugo R, Ochoa JL. Quantitative somatosensory thermotest. A key method for functional evaluation of small caliber afferent channels. Brain 1992;115:893–913.

Verrillo RT. Age related changes in the sensitivity to vibration. J. Gerontol. 1980;3S:185–93.

Wahrén LK, Torebjörk E, Jörum E. Central suppression of cold-induced C fibre pain by myelinated fibre input. Pain 1989; 38:313–19.

Werner RA, Franzblau A, Johnston E. Comparison of multiple frequency vibrometry testing and sensory nerve conduction measures in screening for carpal tunnel syndrome. Arch. Phys. Med. Rehabil. 1994;75:1228–32.

Winn FJ, Morrissey SJ, Huechtker ED. Cross-sectional comparison of nerve conduction and vibration threshold testing: do screening tools for occupationally induced cumulative trauma disorders result in differing outcomes? Disability and Rehabilitation 2000;22:627–32.

Yarnitsky D, Ochoa JL. Release of cold-induced burning pain by block of cold-specific afferent input. Brain 1990;113: 893–902.

Yarnitsky D. Quantitative sensory testing. Muscle Nerve 1997; 20,198–204.

Chapter 10
Thermography

Conventional nerve conduction studies (see Chapters 7 and 8) exclusively test nerve impulse conduction in large-caliber myelinated sensory and motor fibers. Thermography provides noninvasive insights into the functional status of small-caliber, mostly unmyelinated, nociceptor and sympathetic vasomotor nerve fibers. Thermography is not well suited for routine diagnosis of nerve entrapment at the carpal tunnel or elsewhere, because nerve compression predominantly affects myelinated fibers. However, the method is useful in evaluating painful diseases of peripheral nerves of all kinds. Thermography sensitively detects and precisely delineates the status and distribution of skin temperature. When used in conjunction with local anesthetic nerve blocks, thermography can objectively document the cutaneous distribution of nerve fibers from specific nerve trunks, thus providing data that may be critical in clinical assessment (see Color Plate 10-1A; Color Plates 16-2 and 16-4).

Thermography is best combined with quantitative sensory testing of function of small-caliber sensory channels (see Chapter 9), so that function of small-caliber sensory fibers and small-caliber sympathetic fibers can be correlated. Details of methodology and general interpretation of thermography are beyond the scope of this chapter (for reviews, see Aarts, Gautherie & Ring, 1975; Houdas & Ring, 1982; Engel, Flesch & Stüttgen, 1985; Abernathy & Uematsu, 1986).

Abnormal Patterns

Abnormal thermographic patterns may result from neuropathic abnormalities and also, of course, from focal inflammation or vascular disease. Four elementary thermographic patterns of neuropathic origin can be defined: two are "hot," and two are "cold" (Ochoa, 1986b).

1. *Hot pattern I: sympathoparalytic vasodilatation.* If sympathetic vasomotor tone is acutely removed, for example, through sympathetic blockade, sympathectomy, somatic nerve block, or neurectomy, the skin acutely warms. The mechanism is increased blood flow as a consequence of arteriolar vasodilatation after removal of sympathetic-mediated vasoconstrictor tone. Color Plate 10-1A [found facing page 316] is an infrared thermogram displaying hyperthermia in the median nerve territory of the palm and digits during local anesthetic median nerve block).

2. *Cold pattern I: denervation supersensitivity vasospasm.* Chronic interruption of the postganglionic sympathetic neuron that supplies skin eventually leads to reduced blood flow, resulting in hypothermia of the denervated areas. The blood flow reduction by vasospasm in arteriolar smooth muscle is caused by sympathetic denervation supersensitivity (Cannon & Rosenblueth, 1949). Because cold pattern I results from a postsynaptic abnormality in the smooth muscle proper, the vasospasm and the resulting skin cooling cannot be reversed by conventional sympathetic ganglion blocks, sympathectomy, nerve blocks, or neurectomy (Color Plate 10-1B is an infrared thermogram displaying hypothermia in the median nerve territory of the palm and digits present chronically, corresponding to denervation supersensitivity after severe injury to the median nerve at the forearm level).

3. *Cold pattern II: somatosympathetic reflex vasoconstriction.* Excitation of sensory receptors (at least from the skin), or "irritation" of a sensory nerve, normally elicit rapid cooling of the skin, mostly in the territory from which afferent input emanates. This phenomenon is easily reproduced by electrical stimulation of a nerve trunk. It is a reflex, like a tendon reflex, but the afferent input activates sympathetic rather than lower motor units in the efferent limb of the reflex arc. In the clinic, sympathetic denervation supersensitivity vasospasm can be distinguished from neurally sustained somatosympathetic reflex vasoconstriction through somatic local nerve block. Vasodilatation after nerve block attests to neural mediation of the vasoconstriction. (See Color Plate 16-4D where baseline hypothermia [see Color Plate 16-4B] is reversed after median nerve block [see Color Plate 16-4D], indicating maintenance of the vasoconstriction through sympathetic neural outflow, even in the partially denervated half of the index finger.) However, this does not resolve whether the exaggerated vasoconstrictor tone is an innocent sympathetic response to abnormal afferent input or whether it depends on primarily up-modulated central sympathetic control. An experimental animal preparation illustrates that abnormal afferent activity generated in myelinated fibers proximal to a local nerve lesion elicits, via spinal reflex connections, sympathetic efferent activity that reaches peripheral targets along uninjured small-caliber fibers. Under these circumstances, neurectomy immediately reverses the local vasoconstriction (see Figure 2 in Bennett & Ochoa, 1991).

4. *Hot pattern II: antidromic vasodilatation.* This interesting pattern is also caused by changes in neurosecretory function of peripheral nerve fibers. However, here the hyperthermia resulting from vasodilatation is independent of sympathetic activity. The pattern relates to enhanced neurosecretion of vasodilator substances, chiefly calcitonin gene-related peptide (Brain, Escott, Hughes & Kajekar, 1994), released from nerve endings of sensory nociceptor units in response to nerve action potentials. These nerve impulses are either conducted antidromically from parent axon, or reflected antidromically when afferent impulses initiated in dichotomized nerve terminals of nociceptor endings reach branching points.

A familiar example of this phenomenon is the flare component of the triple response of Lewis (1927) elicitable by intradermal injection of histamine. The chemical agent stimulates chemoreceptors in the excitable membrane of C nociceptor units and fires afferent orthodromic volleys of nerve impulses. Impulses that reflect at branching points, under normal circumstances, trigger cutaneous neurosecretion and vasodilatation.

Stimulation of nerve trunks at intensity sufficient to excite propagated nerve impulses in midaxons of nociceptors endowed with this neurosecretory property elicit antidromic vasodilatation. This is strikingly confined to the skin territory supplied by the nerve trunk or the individual nerve fascicles stimulated (Ochoa, Comstock, Marchettini & Nizamuddin, 1987). Color Plate 10-1D is an infrared thermogram displaying hyperthermia in the cutaneous territory of a median nerve fascicle. The hatched area of skin shown in Color Plate 10-1C marks the territory of projection of painful paresthesias induced by intense repetitive intrafascicular stimulation of the median nerve at elbow level. This thermogram was taken shortly after prolonged stimulation was stopped. If stimulation were resumed, the focal hyperthermia would be replaced by hypothermia, because during stimulation, the evoked somatosympathetic reflex vasoconstriction [cold pattern II] overrides antidromic vasodilatation.

Direct evidence that cutaneous vasodilatation in a particular case is caused by antidromic neurosecretion rather than by sympathoparalytic vasodilatation is often unavailable. An indirect differential strategy is to demonstrate that the symptomatic vasodilated skin retains capacity for reflex sympathetic vasoconstriction. This clinical stratagem is viable because sympathetic-mediated vasoconstriction overrides nociceptor-mediated antidromic vasodilatation (Ochoa, Yarnitsky, Marchettini, Dotson & Cline, 1990). This occurrence also warns the clinician about the possibility that states of abnormal primary nociceptor activity, leading to pain and associated antidromic vasodilatation, might be partially masked by superimposed and predominant sympathetic reflex vasoconstriction.

In certain natural disease states, antidromic neurogenic vasodilatation, either localized or diffuse, may be prominent and is best detected by thermographic monitoring (Ochoa, 1986a; Cline, Ochoa & Torebjörk, 1989).

In summary, patients with hyperthermic symptomatic limbs do not necessarily have paralysis of sympathetic efferent activity. Conversely, patients with hypothermic symptomatic limbs do not necessarily have exaggerated neural sympathetic outflow; they may actually have ablated sympathetic postganglionic outflow.

Objective Thermographic Delineation of Cutaneous Innervations

Figure 16-3 and Color Plate 16-4 illustrate the cutaneous innervation pattern, as reflected in the thermogram, following local anesthetic block of the median nerve in patients. The block causes acute paralysis of sympathetic vasomotor fibers and results in vasodilatation in the cutaneous distribution of the blocked fibers. The thermogram shows increased temperature in this distribution (hot pattern I). Both sympathetic sudomotor (Guttmann, 1940) and vasomotor fibers distribute over the same area of skin as cutaneous sensory fibers, so determination of the area of sympathetic supply provides a valid measure of the area of sensory distribution.

This technique is more objective than other methods of measuring sensory patterns such as mapping paresthesias following percutaneous electrical stimulation or mapping sensory deficit after nerve block, which rely on the patient for subjective sensory witnessing (Highet, 1942; Schady, Ochoa, Torebjörk & Chen, 1983; Marchettini, Cline & Ochoa, 1990). Similar data can be obtained by the relatively more cumbersome technique of measuring sympathetic sudomotor function with a "sweat test" (Moberg, 1958).

Thermography and Positive Sensory Symptoms

Thermography is very useful in the evaluation of patients expressing positive sensory symptoms, specifically pains and hyperalgesias, that originate from dysfunction of nerve fibers. In painful median mononeuropathy, including rare instances of painful carpal tunnel syndrome, any of the four abnormal patterns described earlier may be seen, depending on the acuteness and mechanism of the neuropathy.

Ill-conceived use of thermography can prove misleading. The most common level of misuse is considering the simple physical sign that is quantified by thermography as if it were diagnostic of a syndrome. An unfortunate example is diagnosing "reflex sympathetic dystrophy" or complex regional pain syndrome simply by documenting a hypothermic symptomatic limb; this may condemn the patient to repetitive sympathetic blocks and sometimes to ultimate sympathectomy, an itinerary that characteristically meets therapeutic failure. This ill-advised practice stems from misperceiving in thermography an illusion of pathophysiology, when in reality it only records spectacularly a clinical sign: deviation of temperature.

Thermography in Carpal Tunnel Syndrome

Thermography is not useful for the routine diagnosis of carpal tunnel syndrome. Like other entrapment neuropathies, carpal tunnel syndrome primarily affects larger myelinated fibers (see Chapter 12). Fowler and Ochoa (1975), using a baboon model of *acute* focal compression neuropathy, found pathologic damage in unmyelinated fibers only if wallerian degeneration was occurring in myelinated fibers. Marotte (1974) found that unmyelinated fiber structure remained intact until late in the course of *chronic* animal nerve entrapment. Thus, the pathophysiology of carpal tunnel syndrome is such that thermographic determination of small-fiber function is a relatively insensitive test for its diagnosis. Clinical data support this conclusion. Median nerve autonomic vasomotor dysfunction is demonstrable in only a minority of cases of carpal tunnel syndrome (Aminoff, 1979). Thermography may show abnormalities in median nerve distribution in severe cases of carpal tunnel syndrome (Harway, 1986). However, in clinical series, many patients with carpal tunnel syndrome diagnosed on clinical and electrophysiologic criteria have normal thermographic studies; for example, So et al. (1989) found abnormal thermograms in only 55% of their patients with carpal tunnel syndrome. Another series reported similar results (Myers, Vermeire, Sherry & Cros, 1988).

In the 1990s, some authors remained highly enthusiastic about thermography for diagnosis of carpal tunnel syndrome. Tchou et al. (1992) compared thermograms of 61 patients with "diagnosed carpal tunnel syndrome" (clinical and electrodiagnostic criteria) and 40 symptom-free volunteers. They diagnosed thermographic abnormality when more than 25% of the measured areas within median nerve territory displayed a temperature increase of at least 1°C when compared with the symptom-free hand. A sensitivity of 93% and a specificity of 98% were reported, but the authors cautioned that usefulness of the method could not embrace bilateral disorders. In turn, Giordano et al. (1992) evaluated clinically, electrodiagnostically, and thermographically 40 cases of idiopathic carpal tunnel syndrome, compared with 30 healthy control subjects. Abnormal hypothermia and hyperthermia were often found and attributed to increase or decrease of unmyelinated sympathetic vasoconstrictor tone. Changes were described as most prominent in the territory of the palmar cutaneous branch, in the thenar region.

When thermographic abnormalities are present in patients with carpal tunnel syndrome, interpretation is complicated by the nonspecific nature of the abnormalities. In a given patient, the thermogram may not distinguish which side is abnormal and may not differentiate between ulnar and median nerve dysfunction (Reilly, Clarke & Ring, 1989; So, Olney & Aminoff, 1989).

References

Aarts NJM, Gautherie M, Ring EFJ, eds. Thermography. Proceedings of the 1st European Congress on Thermography, organized by the European Thermographic Association with the collaboration of the American Thermographic Society, Amsterdam, June 1974. Basel, Switzerland: Karger, 1975.

Abernathy M, Uematsu S, eds. Medical thermology. Washington, DC: American Academy of Thermology, 1986.

Aminoff MJ. Involvement of peripheral vasomotor fibres in carpal tunnel syndrome. J. Neurol. Neurosurg. Psychiatry 1979;42:649–55.

Bennett GJ, Ochoa JL. Thermographic observations on rats with experimental neuropathic pain. Pain 1991;45:61–67.

Brain SD, Escott KJ, Hughes SR, Kajekar R. Calcitonin gene-related peptide (CGRP): responsible for the increased blood flow induced by the stimulation of sensory nerves. Agents Actions 1994;41[Suppl C, 2]:C262–63.

Cannon WB, Rosenblueth A. The Supersensitivity of Denervated Structures: a Law of Denervation. New York: Macmillan, 1949.

Cline MA, Ochoa JL, Torebjörk HE. Chronic hyperalgesia and skin warming caused by sensitized C nociceptors. Brain 1989;112:621–47.

Engel JM, Flesch U, Stiittgen G. Applied Thermology. Thermological Methods. Weinheim, Germany: VCH Verlagsgesellschaft, 1985.

Fowler TJ, Ochoa JL. Unmyelinated fibres in normal and compressed peripheral nerves of the baboon; a quantitative electron microscopic study. Neuropathol. Appl. Neurobiol. 1975;1:247–65.

Giordano N, Battisti E, Franci A, et al. Telethermographic assessment of carpal tunnel syndrome. Scand. J. Rheumatol. 1992;21:42–5.

Guttmann L. Topographic studies of disturbances of sweat secretion after complete lesions of peripheral nerves. J. Neurol. Psychiatry 1940;3:197–210.

Harway RA. Precision thermal imaging of the extremities. Orthopedics 1986;9:379–82.

Highet WB. Procaine nerve block in the investigation of peripheral nerve injuries. J. Neurol. Psychiatry 1942;5:101–16.

Houdas Y, Ring EFJ. Human body temperature. Its measurement and regulation. New York: Plenum Press, 1982.

Lewis T. The Blood Vessels of the Human Skin and Their Responses. London: Shaw & Sons, 1927.

Marchettini P, Cline M, Ochoa JL. Innervation territories for touch and pain afferents of single fascicles of the human ulnar nerve. Mapping through intraneural microrecording and microstimulation. Brain 1990;113:1491–1500.

Marotte LR. An electron microscope study of chronic median nerve compression in the guinea-pig. Acta. Neuropathol. (Berl.) 1974;27:69–82.

Moberg E. Objective methods for determining the functional value of sensibility in the hand. J. Bone Joint Surg. 1958; 40B:454–76.

Myers S, Vermeire P, Sherry B, Cros D. Liquid crystal thermography: quantitative studies of abnormalities in the carpal tunnel syndrome. Neurology (Minneap.) Suppl. 1988; 38:200.

Ochoa JL. The newly recognized painful ABC syndrome: thermographic aspects. Thermology 1986a;2:65–107.

Ochoa JL. Unmyelinated fibers, microneurography, thermography and pain. American Association of Electromyography and Electrodiagnosis; ninth annual continuing education course B. Rochester, NY: AAEE., 1986b;29–34.

Ochoa JL, Comstock WJ, Marchettini P, Nizamuddin G. Intrafascicular nerve stimulation elicits regional skin warming that matches the projected field of evoked pain. In:

Schmidt RF, Schaible H-G, Vahle-Hinz C, eds. Fine Afferent Nerve Fibers and Pain. Weinheim, Germany: VCH Verlagsgesellschaft, 1987.

Ochoa JL, Yarnitsky D, Marchettini P, Dotson R, Cline M. Antidromic vasodilatation overridden by somatosympathetic reflexes in man. Intraneural stimulation and thermography (abst). Soc. Neurosci. 1990;16:1280.

Reilly PA, Clarke AK, Ring EF. Thermography in carpal tunnel syndrome (CTS). Br. J. Rheumatol. 1989;28:553–54.

Schady W, Ochoa JL, Torebjörk HE, Chen LS. Peripheral projections of fascicles in the human median nerve. Brain 1983;106:745–60.

So YT, Olney RK, Aminoff MJ. Evaluation of thermography in the diagnosis of selected entrapment neuropathies. Neurology 1989;39:1–5.

Tchou S, Costich JF, Burgess RC, et al. Thermographic observations in unilateral carpal tunnel syndrome: report of 61 cases. J. Hand Surg. 1992;17A:631–37.

Chapter 11
Imaging the Carpal Tunnel and Median Nerve

Radiographs, computed tomographic (CT) scans, magnetic resonance imaging (MRI) scans, and ultrasonography (US) have all been used to image the wrists of patients with carpal tunnel syndrome. Each imaging technique can sometimes show abnormalities in patients with carpal tunnel syndrome, but none of these techniques has established diagnostic accuracy sufficient to be make it useful for routine evaluation of patients with suspected carpal tunnel syndrome. This chapter reviews the different techniques. The value of imaging for specific problems such as postoperative assessment (Chapter 15), carpal tunnel tumors (Chapter 19), or unusual causes of carpal tunnel syndrome (Chapter 6) are discussed in other chapters.

Wrist Radiography

Wrist radiography is not needed for evaluation of most patients with carpal tunnel syndrome. Table 11-1 shows the results of radiographs of 447 wrists with definite carpal tunnel syndrome by both clinical and electrodiagnostic criteria (Bindra, Evanoff, Chough, Cole, Chow & Gelberman, 1997). Only two wrists showed abnormalities that theoretically might affect therapy (one calcified mass in the carpal tunnel and one soft tissue shadow in the carpal tunnel), but the patients with these findings underwent successful endoscopic carpal tunnel surgery without attention to the radiographic abnormalities.

Wrist radiography provides a rough estimate of size of the carpal tunnel. Gelmers (1981) took vertical wrist radiographs of the boundaries of the tunnel, approximating the flexor retinaculum as a straight line from the navicular tuberosity to the pisiform bone. Table 11-2 shows his data that compare a cross-sectional area of the carpal tunnel in women who have carpal tunnel syndrome and in controls. The symptomatic women had a statistically significant smaller mean cross-sectional area of the carpal tunnel. Another small series did not find differences in canal dimensions, estimated from plain radiographs, between patients with carpal tunnel syndrome and control subjects matched for age, weight, stature, and sex (Cobb, Bond, Cooney & Metcalf, 1997).

Hand Radiography

Hand radiographs are normal in patients with carpal tunnel syndrome unless there is an associated disease affecting the hand, such as rheumatoid arthritis or acromegaly. An exception to this generalization is the presence of acroosteolysis of the terminal phalange of the index or middle fingers, often associated with ischemic changes in overlying skin, in exceptionally rare patients with severe carpal tunnel syndrome (Tosti, Morelli, D'Alessandro & Bassi, 1993).

Computed Tomographic Scanning

The anatomy of the carpal canal can be imaged *in vivo* by CT (see Figures 1-15 and 1-16). Serial cross sections show the carpal bones, flexor tendons, flexor retinaculum, and median nerve (Zucker-Pinchoff, Hermann & Srinivasan, 1981). Good detail

Table 11-1. Findings in Routine Wrist Radiographs in 447 Instances of Carpal Tunnel Syndrome

Findings on Wrist Radiographs	Percent of Wrists
Normal	67
Irrelevant abnormalities (osteopenia, carpal cysts, vascular calcification, etc.)	14
Abnormalities possibly related to carpal tunnel syndrome:	19
Degenerative changes, basal thumb joint	11
Degenerative changes, radiocarpal or intercarpal joints	10
Malunited distal radial fracture	2
Other carpal abnormalities such as nonunion of fractures	5
Abnormalities of theoretic therapeutic import (see text)	0.4

Data from RR Bindra, BA Evanoff, LY Chough, RJ Cole, JC Chow, RH Gelberman. The use of routine wrist radiography in the evaluation of patients with carpal tunnel syndrome. J. Hand Surg. 1997;22A:115–19.

is obtained with 3-mm thick slices. The flexor tendons (attenuation coefficient approximately 100 Hounsfield units) have higher attenuation than their surrounding synovial fluid. The median nerve blends with the synovium. The flexor retinaculum is visible as a thin soft tissue line (Merhar, Clark, Schneider & Stern, 1986). Three-dimensional CT reconstruction can provide images of relationships of bones, median nerves, and other soft tissues (Cartolari, Sozio, Boni, Capoccia & Vocino, 1994; Buitrago-Téllez, Horch, Allmann, Stark & Langer, 1998).

Measurements by CT of the cross-sectional area of the canal have given conflicting results in patients

Table 11-2. Carpal Tunnel Cross-Sectional Area by Wrist Radiography

	Area (mm²)	Standard Error
Female controls (19)	206.6	12.4
Female subjects with carpal tunnel syndrome (11)	153.8*	11.8
Male controls (17)	234.1	14.3

*$P < .001$ compared with female controls.
Data from HJ Gelmers. Primary carpal tunnel stenosis as a cause of entrapment of the median nerve. Acta. Neurochir. (Wien.) 1981;55:317–20.

with carpal tunnel syndrome. Table 11-3 compares carpal canal cross-sectional area measured by CT in women who have carpal tunnel syndrome and in controls (Dekel, Papaioannou, Rushworth & Coates, 1980; Dekel & Rushworth, 1993).

The symptomatic women had a statistically significant smaller mean cross-sectional area of the carpal tunnel. Male controls had larger tunnel cross-sectional areas. There was a large overlap between the areas for individual patients and individual controls, so this technique does not provide a diagnostic test for individual patients. There was no correlation between patient age and tunnel area, suggesting that tunnel area is determined by age 20 and does not decline with age.

Bleecker and colleagues (1985) studied all 14 male electricians in an electrical shop. They classified the condition of the workers as (1) symptomatic carpal tunnel syndrome, (2) asymptomatic with abnormal median nerve conduction, or (3) normal. Using 5-mm contiguous CT slices through the canal, they identified the slice in each patient with the smallest cross-sectional area. In most cases the smallest area was 2.0 to 2.5 cm distal to the distal wrist crease, but in four cases the minimum area was more proximal. For both the workers with carpal tunnel syndrome and the workers with asymptomatic median nerve conduction abnormalities, the mean of the smallest tunnel cross-sectional area was lower than for the normal workers.

In contrast, Merhar and colleagues (1986) found no significant difference in canal areas comparing patients with controls. They used a 3-mm section technique that visualized the flexor retinaculum. Dekel and colleagues (1980) had not visualized the retinaculum and approximated it for measurement purposes by a straight line connecting the scaphoid tubercle to the pisiform or trapezium to the hook of the hamate. The flexor retinaculum is actually slightly curved so that the canal is oval. As expected, the areas reported by Merhar and colleagues were slightly larger than those reported by Dekel and colleagues. Merhar and colleagues also measured the relative amount of synovium in the canal, the attenuation coefficient of the canal, and the thickness of the flexor retinaculum and found that these did not differ significantly between patients and controls.

Table 11-3. Carpal Tunnel Cross-Sectional Area by Computed Tomographic Scan

	Proximal Area (mm²)	Standard Error	Distal Area (mm²)	Standard Error
Female controls (19)	213.7	4.8	209.3	7.7
Female subjects with carpal tunnel syndrome (26) (42 hands)	184.1[a]	4.0	188.0[b]	6.5
Male controls (14)	279.9	8.3	254.1	7.8

[a]$P < .001$.
[b]$P < .05$ compared with female controls.
Data from S Dekel, T Papaioannou, G Rushworth, R Coates. Idiopathic carpal tunnel syndrome caused by carpal stenosis. BMJ. 1980;280:1297–99.

Jessurun and colleagues (1987) compared CT scans of the carpal tunnel in patients and controls with the wrist neutral, flexed 70 degrees, or extended 70 degrees. They found that the normal median nerve moves away from the flexor retinaculum during wrist flexion. In one-fifth of hands with carpal tunnel syndrome, this nerve movement relative to the flexor retinaculum did not occur with flexion. The cross-sectional areas of the tunnel did not change significantly among the three positions in patients or controls. There was no significant difference in the areas of the tunnels between patients and controls. The tunnel area was smallest 6 mm proximal to the distal border of the hook of the hamate. At this level the fraction of the tunnel occupied by tendons was larger in female patients than in female controls; however, male patients and controls matched female patients in the fraction of their tunnels occupied by tendons. Winn and Habes (1990) found that patients who had carpal tunnel syndrome had *larger* minimum tunnel areas as measured by CT than did sex-matched controls.

In summary, there are conflicting data on the relationship between tunnel size, as measured by CT scan, and the development of carpal tunnel syndrome. Even in the studies that found smaller mean tunnel sizes in groups of patients with carpal tunnel syndrome, the differences are insufficient to provide useful diagnostic information in most individual patients.

On rare occasions, CT scan of the wrist might reveal other wrist pathology or anomalies of diagnostic importance (Hindman, Kulik, Lee & Avolio, 1989). Nonetheless, in most cases of carpal tunnel syndrome, wrist CT scan is not a necessary part of the diagnostic evaluation. Currently, on those exceptional occasions when wrist cross-sectional imaging is needed in patients with carpal tunnel syndrome, MRI is usually preferable to CT.

Magnetic Resonance Imaging Scanning

MRI of the wrist using surface coils can give excellent high-resolution images of the hands and wrists (see Figures 1-16 and 1-17) (Weiss, Beltran, Shamam, Stilla & Levey, 1986; Middleton, Kneeland, Kellman, Cates, Sanger, Jesmanowicz & Froncisz, 1987; Mesgarzadeh, Schneck & Bonakdarpour, 1989a). Normal anatomy varies with wrist position (Zeiss, Skie, Ebraheim & Jackson, 1989; Skie, Zeiss, Ebraheim & Jackson, 1990). Newer, less validated, approaches include using surface coils, a 1.5-Tesla magnet, and imaging sequences with fat and flow suppression and T2 weighting to perform MR neurography that increases the conspicuity of the median nerve (Howe, Saunders, Filler, McLean, Heron, Brown & Griffiths, 1994) or using low-field (0.2 Tesla) MRI, emphasizing T2-weighted turbo spin echo and magnetization transfer sequences (Bonel, Heuck, Frei, Herrmann, Scheidler, Srivastav & Reiser, 2001).

Details of a variety of hand pathologies, such as ganglia and other masses, fractures, osteonecrosis, tendon abnormalities, ligamentous injuries, vascular malformations, and rheumatoid deformities, are visible by MRI (Siegel, White & Brahme, 1996).

A variety of MRI abnormalities can be found in some patients with carpal tunnel syndrome:

1. Swelling of the median nerve
2. Flattening of the median nerve

3. Abnormal signal intensity of the median nerve on T2-weighted images
4. Palmar bowing of the flexor retinaculum
5. Abnormalities of tendons or deep palmar bursa in the carpal tunnel
6. Abnormal structures within the carpal tunnel
7. Abnormal signal in thenar muscles

Swelling of the Median Nerve

MRI scans of the median nerve in hands with carpal tunnel syndrome typically show that the nerve is larger as it enters the tunnel than it is in the distal forearm (Mesgarzadeh, Schneck, Bonakdarpour, Mitra & Conaway, 1989). In the tunnel it has an hourglass appearance, tapering as it runs from the level of the pisiform bone to the level of the hook of the hamate. Even at the hook of the hamate, it is larger than it is in the distal forearm.

The value of median nerve size as a diagnostic parameter is debated, partly because studies differ in the definition of median nerve swelling. A non-quantitative visual evaluation of the nerve found that the nerve was enlarged at the level of the pisiform compared with its size at the level of the hook of the hamate in 23% of patients who had carpal tunnel syndrome and 24% of controls (Radack, Schweitzer & Taras, 1997). A quantitative study found that in 90% of patients who had carpal tunnel syndrome, the median nerve was enlarged at least at one level, usually the level of the pisiform (Seyfert, Boegner, Hamm, Kleindienst & Klatt, 1994). In patients with more advanced carpal tunnel syndrome (corresponding approximately to our class 3, Chapter 3) the swelling may also be seen at the level of the radius, whereas in mild carpal tunnel syndrome (class 1) the swelling is more likely to be localized to the levels of the pisiform and hamate (Kleindienst, Hamm & Lanksch, 1998). Swelling that is visualized by MRI is often not evident at surgery after the flexor retinaculum has been sectioned (Seyfert et al., 1994).

Flattening of the Median Nerve

The median nerve is oval in the carpal tunnel and becomes flatter (higher ratio of antero-posterior width to thickness) as the nerve progresses distally through the tunnel. The MRI of the median nerve infrequently appears excessively flattened in patients who have carpal tunnel syndrome, but flattening can also be seen in occasional control subjects (Radack et al., 1997). In quantitative studies, significantly increased flattening was found at the level of the pisiform in a group of patients who had advanced (class 3) carpal tunnel syndrome, but neither in patients who had milder carpal tunnel syndrome nor at hamate or radius levels in patients who had advanced carpal tunnel syndrome (Kleindienst et al., 1998).

Abnormal Signal Intensity of the Median Nerve on T2-Weighted Images

The median nerve of patients who have carpal tunnel syndrome can show increased signal intensity on T2-weighted MRI (Mesgarzadeh, Schneck, Bonakdarpour, Mitra & Conaway, 1989). The signal is increased in comparison with the signal intensity of thenar muscles and is visible in the nerve throughout its course within the carpal tunnel but rarely extends proximal to the distal radio-ulnar joint (Mesgarzadeh, Schneck, Bonakdarpour, Mitra & Conaway, 1989). At times the signal is most intense circumferentially, suggesting epineurial edema. Increased nerve signal intensity can be seen in clinically early carpal tunnel syndrome (corresponding approximately to our class 1) and can be present in the absence of median nerve flattening or swelling (Kleindienst, Hamm, Hildebrandt & Klug, 1996). The incidence of increased median nerve signal intensity varies—20% in one series, 59% in another (Seyfert et al., 1994; Radack et al., 1997). In the later series, however, median nerve signal was also increased in 49% of wrists with clinical syndromes other than well-defined carpal tunnel syndrome.

The signal intensity in the nerve is more likely to be normal in patients with more advanced carpal tunnel syndrome (class 3) than in patients with mild or moderate (classes 1 or 2) carpal tunnel syndrome (Kleindienst et al., 1998). A less common finding in wrists of patients with carpal tunnel syndrome is abnormally low signal intensity of the median nerve on T2-weighted images (Reicher & Kellerhouse, 1990). In these instances, the nerve appears inhomogeneous, smaller in cross section, and less distinct from surrounding structures. This occurs in late carpal tunnel syndrome, correlating with clinical and electrodiagnostic findings of axonal degeneration (class 3) (Kleindienst et al., 1996).

Palmar Bowing of the Flexor Retinaculum

Patients who have carpal tunnel syndrome sometimes have abnormal volar bowing of the flexor retinaculum that is detectable by MRI (Mesgarzadeh, Schneck, Bonakdarpour, Mitra & Conaway, 1989). This is a relatively insensitive finding, present in less than one-third of patients with carpal tunnel syndrome (Seyfert et al., 1994; Radack et al., 1997). In contrast, palmar bowing was present in 6% of patients who were referred for wrist MRI and did not have clinically and electrodiagnostically proven carpal tunnel syndrome (Radack et al., 1997).

Carpal Tunnel Flexor Tenosynovitis

Carpal tunnel MRI can demonstrate patchy thickening of the flexor tenosynovium, most easily seen on transverse proton-density or fast (T2-weighted) spin echo images (Middleton et al., 1987; Healy, Watson, Longstaff & Campbell, 1990; Seyfert et al., 1994). Pathologically this tissue can be edematous or fibrotic. These changes are found in little more than one-third of wrists with carpal tunnel syndrome and in nearly one-fifth of wrists imaged for other diagnoses, so these changes are neither sensitive nor specific for carpal tunnel syndrome (Radack et al., 1997). Another soft tissue abnormality that is occasionally present in the wrists of patients with carpal tunnel syndrome is deep palmar bursitis, which appears as a well-defined fluid collection (bright and homogeneous on T2-weighted images) within the tunnel, dorsal to the flexor tendons (Radack et al., 1997).

Abnormal Structures within the Carpal Tunnel

MRI often demonstrates asymptomatic anatomic variations in the tunnel such as proximal extension of lumbricals into the tunnel, persistent median artery, or anomalous relation of the median nerve to the flexor tendons (Middleton et al., 1987).

Carpal Canal Size

A number of attempts have been made to compare MRI measurements of carpal tunnel size between patients with carpal tunnel syndrome and control subjects (Cobb, Dalley, Posteraro & Lewis, 1992; Bak, Bak, Gaster, Mathiesen, Ellemann, Bertheussen & Zeeberg, 1997; Cobb, Bond, Cooney & Metcalf, 1997; Horch, Allmann, Laubenberger, Langer & Stark, 1997; Pierre-Jerome, Bekkelund, Mellgren & Nordstrom, 1997; Monagle, Dai, Chu, Burnham & Snyder, 1999). The studies vary in technical details (e.g., magnet size or imaging sequences) and in parameters used to estimate size of the canal (volume alone or corrected for volume of canal contents, cross-sectional area at varied levels, transverse and anteroposterior diameters, changes in carpal measurements after flexion or extension). There is no consensus on an MRI technique that correlates a measure of carpal canal configuration with the risk of developing or of having carpal tunnel syndrome. Even in those studies that find a statistically significant difference between mean values of a size parameter for control subjects versus patients with carpal tunnel syndrome, the overlap between groups is such that the parameter does not provide a sensitive diagnostic test for carpal tunnel syndrome (Cobb et al., 1997).

Abnormal Signal in Thenar Muscles

When carpal tunnel syndrome is severe enough to cause interruption of axons to the thenar muscles, these muscles can be abnormally bright on T2-weighted or STIR (short time to inversion recovery) MRI (Jarvik, Kliot & Maravilla, 2000). STIR images can also be abnormally bright if the muscle is edematous owing to other causes such as blunt trauma, acute myositis, or severe strains (McDonald, Carter, Fritz, Anderson, Abresch & Kilmer, 2000). STIR images of the thenar muscles are an insensitive test for carpal tunnel syndrome both because most cases of carpal tunnel syndrome are not severe enough to cause interruption of motor axons and

Table 11-4. Cross-Sectional Areas of the Median Nerve by Magnetic Resonance Imaging

Cross-Sectional Area (mm²)	Carpal Tunnel Syndrome (72 Hands)*	Controls (39 Hands)
Level of hook of the hamate	7.7 ± 2.1	5.5 ± 1.4
Level of pisiform	15.0 ± 3.5	7.5 ± 1.8
Level of distal radius	10.5 ± 2.8	6.8 ± 1.8

*$P <.01$ or better compared with control group.
Data of S Seyfert, F Boegner, B Hamm, A Kleindienst, C Klatt. The value of magnetic resonance imaging in carpal tunnel syndrome. J. Neurol. 1994;242:41–46.

Table 11-5. Ultrasound Measurements of Median Nerve Size in Symptomatic Wrists of Patients with Carpal Tunnel Syndrome and in Wrists of Control Patients

	Carpal Tunnel Syndrome*	Controls
Major axis (mm)		
Distal edge flexor retinaculum	6.8 ± 1.3	6.0 ± 0.8
Hook of the hamate	5.6 ± 0.7	5.2 ± 0.6
Distal wrist crease	7.1 ± 1.5	5.4 ± 0.4
Minor axis (mm)		
Distal edge flexor retinaculum	2.3 ± 0.4	1.8 ± 0.3
Hook of the hamate	2.2 ± 0.3	1.8 ± 0.3
Distal wrist crease	2.6 ± 0.5	2.1 ± 0.3
Cross-sectional area (mm²)		
Distal edge flexor retinaculum	14.1 ± 4.7	10.0 ± 2.6
Hook of the hamate	11.0 ± 2.4	8.8 ± 1.6
Distal wrist crease	16.8 ± 6.4	10.2 ± 2.5
Flattening ratio (minor axis/major axis)		
Distal edge flexor retinaculum	3.09 ± 0.69	3.39 ± 0.79
Hook of the hamate	2.57 ± 0.48	2.81 ± 0.54

*All differences between carpal tunnel syndrome and control wrists were significant at $P <.0001$. In contrast, nerve size in the distal forearm was not significantly different for carpal tunnel syndrome and control wrists.
Data from KI Nakamichi, S Tachibana. Enlarged median nerve in idiopathic carpal tunnel syndrome. Muscle Nerve 2000;23:1713–18.

because STIR MRI is slightly less sensitive than needle electromyographic studies in detecting axonal interruption (McDonald et al., 2000).

Ultrasonography

High-frequency (7.5 to 13.0 MHz) longitudinal and axial US of the wrist can image the median nerve, flexor tendons, and other wrist and hand structures and demonstrates abnormalities in some patients with carpal tunnel syndrome. US imaging is faster and less expensive than MRI and has many similarities to MRI in the types and diagnostic accuracy of abnormal findings.

Median Nerve

The median nerve is usually easily identified as a hypoechogenic structure underneath the flexor retinaculum. It can be distinguished from the surrounding flexor tendons by watching tendons glide with passive or active finger motion. The median nerve can be traced on longitudinal scans; the normal nerve often has a somewhat "hourglass" outline, appearing wider at the distal wrist crease, thinner at the level of the hook of the hamate, and wider again at the distal edge of the flexor retinaculum. The oval cross section of the median nerve can be seen and measured on axial scans. Cadaver studies suggest that these measurements are reliable and reproducible (Nakamichi & Tachibana, 2000).

Wrists with carpal tunnel syndrome have greater median nerve cross-sectional area within the carpal tunnel than do wrists of control subjects (Duncan, Sullivan & Lomas, 1999; Nakamichi & Tachibana, 2000). At the levels of the distal edge of the flexor retinaculum or the hook of the hamate, the median nerve is flatter in symptomatic wrists of patients with carpal tunnel syndrome than in control wrists.

Comparison of Tables 11-4 and 11-5 shows that MRI and US support the evidence that the median nerve is enlarged throughout the carpal tunnel in groups of patients with carpal tunnel syndrome. The US and MRI measurements of nerve size can differ, however.

When US is used as a diagnostic test in wrists with a diagnosis of carpal tunnel syndrome established by clinical presentation and abnormal median nerve conduction studies, 80% of median nerves show abnormal swelling of the median nerve in the proximal carpal tunnel and 65% show abnormal flattening of the median nerve at the level of the hook of the hamate (Buchberger, Judmaier, Birbamer, Lener & Schmidauer, 1992).

Flexor Retinaculum

US can also visualize abnormal (>4 mm) palmar bowing of the flexor retinaculum in some patients who have carpal tunnel syndrome. In one study this was demonstrated in 45% of wrists with clinically and electrodiagnostically confirmed carpal tunnel syndrome (Buchberger et al., 1992). Palmar bowing is usually more accurately assessed by MRI than by US.

The sensitivity of US as a diagnostic test for carpal tunnel syndrome is increased by combining bowing of the flexor retinaculum, median nerve swelling, and median nerve flattening; 95% of the wrists with definite carpal tunnel syndrome show at least one of these abnormalities (Buchberger, Judmaier, Birbamer, Hasenohrl & Schmidauer, 1993). However, validation of these parameters in large series and extrapolation of the findings to patients with symptoms but normal nerve conduction studies are still unavailable.

Flexor Tendons

The US appearance of the flexor tendons in the carpal tunnel is normal in most patients who have carpal tunnel syndrome (Nakamichi & Tachibana, 1993). In some patients the tendons appear enlarged, inhomogeneous, hyperechogenic, or surrounded by hypoechogenic tissue (Nakamichi & Tachibana, 1993; Missere et al., 1998). The tendon changes are sometimes seen in patients who have mild carpal tunnel syndrome or in patients who have flexor tenosynovitis and do not have carpal tunnel syndrome. When the hypogenic area is particularly enlarged, inflammatory synovitis, such as that of rheumatoid arthritis or granulomatous infection

should be more strongly considered in the differential diagnosis (Nakamichi & Tachibana, 1993).

Other Structures

US can demonstrate structural abnormalities within the carpal tunnel such as ganglion cysts, lipomas, or other abnormal masses, but in general MRI is more sensitive than US for detecting and characterizing abnormal contents of the canal.

Summary: Diagnostic Value of Imaging in Evaluation of Suspected Carpal Tunnel Syndrome

The studies mentioned previously report varied sensitivities and specificities of imaging findings in carpal tunnel syndrome. The diagnostic sensitivity can be increased if the diagnosis of carpal tunnel syndrome is supported when a single abnormality is present, but, of course, this decreases specificity (Seyfert et al., 1994). The diagnostic sensitivity is decreased, but the specificity is increased if pairs of findings are used as the diagnostic criteria (Radack et al., 1997). The specificity and sensitivity can also be shifted by slight adjustments in the normal limits. Repeating the wrist MRI after the patient does 10 minutes of wrist exercises has been proposed as another way to increase sensitivity (Brahme, Hodler, Braun, Sebrechts, Jackson & Resnick, 1997).

Unfortunately, there are few series that carefully compare imaging abnormalities in patients with verified carpal tunnel syndrome with findings in controls. In patients with carpal tunnel syndrome confirmed by electrodiagnostic testing, the individual imaging abnormalities have relatively low sensitivity; the highest specificities are for findings with low sensitivity (Table 11-6) (Radack et al., 1997; Jarvik et al., 2000). There is good intrarater and interrater reliability for these findings.

There are few data on the use of MRI scanning in patients who have symptoms suggestive of carpal tunnel syndrome but have normal electrodiagnostic test results. A small series examined wrist MRI in patients who had symptoms of

Table 11-6. Accuracy of Magnetic Resonance Imaging Signs for Diagnosis of Carpal Tunnel Syndrome

Abnormal Magnetic Resonance Imaging Finding	Sensitivity		Specificity	
	Radack	Jarvik	Radack	Jarvik
Increased median nerve signal	0.59	0.58	0.51	0.59
Swelling of the median nerve	0.23	—	0.76	—
Bowing of the flexor retinaculum	0.32	0.16	0.94	0.91
Flattening of the median nerve	0.05	0.27	0.97	0.70
Flexor tenosynovitis	0.36	0.19	0.82	0.93
Deep palmar bursitis	0	0.19	0.94	0.93

Adapted from JG Jarvik, M Kliot, KR Maravilla. MR nerve imaging of the wrist and hand. Hand Clin. 2000;16:13–24; and DM Radack, ME Schweitzer, J Taras. Carpal tunnel syndrome: are the MR findings a result of population selection bias? AJR. Am. J. Roentgenol. 1997;169:1649–53.

carpal tunnel syndrome during wrist use, no symptoms at rest, normal electrodiagnostic tests, and relief of symptoms after carpal tunnel surgery (Brahme et al., 1997). In all symptomatic wrists there were four or more abnormalities suggestive of carpal tunnel syndrome, whereas no wrist of a control subject had more than three abnormalities. In contrast, another study compared wrist MRI scans in patients with electrodiagnostically confirmed carpal tunnel syndrome and in patients with suspected carpal tunnel syndrome who had negative electrodiagnostic studies and concluded that "neither symptoms nor electrophysiologic findings in carpal tunnel syndrome were related to specific MRI parameters" (Bak et al., 1997).

In summary, wrist imaging is not a routine part of evaluation of patients with suspected carpal tunnel syndrome (Rosenbaum, 1993; Seyfert et al., 1994; Radack et al., 1997). Whereas many patients with carpal tunnel syndrome do have abnormalities

that are visible, particularly with US or MRI, there is still little consensus on the accuracy of various imaging findings and little validation of imaging findings in the most difficult diagnostic cases that is those with symptoms that might be due to carpal tunnel syndrome but normal neurologic and electrodiagnostic evaluations.

References

Bak L, Bak S, Gaster P, Mathiesen F, Ellemann K, Bertheussen K, Zeeberg I. MR imaging of the wrist in carpal tunnel syndrome. Acta Radiol. 1997;38:1050–52.

Bindra RR, Evanoff BA, Chough LY, Cole RJ, Chow JC, Gelberman RH. The use of routine wrist radiography in the evaluation of patients with carpal tunnel syndrome. J. Hand Surg. 1997;22A:115–19.

Bleecker ML, Bohlman M, Moreland R, Tipton A. Carpal tunnel syndrome: role of carpal canal size. Neurology 1985;35:1599–1604.

Bonel HM, Heuck A, Frei KA, Herrmann K, Scheidler J, Srivastav S, Reiser M. Carpal tunnel syndrome: assessment by turbo spin echo, spin echo, and magnetization transfer imaging applied in a low-field MR system. J. Comput. Assist. Tomogr. 2001;25:137–45.

Brahme SK, Hodler J, Braun RM, Sebrechts C, Jackson W, Resnick D. Dynamic MR imaging of carpal tunnel syndrome. Skeletal Radiol. 1997;26:482–87.

Buchberger W, Judmaier W, Birbamer G, Hasenohrl K, Schmidauer C. The role of sonography and MR tomography in the diagnosis and therapeutic control of the carpal tunnel syndrome. Fortschr. Röntgenstr. 1993;159:138–43.

Buchberger W, Judmaier W, Birbamer G, Lener M, Schmidauer C. Carpal tunnel syndrome: diagnosis with high-resolution sonography. AJR. Am. J. Roentgenol. 1992; 159: 793–98.

Buitrago-Téllez CH, Horch R, Allmann KH, Stark GB, Langer M. Three-dimensional computed tomography reconstruction of the carpal tunnel and carpal bones. Plast. Reconstr. Surg. 1998;101:1060–64.

Cartolari R, Sozio A, Boni S, Capoccia R, Vocino L. Carpal tunnel syndrome: the role of tridimensional computerized tomography. Chir. Organi Mov. 1994;79:157–62.

Cobb TK, Bond JR, Cooney WP, Metcalf BJ. Assessment of the ratio of carpal contents to carpal tunnel volume in patients with carpal tunnel syndrome: a preliminary report. J. Hand Surg. 1997;22A:635–39.

Cobb TK, Dalley BK, Posteraro RH, Lewis RC. Establishment of carpal contents/canal ratio by means of magnetic resonance imaging. J. Hand Surg. 1992;17A:843–49.

Dekel S, Papaioannou T, Rushworth G, Coates R. Idiopathic carpal tunnel syndrome caused by carpal stenosis. BMJ. 1980;280:1297–99.

Dekel S, Rushworth G. The etiology of idiopathic carpal tunnel syndrome. In: Tubiana R, ed. The Hand. Philadelphia: WB Saunders, 1993;450–62.

Duncan I, Sullivan P, Lomas F. Sonography in the diagnosis of carpal tunnel syndrome. AJR. Am. J. Roentgenol. 1999; 173:681–84.

Gelmers HJ. Primary carpal tunnel stenosis as a cause of entrapment of the median nerve. Acta Neurochir. (Wien) 1981;55:317–20.

Healy C, Watson JD, Longstaff A, Campbell MJ. Magnetic resonance imaging of the carpal tunnel. J. Hand Surg. 1990; 15B:243–48.

Hindman BW, Kulik WJ, Lee G, Avolio RE. Occult fractures of the carpals and metacarpals: demonstration by CT. AJR. Am. J. Roentgenol. 1989;153:529–32.

Horch RE, Allmann KH, Laubenberger J, Langer M, Stark GB. Median nerve compression can be detected by magnetic resonance imaging of the carpal tunnel. Neurosurgery 1997; 41:76–82.

Howe FA, Saunders DE, Filler AG, McLean MA, Heron C, Brown MM, Griffiths JR. Magnetic resonance neurography of the median nerve. Br. J. Radiol. 1994;67:1169–72.

Jarvik JG, Kliot M, Maravilla KR. MR nerve imaging of the wrist and hand. Hand Clin. 2000;16:13–24.

Jessurun W, Hillen B, Zonneveld F, Huffstadt AJ, Beks JW, Overbeek W. Anatomical relations in the carpal tunnel: a computed tomographic study. J. Hand Surg. 1987;12B: 64–67.

Kleindienst A, Hamm B, Hildebrandt G, Klug N. Diagnosis and staging of carpal tunnel syndrome: comparison of magnetic resonance imaging and intra-operative findings. Acta Neurochir. (Wien.) 1996;138:228–33.

Kleindienst A, Hamm B, Lanksch WR. Carpal tunnel syndrome: staging of median nerve compression by MR imaging. J. Magn. Reson. Imaging 1998;8:1119–25.

McDonald CM, Carter GT, Fritz RC, Anderson MW, Abresch RT, Kilmer DD. Magnetic resonance imaging of denervated muscle: comparison to electromyography. Muscle Nerve 2000;23:1431–34.

Merhar GL, Clark RA, Schneider HJ, Stern PJ. High-resolution computed tomography of the wrist in patients with carpal tunnel syndrome. Skeletal Radiol. 1986;15:549–52.

Mesgarzadeh M, Schneck CD, Bonakdarpour A. Carpal tunnel: MR imaging. Part I. Normal anatomy. Radiology 1989; 171:743–48.

Mesgarzadeh M, Schneck CD, Bonakdarpour A, Mitra A, Conaway D. Carpal tunnel: MR imaging. Part II. Carpal tunnel syndrome. Radiology 1989;171:749–54.

Middleton WD, Kneeland JB, Kellman GM, Cates JD, Sanger JR, Jesmanowicz A, Froncisz W, Hyde JS. MR imaging of the carpal tunnel: normal anatomy and preliminary findings in the carpal tunnel syndrome. AJR. Am. J. Roentgenol. 1987;148:307–16.

Missere M, Lodi V, Naldi M, Caso MA, Prati F, Raffi GB. Use of ultrasonography in monitoring work-related carpal tunnel syndrome: a case report. Am. J. Ind. Med. 1998;33: 560–64.

Monagle K, Dai G, Chu A, Burnham RS, Snyder RE. Quantitative MR imaging of carpal tunnel syndrome. AJR. Am. J. Roentgenol. 1999;172:1581–86.

Nakamichi K, Tachibana S. The use of ultrasonography in detection of synovitis in carpal tunnel syndrome. J. Hand Surg. 1993;18B:176–79.

Nakamichi KI, Tachibana S. Enlarged median nerve in idiopathic carpal tunnel syndrome. Muscle Nerve 2000;23: 1713–18.

Pierre-Jerome C, Bekkelund SI, Mellgren SI, Nordstrom R. Quantitative MRI and electrophysiology of preoperative carpal tunnel syndrome in a female population. Ergonomics 1997;40:642–49.

Radack DM, Schweitzer ME, Taras J. Carpal tunnel syndrome: are the MR findings a result of population selection bias? AJR. Am. J. Roentgenol. 1997;169:1649–53.

Reicher MA, Kellerhouse LE. Carpal tunnel disease, flexor and extensor tendon disorders. In: Reicher MA, Kellerhouse LE, eds. MRI of the Wrist and Hand. New York: Raven Press, 1990;49–68.

Rosenbaum RB. The role of imaging in the diagnosis of carpal tunnel syndrome. Invest. Radiol. 1993;28:1059–62.

Seyfert S, Boegner F, Hamm B, Kleindienst A, Klatt C. The value of magnetic resonance imaging in carpal tunnel syndrome. J. Neurol. 1994;242:41–46.

Siegel S, White LM, Brahme S. Magnetic resonance imaging of the musculoskeletal system. Part 5. The wrist. Clin. Orthop. 1996;332:281–300.

Skie M, Zeiss J, Ebraheim NA, Jackson WT. Carpal tunnel changes and median nerve compression during wrist flexion and extension seen by magnetic resonance imaging. J. Hand Surg. 1990;15A:934–39.

Tosti A, Morelli R, D'Alessandro R, Bassi F. Carpal tunnel syndrome presenting with ischemic skin lesions, acroosteolysis, and nail changes. J. Am. Acad. Dermatol. 1993; 29:287–90.

Weiss KL, Beltran J, Shamam OM, Stilla RF, Levey M. High-field MR surface-coil imaging of the hand and wrist. Part I. Normal anatomy. Radiology 1986;160:143–46.

Winn FJ Jr, Habes DJ. Carpal tunnel area as a risk factor for carpal tunnel syndrome. Muscle Nerve 1990;13:254–58.

Zeiss J, Skie M, Ebraheim N, Jackson WT. Anatomic relations between the median nerve and flexor tendons in the carpal tunnel: MR evaluation in normal volunteers. AJR. Am. J. Roentgenol. 1989;153:533–36.

Zucker-Pinchoff B, Hermann G, Srinivasan R. Computed tomography of the carpal tunnel: a radioanatomical study. J. Comput. Assist. Tomogr. 1981;5:525–28.

Chapter 12

Acute and Chronic Mechanical Nerve Injury: Pathologic, Physiologic, and Clinical Correlations

The pathophysiology of mechanical nerve injury is more complex than often assumed, even by skilled practitioners. Substantial scientific data are available on the basic underlying structural and functional derangements and permit intelligible clinical, pathologic, and electrophysiologic correlations.

Among the multiple types of physical injury to nerves, the incidence of mechanical trauma far exceeds electrical, cold, heat, injection, or radiation nerve damage. Particularly in the median nerve, chronic local mechanical compression and entrapment are much more common than transection, percussion and stretch injury, or acute neurapraxia.

To explain the pathophysiology of carpal tunnel syndrome, the archetype of chronic focal nerve entrapment, we begin with a general discussion of the consequences of acute and chronic nerve ischemia and acute and chronic nerve compression.

Acute Ischemia and Nerve Fiber Dysfunction

Acute episodes of nerve compression and ischemia are dynamically intertwined in chronic entrapment of the median nerve at the carpal tunnel. This pathogenic overlap probably applies to mechanically entrapped nerves in general. Both acute and chronic local compression cause direct mechanical distorsion of nerve fibers and disrupt nerve microcirculation. Acute ischemia provokes transient clinical manifestations similar to those commonly experienced by patients with carpal tunnel syndrome. However, as clarified in this discussion, ischemia does not cause the distinctive chronic pathology of myelinated fibers found in locally entrapped nerves.

Acute compression of a limb above systolic pressure leads to a stereotyped sequence of sensory and motor, negative and positive manifestations (for general review, see Sivak & Ochoa, 1987). Paresthesias and mild fasciculations usually develop within a few minutes of onset of ischemia. Acroparesthesias are central to this topic, because they are commonplace in carpal tunnel syndrome and other entrapment neuropathies. The *intraischemic* paresthesias reflect ectopic impulse generation in sensory fibers caused by transient disruption of membrane excitability (Kugelberg, 1944; Merrington & Nathan, 1949; Nathan, 1958; Bergmans, 1973, 1982a, 1982b). Fasciculations, from ectopic impulse generation in motor nerve fibers, are less common than paresthesias because motor fibers accommodate better than sensory fibers to deviations in membrane potential (Erlanger & Blair, 1938). This difference in accommodation is a reflection of differences in concentration of potassium channels found in those two types of fibers (Culp & Ochoa, 1982).

Approximately 20 minutes after onset of ischemia, muscle weakness and sensory loss ensue, following a characteristically centripetal pattern. These are expressions of nerve conduction block in motor and sensory nerve fibers. Initially, nerve impulse conduction falls selectively in large-caliber myelinated fibers. Indeed, whereas light touch is lost, sympathetic function and "temperature sensation" remain unaffected (Lewis, Pickering & Rothschild, 1931; Gasser, 1935; Sinclair & Hinshaw, 1950). Preferential involvement of large-caliber fiber functions is a reflection of differential susceptibility of nerve fibers to anoxia (Lewis et al., 1931; Gasser & Grundfest, 1936).

Quantitative measurement of thermal thresholds allows specific testing of submodalities of temperature sensation (see Chapter 9). Warm sensation, mediated by unmyelinated fibers, is relatively resistant to ischemia (Yarnitsky & Ochoa, 1991), whereas cold sensation, mediated by small-caliber myelinated fibers, fails much earlier (Figure 12-1) (Yarnitsky & Ochoa, 1990). Furthermore, warm sensation behaves differently from pain induced by

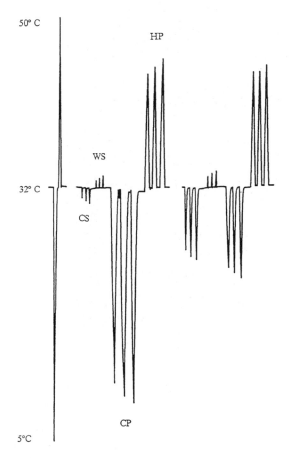

Figure 12-1. Quantitative Marstock thermotest comparing normal profile (*left*) against dissociated loss of cold sensation (CS) with sparing of warm sensation (WS) during ischemia (*right*). Note that, together with increased thresholds for cold sensation, there are lowered thresholds for pain induced by low temperature, due to disinhibition as reported by Yarnitsky and Ochoa (1990). (CP = cold pain; HP = heat pain.)

heat, which is much more resistant to ischemia, even though both sensations are served by subsets of unmyelinated fibers. The explanation for this puzzling phenomenon is that warm sensation requires much spatial summation; that is, a critical population of nerve fibers must be activated for warmth to be perceptible. Pain induced by heat requires a lesser degree of spatial summation (Yarnitsky & Ochoa, 1991).

Deficit of motor and sensory nerve fiber function recovers almost immediately on reestablishment of circulation, provided ischemia is not sustained beyond approximately 2 hours. In the case of acute ischemia induced by local limb compression above systolic pressure, the situation is complicated by the possibility that local compression might mechanically deform and thus affect function of nerve fibers. Lewis et al. (1931) discounted the role of acute local mechanical compression in an ingeniously simple experiment: Once ascending paralysis and sensory loss were established after application to the arm of a pneumatic cuff inflated above systolic pressure, the authors placed a second suprasystolic cuff proximally and then released the first one. Although pressure on the first site was relieved by removal of the first cuff, anesthesia and paralysis did not recover until after the second site of compression had been released, indicating that the neural deficits were sustained by unrelieved ischemia rather than by direct nerve fiber compression.

During acute ischemia, nerve fiber functions served by unmyelinated fibers are retained for about an hour, much longer than functions of myelinated fibers. The "neurapraxia" of severe local nerve compression also strikingly spares not only function but also structure of small-caliber nerve fibers (Fowler & Ochoa, 1975). This and other coincidences misled pioneers to attribute erroneously to ischemia the pathology of neurapraxia (Denny-Brown & Brenner, 1944b).

Postischemic paresthesias typically occur after ischemia is released and motor and sensory deficit have resolved. In a classic study, Merrington and Nathan (1949) offered indirect evidence that postischemic paresthesias are caused by ectopic generation of nerve impulses. Microneurography directly confirms Merrington and Nathan's conclusion. Figure 12-2 shows recordings of paroxysmal ectopic nerve discharges from single sensory fibers in one of the authors (JO); these occurred at the

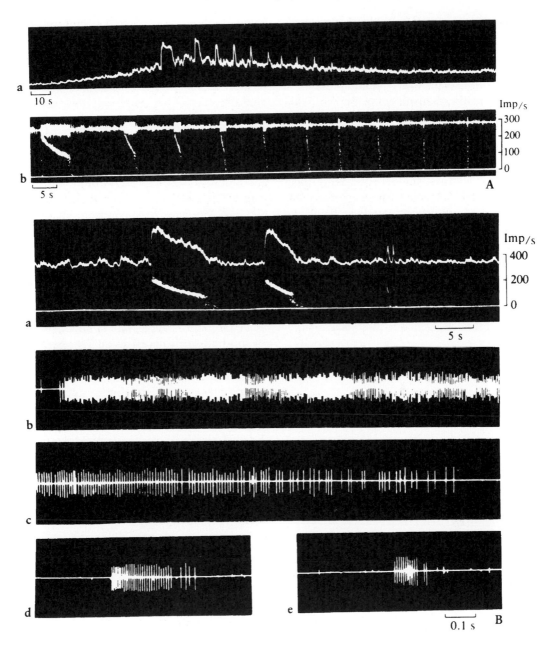

Figure 12-2. (A) Series of 10 high-frequency postischemic discharges in a single unit recorded from the ulnar nerve at elbow level. **(a)** Integrated neurogram, dominated by single unit bursts. Recording started on release of cuff in upper arm after 15 minutes of ischemia. **(b)** Discriminated neurogram of part of the sequence shown in **a** displayed at an extended time scale. Upper trace is original neurogram; lower trace displays "instantaneous" firing frequency of the unit. Note the fairly regular repeat of bursts and their decreasing duration. Note also the uniform impulse frequency at the onset of bursts and the progressive steepness of the frequency decay in subsequent bursts. There seems to be a critical firing frequency of approximately 130 Hz, below which the impulse frequency drops abruptly. **(B)** Prolonged high-frequency postischemic discharges in a single unit recorded from the median nerve at elbow level. Unitary bursts appeared during the second minute after release of cuff compression around forearm, maintained for 25 minutes. **(a)** Integrated neurogram (*upper trace*) shows four abrupt deflections, representing single unit discharges, also displayed in **b** through **e**. "Instantaneous" frequency plot (*lower trace*) shows initial frequency of approximately 220 Hz with exponential fall to approximately 150 Hz and subsequent breakdown. Duration of consecutive bursts diminished from an initial maximum of 7 seconds. Part **b** displays the beginning and **c** the end of first unitary burst shown in **a**. Note regular firing frequency at the beginning and missing beats toward the end. Last two bursts in **a** are displayed in **d** and **e**. (Reproduced with permission from JL Ochoa, HE Torebjörk. Paresthesiae from ectopic impulse generation in human sensory nerves. Brain 1980;103:835–53.)

same time as the abnormal postischemic sensations (Ochoa & Torebjörk, 1980).

Nocturnal acroparesthesias in patients with chronic nerve entrapment may be induced by ischemia developed during transient local compression in sleep (presumably of positional origin). Alternatively, those paresthesias might be caused by increased mechanical deformation of nodes of Ranvier, possibly by sustained abnormal posture and further pressure during sleep.

Notably, nocturnal acroparesthesias largely involve tingling and buzzing. These are sensations that correspond to afferent activity in tactile, large-caliber mechanoreceptors (Ochoa & Torebjörk, 1983). Patients with carpal tunnel syndrome are less likely to experience pains or thermal sensations, which are mediated by small-caliber nerve fibers (Ochoa & Torebjörk, 1989). Small-caliber fibers tend not to engage in ectopic discharge during postischemic paresthesias (Ochoa & Torebjörk, 1980).

Pathophysiology of Vasa Nervorum

Key aspects of the structure and pathophysiology of the delicate intraneural microcirculatory apparatus were elucidated in the 1970s and 1980s (Lundborg, 1970, 1975, 1979, 1980; Olsson & Reese, 1971; Olsson, 1972; Lundborg & Rydevik, 1973; Lundborg, Nordborg, Rydevik & Olsson, 1973; Lundborg, Myers & Powell, 1983; Olsson & Kristensson, 1973; Rydevik, 1979; Myers, Murakami & Powell, 1986; Powell & Myers, 1986). A vascular plexus of small vessels courses longitudinally at various depths in the epineurium, feeding smaller vessels running on the perineurial surface of nerve fascicles. These obliquely pierce the multicellular and collagenous layers of perineurium, to connect with endoneurial vessels of even smaller caliber. The anastomotic system supplying the endoneurial surface is relatively independent of the blood supply of the fascicular core. Thus, transperineurial vascular occlusion during nerve compression causes subperineurial nerve fiber pathology, whereas thrombosis of microcirculation causes necrosis of the central core of the fascicles (Figure 12-3) (Parry & Brown, 1981; Powell & Myers, 1986).

Once it reaches critical levels, ischemia sets off a pathophysiologic sequence. The resulting increased microvascular permeability leads to endoneurial edema and increased intrafascicular fluid pressure. The perineurium, relatively resistant to anoxia, remains comparatively stiff and impermeable. The resulting "microcompartment" state restricts endoneurial blood flow and is believed to promote nerve fiber pathology and endoneurial fibrosis (Lundborg, 1988).

Whereas critical disruption of intraneural circulation through nerve compression may eventually cause local demyelinating nerve fiber damage, acute compression of nerve may additionally induce blockage of axoplasmic transport (Rydevik, McLean, Sjöstrand & Lundborg, 1980). Impaired axoplasmic transport conceivably results in anterograde axonal atrophy or degeneration.

Acute Ischemia and Nerve Infarction

Acute prolonged suppression of arterial blood supply to a limb leads to cell death. The characteristics of ischemic nerve infarctions have been well defined in animals and vary depending on the experimental approach (Korthals & Wisniewski, 1975; Hess, Eames, Darveniza & Gilliatt, 1979; Parry & Brown, 1981; Nukada & Dyck, 1984). Detailed neuropathologic examination of selected human cases has allowed definition of typical patterns of distribution of the pathology in naturally occurring nerve infarctions and of the kind and degree of pathologic reactions in subtypes of nerve fibers (Raff, Sangalang & Asbury, 1968; Asbury, 1970; Asbury & Johnson, 1978).

The subject of nerve infarction is somewhat tangential to the pathology of carpal tunnel syndrome. However, even in infarction after severe acute nerve ischemia, unmyelinated fibers tend to be spared, while myelinated fibers are degenerating (Fujimura, Lacroix & Said, 1991).

Chronic Ischemia and Nerve Pathology

Chronic nerve ischemia may also lead to pathologic changes in nerve trunks and clinical nerve fiber dysfunction. Early reports on pathology of human nerves in chronic ischemic conditions described concrete dropout of nerve fibers (Joffroy & Achard, 1889; Gairns, Garven & Smith, 1960; Garven, Gairns & Smith, 1962). Later, longitudinal

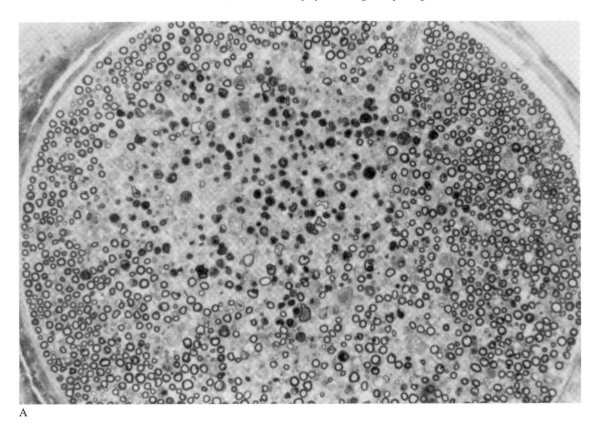

A

Figure 12-3. (**A**) Light micrograph of cross section of tibial nerve of rat showing striking centrofascicular degeneration of nerve fibers owing to experimentally induced partial nerve infarction. (Reproduced with permission from Gareth J. Parry, MD, unpublished material. See: GJ Parry, MJ Brown. Arachidonate-induced experimental nerve infarction. J. Neurol. Sci. 1981;50:123.)

microdissection of nerve fibers revealed that demyelination, not highlighted on nerve trunk cross sections, is commonplace in chronic ischemia (Eames & Lange, 1967). Electron microscopy of these nerves has shown that, just as for acute nerve infarction, chronic ischemia tends to spare unmyelinated fibers in human nerves (Asbury & Johnson, 1978). Development of animal experimental models of chronic nerve ischemia is still needed.

Acute Severe Local Mechanical Trauma to Nerve

Cajal (1928) described the pathologic events that follow acute axonal transaction ("axonotmesis" and "neurotmesis"; Seddon, 1943) through the degenerative and regenerative stages. An acute mechanical injury to the median nerve leading to interruption of

a population of axons might be delayed in its regenerative progress if the new axons must grow through an area of pre-existing nerve pathology at the carpal tunnel. At usual sites of entrapment, common pathologic changes are endoneurial fibrosis, thickening of the perineurium and epineurium, formation of space-occupying Renaut bodies, and probably local disruption of microcirculation.

Severe acute mechanical trauma to median nerve at the wrist may be complicated by impaired regeneration, such as formation of a post-traumatic neuroma. The acute injury may thus result in chronic symptoms. The clinical picture might be misinterpreted as reflecting chronic nerve entrapment deserving surgical decompression at the carpal tunnel. However, the pathology of chronic entrapment, featuring slowly acquired nerve fiber distortion and dropout, concurrent

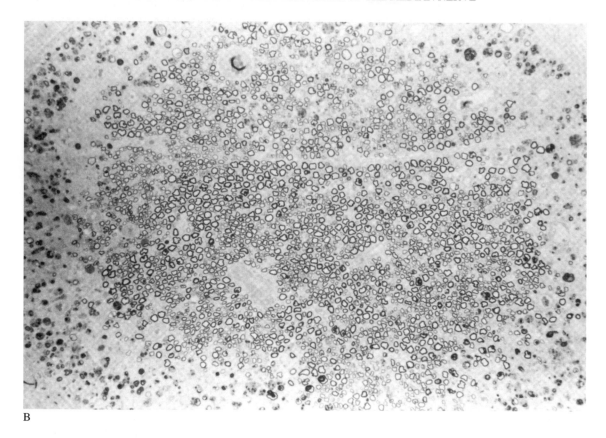

B

Figure 12-3. *Continued.* **(B)** Light micrograph of cross section of tibial nerve of rat showing striking subperineurial demyelination due to interference with transperineurial blood supply caused by local external compression. (Reproduced with permission from Henry Powell, PhD, unpublished material. See: HC Powell, RR Myers. Pathology of experimental nerve compression. Lab. Invest. 1986;55:91.)

attempts at repair, and recurrent damage of old and new structures, is different from the stable pathology that may persist after an isolated traumatic episode. Appropriate therapy varies with the pathology; chronic compression does benefit from carpal tunnel decompression, but direct mechanical nerve trauma may require microneurosurgery (Figure 12-4).

Percussion Injury

Like acute compression injury, a single percussive episode to peripheral nerve causes different types of histopathologic consequences, depending on the force applied. S. Weir Mitchell is quoted by Richardson and Thomas (1979): "In some cases where I struck the nerve sharply with a smooth broad whalebone slip, allowing a thin layer of muscle to intervene, the paralysis which ensued, although temporary, was in degree complete. Within a few days, the rabbit showed no discernible paralysis." In turn, Denny-Brown and Brenner (1944a) state that, after percussion injury to cat sciatic nerve, paralysis completely recovered within 1 week. The eventual histopathologic correlate was focal demyelination with distal axonal degeneration in less than 2% of the fibers. More forceful blows by Richardson and Thomas (1979) caused increasing incidence of axonal degeneration.

The woodwind musician in Figure 12-4 violently percussed his median nerve at wrist level when he spanked a protruding piece of metal decorating his son's belt. Clinical and electrophysiologic evaluation showed definite axonal degeneration. Arrested recovery suggested neuroma formation, which was confirmed and treated microsurgically by fascicular repair.

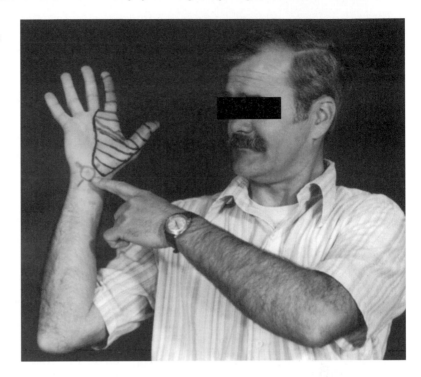

Figure 12-4. Patient points at site of previous mechanical injury that coincides with stationary point of Tinel's sign. Note involvement of palmar cutaneous branch. After fascicular repair, there was additional early postoperative numbness of digits III and IV before eventual progressive recovery.

Neurapraxia

The median nerve, like any other, can undergo an acute primary deformation of nerve fibers that leads to the clinical electrophysiologic state of "neurapraxia" (Seddon, 1943). Whereas clinical neurapraxia is best exemplified by injury to the radial nerve in "Saturday night paralysis," it may also affect the median nerve at the carpal tunnel under unusual circumstances. Figure 12-5 illustrates a rare microscopic example of the primary neurapraxic lesion of myelinated fibers caused by acute local compression of the median nerve in the carpal canal (Neary, Ochoa & Gilliatt, 1975). In terms of duration of the clinical abnormalities, severity of the structural changes, and nature of the electrophysiologic correlates, neurapraxia represents an intermediate state between rapidly reversible ischemic nerve block and the devastating local lesion caused by severe mechanical trauma leading to interruption of nerve fibers (axonotmesis) or whole nerve trunks (neurotmesis) (Seddon, 1943).

Clinically, in both neurapraxia and acute reversible ischemia there is a deficit of motor nerve function and of those sensory nerve functions served by large-caliber myelinated fibers, with sparing of sensory and autonomic functions served by small-caliber nerve fibers (Moldaver, 1954; Bolton & McFarlane, 1978). Thus, neurapraxic sensory loss differs from the multimodality sensory loss that correlates with gross interruption of axons. Whereas functional recovery after transaction of axons may take many months or years, recovery of neurapraxia usually takes weeks or a few months at most. Distal to a site of neurapraxic injury, a nerve remains electrically excitable (Erb, 1876). In contrast, within days of axonal interruption, the fibers distal to the injury are no longer electrically excitable. Nerve conduction studies can often use this difference in physiology to distinguish neurapraxia from axonotmesis early after nerve injury, before muscle atrophy or electromyographic signs of denervation are evident.

The pathology of neurapraxia changes depending on the time after injury at which the nerve is examined. The pathologic characteristics of the lesion underlying neurapraxia also differ, depending on the power of the examiner's microscope. The pioneering study by Denny-Brown and Brenner (1944b) emphasized late observations, by which time demyelination was present. Furthermore, the observations were limited to optic

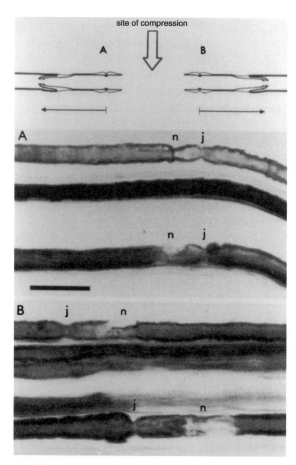

Figure 12-5. Fresh postmortem median nerve specimen obtained from the carpal tunnel of a 30-year-old man. He died after being in a state for several hours of decorticate rigidity with marked flexion of the wrists, maintained after death. This caused pressure on the nerve under the distal part of the flexor retinaculum. Microscopic abnormalities indicative of mechanical distortion of axons and myelin were found over a distance of ±7 mm. The figure reproduces single fibers to show displacement of the nodes of Ranvier in opposite directions: A = proximal, B = distal. Bar = 30 μm. (j = Schwann cell junction; n = new position of node.) (Reproduced with permission from D Neary, JL Ochoa, RW Gilliatt. Subclinical entrapment neuropathy in man. Neurol. Sci. 1975;24:283–98.)

microscopy, preventing recognition of telltale fine structural changes that are a signature of their mechanical origin. Over and above the optical resolution handicap, Denny-Brown and Brenner were further constrained by the limitations of contempo-

rary knowledge. Indeed, local constriction of a limb by cuff leads to immediately reversible sensorimotor dysfunction caused by ischemia, and not by direct mechanical pressure (Lewis et al., 1931). Because simple prolongation of local constriction time may lead to neurapraxia, neurapraxic demyelination logically seemed to result from sustained ischemia. However, as illustrated in Figures 12-6 and 12-7, finer methods for nerve histology show a characteristic early lesion of myelinated fibers in experimental neurapraxia.

Critical supporting evidence for the mechanical origin of this primary lesion underlying neurapraxia came from analysis of the ultrastructural features of single abnormal myelinated fibers. Single fibers were selected by light microscopy and then subjected to ultrathin longitudinal sections for electron microscopy (Ochoa, 1972). This kind of study has not been reconfronted over the past three decades.

This lesion is unquestionably mechanical in origin, as it involves displacement of structures in the direction of, and proportional to, abnormally operant forces (Ochoa, Danta, Fowler & Gilliatt, 1971; Ochoa, Fowler & Gilliatt, 1972). Demyelination is a secondary event after this lesion. Further evidence for the mechanical origin of this lesion is that it occurs in duplicate at either edge of the site of compression rather than under the whole area of compression (Figure 12-8). Moreover, the direction of displacement of structures is reversed at either edge, in keeping with the development of extruding forces generated from pressure gradients between compressed and uncompressed tissue. This occurrence, which establishes the mechanical nature of the lesion, also explains the lack of pertinence of another experiment that Denny-Brown and Brenner (1944b) cited in support of the ischemic hypothesis. This was a striking experiment by Grundfest (1936) who had shown that nerve segments, contained within pressure chambers, may continue to conduct nerve impulses even under huge pressures, provided oxygen is present in the chamber. This observation was misconstrued as indicating that nerve fibers are relatively indifferent to the effects of pressure; instead, in the lesion shown in Figures 12-6 through 12-8 at the edges of local

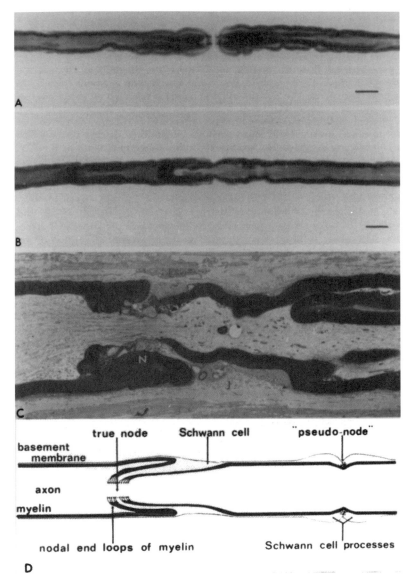

Figure 12-6. Pathology of neurapraxia caused by acute local external compression in limb of a baboon. **(A)** Normal microdissected myelinated fiber showing node of Ranvier. Baboon tibial nerve. Bar = 10 μm. **(B)** Abnormal fiber, early after acute compression. The nodal gap is occluded due to intussusception from right to left. An indentation (pseudonode) marks the original site of the node. Bar = 10 μm. **(C)** Low-power electron micrograph of abnormal myelinated fiber, cut longitudinally after microdissection. Note indentation at Schwann cell junction (J) and new position of the node (N) under infolded myelin. (Reproduced with permission from P Rudge, JL Ochoa, RW Gilliatt. Acute peripheral nerve compression in the baboon. Anatomical and physiological findings. J. Neurol. Sci. 1974;23:403–20.) **(D)** Diagram of affected fiber showing invagination of one paranode by the adjacent one, movement occurring from right to left. (Reproduced with permission from JL Ochoa, TJ Fowler, RW Gilliatt. Changes produced by a pneumatic tourniquet. In: JE Desmedt, ed. New Developments in Electromyography and Clinical Neurophysiology. Basel: Karger, 1973;2:166–73.)

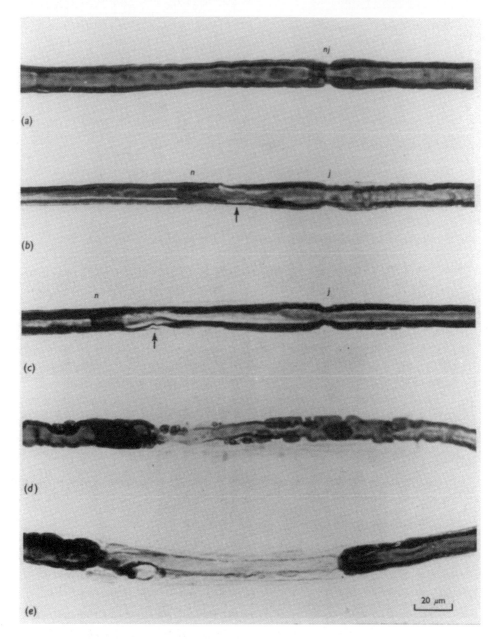

Figure 12-7. Pathology of neurapraxia caused by acute local external compression in limb of a baboon. (**A–C**) Abnormal fibers, 4 days after compression, showing different degrees of nodal displacement (reaching 120 μm in **C**). Note thinning of myelin at arrows. (**D**) A fiber, 15 days after compression, undergoing demyelination of the paranodal region. There is tapering of the myelin of the paranode on the right. (**E**) A thinly myelinated intercalated segment, 61 days after compression. (j = Schwann cell junction; n = new position of node.) (Reproduced with permission from JL Ochoa, TJ Fowler, RW Gilliatt. Anatomical changes in peripheral nerves compressed by a pneumatic tourniquet. J. Anat. 1972;113:433–55.)

compression of nerves in limbs, dependence on pressure gradients is self-evident. In Grundfest's chamber, the nerve segments were subjected to uniform pressures; no pressure gradients could develop there. This primary mechanical lesion affecting myelinated fibers was also shown to occur under conditions of much more focal compression, as caused by a weighted string in baboons (Figures 12-9 through 12-11) (Rudge, Ochoa & Gilliatt, 1974) or by 5-mm wide rubber

Figure 12-8. Pathology of neurapraxia caused by acute local external compression in limb of a baboon. Diagram describing the direction of displacement of the nodes of Ranvier in relation to the compressed zone. (Reproduced with permission from JL Ochoa, TJ Fowler, RW Gilliatt. Anatomical changes in peripheral nerves compressed by a pneumatic tourniquet. J. Anat. 1972;113:433–55.)

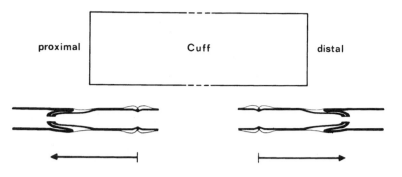

Figure 12-9. Successive nodes from a single fiber in left anterior tibial nerve 24 hours after compression (externally with string) (750 g for 90 minutes) to show extent of the lesion. The proximal end of the fiber is at the top. Note two normal nodes in center of lesion and nodal displacement in opposite directions on either side (new positions of nodes marked by *arrows*). Beyond these, the nodes are again normal. Bar = 20 μm. (Reproduced with permission from P Rudge, JL Ochoa, RW Gilliatt. Acute peripheral nerve compression in the baboon. Anatomical and physiological findings. J. Neurol. Sci. 1974;23:403–20.)

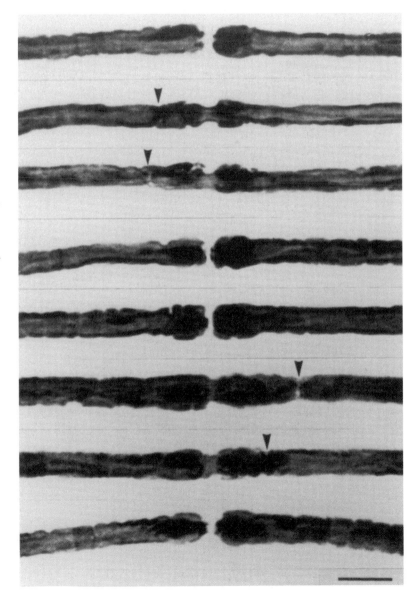

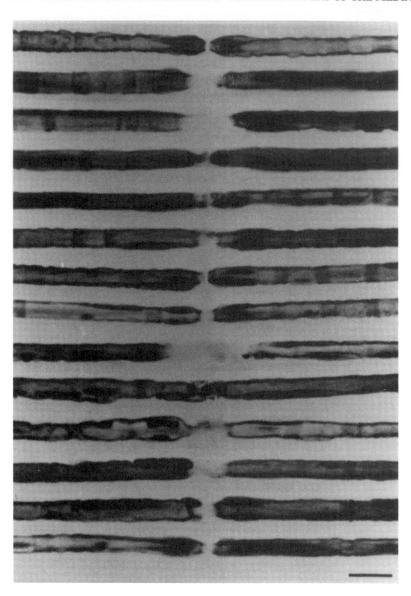

Figure 12-10. Successive nodes from a single fiber in the right anterior tibial nerve 8 days after compression (with string) to show extent of lesion. Early demyelination is present. Note normal nodes at center (retouched) and at each edge of lesion. Bar = 20 μm. (Reproduced with permission from P Rudge, JL Ochoa, RW Gilliatt. Acute peripheral nerve compression in the baboon. Anatomical and physiological findings. J. Neurol. Sci. 1974;23:403–20.)

bands applied to the thinner limbs of rodents (Ochoa, unpublished data).

Unmyelinated fibers, and even small-caliber myelinated fibers, escape damage in neurapraxia. Whereas functional sparing of small-caliber fibers during *acute* ischemia is explainable by differential susceptibility to anoxia; sparing of structure of small fibers in the mechanical lesion underlying neurapraxia has a different mechanism (Ochoa et al., 1972). However, the common feature was another reason why Denny-Brown and Brenner (1944b) mistakenly concluded that ischemia was the cause of the late demyelinating nerve lesion underlying neurapraxia.

In humans, local mechanical nerve lesions often combine elements of neurapraxia and axonotmesis. This admixture is not at all surprising, as the experimental requirements to achieve relatively pure neurapraxia are stringent and demand rigorous titration of severity of the mechanical insult (Fowler, Danta & Gilliatt, 1972; Fowler, 1975). Naturally, less controlled experiments on acute nerve compression tend to yield a mixed pathology of axons and myelin sheaths (as they do in nerve percussion injury).

Clinical and electrophysiologic recovery from genuine neurapraxia may be substantially delayed in instances of particularly severe nerve compression (Rudge, 1974; Harrison, 1976). This protracted course correlates with the development of a component of intracellular edema of nerve fibers and necrosis of Schwann cells, affecting particularly the ad-axonal loops of Schwann cell cytoplasm. Such pathology is almost certainly a consequence of anoxia. Somehow, these aberrant structures that interfere with transmission of nerve impulses are tolerated by the organism, their scavenging and repair through remyelination being delayed (Figures 12-12 and 12-13) (Ochoa et al., 1972; Ochoa, 1981).

In addition to this well-defined and electrophysiologically matched mechanical lesion underlying neurapraxia, acute or chronic local nerve compression can, under special circumstances, cause demyelination that is strikingly confined to subperineurial nerve fibers (Aguayo, Nair & Midgley, 1971). The distinctive, strictly subperincurial localization of the demyelination suggests that impaired blood flow in transperineurial vessels causes the lesion through ischemia (Powell & Myers, 1986). As discussed previously, a separate microvascular system supplies nerve fibers in the core of the fascicles; these core fibers are selectively infarcted in certain conditions (Parry & Brown, 1981), but are spared in the perineural demyelination (see Figure 12.3A and B) (Hess et al., 1979; Powell & Myers, 1986).

The application of constricting devices directly on the surface of nerve trunks can also lead to nerve pathology (Dyck, 1969; Aguayo et al., 1971). In the 1980s, Bennett and Xie (1988) standardized a nerve constriction lesion caused by snug application of a series of ligatures along the sciatic nerve in rats. The ligatures lead predominantly to axonal degeneration of myelinated fibers and a thoroughly characterized set of peripheral and central physiologic consequences dominated by irritative sensory phenomena, overshadowing sensorimotor deficit.

Chronic Nerve Entrapment

Chronic nerve entrapment causes distinct pathologic changes. These have been described in animal models of natural local nerve entrapment and also in archetypical syndromes of chronic nerve

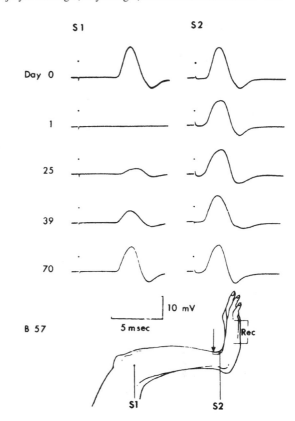

Figure 12-11. Evoked muscle action potentials from extensor digitorum brevis at different intervals after compression of the right anterior tibial nerve (externally with string at *arrow*) (1.5 kg for 90 minutes). Sites of stimulating and recording electrodes shown at bottom of figure. (Reproduced with permission from P Rudge, JL Ochoa, RW Gilliatt. Acute peripheral nerve compression in the baboon. Anatomical and physiological findings. J. Neurol. Sci. 1974;23:403–20.)

entrapment in humans. However, these pathologic lesions have not been reproduced through experimental local nerve constriction. The pathogenesis of the natural lesions is more complex than steady constriction. For example, at the carpal tunnel the pressure on the median nerve varies during the day, and compression may be accompanied by intermittent local nerve stretching and friction from movement of adjacent structures. Marie and Foix (1913) provided a notable early description of the histopathologic correlates of local nerve entrapment. They documented that some forms of chronic thenar atrophy were caused by a lesion of the median nerve in the region of the carpal tunnel. Using classic myelin stains, they showed that

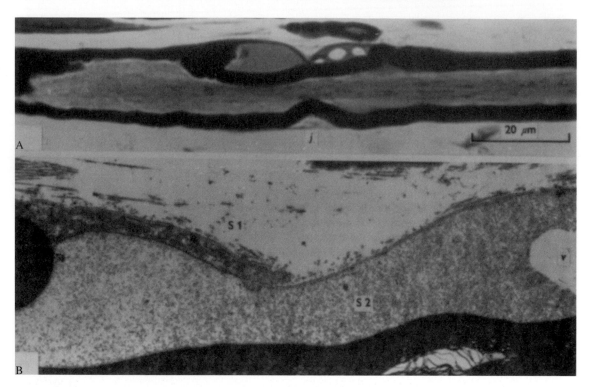

Figure 12-12. Pathology of neurapraxia caused by acute local external compression in limb of a baboon. **(A)** Longitudinal section of fiber 4 days after compression, showing indented myelin at the Schwann cell junction (j) and swollen Schwann cell cytoplasm containing vacuoles. Epon-toluidine blue. **(B)** Electron micrograph showing detail of the fiber shown in **A**. The thin tongue of paranodal Schwann cell cytoplasm on the left (S1) has been dissected from the myelin by a swollen cell process intruding from the Schwann cell on the right (S2). In the latter, cytoplasmic differentiation is lost, and there is a vacuole (v). (Magnification 8,700×.) (Reproduced with permission from JL Ochoa, TJ Fowler, RW Gilliatt. Anatomical changes in peripheral nerves compressed by a pneumatic tourniquet. J. Anat. 1972;113:433–55.)

myelinated fibers, traced from the forearm, disappeared at wrist level. Some 50 years later, in a clinical, electrophysiologic, and autopsy human study of proven carpal tunnel syndrome at Queen Square, Thomas and Fullerton (1963) confirmed the presence of local pathology in median nerve at the wrist. They found in nerve cross sections that density of myelinated fibers was partially preserved distal to the wrist, indicating that the dropout of

myelin at the wrist was not invariably due to axonal interruption. At that time, demonstration of local demyelinating pathology carried no challenge to the prevailing assumption that local nerve demyelination associated with mechanical trauma must be ischemic in origin. Later, animals with chronic nerve entrapment were shown to exhibit similar changes (Figure 12-14) (Fullerton & Gilliatt, 1967), and shortly after, a distinctive morphologic

▶ **Figure 12-13.** Pathology of neurapraxia caused by acute local external compression in limb of a baboon. **(A)** Low-power electron micrograph of a nerve fiber swelling 6 weeks after compression. The swollen inner tongue of Schwann cell cytoplasm (v) separates most of the surface of the axon (ax) from the myelin sheath. A sector remains attached to the sheath. (Magnification 3,000×.) **(B)** Enlargement of area arrowed in **A**. The mesaxon (m) is seen with swollen Schwann cell cytoplasm (v) on either side of it. (Magnification 44,000×.) **(C)** A myelinated fiber from the same nerve, showing axon (ax) and a pocket of edema (v). A macrophage (ma) has penetrated the basement membrane and broken into the myelin sheath. (Magnification 4,600×.) (Reproduced with permission from JL Ochoa, TJ Fowler, RW Gilliatt. Anatomical changes in peripheral nerves compressed by a pneumatic tourniquet. J. Anat. 1972;113:433–55.)

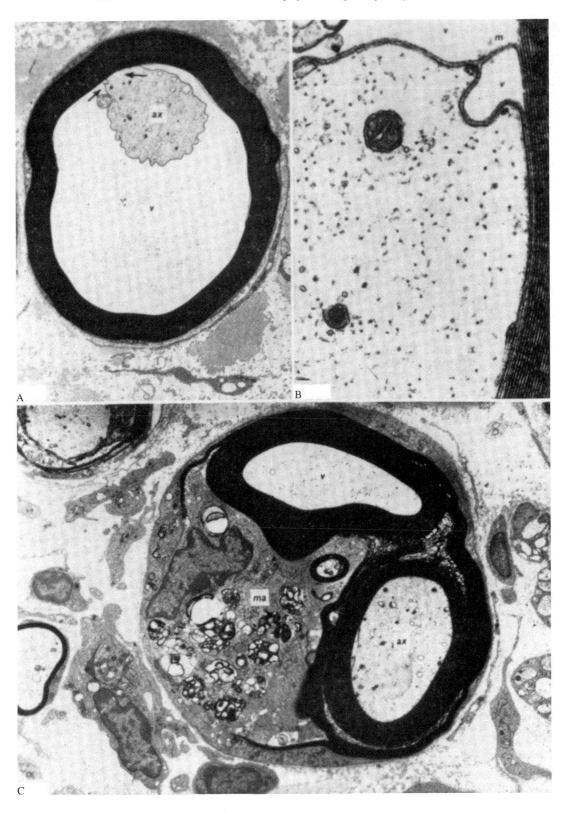

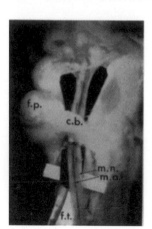
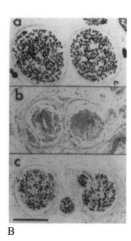

A   B

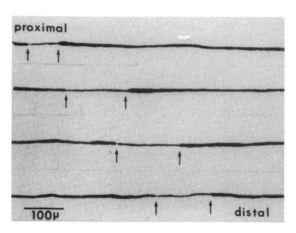

Figure 12-14. (A) Chronic nerve entrapment in the guinea pig. A dissection of the palmar surface of the right wrist and forefoot of a young guinea pig. A piece of black card has been placed behind the median nerve (m.n.) and its accompanying artery (m.a.). The transverse cartilaginous bar (c.b.), which supports the footpad (f.p.), can be seen. Proximal to the wrist, a card marked with 1-mm squares has been inserted in front of the flexor tendons (f.t.). (Courtesy of Dr. J. E. C. Hern.) (B) Two fascicles of the median nerve from transverse sections taken (a) above, (b) at, and (c) below the wrist. The distance between **a** and **b** was 2 mm and between **b** and **c** 3 mm. Sections fixed in Flemming's solution and stained by modified Weigert method to show myelin sheaths. Bar = 200 μm. (Reproduced with permission from PM Fullerton, RW Gilliatt. Median and ulnar neuropathy in the guinea pig. J. Neurol. Neurosurg. Psychiatry 1967;30: 393–402.)

Figure 12-15. Pathology of chronic nerve entrapment in the guinea pig. Consecutive lengths of a single fiber from the median nerve in the midforearm to show intercalated segments (*arrows*) occurring at regular intervals along the fiber (1% osmium tetroxide). (Reproduced with permission from MH Anderson, PM Fullerton, RW Gilliatt, JEC Hern. Changes in the forearm associated with median nerve compression at the wrist in the guinea pig. J. Neurol. Neurosurg. Psychiatry 1970;33:70–79.)

change was described in microdissected myelinated fibers: peculiar deformities of the myelin sheaths with thickening of proximal paranodal myelin and thinning of distal paranodal myelin. The deformities were consistently polarized in consecutive myelin segments (Figure 12-15) (Anderson, Fullerton, Gilliatt & Hern, 1970). This finding was not understood until the same polarized deformity was shown to be present in reverse, distal to the wrist (Figure 12-16) (Ochoa & Marotte, 1973). The symmetry of the myelin changes suggested a mechanical origin in analogy to the distinct mechanical deformity, also polarized symmetrically around the compression, that had been described as a correlate of acute neurapraxia in experimentally compressed nerves (Ochoa et al., 1972). Certainly, the tapered paranodes of myelin segments and the buckled paranodes on the opposite ends result from displacement of inner myelin

lamellae away from the entrapped site (Figure 12-17). Such a pathologic profile of myelinated fibers in entrapped nerves disproves the hypothesis that local nerve anoxia is its cause. Local anoxia explains neither the tapering of myelin sheaths nor the focal demyelination that is so capriciously localized to the distal ends of internodes proximal to the entrapment and to the proximal end of internodes distal to the entrapment. Rather, compression causes myelin lamellae to slip because of mechanical stresses operating in opposite directions at the sites of nerve entrapment.

The dynamics of development of distortion of myelin segments in chronically entrapped nerve fibers, in a polarized and mirror-image fashion, are not precisely known. Our explanation of why the myelin lamellae closest to the axon are most affected has been speculative: Mechanical friction or stretching of the entrapped fibers may strain the specialized subcellular attachments of myelin to axon; eventually, detached inner portions of myelin spiral may suffer progressive slippage following mechanical pressure waves propagated away from the site of entrapment; redundant inner myelin lamellae may be pushed into the envelope of outer myelin lamellae attached to the down-

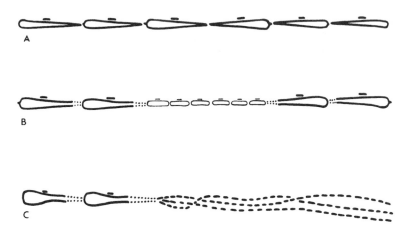

Figure 12-16. Pathology of chronic nerve entrapment in the guinea pig. (**A**) Diagram showing distorted myelin segments from median nerve of young guinea pig. Note reversal of polarity at the wrist. (**B**) Further distortion and exposure of the axon proximal and distal to the site of entrapment. The median nerve under the carpal tunnel has lost its original myelin segments: Multiple, short remyelinated internodes repair the lesion. (**C**) Advanced lesion with massive bulbs and axonal wallerian degeneration and regeneration. (Reproduced with permission from Ochoa JL. Nerve fiber pathology in acute and chronic compression. In: GE Omer Jr., M Spinner, eds. Management of Peripheral Nerve Problems. Philadelphia: WB Saunders, 1980;495.)

stream paranode (Figure 12-18) (Ochoa, 1980). When all myelin lamellae drift away, paranodal axons become obviously exposed, "demyelinated." Redundant myelin lamellae at the distended paranodes may progressively compress the axon. This should alter electrical axonal resistance and axoplasmic flow and eventually lead to axonal degeneration. Probably, critically narrowed axons distal to the site of entrapment undergo reversible partial atrophy before they degenerate. This "axon cachexia" explains subtle dysfunctions detectable electrophysiologically distal to sites of entrapment.

This distinctive pathology in chronic entrapment of animal nerves has been confirmed as a subclinical finding in human nerve trunks at common sites of entrapment (Figures 12-19 and 12-20) (Neary & Eames, 1975; Neary et al., 1975; Jefferson & Eames, 1979).

The myelin distortions that support a mechanical origin for the pathologic changes observed in local nerve entrapment cannot be naïvely taken to indicate that primary mechanical phenomena alone participate in the genesis of structural and physiologic abnormalities related to local nerve entrapment. As mentioned earlier, transient positive sensory phenomena in local nerve entrapment probably reflect nerve fiber hyperexcitability caused by ischemia. Prolonged ischemia might

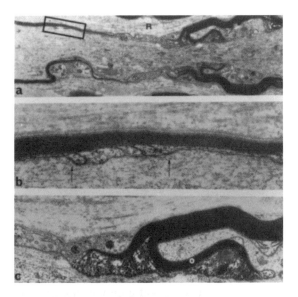

Figure 12-17. Pathology of chronic nerve entrapment in the guinea pig. (**A**) Low-power electron micrograph of a moderately abnormal fiber taken from the median nerve of a guinea pig above the wrist. The paranode on the left is tapered. The bulbous paranode on the right shows inturning of a group of inner lamellae. (Magnification 7,000×.) (**B**) Enlargement of the area enclosed; in the rectangle in **A**. Six myelin lamellae end in cytoplasmic loops between the arrows. (Magnification 48,000×.) (**C**) Detail of the bulbous paranode. (Magnification 20,000×.) (R = node of Ranvier.) (Reproduced with permission from JL Ochoa, L Marotte. The nature of the nerve lesion underlying chronic entrapment. J. Neurol. Sci. 1973;19:491–95.)

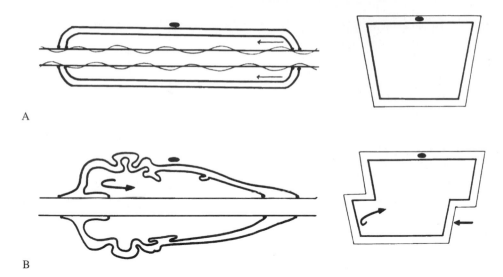

Figure 12-18. Pathology of chronic nerve entrapment in the guinea pig. **(A)** Normal myelin segment and unrolled myelin sheath *(right)*, which is trapezoid shaped. Hypothetical pressure waves in the direction of the arrows along the axon. **(B)** Distorted segment with tapered end caused by myelin slippage and bulbous end containing inturned redundant myelin lamellae. If the myelin were unrolled, it would be altered as indicated *(right)*. (Reproduced with permission from Ochoa JL. Nerve fiber pathology in acute and chronic compression. In: GE Omer Jr., M Spinner, eds. Management of Peripheral Nerve Problems. Philadelphia: WB Saunders, 1980;497.)

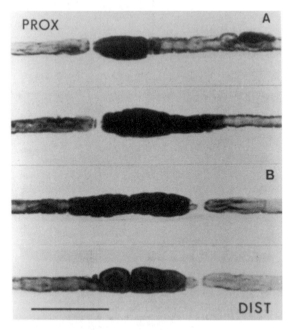

Figure 12-19. Pathology of chronic entrapment of human median nerve. **(A)** Two consecutive nodes from a single fiber proximal (PROX) to the flexor retinaculum. **(B)** Two consecutive nodes from a (different) single fiber distal (DIST) to the upper border of the retinaculum. In each case, the fibers are mounted with their proximal portions to the left. Bar = 50 μm. (Reproduced with permission from D Neary, JL Ochoa, RW Gilliatt. Subclinical entrapment neuropathy in man. J. Neurol. Sci. 197S;24:283–98.)

cause nerve fiber hypoexcitability even in the absence of substantial morphologic changes (Sladsky, Tschoepe, Greenberg & Brown, 1991). Furthermore, subperineurial demyelination, if eventually demonstrated in human nerve fascicles at sites of chronic entrapment, would not be surprising as the consequence of ischemia due to impaired transperineurial circulation (Powell & Myers, 1986). Finally, chronic endoneurial edema in entrapped nerves is a likely consequence of hemodynamic derangement (Sunderland, 1976). Thus, both primarily mechanical and primarily ischemic events probably contribute to the development of structural abnormalities of nerve fibers, particularly of myelinated fibers, and to biophysical abnormalities leading to ectopic impulse generation, conduction block, and their clinical correlates.

Tinel's Sign in Carpal Tunnel Syndrome

Tinel's sign highlights a possible role of primary mechanical factors underlying the development of paresthesias in carpal tunnel. For this sign, a gentle mechanical force—tapping on the nerve—generates ectopic discharges (see Ochoa et al., 1982, for electrophysiologic evidence). The presence of

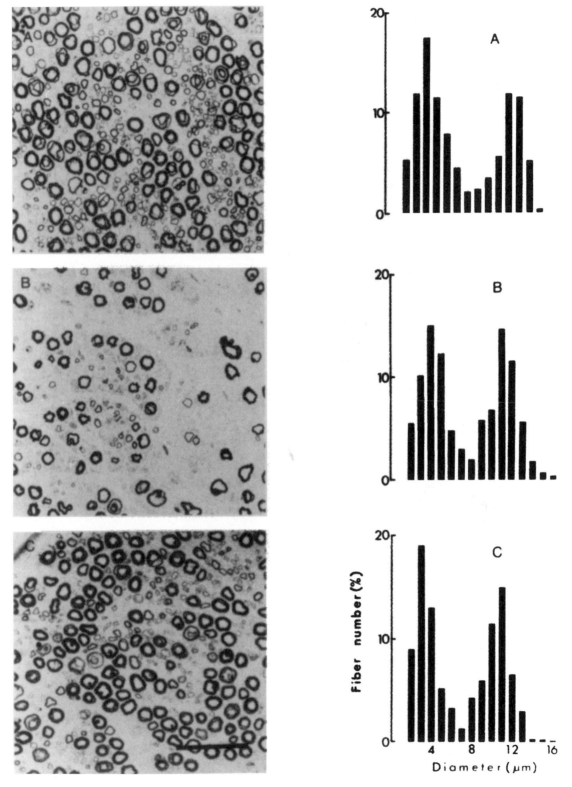

Figure 12-20. Pathology of chronic entrapment of human nerve. On the left, enlarged portions of transverse sections of ulnar nerve. On the right, histograms of fiber diameter from the same sections. (**A**) Proximal to the elbow. (**B**) In the ulnar groove. (**C**) Distal to the elbow. Bar = 50 μm. (Reproduced with permission from D Neary, JL Ochoa, RW Gilliatt. Subclinical entrapment neuropathy in man. J. Neurol. Sci. 1975;24:283–98.)

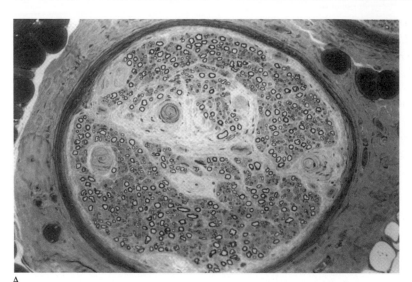

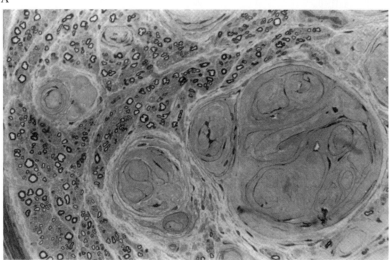

Figure 12-21. Chronic entrapment of human nerve. **(A)** Cross section of fascicle obtained from the lateral femorocutaneous nerve at the site of entrapment in a patient with meralgia paresthetica. Half a dozen Renaut bodies occur. **(B)** Higher-power view of cross section of Renaut bodies from an adjacent level in the same nerve as **A**.

hyperexcitable nerve sprouts or hyperexcitable dysmyelinated stretches of nerve fibers predisposes to the ectopic discharges (Konorski & Lubinska, 1946; Brown & Iggo, 1963; Smith & McDonald, 1980, 1982). Therefore, conceivably, over and above ischemic and postischemic ionic phenomena, mechanical factors might operate on abnormal nerve fibers at sites of chronic entrapment to generate intermittent paresthesias, because the physiologic basis of Tinel's sign and of "spontaneous" paresthesias is basically equivalent (Diamond, Ochoa & Culp, 1982).

Renaut Bodies

After an original description by Renaut (1881), the peculiar bodies shown in Figure 12-21 became "forgotten endoneurial structures" (Asbury, 1973). These Renaut bodies are conspicuous at sites of chronic nerve entrapment but are not exclusive to that pathologic state. We have found them in many locally entrapped nerve segments, particularly in the median and ulnar nerves at wrist and elbow, respectively. Jefferson et al. (1981) demonstrated that more than half of their

74 autopsied nerves showed these structures at sites of common entrapment but not in adjacent segments of the same nerves. They concluded that these bodies are pathologic formations without protective function.

Renaut bodies can be microdissected out of entrapped nerves. They are spindle-shaped structures measuring up to 2 mm or more in length. While they do occupy endoneurial space, their pathophysiologic significance is unknown. They might be organized remnants of endoneurial vessels. Their formation, featuring an early stage of endoneurial clefting, has been followed sequentially in experimental animals subjected to repeated mechanical trauma of plantar nerves (Ortman, Sahenk & Mendell, 1983).

Some Pathologic, Physiologic, and Clinical Correlations in Chronic Nerve Entrapment

The pathology of local nerve compression ranges from microscopically undetectable molecular disruption of the excitable biophysical apparatus, through demyelination and remyelination, to axonal degeneration and regeneration. Understandably, the clinical expression of nerve entrapment pathology includes positive and negative motor and sensory and sympathetic phenomena. Regardless of whether mechanical or ischemic in origin, and regardless of whether stable or intermittent, derangements in nerve membrane excitability in local entrapment underlie the development of paresthesias and occasional myokymia and other positive phenomena traceable to motor nerve fibers. Muscle weakness associated with atrophy is obviously due to axonal interruption. Weakness may also occur when fibers with pathologic myelin sheaths develop conduction block. Moreover, weakness and muscle fatigue develop when those fibers are unable to sustain high rates of impulse discharge (McDonald, 1982). Sensory deficit, when present, most commonly consists of diminished tactile acuity. Subtle sensory deficits may be expressed as clumsiness of manipulation and may be misconstrued as muscle weakness. Tactile proprioceptive deficits may interfere with performance of highly refined finger movements, such as those of skilled musicians (Johansson & Westling, 1987).

Deficits in cold and warm perception and pain are inconspicuous manifestations of nerve entrapment partly because these pain and temperature modalities are served by small-caliber fibers that are affected late by pathology in local entrapment. Furthermore, patients are likely to be aware of deficits of tactile, discriminative ability of the hand, while overlooking mild deficits in protective nociception.

Similarly, sympathetic dysfunction tends not to be a prominent aspect of the clinical expression of chronic nerve entrapment (Aminoff, 1979). However, in severe nerve pathology there may be clear signs of sympathetic deficit, in the form of anhydrosis and vasomotor denervation. Signs of irritation of sympathetic efferent nerve fibers in the form of excessive sweating and vasospasm are decidedly uncommon in chronic nerve entrapment and rarely reported in acute neurapraxia (Bolton & McFarlane, 1978). The hypothermia related to vasospasm commonly observed in "causalgiform syndromes" usually represents a somatosympathetic reflex response rather than ectopic discharge in sympathetic fibers. Alternatively, a chronically vasoconstricted limb, a common consequence of local nerve injury, results from sympathetic denervation supersensitivity rather than from increased sympathetic neural activity.

The pathophysiology of pain in nerve injury and entrapment is treated in Chapter 16.

Pressure Studies

Measurement of physical pressure within body compartments, and even within a microenvironment such as the endoneurium, has helped in the understanding of the pathogenesis of acute nerve compression and chronic entrapment. In the mid-1970s, wick catheters became a new research and clinical tool (Whitesides, Haney, Morimoto & Harada, 1975; Mubarak, Hargens, Owen, Garetto & Akeson, 1976). Measurements with these fine catheters inserted into limb compartments yield a range of normal interstitial intramuscular fluid pressures of 7 to 8 mm Hg in humans. Pressures greater than 30 mm Hg presage complications such as neural deficit, Volkmann's contracture, or in extreme cases, gangrene (Mubarak, Owen, Hargens, Garetto & Akeson, 1978). At pressures above 30 mm Hg, pain and paresthesias first appear (Mubarak et al., 1976; Lundborg, Gelberman, Minteer-Convery, Lee & Hargens, 1982; Gelberman, Szabo, Williamson & Dimick, 1983). Normal capillary pressure in muscle is 20 to 30 mm Hg in cats (Fronek & Zweifach, 1975) and dogs (Hargens, Akeson, Mubarak, Owen, Evan, Garetto & Schmidt, 1978). The need for dermotomy, fasciotomy, and epimysiotomy can be monitored by measuring intracompartmental fluid pressure. The most reliable clinical indication of increased tissue pressure within a closed fascial space is sensory dysfunction, because all compartments in forearm and leg contain a nerve and, under the circumstances of pain and muscle swelling, motor performance is not a reliable measure. Compartment pressure sufficient to damage nerves and muscles is seldom sufficient to occlude a major artery, and thus common clinical signs of vascular dysfunction are a late manifestation.

The micropipette method allows direct measurement of endoneurial fluid pressure (Low & Dyck, 1977; Myers, Powell, Costello, Lambert & Zweifach, 1978). Exposed rat sciatic nerves directly compressed within a special chamber for 2 to 8 hours, at 30 mm Hg to interfere with venular flow, or at 80 mm Hg to cause circulatory arrest in the nerve, were found to have developed a three- to fourfold increase in endoneurial fluid pressure and endoneurial edema (Lundborg et al., 1983). Endoneurial edema becomes associated with progressive deposition of endoneurial collagen and may close a vicious cycle of nerve ischemia by interfering with nerve blood flow (Myers, Mizisin, Powell & Lampert, 1982; Lundborg, 1988). The hypertonic quality of endoneurial edema fluid may impair ionic equilibrium and interfere with excitable membrane function (Myers et al., 1978). As predicted from the distribution of nerve fiber damage in acute compression with tourniquet (Ochoa et al., 1972), the distribution of edema is at the edges of the microcuff used by Lundborg, Myers, and Powell, as strikingly illustrated to the naked eye by Evans blue extravasation (Lundborg, 1988).

Findings and mechanisms analogous to those documented for nerve seem to apply to compression of dorsal root ganglia (Rydevik, Myers & Powell, 1989).

Pressure studies in the carpal tunnel have revealed striking correlations with clinical and electrophysiologic parameters in symptomatic patients with carpal tunnel syndrome. Increased canal pressures have been recorded in several independent studies (Gelberman, Hergenroeder, Hargens, Lundborg & Akeson, 1981; Lundborg et al., 1982; Werner, Elmquist & Ohlin, 1983; Chaise & Witvoet, 1984; Szabo & Chidgey, 1989). Patients often have pressures of approximately 30 mm Hg with the wrist in the neutral position. This is just below the level needed to induce symptoms of nerve compression. The canal pressure in both healthy subjects and patients with carpal tunnel syndrome increases significantly with wrist flexion and extension so that pressure in the carpal tunnel fluctuates continually during normal daily activities (Smith, Sonstegard & Anderson, 1977; Werner et al., 1983). Increase in pressure with wrist flexion explains the effect of Phalen's wrist flexion test. Therapeutic wrist splinting prevents some of these recurring daily increases in canal pressure.

In patients with carpal tunnel syndrome, the pressure is usually highest in the distal third of the tunnel (Luchetti, Schoenhuber, De Cicco, Alfarano, Deluca & Landi, 1989; Luchetti, Schoenhuber, Alfarano, Deluca, De Cicco & Landi, 1990). Intraoperative sensory nerve conduction studies show the greatest slowing of nerve conduction and decrement of sensory nerve action potential amplitude along the nerve in this distal portion of the canal (Luchetti et al., 1990).

Carpal tunnel pressure measurements are not useful as a routine diagnostic test for carpal tunnel syndrome. In addition to their invasive nature, they do not reliably distinguish symptomatic from asymptomatic patients.

References

Aguayo AJ, Nair CPV, Midgley R. Experimental progressive compression neuropathy in the rabbit. Histologic and electrophysiologic studies. Arch. Neurol. 1971;24:358–64.

Aminoff MJ. Involvement of peripheral vasomotor fibres in carpal tunnel syndrome. J. Neurol. Neurosurg. Psychiatry 1979;42:649–55.

Anderson MH, Fullerton PM, Gilliatt RW, Hern JEC. Changes in the forearm associated with median nerve compression at the wrist in the guinea pig. J. Neurol. Neurosurg. Psychiatry 1970;33:70–79.

Asbury AK. Ischemic disorders of peripheral nerve. In: Vinken PJ, Bruyn GW, eds. Handbook of Clinical Neurology. Amsterdam: North-Holland, 1970;8:154–64.

Asbury AK. Renaut bodies: a forgotten endoneurial structure. J. Neuropathol. Exp. Neurol. 1973;32:334–43.

Asbury AK, Johnson PC. Pathology of Peripheral Nerve. Philadelphia: WB Saunders, 1978.

Bennett GJ, Xie Y-K. A peripheral mononeuropathy in rat that produces disorders of pain sensation like those seen in man. Pain 1988;33:87–107.

Bergmans J. Physiological observations on single human nerve fibres. In: Desmedt JE, ed. New Developments in Electromyography and Clinical Neurophysiology. Basel: S Karger, 1973;2:89–127.

Bergmans J. Modifications induced by ischemia in the recovery of human motor axons from activity. In: Culp WJ, Ochoa JL, eds. Abnormal Nerves and Muscles as Impulse Generators. New York: Oxford University Press, 1982a;419–42.

Bergmans J. Repetitive activity induced in single human motor axons: a model for pathological repetitive activity. In: Culp WJ, Ochoa JL, eds. Abnormal Nerves and Muscles as Impulse Generators. New York: Oxford University Press, 1982b;393–418.

Bolton FB, McFarlane RM. Human pneumatic tourniquet paralysis. Neurology (Minneap.) 1978;28:787–93.

Brown AG, Iggo A. The structure and function of cutaneous "touch corpuscles" after nerve crush. J. Physiol. (Lond.) 1963;165:28–29P.

Cajal SR. Degeneration and Regeneration of the Nervous System. Vols. 1–2. London: Oxford University Press, 1928.

Chaise F, Witvoet J. Mesures des pressions intracanalaires dans le syndrome du canal carpien idiopathique non déficitaire. Rev. Chir. Orthop. 1984;70:75–78.

Culp WJ, Ochoa JL, eds. Abnormal nerves and muscles as impulse generators. New York: Oxford University Press, 1982.

Denny-Brown D, Brenner C. The effect of percussion of nerve. J. Neurol. Neurosurg. Psychiatry 1944a;7:76–95.

Denny-Brown D, Brenner C. Paralysis of nerve induced by direct pressure and by tourniquet. Arch. Neurol. Psychiatry 1944b;51:1–26.

Diamond J, Ochoa JL, Culp WJ. An introduction to abnormal nerves and muscles as impulse generators. In: Culp WJ, Ochoa JL, eds. Abnormal Nerves and Muscles as Impulse Generators. New York: Oxford University Press, 1982;3–24.

Dyck PJ. Experimental hypertrophic neuropathy: pathogenesis of onion bulb formations produced by repeated tourniquet applications. Arch. Neurol. 1969;21:73–95.

Eames RA, Lange LS. Clinical and pathological study of ischaemic neuropathy. J. Neurol. Neurosurg. Psychiatry 1967;30:215–26.

Erb W. Diseases of the peripheral cerebrospinal nerves. In: Ziemssen H von, ed. Cyclopedia of the Practice of Medicine. Vol. 11. London: Samson Low, Marston, Searle and Rivington, 1876.

Erlanger J, Blair EA. Comparative observations on motor and sensory fibers with special reference to repetitiousness. Am. J. Physiol. 1938;121:431–53.

Fowler TJ. Tourniquet paralysis in the baboon. DM thesis, University of Oxford, 1975.

Fowler TJ, Danta G, Gilliatt RW. Recovery of nerve conduction after a pneumatic tourniquet: observations on the hind limb of the baboon. J. Neurol. Neurosurg. Psychiatry 1972;35:638–47.

Fowler TJ, Ochoa JL. Unmyelinated fibres in normal and compressed peripheral nerves of the baboon: a quantitative electron microscopic study. Neuropathol. Appl. Neurobiol. 1975;1:247–65.

Fronek K, Zweifach BW. Microvascular pressure distribution in skeletal muscle and the effect of vasodilatation. Am. J. Physiol. 1975;228:791–96.

Fujimura H, Lacroix C, Said G. Vulnerability of nerve fibres to ischaemia. A quantitative light and electron microscope study. Brain 1991;114:1929–42.

Fullerton PM, Gilliatt RW. Median and ulnar neuropathy in the guinea pig. J. Neurol. Neurosurg. Psychiatry 1967;30:393–402.

Gairns FW, Garven HSD, Smith G. The digital nerves and the nerve endings in progressive obliterative vascular disease of the leg. Scott. Med. J. 1960;5:382–91.

Garven HSD, Gairns FW, Smith G. The nerve fibre populations of the nerves of the leg in chronic occlusive arterial disease in man. Scott. Med. J. 1962;7:250–65.

Gasser HS. Conduction in nerves in relation to fiber types. Assoc. Res. Nervous Mental Dis. 1935;15:35–59.

Gasser HS, Grundfest H. Action and excitability in mammalian A fibers. Am. J. Physiol. 1936;117:113–33.

Gelberman R, Hergenroeder P, Hargens A, Lundborg G, Akeson W. The carpal tunnel syndrome. A study of carpal tunnel pressures. J. Bone Joint Surg. 1981;61A:380–83.

Gelberman R, Szabo RM, Williamson RV, Dimick MP. Sensibility testing in peripheral nerve compression syndromes. An experimental study in humans. J. Bone Joint Surg. 1983; 65A:632–38.

Grundfest H. Effects of hydrostatic pressures upon the excitability, the recovery, and the potential sequence of frog nerve. Cold Spring Harbor Symp. Quant. Biol. 1936;4: 179–87.

Hargens AR, Akeson WH, Mubarak SJ, Owen CA, Evans KL, Garetto LP, Schmidt DA. Fluid balance within the canine anterolateral compartment and its relationship to compartment syndromes. J. Bone Joint Surg. 1978;604:499–505.

Harrison MJG. Pressure palsy of the ulnar nerve with prolonged conduction block. J. Neurol. Neurosurg. Psychiatry 1976; 39:96–99.

Hess K, Eames RA, Darveniza P, Gilliatt RW. Acute ischaemic neuropathy in the rabbit. J. Neurol. Sci. 1979;44:19–43.

Jefferson D, Eames RA. Subclinical entrapment of the lateral femoral cutaneous nerve: an autopsy study. Muscle Nerve 1979;2:145–54.

Jefferson D, Neary D, Eames RA. Renaut body distribution at sites of human peripheral nerve entrapment. J. Neurol. Sci. 1981;49:19–29.

Joffroy A, Achard C. Nevrite périphérique d'origine vasculaire. Arch. Med. Exp. 1889;1:229–40.

Johansson RS, Westling G. Significance of cutaneous input for precise hand movements. Electroencephalogr. Clin. Neurophysiol. 1987;39:[Suppl.]:53–57.

Konorski J, Lubinska L. Mechanical excitability of regenerating nerve fibers. Lancet 1946;1:609–10.

Korthals JK, Wisniewski HM. Peripheral nerve ischemia. Part 1. Experimental model. J. Neurol. Sci. 1975;24:65–76.

Kugelberg E. Accommodation in human nerves and its significance for the symptoms in circulatory disturbances and tetany. Acta. Physiol. Scand. 1944;8:[Suppl. XXIV]:1–105.

Lewis T, Pickering GW, Rothschild P. Centripetal paralysis arising out of arrested blood flow to the limb, including notes on a form of tingling. Heart 1931;16:1–32.

Low PA, Dyck PJ. Increased endoneurial fluid pressure in experimental lead neuropathy. Nature 1977;269:427–28.

Luchetti R, Schoenhuber R, Alfarano M, Deluca S, De Cicco G, Landi A. Carpal tunnel syndrome: correlations between pressure measurement and intraoperative electrophysiological nerve study. Muscle Nerve 1990;13:1164–68.

Luchetti R, Schoenhuber R, De Cicco G, Alfarano M, Deluca S, Landi A. Carpal-tunnel pressure. Acta Orthop. Scand. 1989; 60:396–99.

Lundborg G. Ischemic nerve injury. Experimental studies on intraneural microvascular pathophysiology and nerve function in a limb, subjected to temporary circulatory arrest. Scand. J. Plast. Reconstr. Surg. Suppl. 1970;6:1–113.

Lundborg G. Structure and function of the intraneural microvessels as related to trauma, edema formation and nerve function. J. Bone Joint Surg. 1975;57A:938–48.

Lundborg G. The intrinsic vascularization of human peripheral nerves. Structural and functional aspects. J. Hand Surg. 1979;4:34–41.

Lundborg G. Intraneural microcirculation and peripheral nerve barriers. In: Omer G, Spinner M, eds. Management of Peripheral Nerve Problems. Philadelphia: WB Saunders, 1980;903–16.

Lundborg G. Nerve Injury and Repair. New York: Churchill Livingstone, 1988.

Lundborg G, Gelberman R, Minteer-Convery M, Lee VF, Hargens A. Median nerve compression in the carpal tunnel: the functional response to experimentally induced controlled pressure. J. Hand Surg. 1982;7:252–59.

Lundborg G, Myers R, Powell H. Nerve compression injury and increase in endoneurial fluid pressure: "miniature compartment syndrome." J. Neurol. Neurosurg. Psychiatry 1983; 46:1119–24.

Lundborg G, Nordborg C, Rydevik B, Olsson Y. The effect of ischemia on the permeability of the perineurium to protein tracers in rabbit tibial nerve. Acta. Neurol. Scand. 1973; 49:287–94.

Lundborg G, Rydevik B. Effects of stretching the tibial nerve of the rabbit. A preliminary study of the intraneural circulation and the barrier function of the perineurium. J. Bone Joint Surg. 1973;55B:390–401.

Marie P, Foix C. Atrophic isolée de l'éminence thénar d'origine névritique. Rôle du ligament annulaire antérieur du carpe dans la pathogénie de la lésion. Rev. Neurol. (Paris) 1913;26:647.

McDonald WI. Clinical consequences of conduction defects produced by demyelination. In: Culp WJ, Ochoa JL, eds. Abnormal Nerves and Muscles as Impulse Generators. New York: Oxford University Press, 1982;253–70.

Merrington WR, Nathan PW. A study of post-ischaemic paresthesiae. J. Neurol. Neurosurg. Psychiatry 1949;12:1–18.

Moldaver J. Tourniquet paralysis syndrome. Arch. Surg. 1954;68:136–44.

Mubarak SJ, Hargens AR, Owen CA, Garetto LP, Akeson WH. The wick catheter technique for measurement of intramuscular pressure. A new research and clinical tool. J. Bone Joint Surg. 1976;58A:1016–20.

Mubarak SJ, Owen CA, Hargens AR, Garetto LP, Akeson WH. Acute compartment syndromes: diagnosis and treatment with the aid of the wick catheter. J. Bone Joint Surg. 1978;60A:1091–95.

Myers RR, Mizisin AP, Powell HC, Lampert PW. Reduced nerve blood flow in hexachlorophene neuropathy. Relationship to elevated endoneurial fluid pressure. J. Neuropathol. Exp. Neurol. 1982;41:391–99.

Myers RR, Powell HC, Costello ML, Lambert PW, Zweifach BW. Endoneurial fluid pressure: direct measurement with micropipettes. Brain Res. 1978;148:510–15.

Myers RR, Murakami H, Powell HC. Reduced nerve blood flow in edematous neuropathies—a biochemical mechanism. Microvasc. Res. 1986;32:145–51.

Nathan PW. Ischaemic and post-ischaemic numbness and paraesthesiae. J. Neurol. Neurosurg. Psychiatry 1958;21: 12–23.

Neary D, Eames RA. The pathology of ulnar nerve compression in man. Neuropathol. Appl. Neurobiol. 1975;1:69–88.

Neary D, Ochoa JL, Gilliatt RW. Subclinical entrapment neuropathy in man. J. Neurol. Sci. 1975;24:283–98.

Nukada H, Dyck PJ. Microsphere embolization of nerve capillaries and fiber degeneration. Am. J. Pathol. 1984; 115:275–87.

Ochoa JL. Ultrathin longitudinal sections of single myelinated fibres for electron microscopy. J. Neurol. Sci. 1972; 17:103–6.

Ochoa JL. Nerve fiber pathology in acute and chronic compression. In: Omer GE Jr., Spinner M, eds. Management of Peripheral Nerve Problems. Philadelphia: WB Saunders, 1980;487–501.

Ochoa JL. Some aberrations of nerve repair. In: Gorio A, Millesi H, Mingrino S, eds. Post Traumatic Peripheral Nerve Regeneration: Experimental Basis and Clinical Implications. New York: Raven Press, 1981;147–55.

Ochoa JL, Danta G, Fowler TJ, Gilliatt RW. Nature of the nerve lesion caused by a pneumatic tourniquet. Nature 1971; 233:265–66.

Ochoa JL, Fowler TJ, Gilliatt RW. Anatomical changes in peripheral nerves compressed by a pneumatic tourniquet. J. Anat. 1972;113:433–55.

Ochoa JL, Fowler TJ, Gilliatt RW. Changes produced by a pneumatic tourniquet. In: Desmedt JE, ed. New Developments in Electromyography and Clinical Neurophysiology. Basel: Karger, 1973;2:166–73.

Ochoa JL, Marotte L. The nature of the nerve lesion underlying chronic entrapment. Neurol. Sci. 1973;19:491–95.

Ochoa JL, Torebjörk HE. Paresthesiae from ectopic impulse generation in human sensory nerves. Brain 1980;103: 835–53.

Ochoa JL, Torebjörk HE. Sensations evoked by intraneural microstimulation of single mechanoreceptor units innervating the human hand. J Physiol. 1983;342:633–54.

Ochoa JL, Torebjörk HE. Sensations evoked by intraneural microstimulation of C nociceptor fibres in human skin nerves. J. Physiol. (Lond.) 1989;415:583–99.

Ochoa JL, Torebjörk HE, Culp WJ, Schady W. Abnormal spontaneous activity in single sensory nerve fibers in humans. Muscle Nerve 1982;5574–77.

Olsson Y. The involvement of vasa nervorum in diseases of peripheral nerves. In: Vinken, PJ and Bruyn V, eds. Handbook of Clinical Neurology, part II. Vol 12. Vascular Diseases of the Nervous System. Amsterdam: North-Holland., 1972;641–64.

Olsson Y, Kristensson K. The perineurium as a diffusion barrier to protein tracers following trauma to nerves. Acta Neuropathol. (Berl.) 1973;23:105–11.

Olsson Y, Reese TS. Permeability of vasa nervorum and perineurium in mouse sciatic nerve studied by fluorescence and electron microscopy. J. Neuropathol. Exp. Neurol. 1971;30:105–19.

Ortman JA, Sahenk Z, Mendell JR. The experimental production of Renaut bodies. J. Neurol. Sci. 1983;62:233–41.

Parry GJ, Brown MJ. Arachidonate-induced experimental nerve infarction. J. Neurol. Sci. 1981;50:123–33.

Powell HC, Myers RR. Pathology of experimental nerve compression. Lab. Invest. 1986;55:91–100.

Raff MC, Sangalang V, Asbury AK. Ischemic mononeuropathy multiplex associated with diabetes mellitus. Arch. Neurol. 1968;18:487–99.

Renaut J. Système hyalin de soutènement des centres nerveux et de quelques organes des sense. Arch. Physiol. Norm. Pathol. 1881;8:846–59.

Richardson PM, Thomas PK. Percussive injury to peripheral nerve in rats. J. Neurosurg. 1979;51:178–87.

Rudge P. Tourniquet paralysis with prolonged conduction block: electrophysiological study. J. Bone Joint Surg. 1974;56B:716–20.

Rudge P, Ochoa JL, Gilliatt RW. Acute peripheral nerve compression in the baboon. Anatomical and physiological findings. J. Neurol. Sci. 1974;23:403–20.

Rydevik B. Compression injury of peripheral nerve. Experimental studies on microcirculation, oedema formation, axonal transport, fibre structure and function in nerves subjected to acute, graded compression. Thesis, University of Göteborg, Göteborg, 1979.

Rydevik B, McLean WG, Sjöstrand J, Lundborg G. Blockage of axonal transport induced by acute graded compression of the rabbit vagus nerve. J. Neurol. Neurosurg. Psychiatry 1980;43:690–98.

Rydevik BL, Myers RR, Powell HC. Pressure increase in the dorsal root ganglion following mechanical compression. Closed compartment syndrome in nerve roots. Spine 1989;14:574–76.

Seddon HJ. Three types of nerve injury. Brain 1943;66:237–88.

Sinclair DC, Hinshaw JR. A comparison of the dissociation produced by procaine and by limb ischaemia. Brain 1950;73:480–98.

Sivak M, Ochoa JL. Positive manifestations of nerve fiber dysfunction: clinical, electrophysiologic, and pathologic correlates. In: Brown WF, Bolton CF, eds. Clinical Electromyography: Boston: Butterworth–Heinemann, 1987;1–30.

Sladsky JT, Tschoepe RL, Greenberg JH, Brown MJ. Peripheral neuropathy after chronic endoneurial ischemia. Ann. Neurol. 1991;29:272–78.

Smith EM, Sonstegard DA, Anderson WH Jr. Carpal tunnel syndrome: contribution of flexor tendons. Arch. Phys. Med. Rehabil. 1977;58:379–85.

Smith KJ, McDonald WI. Spontaneous and mechanically evoked activity due to central demyelinating lesion. Nature 1980;286:154–55.

Smith KJ, McDonald WI. Spontaneous and evoked electrical discharges from a central demyelinating lesion. J. Neurol. Sci. 1982;55:39–47.

Sunderland S. The nerve lesion in the carpal tunnel syndrome. J. Neurol. Neurosurg. Psychiatry 1976;39:615–26.

Szabo RM, Chidgey LK. Stress carpal tunnel pressure in patients with carpal tunnel syndrome and normal patients. J. Hand Surg. 1989;14A:624–27.

Thomas PK, Fullerton PM. Nerve fiber size in the carpal tunnel syndrome. J. Neurol. Neurosurg. Psychiatry 1963; 26:520–27.

Werner CO, Elmquist D, Ohlin P. Pressure and nerve lesion in the carpal tunnel. Acta. Orthop. Scand. 1983;54: 312–16.

Whitesides TE Jr., Haney TC, Morimoto K, Harada H. Tissue pressure measurements as a determinant for the need of fasciotomy. Clin. Orthop. 1975;113:43–51.

Yarnitsky D, Ochoa JL. Release of cold-induced burning pain by block of cold-specific afferent input. Brain 1990; 113:893–902.

Yarnitsky D, Ochoa JL. Differential effect of compression-ischaemia block on warm sensation and heat-induced pain. Brain 1991;114:907–13.

Chapter 13
Activity, Occupation, and Carpal Tunnel Syndrome

Activities that can cause carpal tunnel syndrome include sustained wrist or palmar pressure, prolonged wrist extension and flexion, repetitive hand and wrist use, work with vibrating tools, and possibly hand use in the cold. At least one-half of all cases of carpal tunnel syndrome in North America appear attributable to occupational hand activities (Hagberg, Morgenstern & Kelsh, 1992; Rossignol, Stock, Patry & Armstrong, 1997). In 1999, there were an estimated 27,900 instances of carpal tunnel syndrome leading to time loss from work among workers in private American industries, reflecting an annual incidence of 31 per 100,000 full-time workers (Bureau of Labor Statistics, 2001). These cases resulted in a median annual work loss of 27 days.

Carpal tunnel syndrome that is not severe enough to result in time loss is much more common; the Occupational Health Supplement of the 1988 National Health Interview Survey found that 530 workers per 100,000 had been told within the previous year by a physician that they had carpal tunnel syndrome (Tanaka, Wild, Seligman, Halperin, Behrens & Putz-Anderson, 1995; Tanaka, Wild, Cameron & Freund, 1997). Among adults who had been employed at least part of the year preceding the survey, 670 per 100,000 women and 420 per 100,000 men had carpal tunnel syndrome by this definition. The prevalence of carpal tunnel syndrome varied from industry to industry, and repetitive bending or twisting of hands or wrists and use of vibrating tools were important risk factors for the presence of carpal tunnel syndrome, even after adjustment of wrist for personal factors such as body mass index, gender, and age.

For the 1.5 million workers covered by the Washington State workers' compensation system, the incidence of accepted claims for carpal tunnel syndrome was 170 cases per 100,000 workers per year from 1984 to 1988 and 290 cases per 100,000 workers per year from 1992 to 1994 (Table 13-1) (Franklin, Haug, Heyer, Checkoway & Peck, 1991; Daniell, Fulton-Kehoe, Bradley & Franklin, 1998). The diagnosis of carpal tunnel syndrome was based on physicians' diagnoses submitted on workers' compensation claims, a standard that can lead to some diagnostic misclassification. Some industries had yearly incidences exceeding 1,000 cases per 100,000 workers; oyster, crab, and clam packers had the highest incidence with 2,600 cases per 100,000 workers (Franklin, Haug, Peck, Heyer & Checkoway, 1990; Franklin et al., 1991). The incidence of carpal tunnel syndrome varied markedly from one industry to the next.

The reported incidence of carpal tunnel syndrome in workers varies greatly from state to state. The annual incidence for Massachusetts from 1992 to 1997 was 40 cases of carpal tunnel syndrome per 100,000 workers (Davis, Wellman & Punnett, 2001). In Oregon in 1991 there were 115 accepted workers' compensation disability claims for carpal tunnel syndrome per 100,000 workers (Oregon Department of Insurance and Finance, 1992). In Wisconsin in the early 1990s, the annual rate of carpal tunnel surgery under workers' compensation was 92 per 100,000 women and 54 per 100,000 men (Hanrahan, Higgins, Anderson & Smith, 1993). These statistical variations reflect differences in medical, industrial, and regulatory practice, including accuracy of reporting, diagnos-

Table 13-1. Annual Incidence of Carpal Tunnel Syndrome in Selected Washington State Industries, 1984 to 1988

Industrial Class Description	Rate per 100,000 Full-Time Workers
Oyster, crab, clam packing	2,570
Meat, poultry dealers	2,390
Logging operations	890
Grocery stores	370
Higher education institutions	40

Data from GM Franklin, J Haug, N Heyer, H Checkoway, N Peck. Occupational carpal tunnel syndrome in Washington State, 1984–1988. Am. J. Public Health 1991;81:741–46.

tic criteria, and treatment approaches for carpal tunnel syndrome.

Historical Background

Insight into the role of activities or occupations in causing median neuropathy has a long tradition. Before the recognition of the pathogenic importance of the carpal tunnel, Oppenheim's *Textbook of Nervous Diseases* (1911) listed laundry women, joiners, locksmiths, milkers, cigar makers, carpetbeaters, and dentists among those prone to occupational median nerve pareses. In their seminal report on carpal tunnel syndrome in six women, Brain and colleagues (1947) characterized median nerve compression in the carpal tunnel as "spontaneous," but thought that manual work was a contributing factor to the development of the syndrome. Kendall (1950) described five cases of carpal tunnel syndrome that he attributed to "unusually heavy household duties rather late in life." Tanzer (1959) stressed the role of increased hand use before the onset of symptoms. Over the years numerous reports have associated carpal tunnel syndrome with various professions. Most of these reports have been based on single cases or clusters of cases, and skeptics have pointed to the high incidence of carpal tunnel syndrome in the general population as evidence that these associations are fortuitous. For example, Phalen (1966) emphasized that the largest group of his patients were housewives and concluded that, "common, typical carpal tunnel syndrome—spontaneous compression neu-

ropathy of the median nerve in the carpal tunnel—is not an occupational disease." He thus evaded the issue of whether the activities of a housewife might be a contributing factor to pathogenesis. He did, however, concede that excessive hand use is a contributing factor in some cases.

Birkbeck and Beer (1975) surveyed the activities of 588 patients who had symptoms of carpal tunnel syndrome and abnormal median nerve conduction studies. Of the employed patients without medical conditions that might predispose to development of carpal tunnel syndrome, 79% worked in occupations requiring repetitive hand movements. Of the 72 housewives, 51% were knitters. The study made no attempt to quantify or better define "repetitive hand movement" and provided no control data on the activities or hobbies of a nonaffected peer group.

The concept that carpal tunnel syndrome is an occupational illness is strongly ingrained in popular American culture. For example, many papers in the dental literature warn dentists and dental hygienists of the occupational risk of carpal tunnel syndrome, a risk that is plausible given the repetitive hand use, awkward wrist postures, and use of vibrating tools inherent in their work, yet we are unaware of a well-controlled study that confirms the association (Osborn, Newell, Rudney & Stoltenberg, 1990; Conrad, Conrad & Osborn, 1992, 1993; Gerwatowski, McFall & Stach, 1992; Stockstill, Harn, Strickland & Hruska, 1993; Nakladalova, Fialova, Korycanova & Nakladal, 1995; Lalumandier, McPhee, Riddle, Shulman & Daigle, 2000; Hamann, Werner, Franzblau, Rodgers, Siew & Gruninger, 2001). Tables 13-2 and 13-3 illustrate the wide variety of activities and occupations that have been purported to cause carpal syndrome.

Epidemiology

Armstrong and Silverstein (1987) have urged use of a formal epidemiologic analysis to clarify the relation of carpal tunnel syndrome to occupation. Epidemiologic evidence for a causal relationship includes (1) a strong and consistent statistical correlation between activities and the occurrence of carpal tunnel syndrome, (2) a dose-response relation between reputed cause and effect, (3) a temporal relation between reputed cause and effect, and

(4) biological plausibility supporting the causal nature of the association (MacMahon & Pugh, 1970; Fletcher, Fletcher & Wagner, 1982; Mausner & Kramer, 1985).

Cross-Sectional and Case-Control Studies on Relation between Manual Activity and Carpal Tunnel Syndrome

Over 30 epidemiologic case-control and cross-sectional studies have investigated the relationship between carpal tunnel syndrome and occupation or specific hand activities, and many have found an association (see Table 13-3). Reviews and meta-analyses have critiqued the quality of these studies and summarized these data (Stock, 1991; Kuorinka, Forcier, Hagberg, Silverstein, Wells, Smith, Hendrick & Carayon, 1995; Bernard, 1997; Abbas, Afifi, Zhang & Kraus, 1998).

Despite widespread recognition of the relationship between hand and wrist use and symptoms of carpal tunnel syndrome, some authors still debate whether activities are a cause of the basic pathology of the syndrome (Nathan, Meadows & Doyle, 1988a; Schottland, Kirschberg, Fillingim, Davis & Hogg, 1991; Kasdan, Wolens, Leis, Kasdan & Stallings, 1994; Radecki, 1995; Vender, Kasdan & Truppa, 1995; Hadler, 1997). Their doubts concerning epidemiologic studies in which diagnostic criteria and measures of exposure vary have been cogently critiqued (Silverstein, Silverstein & Franklin, 1996).

Various epidemiologic studies use different research definitions of carpal tunnel syndrome. Subtle abnormalities of median nerve conduction can frequently be detected in workers, whether or not they use their hands for heavy or repetitive work. Because median nerve conduction abnormalities can be asymptomatic, these observations do not resolve the issue of whether certain activities can cause carpal tunnel syndrome (Nathan, Meadows & Doyle, 1988a; Schottland et al., 1991). Many of the epidemiologic studies use case definitions for carpal tunnel syndrome that would not be precise enough for clinical patient care and are apt to overdiagnose carpal tunnel syndrome in the workplace; as this misclassification applies to both low-exposure and high-exposure workers, it is likely

Table 13-2. Examples of Case Reports and Case Clusters of Carpal Tunnel Syndrome Associated with Occupations, Activities, or Postures

Setting	Reference
Automotive worker	Rothfleisch & Sherman, 1976; Gordon, Bowyer & Johnson, 1987
Bicycle rider	Mellion, 1991; Braithwaite, 1992
Cardiologist	Stevens, 1990
Cornhusker	Jones & Scheker, 1988
Central nervous system disease causing sustained abnormal wrist posture	Alvarez, Larkin & Roxborough, 1982; Orcutt, Kramer, Howard, Keenan, Stone, Waters & Gellman, 1990
Electrician	Bleecker, Bohlman, Moreland & Tipton, 1985
Musician	Hochberg, Leffert, Heller & Merriman, 1983; Charness, 1992; Dent & Hadden, 1992; Lederman, 1994
Paraplegic	Aljure, Eltorai, Bradley, Lin & Johnson, 1985; Gellman, Sie & Waters, 1988; Davidoff, Werner & Waring, 1991; Dozono, Hachisuka, Hatada & Ogata, 1995; Nemchausky & Ubilluz, 1995; Oesterling, Morgan, Edlich & Steers, 1995; Jackson, Hynninen, Caborn & McLean, 1996
Polio victim	Waring & Werner, 1989; Werner, Waring & Davidoff, 1989;
Rock climber	Hochholzer, Krause & Heuk, 1993
Sign language interpreter	Stedt, 1989; Podhorodecki & Spielholz, 1993; Smith, Kress & Hart, 2000
Staple gun user	Hoffman & Hoffman, 1985

to bias studies against finding true associations (Silverstein et al., 1996).

The National Institute for Occupational Safety and Health review of epidemiologic studies on occupational carpal tunnel syndrome concluded that there was evidence of positive associations between highly repetitive work, forceful work, or exposure to vibration and the development of carpal tunnel syndrome (Bernard, 1997). There was insufficient evidence to associate specific postures or hand or wrist positions to development of carpal tunnel syndrome. There was strong evidence that combined factors such as force and repetition or force and posture were associated with development of carpal tunnel syndrome.

Table 13-3. Controlled Epidemiologic Studies on Occupation and Carpal Tunnel Syndrome

Reference	Method	Workers
Abbas, Faris, Harber, Mishriky, El-Shahaly, Waheeb & Kraus, 2001	Cross-sectional	Electronics assemblers
Armstrong & Chaffin, 1979	Case-control	Sewing machine operators
Barnhart, Demers, Miller, Longstreth & Rosenstock, 1991	Cross-sectional	Ski manufacturing workers
Baron, Milliron, Habes & Fidler, 1991	Cross-sectional	Grocery checkers
Bovenzi, Zadini, Franzinelli & Borgogni, 1991	Cross-sectional	Foresters using chain saws
Bovenzi & Italian Study Group on Physical Hazards in the Stone Industry, 1994	Cross-sectional	Stone and quarry workers
Cannon, Bernacki & Walter, 1981	Case-control	Aircraft engine workers
Chatterjee, Barwick & Petrie, 1982[a]	Case-control	Rock drillers
Chiang, Chen, Yu & Ko, 1990; Chiang, Ko, Chen, Yu, Wu & Chang, 1993[a]	Cross-sectional	Frozen fish processors
De Krom, Kester, Knipschild & Spaans, 1990	Nested case-control	Community and hospital sample
English, Maclaren, Court-Brown, Hughes, Porter, Wallace & Graves, 1995	Case-control	—
Farkkila, Pyykko, Jantti, Aatola, Starck & Korhonen, 1988	Cross-sectional	Forestry workers using chain saws
Feldman, Travers, Chirico-Post & Keyserling, 1987	Cross-sectional	Electronics workers
Giersiepen, Eberle & Pohlabeln, 2000	Case-control	—
Koskimies, Farkkila, Pyykko, Jantti, Aatola, Starck & Inaba, 1990	Cross-sectional	Forestry workers using chain saws
Leclerc, Franchi, Cristofari, Delemotte, Mereau, Teyssier-Cotte & Touranchet, 1998	Cross-sectional	Assembly line, clothing, food, and shoe workers
Liss, Jesin, Kusiak & White, 1995	Cross-sectional	Dental hygienists
Loslever & Ranaivosoa, 1993	Cross-sectional	Varied jobs
Marras & Schoenmarklin, 1993	Cross-sectional	Industrial workers
Moore & Garg, 1994[a]	Cross-sectional	Pork processors
Morgenstern, Kelsh, Kraus & Margolis, 1991	Cross-sectional	Grocery checkers
Nathan, Meadows & Doyle, 1988[a,b,c]	Cross-sectional	Varied industrial workers
Nilsson, Hagberg, Burström & Lundströmj, 1990	Cross-sectional	Platers using vibrating tools
Nordstrom, Vierkant, DeStefano & Layde, 1997	Case-control	—
Osorio, Ames, Jones, Castorina, Rempel, Estrin & Thompson, 1994[a]	Cross-sectional	Supermarket workers
Park, Nelson, Silverstein & Mirer, 1992	Cross-sectional	Auto manufacturing workers
Pocekay, McCurdy, Samuels, Hammond & Schenker, 1995	Cross-sectional	Semiconductor workers
Punnett, Robins, Wegman & Keyserling, 1985	Cross-sectional	Garment workers
Roquelaure, Mechali, Dano, Fanello, Benetti, Bureau, Mariel, Martin, Derriennic & Penneau-Fontbonne, 1997	Case-control	—
Schottland, Kirschberg, Fillingim, Davis & Hogg, 1991	Cross-sectional	Poultry workers
Silverstein, BA, Fine & Armstrong, 1987[a,b]	Cross-sectional	Varied industrial workers
Stetson, Silverstein, Keyserling, Wolfe & Albers, 1993[d]	Cross-sectional	Varied industrial workers
Tanaka, Wild, Seligman, Behrens, Cameron & Putz-Anderson, 1994; Tanaka, Wild, Seligman, Halperin, Behrens & Putz-Anderson, 1995; Tanaka, Wild, Cameron & Freund, 1997	Cross-sectional	Data from Occupational Health Supplement of National Health Interview Survey
Werner, RA, Franzblau, Albers & Armstrong, 1997[d]	Cross-sectional	Varied industrial workers
Wieslander, Norback, Gothe & Juhlin, 1989	Case-control	—

[a]Study meets criteria of Bernard (1997) for study design and definition of population, exposure, and outcome.

[b]Study meets criteria of Stock (1991) for study design and definition of population, exposure, and outcome.

[c]Data have been re-analyzed extensively. See, for example, Stock, 1991; Bernard, 1997; Szabo, 1998; and the author's reply, Nathan, 1992.

[d]Study examines median nerve conduction without regard to symptoms of carpal tunnel syndrome.

Vibration Exposure and Carpal Tunnel Syndrome

Occupational exposure to vibration can cause carpal tunnel syndrome. In a case-control study in four plants of the Pratt and Whitney Aircraft Company, 30 workers who had carpal tunnel syndrome were identified from workers' compensation and medical department records and retrospectively compared with 90 control employees who did not have carpal tunnel syndrome (Cannon, Bernacki & Walter, 1981). Some 70% of those who had carpal tunnel syndrome, but only 14% of the controls, worked with vibrating hand tools (surface grinders, polisher/buffers, and small hand tools), giving a statistically significant association between vibrating tool use and carpal tunnel syndrome ($P < .01$ by Chi-square). A nonstatistically significant association was found with "performance of repetitive motion tasks." The results are illustrated in Figure 13-1.

Among forestry workers who were exposed to the vibration of chain saws, 20% had symptoms and nerve conduction studies consistent with carpal tunnel syndrome (Koskimies, Farkkila, Pyykko, Jantti, Aatola, Starck & Inaba, 1990). In another group of foresters, the odds ratio for having carpal tunnel syndrome, adjusted for body mass index and age, was 21.3 for foresters compared with controls (Bovenzi, Zadini, Franzinelli & Borgogni, 1991). In a Swedish case-control study, vibration exposure from use of hand-held tools was a clear-cut risk factor for development of carpal tunnel syndrome (Wieslander, Norback, Gothe & Juhlin, 1989).

A cross-sectional study compared the prevalence of carpal tunnel syndrome in platers who worked with vibrating tools and in office workers (Nilsson, Hagberg, Burström & Lundströmj, 1990). The prevalence of carpal tunnel syndrome for platers was 13.5%, and the odds ratio for having carpal tunnel syndrome was 11.0 for platers compared with office workers.

A case-control study used hospital records to match patients who had undergone carpal tunnel surgery to randomly chosen controls (Wieslander et al., 1989). The patients who had undergone carpal tunnel surgery were more likely than controls to use vibrating hand tools (odds ratio, 3.3; $P <.002$); repetitive wrist movements (odds ratio, 2.7; $P <.006$) and work that placed a heavy load on

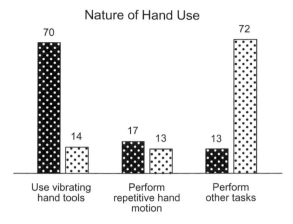

Figure 13-1. Development of carpal tunnel syndrome (CTS) in aircraft builders. Numbers indicate percentage of workers with CTS or of control workers in each category. Use of vibrating tools was a statistically significant risk factor ($P <.01$) for developing CTS. The relationship between performing repetitive motion tasks and development of CTS was not statistically significant in this study. (Data from LJ Cannon, EJ Bernacki, SD Walter. Personal and occupational factors associated with carpal tunnel syndrome. J. Occup. Med. 1981;23:255–58.)

wrists (odds ratio, 1.8; P not significant) were also evaluated in this study.

Exposure to vibration is also associated with mild asymptomatic abnormalities of nerve conduction across the carpal tunnel. Nathan and colleagues (1988a) found that 61% of grinder workers but only 28% of administrative or clerical workers had focal median nerve sensory conduction slowing on the serial sensory latency test. Among rock drillers exposed to low-frequency vibration, 44% had decreased amplitude of median sensory nerve action potentials from the index finger compared with ulnar sensory nerve action potentials from the little finger, whereas only 7% of controls had this abnormality (Chatterjee, Barwick & Petrie, 1982). Platers and truck assemblers working with vibrating tools and forceful grips were more likely than office workers to have impaired median nerve conduction (Nilsson, Hagberg, Burstrom & Kihlberg, 1994).

Carpal tunnel syndrome accounts for only a fraction of the hand and arm symptoms experienced by workers who are exposed to vibration (Figure 13-2). *Hand-arm vibration syndrome* is a constellation of

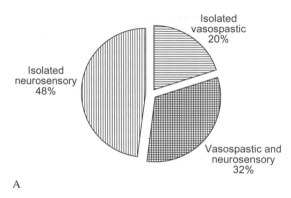

A

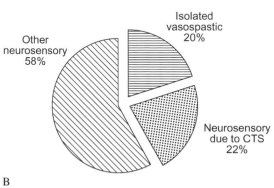

B

Figure 13-2. Hand problems in 100 vibration-exposed symptomatic male workers. **(A)** Distribution of vasospastic versus neurosensory symptoms. **(B)** Only 22% of hand symptoms were attributed to carpal tunnel syndrome (CTS) based on symptom pattern and physical examination. (Data from T Stromberg, G Lundborg, LB Dahlin, Anatomy, function, and pathophysiology of peripheral nerves and nerve compression. Hand Clin. 1996;12[2]:185–93.)

upper-extremity disorders caused by vibration exposure (Brammer & Taylor, 1988; Taylor & Wasserman, 1988; Noel, 2000). Symptoms include finger blanching, numbness, tingling, hand pain, grip weakness or fatigue, and joint stiffness. Vibration-induced vascular disorders, including digital organic microangiopathy, digital vasospasm, and upper-extremity arterial thrombosis, can cause *vibration white finger*. Damage to Pacinian corpuscles, digital sensory neuropathy, carpal tunnel syndrome, and musculoskeletal changes can all contribute to the symptom complex (Taylor, 1988).

Prolonged occupational exposure to low-frequency vibration can also cause a distal neuropathy in the hands, particularly affecting function in digital branches of median and ulnar nerves (Bram-

mer & Pyykko, 1987). Two-point discrimination and sensitivity to vibration can be impaired (Haines & Chong, 1987; Lundborg, Dahlin, Lundstrom, Necking & Stromberg, 1992; Rosén, Stromberg & Lundborg, 1993; Sakakibara, Hirata, Hashiguchi, Toibana, Koshiyama, Zhu, Kondo, Miyao & Yamada, 1996). Patients often have impaired warm and cold sensitivity in the fingers, even with normal nerve conduction studies, suggesting dysfunction of unmyelinated and small myelinated fibers (Ekenvall, Nilsson & Gustavsson, 1986). Ulnar and median digital nerve conduction is often impaired in the hands of those exposed to prolonged vibration; less frequently, median nerve conduction is impaired across the carpal tunnel (Sakakibara, Kondo, Miyao & Yamada, 1994; Sakakibara, Hirata, Hashiguchi, Toibana, Koshiyama, Zhu & Yamada, 1995). Even when digital or transcarpal conduction is slowed, nerve conduction velocity between the palm and proximal digit usually remains normal (Sakakibara, Hirata, Hashiguchi, Toibana & Koshiyama, 1998). Using special techniques to measure conduction in slower motor fibers, abnormal conduction in motor fibers, such as in the ulnar nerve in the forearm, is demonstrable in some of those who have been chronically exposed to vibration (Alaranta & Seppalainen, 1977). Digital nerve biopsy can show evidence of demyelination, decreased number of myelinated fibers, and perineural fibrosis (Takeuchi, Futatsuka, Imanishi & Yamada, 1986; Takeuchi, Takeya & Imanishi, 1988). In vibration-exposed workers, biopsies of the dorsal interosseous nerve proximal to the wrist have shown similar pathology (Stromberg, Dahlin, Brun & Lundborg, 1997).

Among patients with hand-arm vibration syndrome, the presence of nocturnal hand paresthesias is a clue that carpal tunnel syndrome might be contributing to symptoms. Boyle and colleagues (1988) described 19 patients who had worked for years with vibrating tools and who had episodic finger blanching, usually associated with hand tingling or numbness. Table 13-4 shows the relationship in these patients between presence of hand tingling at night (unassociated with blanching) and occurrence of abnormal nerve conduction across the carpal tunnel.

A study of Minnesota workers who had undergone carpal tunnel surgery suggested that hand-arm vibration syndrome had been insufficiently recog-

Table 13-4. Symptoms versus Nerve Conduction in 19 Patients Affected by Hand-Arm Vibration Syndrome

Median Nerve Conduction Across the Carpal Tunnel	Nocturnal Hand Paresthesias	
	Present	Absent
Abnormal	10	2
Normal	2	5

Data from JC Boyle, NJ Smith, FD Burke. Vibration white finger. J. Hand Surg. 1988;13B:171–76.

nized as a potential cause of hand symptoms in these patients (Miller, Lohman, Maldonado & Mandel, 1994). Patients who have carpal tunnel syndrome and have had vibration exposure usually improve after carpal tunnel surgery, but they are more likely than those who have not been exposed to vibration to have residual postoperative symptoms (Hagberg, Nystrom & Zetterlund, 1991; Bostrom, Gothe, Hansson, Lugnegard & Nilsson, 1994).

Repetitive or Forceful Activity and Carpal Tunnel Syndrome

Highly repetitive hand and wrist activity is often defined as working with a cycle time of less than 30 seconds or with at least 50% of the work cycle performing the same fundamental movement (Silverstein, Fine & Armstrong, 1987). This type of repetitive activity is associated with an increased risk of developing carpal tunnel syndrome. Forceful hand and wrist activity is less important than repetitiveness as a cause of carpal tunnel syndrome, but forceful activity combined with repetitive activity is more strongly associated with carpal tunnel syndrome than is repetitive activity alone.

Silverstein and colleagues (1987) surveyed 652 workers in six industries (electronics assembly, major appliance manufacture, metal casting, apparel sewing, ductile iron foundry, and bearing manufacture). They inspected each job and classified it for high or low repetitiveness and high or low force. The classifications were carefully defined and confirmed by videotape and electromyographic analysis of the job activity. As shown in Figure 13-3, the prevalence of carpal tunnel syndrome was lowest among workers on "low force–low repetitiveness" jobs and highest among workers on "high force–high repetitiveness" jobs. Highly repetitive wrist movement was a greater risk factor for development of carpal tunnel syndrome than was forceful wrist use. The odds ratio for development of carpal tunnel syndrome was 5.5

Figure 13-3. "Dose" of wrist activity and risk of developing carpal tunnel syndrome (CTS). (Data from BA Silverstein, LJ Fine, TJ Armstrong. Occupational factors and carpal tunnel syndrome. Am. J. Ind. Med. 1987;11:343–58.)

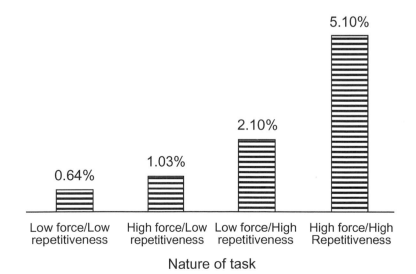

Percentage of Workers at Each Task Who Have CTS

5.10%

2.10%

1.03%

0.64%

Low force/Low repetitiveness   High force/Low repetitiveness   Low force/High repetitiveness   High force/High Repetitiveness

Nature of task

comparing jobs with high repetition with jobs with low repetition and adjusting for age, gender, years on the job, and plant.

Two cross-sectional studies have surveyed workers in Taiwanese frozen food processing plants. In the first, basing the diagnosis of carpal tunnel syndrome on both clinical and electrodiagnostic abnormalities, those whose work required repetitive wrist movement were more likely than other workers to develop carpal tunnel syndrome (odds ratio 7.4 after adjustment for gender, age, and length of employment) (Chiang, Chen, Yu & Ko, 1990). Hand exposure to cold during work was also associated with an increased risk of developing carpal tunnel syndrome. In the second study, basing the diagnosis of carpal tunnel syndrome on history and examination by an occupational physician, carpal tunnel syndrome was more common in women who did forceful arm work, but no effect of repetitive arm work on prevalence of carpal tunnel syndrome was demonstrable (Chiang, Ko, Chen, Yu, Wu & Chang, 1993).

A cross-sectional study of grocery store workers assessed job repetitiveness based on work tasks and hours per week spent performing those tasks (Osorio, Ames, Jones, Castorina, Rempel, Estrin & Thompson, 1994). Comparing high-risk with low-risk jobs, the relative risk for having symptoms suggestive of carpal tunnel syndrome was 8.3 for the high-risk jobs. The relative risk for having carpal tunnel syndrome diagnosed by clinical and nerve conduction criteria was 6.18 after adjustment for age, sex, alcohol exposure, and adverse medical history, but did not reach statistical significance. In another cross-sectional study of supermarket workers, carpal tunnel syndrome was diagnosed in 11% of female checkers but in only 4% of female noncheckers (adjusted odds ratio 3.7, 95% confidence interval 0.7 to 16.7) (Baron, Milliron, Habes & Fidler, 1991). The checkers did between 1,432 and 1,782 repetitions per hour with their right hands and between 832 and 1,260 with their left hands, often moving their wrists through awkward postures.

Feldman and colleagues (1987) studied an electronics assembly plant with 700 employees. The plant came to their attention because 52 workers' compensation claims for carpal tunnel syndrome had been filed among its employees within 5 years. The authors divided the plant into high-risk and low-risk jobs. The high-risk jobs (shaker bar welding, radial welding, axial welding, and integrated line work) were reviewed and found to require highly repetitive "exertional flexion-extension-pinching motions." Workers from the high-risk jobs were more likely than workers from the low-risk jobs to have hand symptoms, positive Phalen's signs, or hand weakness.

Punnett and colleagues (1985) did a cross-sectional survey of women working in a garment sewing shop near Boston; women working in a hospital (nurses, laboratory technicians, food and laundry workers, and administrative personnel, but not typists) served as controls. Using a case definition based on a symptom questionnaire and physical examination, the prevalence of carpal tunnel syndrome was 18% in the garment workers, but only 6% in the hospital workers. Garment workers were three times more likely than hospital workers to have carpal tunnel syndrome diagnosed (95% confidence limits of relative risk were 1.2 to 7.6). Among the garment workers, incidence of carpal tunnel syndrome varied with task. The highest incidence, 5.6 times higher than hospital workers, was among lining stitchers. This job required repetitive low force wrist and fine finger movements. Underpressers, who did hand ironing requiring arm pressure but less movement at the wrists and fingers, were only 1.5 times more likely than hospital workers to develop carpal tunnel syndrome.

A cross-sectional study of workers in a ski manufacture plant compared those doing repetitive or sustained wrist flexion, extension, or radial or ulnar deviation or pinch-type grip with those not doing repetitive activity (Barnhart, Demers, Miller, Longstreth & Rosenstock, 1991). Workers in repetitive tasks were 3.95 times more likely to develop carpal tunnel syndrome than those in nonrepetitive tasks (confidence interval 1.0 to 15.8). This conclusion was based on a definition of carpal tunnel syndrome using nerve conduction results plus an abnormal Phalen's or Tinel's sign. However, when the definition of carpal tunnel syndrome that required symptoms was used, the relative risk was only 1.63 and was not statistically significant.

A case-control study, discussed previously regarding vibration, also supported the role of repetitive activity in causation of carpal tunnel syndrome (Wieslander et al., 1989).

Temporal Relationship—Activity and Carpal Tunnel Syndrome

Those who have carpal tunnel syndrome commonly observe that symptoms are closely related in time to certain hand activities. Symptoms routinely occur with rest or sleep after those activities. Frequently, workers who have carpal tunnel syndrome can identify job tasks that are likely to make them symptomatic. They often note transient relief of symptoms on weekends or vacations. A job change can lead to complete resolution of symptoms (Gordon, Bowyer & Johnson, 1987).

There are few longitudinal studies of occupational carpal tunnel syndrome (Table 13-5). Some 77 asymptomatic workers who had mildly abnormal transcarpal median nerve conduction were followed for an average of 17 months and compared with asymptomatic age- and sex-matched coworkers who had normal nerve conduction (Werner, Franzblau, Albers, Buchele & Armstrong, 1997). At follow-up, 12% of workers with abnormal median nerve conduction and 10% of workers with normal nerve conduction had hand symptoms that might be due to carpal tunnel syndrome (not significantly different, $P = .73$). Repetition at work was graded from 0 (idle) to 10 (rapid steady motion, difficulty keeping up); each increased unit of repetition had an odds ratio of 1.35 for increased risk of development of hand symptoms.

A cohort of 16 dental hygienists was followed for 3 years after graduation from their dental hygiene training program. All were working 32 hours or more per week. Over 3 years, none had been diagnosed as having carpal tunnel syndrome, but four had hand symptoms, and the mean measures of median nerve function by vibrametry showed slight deterioration, whereas their right hand grip strength had improved (Conrad, Conrad & Osborn, 1993).

Nathan and colleagues (1992, 1998) followed 289 workers from four industries for 11 years. At the 5-year follow-up, there was no apparent relationship between the risk of developing carpal tunnel syndrome in the prior 5 years and the nature of occupational hand use. This issue was not addressed at the 11-year follow-up. Workers who had mild abnormalities of median nerve conduction (prolonged maximum serial sensory latency difference) at entrance into the study had an increased probability of developing clinical carpal

Table 13-5. Longitudinal Studies of Carpal Tunnel Syndrome and Occupation

Reference	Workers
Kearns, Gresch, Weichel, Eby & Pallapothu, 2000	Pork processors
Nathan, Keniston, Myers & Meadows, 1992; Nathan & Keniston, 1998	Varied industrial workers
Werner, Franzblau, Albers, Buchele & Armstrong, 1997	Manufacturing and clerical workers
Conrad, Conrad & Osborn, 1993	Dental hygienists

tunnel syndrome during follow-up. The prevalence of slowing increased over time, but most workers who had mild slowing at the end of the 11 years did not have symptoms of carpal tunnel syndrome, and many workers with mildly symptomatic carpal tunnel syndrome at the beginning of the study had resolution of symptoms over time without undergoing carpal tunnel surgery.

The connection between hand use and *symptoms* of carpal tunnel syndrome is unequivocal. However, whether hand use is the *cause* of the median neuropathy underlying the carpal tunnel syndrome is a more difficult question. For example, the occurrence of symptoms while driving is a common experience, but this no more proves that driving is a cause of pathology than does the prevalence of nocturnal symptoms implicate sleep as a causative factor. Nonetheless, the persuasive temporal patterns of certain activities preceding the appearance of symptoms in many individuals supports the hypothesis that hand usage can cause median nerve pathology and trigger expression of carpal tunnel syndrome. This conclusion is entirely in keeping with the mechanical cause of the nerve fiber deformity in chronic focal nerve compression (see Chapter 12).

Dose-Response Relationship

Many patients with carpal tunnel syndrome are aware of a personal dose-response relationship and can describe activities of specific nature or duration that induce their symptoms. However, only a few studies have formally examined "dose" of hand activity with development of carpal tunnel syndrome. One example of a dose effect is the greater

Table 13-6. Relative Risk of Developing Carpal Tunnel Syndrome Related to Hours per Week Spent in Wrist-Flexing Activities

Hours per Week Spent in Activities with Wrist Flexion	Relative Risk of Developing Carpal Tunnel Syndrome	95% Confidence Interval
0	1.0	—
1–7	1.5	1.3–1.9
8–19	3.0	1.8–4.9
20–40	8.7	3.1–24.1

Data from MCTFM De Krom, ADM Kester, PG Knipschild, F Spaans. Risk factors for carpal tunnel syndrome. Am. J. Epidemiol. 1990;132:1102–10.

detriment of combining forceful and repetitive activities compared with repetitive activities alone (see Figure 13-3).

De Krom and colleagues (1990) asked study participants to estimate the number of hours per week that they had participated in activities that included wrist flexion or extension in the 5 years before developing symptoms of carpal tunnel syndrome. They found that the risk of developing carpal tunnel syndrome increased as the number of hours per week with these activities increased (Table 13-6). The effect was greater for flexion activities than for extension activities.

Among the supermarket checkers, the odds ratio for development of carpal tunnel syndrome increased with more years on the job or more work hours per week (Baron et al., 1991).

Biological Plausibility

The causal relationship between mechanical activities of the hand and development of local median nerve pathology that is expressed as carpal tunnel syndrome is solidly supported by pathophysiologic observations.

Carpal Tunnel Syndrome Is Due to Focal Mechanical Nerve Compression

Carpal tunnel syndrome is a chronic focal compressive neuropathy. Pathologically, the portion of the median nerve contained within the carpal tunnel shows physical slippage of myelin lamellae in opposite directions on either end of the site of entrapment (Ochoa & Marotte, 1973; see Chapter 12 for detailed discussion). This localized nerve pathology shows the focal and mechanical nature of the pathogenic process.

Pressure in the Carpal Tunnel Increases Dynamically with Wrist and Hand Activity

Pressure increases intermittently within the carpal tunnel and often exceeds levels sufficient to injure a nerve. Chapter 12 discusses the role of carpal canal pressure in the pathogenesis of carpal tunnel syndrome. Patients with carpal tunnel syndrome frequently have elevated resting pressures in the carpal canal (Table 13-7). Pressures on the order of 30 mm Hg might not cause steady symptoms of nerve compression but do cause endoneurial edema and pathologic change in nerve (Lundborg, Myers & Powell, 1983). Even in individuals who are asymptomatic, pressures intermittently exceed these levels (same references as Table 13-7). Patients who have classic symptoms of carpal tunnel syndrome yet have normal nerve conductions often have elevated carpal canal pressures (Hamanaka, Okutsu, Shimizu, Takatori & Ninomiya, 1995).

Infrequently, patients who have unequivocal carpal tunnel syndrome by clinical and electrodiagnostic criteria have normal canal pressures (Gelberman, Hergenroeder, Hargens, Lundborg & Akeson, 1981; Rojviroj, Sirichativapee, Kowsuwon, Wongwiwattananon, Tamnanthong & Jeeravipoolvarn, 1990). Perhaps, some of them have more severe median pathology, so that neurologic deficit persists after pathogenic pressure increase has abated (Szabo & Chidgey, 1989). However, measurement technique can also affect pressure recordings; movement of the catheter through the carpal tunnel shows that pressure varies with catheter position (Luchetti, Schoenhuber & Nathan, 1998).

A number of positional and dynamic factors influence carpal canal pressure both in asymptomatic individuals and in patients who have carpal tunnel syndrome. Canal pressure increases with changes in wrist position including flexion, extension, and radial or ulnar deviation and is further affected by changes in finger posture and tendon load (Keir, Wells, Ranney & Lavery, 1997; Keir, Bach & Rempel, 1998a). Power grip can greatly increase the canal pressure in healthy subjects (mean 135 mm Hg in one study) and raise it even higher in patients who have carpal tunnel syndrome (Hamanaka et al., 1995). Regardless of wrist angle, exerting pressure with the tip of the index finger increases pressure within the carpal canal; the canal pressure increases monotonically as the pressure exerted by the finger rises from 0 to 12 N (Rempel, Keir, Smutz & Hargens, 1997). Carpal canal pressures increase more during a pinch-grasp using the tips of the thumb and index finger than during application of an equivalent finger tip pressure without pinching (Keir, Bach & Rempel, 1998b). Pressures also increase during forearm pronation and supination (Werner & Armstrong, 1997; Rempel, Bach, Gordon & So, 1998). Pressures not only increase during repetitive wrist and hand activities but can remain elevated after stopping the activity (Szabo & Chidgey, 1989).

Repetitive hand and wrist activities, such as lifting a 1-lb can out of a box every 3 seconds, typing, or using a computer mouse, can raise pressure in the carpal canal to more than 30 mm Hg, even in subjects who report no symptoms suggestive of carpal tunnel syndrome (Rempel, Manojlovic, Levinsohn, Bloom & Gordon, 1994; Keir, Bach & Rempel, 1999).

Lumbrical excursion into the carpal tunnel during finger flexion occurs commonly in healthy hands and can contribute to carpal canal pressure (Cobb, An, Cooney & Berger, 1994; Cobb, An & Cooney, 1995b). In some workers who use their hands repetitively, hypertrophy of lumbrical muscles might contribute to increases of pressure within the carpal tunnel (Siegel, Kuzma & Eakins, 1995).

The pressure of a tool against the palm of the hand can increase pressure within the carpal tunnel (Cobb, An & Cooney, 1995a). To date, our knowledge of the effect of tool handle design to carpal canal pressures is rudimentary; however, in cadaver studies gripping a 2-in. diameter handle appears to cause higher canal pressure than that generated gripping a 1-in. diameter handle (Cobb, Cooney & An, 1996).

Table 13-7. Carpal Tunnel Pressures Depend on Wrist Position in Patients with Carpal Tunnel Syndrome

Reference	Carpal Tunnel Pressure (mm Hg)		
	Wrist Neutral	Wrist Flexed	Wrist Extended
Gelberman, Hergenroeder, Hargens, Lundborg & Akeson, 1981	32	94	110
Werner, Elmqvist & Ohlin, 1983	31	75	105
Szabo & Chidgey, 1989	10	32	51
Okutsu, Ninomiya, Hamanaka, Kuroshima & Inanami, 1989	43	192	222
Luchetti, Schoenhuber & Nathan, 1998	18	50	96
Rojviroj, Sirichativapee, Kowsuwon, Wongwi-wattananon, Tamnan-thong & Jeeravi-poolvarn, 1990	12	27	33
Hamanaka, Okutsu, Shimizu, Takatori & Ninomiya, 1995	59	—	—
Seradge, Jia & Owens, 1995	44	98	119

Flexor Tenosynovial Edema and Fibrosis Result from Repetitive Activity

Tenosynovial edema and fibrosis of the flexor tendons make major contributions to the chronic increased canal pressure in carpal tunnel syndrome. In most patients who have carpal tunnel syndrome, flexor tenosynovium develops edema and fibrosis without evidence of a cellular inflammatory response (Yamaguchi, Lipscomb & Soule, 1965; Phalen, 1972; Faithfull, Moir & Ireland, 1986; Neal, McManners & Stirling, 1987; Scelsi, Zanlungo & Tenti, 1989; Schuind, Ventura & Pasteels, 1990; Kerr, Sybert & Albarracin, 1992). These histologic changes can be found at the time of carpal tunnel surgery in workers, regardless of pattern of hand use, and in housewives (Chell, Stevens & Davis, 1999). In randomly selected cadavers, fibrous tissue density of tenosynovium and epineurium is greater in the carpal tunnel than just proximal or distal to it and seems to become more prevalent with aging (Armstrong, Castelli, Evans & Diaz-Perez, 1984; Neal, et al., 1987). However, compared with controls who do not have carpal tunnel syndrome, patients who have carpal tunnel syndrome have more extensive tenosynovial pathology within the carpal tunnel (Fuchs, Nathan & Myers, 1991).

A common cause of the flexor tendon edema is probably repetitive finger and wrist use. In rabbits, repetitive wrist and digit flexion induced by median nerve stimulation at 80 Hz for 10 hours led to edema within the carpal tunnel and to slowed median nerve conduction across the carpal tunnel (Andersson, 1970). After 1 day of nerve stimulation, both the edema and the slowing of nerve conduction disappeared within 96 hours. If the flexor retinaculum was sectioned before the period of repetitive stimulation, the mechanical activity still elicited synovial edema, but median nerve conduction was not slowed.

Peripheral nerves are capable of longitudinal gliding in response to joint movement. The median nerve proximal to the carpal tunnel normally glides 1.5 cm or more during the movement from full wrist flexion to full wrist extension (McLellan & Swash, 1976; Wilgis & Murphy, 1986; Wright, Glowczewskie, Wheeler, Miller & Cowin, 1996). The nerve also moves during finger flexion and extension (Bay, Sharkey & Szabo, 1997). The extent of nerve gliding can be estimated by comparing nerve conduction latencies in different joint positions; using this technique, in comparison with asymptomatic individuals, patients who have carpal tunnel syndrome have impaired movement of the median nerve but not of the ulnar nerve (Valls-Solé, Alvarez & Nuñez, 1995). In an experimental cadaver model, changes in carpal canal pressure did not influence median nerve gliding (Bay et al., 1997). However, chronic fibrosis and edema in the canal might account for this impaired nerve gliding and contribute to nerve pathology.

Individuals Vary in Their Susceptibility to Carpal Tunnel Syndrome

Any theory linking carpal tunnel syndrome to job activity needs to consider variations in individual susceptibility to development of carpal tunnel syndrome, the dissociation between the pathology of median nerve compression and the symptoms of carpal tunnel syndrome, and the amount of activity necessary to cause the syndrome.

The guinea pig model of plantar nerve compression, a parallel of median nerve compression in the carpal tunnel, illustrates the combined roles of individual susceptibility and exposure to trauma in development of carpal tunnel syndrome. Guinea pigs characteristically develop electrophysiologic and pathologic evidence of focal compression of the plantar nerves of the hind foot after prolonged housing in cages with wire mesh floors but not after housing on solid floors (Fullerton & Gilliatt, 1965). The animals become more susceptible if injected with an agent that causes demyelination, like diphtheria toxin, but even then the focal compressive neuropathy can be prevented by suspending the animals so that their hind legs do not touch the floors (Hopkins & Morgan-Hughes, 1969).

Among a group of workers performing a task, only a fraction develops carpal tunnel syndrome. In a small percentage of patients, an underlying medical illness or condition such as diabetes, rheumatoid arthritis, acromegaly, hypothyroidism, obesity, or pregnancy helps explain their susceptibility to median nerve compression. In most other patients, the susceptibility is not as readily explained.

Hypothetically, congenitally small carpal canals might predispose to median nerve compression and, with sufficient hand use, to symptomatic carpal tunnel syndrome. Some computed tomographic scan measurements of the cross-sectional area of the carpal tunnel support this hypothesis, but there are contradictory data on the relationship between carpal canal size and risk of development of carpal tunnel syndrome (Bleecker, Bohlman, Moreland & Tipton, 1985; Winn & Habes, 1990; Tan & Tan, 1998).

Gordon and colleagues (1988) have suggested that at least some members of the susceptible subpopulation can be identified by the ratio of wrist anteroposterior diameter to mediolateral diameter measured at the distal wrist crease. New workers in whom this ratio was greater than or equal to 0.70 were more likely to develop carpal tunnel syndrome symptoms within the first year of employment. The value of wrist ratio measurement in pre-

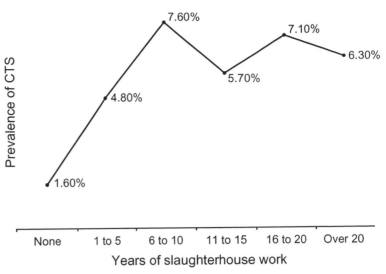

Figure 13-4. Prevalence of carpal tunnel syndrome (CTS) among slaughterhouse workers varies based on years of work exposure. (Data from P Frost, JH Andersen, VK Nielsen. Occurrence of carpal tunnel syndrome among slaughterhouse workers. Scand. J. Work Environ. Health 1998;24:285–92.)

employment screening remains unconfirmed (Wyles & Rodriquez, 1991).

The existence of a subpopulation of workers who are more susceptible to development of carpal tunnel syndrome might explain the finding in some series that the prevalence of carpal tunnel syndrome is higher in workers with fewer years on the job (Falck & Aarnio, 1983; not confirmed in all series, see Cannon et al., 1981; Margolis & Kraus, 1987). In some settings, there is a *survivor effect* or *healthy worker effect*, whereby more susceptible workers become symptomatic and change jobs, whereas less susceptible workers remain asymptomatic and become veteran employees (Morgenstern, Kelsh, Kraus & Margolis, 1991). For example, among slaughterhouse workers, the risk of having carpal tunnel syndrome increases during the early years of employment and then levels off or decreases slightly (Figure 13-4) (Frost, Andersen & Nielsen, 1998).

Pathology versus Symptoms

Asymptomatic median nerve abnormalities at wrist level are common and can be demonstrated both pathologically and by nerve conduction studies (Neary, Ochoa & Gilliatt, 1975; Nathan, Meadows & Doyle, 1988b). Is it possible that those people who have mild nerve conduction abnormalities are the susceptible subpopulation and inevitably

develop carpal tunnel syndrome (barring premature death), and that work activities simply make their condition symptomatic? There are still relatively few long-term data on the natural history of these mild asymptomatic abnormalities, but a few longitudinal nerve conduction studies suggest that these abnormalities are not rapidly progressive (Nathan, Keniston, Myers, Meadows & Lockwood, 1998). The incidence of very mild abnormalities, more than 20% in the series by Nathan et al. (1988b) and more than 40% in the study of pathology by Neary and colleagues (1975), far exceeds the incidence of carpal tunnel syndrome in epidemiologic studies, so many individuals with mild asymptomatic abnormalities remain asymptomatic for years. If they develop persistent symptoms of carpal tunnel syndrome, they usually have nerve injury and dysfunction in excess of the mild pathology.

Occupational Examples

Two different work settings illustrate the quality of data and the uncertainties linking occupation to carpal tunnel syndrome. The meat and poultry processing industry is one with a high prevalence of carpal tunnel syndrome and other upper-extremity disorders. In contrast, keyboard use has a lower risk of causing carpal tunnel syndrome, and in cross-sectional studies, clerical or office personnel often serve as the low-risk group for calculating risk ratios.

Meat and Poultry Processors

Masear and colleagues (1986) described a meat packing plant in Illinois in which 15% of the employees underwent carpal tunnel release over 12 years. Carpal tunnel syndrome, severe enough to require surgical therapy, had developed in 19% of workers boning meat cooled to 3°C, an activity that required bilateral repetitive wrist motions including extreme flexion and ulnar deviation. In comparison, 4% of workers on the loading dock or in sanitation had had carpal tunnel surgery. Of the 117 employees who had carpal tunnel syndrome, 64 had bilateral surgery. Most of the workers who underwent unilateral carpal tunnel syndrome had it in their dominant hand. The authors concluded that wrist motions during meat cutting contributed to the high incidence of carpal tunnel syndrome among the workers.

The study was retrospective and not formally controlled. The authors cited a meat packing plant in a different state with a much lower prevalence of carpal tunnel syndrome than in the plant that they studied. They questioned what roles worker awareness of carpal tunnel syndrome and size of worker's compensation benefits played in explaining differences in prevalence.

Falck and Aarnio (1983) studied 17 butchers in two slaughterhouses in a Finnish town. In these plants, the butchers usually used their knives or other tools in their dominant right hand, while using the left hand to grasp, lift, or tear the carcass. The prevalence of symptomatic carpal tunnel syndrome was 4 of 17 in the right hand and 9 of 17 in the left hand. In the cases with bilateral symptoms, the right hand was always less severely affected. Falck and Aarnio proposed that vigorous use of the nondominant hand explained the paradoxical location of carpal tunnel syndrome in these workers.

In another meat packing plant the prevalence of carpal tunnel syndrome, diagnosed on clinic criteria without obtaining electrodiagnostic studies, was 21% (Gorsche, Wiley, Renger, Brant, Gemer & Sasyniuk, 1999). Workers who did not have carpal tunnel syndrome were followed over a number

of months; the incidence rate of new cases of carpal tunnel syndrome was 9.7 cases per 100 person-years for men and 18.4 for women.

In a cross-sectional comparison between slaughterhouse workers and chemical factory workers, carpal tunnel syndrome was diagnosed based on combined clinical and electrodiagnostic abnormalities or on a history of having undergone carpal tunnel surgery (Frost et al., 1998). Compared with chemical factory workers, slaughterhouse workers who did deboning had an adjusted odds ratio of 5.53 for carpal tunnel syndrome and slaughterhouse workers who did work other than deboning had an adjusted odds ratio of 3.25.

A longitudinal study examined median and ulnar nerve conduction in pork processors before and after 2 months of employment. After 2 months on the job, median distal sensory and motor latencies and median-ulnar latency differences had increased, but ulnar nerve function had not changed significantly (Kearns, Gresch, Weichel, Eby & Pallapothu, 2000). The changes were greater in the dominant than in the nondominant hands.

Keyboarding

Keyboard and mouse use are frequent tasks in the modern computer-intensive office, and the popular perception is that these activities frequently cause carpal tunnel syndrome. The U.S. Department of Labor, Bureau of Labor Statistics reported that in 1996, 29,937 American workers lost time from work due to carpal tunnel syndrome; 586 of these were data-entry keyers (McDiarmid, Oliver, Ruser & Gucer, 2000). The annual incidence of carpal tunnel syndrome was higher among data-entry personnel than for the average worker (Table 13-8).

During typing, carpal tunnel pressures increase, especially if the typing is done with wrists extended 30 degrees or more or flexed 15 degrees (Rempel, 1995). Ulnar deviation while typing can also increase carpal tunnel pressure. Pressure in the carpal tunnel can increase while using a computer mouse (Keir et al., 1999).

Based on workers' compensation surveillance data from Wisconsin, data entry operators had a 12.2 odds ratio for developing carpal tunnel syndrome, but the referent group, other workers' compensation claimants, biases the result (Hanrahan, Higgins, Anderson, Haskins & Tai, 1991).

A study of women doing word processing at a university compared 45 who had carpal tunnel syndrome and 55 who did not (Matias, Salvendy & Kuczek, 1998). After control for anthropometric features and work posture, duration of the day spent at the keyboard predicated probability of having carpal tunnel syndrome; the relationship was monotonic but not linear, so that the risk of developing carpal tunnel syndrome was relatively low for those working at the keyboard less than 2 hours per day and increased most rapidly between 2 and 5 hours per day of keyboard work.

A study compared Japanese women who spent an average of 6 hours per day entering data to age- and sex-matched controls; neither workers nor controls had clinical carpal tunnel syndrome. The data-entry workers had significant slowing of transcarpal median nerve conduction compared with the controls (Murata, Araki, Okajima & Saito, 1996).

Other data are less supportive of an association between keyboarding and development of carpal tunnel syndrome. Some population studies have failed to find a statistically significant association between keyboard use and development of carpal tunnel syndrome (Koller & Blank, 1980; Nordstrom, Vierkant, DeStefano & Layde, 1997). Other surveys of keyboard users have covered varied upper-extremity musculoskeletal complaints but failed to provide sufficient data on the relation of the activity to carpal tunnel syndrome (Bernard, Sauter, Fine, Petersen & Hales, 1994; Hales, Sauter, Peterson, Fine, Putz-Anderson, Schleifer & Ochs, 1994; Tittiranonda, Burastero & Rempel, 1999). Both psychosocial factors in the workplace and local variations in medical practice can affect perceived incidence of carpal tunnel syndrome among workers (Hadler, 1992). A meta-analysis concluded that the relative risk of upper-extremity musculoskeletal disorders was between 2 and 3 for those who used keyboards at least 4 hours per day compared with nonkeyboarding or low-keyboarding clerical workers; the presumably smaller risk of developing carpal tunnel syndrome could not be determined (Punnett, 1995). An uncontrolled survey of Mayo Clinic employees found that the prevalence of carpal tunnel syndrome among frequent computer users was close to that reported in other

Table 13-8. Age-Adjusted 1996 Incidence of Carpal Tunnel Syndrome per 100,000 Full-Time Employees

Occupation	Male Incidence of Carpal Tunnel Syndrome	Female Incidence of Carpal Tunnel Syndrome
Data entry keyers	117	110
All occupations	16	52

Data from M McDiarmid, M Oliver, J Ruser, P Gucer. Male and female rate differences in carpal tunnel syndrome injuries: personal attributes or job tasks? Environ. Res. 2000;83:23–32.

populations (Stevens, Witt, Smith & Weaver, 2001). In summary, prolonged keyboard work is probably a risk factor for development of carpal tunnel syndrome, but the risk appears lower than for other more hand-intensive occupations.

Clinical Care of the Worker Who Has Carpal Tunnel Syndrome

Diagnosis

Treatment of occupational carpal tunnel syndrome begins with precise diagnosis. The principles of diagnosis for workers who have hand and arm symptoms are the same as those for nonworkers and have been reviewed in previous chapters. The diagnostic criteria used for epidemiologic studies cannot be used dogmatically for care of individuals. Nearly 20% of women and a smaller fraction of men frequently experience hand paresthesias, yet most of these neither have carpal tunnel syndrome severe enough to be unequivocally diagnosed nor require aggressive treatment (see Chapter 3 for epidemiology and Chapter 14 for treatment indications). More than 8% of adults had had new onset forearm pain in the week preceding a general population survey; the pain was more common in those who had more diffuse somatic symptoms, were dissatisfied with their colleagues or supervisors, or did repetitive arm or wrist movements (Macfarlane, Hunt & Silman, 2000). There will always be some individuals whose hand symptoms defy precise diagnosis and for whom this diagnostic uncertainty will be a factor in planning treatment. Many workers with carpal tunnel syndrome have additional musculoskeletal upper-extremity conditions, so that diagnosis and treatment of these conditions are important aspects of their care.

Assessing Relationship to Occupation

When a worker has carpal tunnel syndrome, assessing the relationship of the condition to occupation begins with a careful occupational history. In addition to the worker's job title, specific occupational factors, such as nature of hand and arm use on the job, years on the job, hours worked per week, and temporal relationship of symptoms to work and vacation times, should be considered. At times, observation of the job task or ergonomic analysis of the job site is needed. History and physical examination should also encompass other factors that might cause or contribute to the development of carpal tunnel syndrome, including avocational hand and arm use, medical conditions that might predispose to development of carpal tunnel syndrome, and personal factors, such as gender, age, and body mass index (Nathan & Keniston, 1998).

The risk of developing carpal tunnel syndrome varies markedly from industry to industry and task to task. The highest risks for developing carpal tunnel syndrome are for work with vibrating tools and repetitive wrist and finger motion, especially when combined with higher force requirements.

Psychosocial Factors

The symptoms of carpal tunnel syndrome, like those of every medical condition, are modified by psychosocial factors. Workers are more likely to seek medical attention for carpal tunnel syndrome if they are dissatisfied by their work, lack job control, or have little influence at work (Nordstrom et al., 1997; Leclerc, Franchi, Cristofari, Delemotte, Mereau, Teyssier-Cotte & Touranchet, 1998). In part, this reflects the uninspiring nature of repetitive manual work. Workers are more likely to complain of symptoms of carpal tunnel syndrome if they work without breaks

and without task rotation (Roquelaure, Mechali, Dano, Fanello, Benetti, Bureau, Mariel, Martin, Derriennic & Penneau-Fontbonne, 1997). A study of carpal tunnel syndrome in Japanese furniture workers found a much lower prevalence of carpal tunnel syndrome in Japanese than in comparable American workers, despite similarities in median nerve conduction and speculated that cultural differences accounted for this difference (Nathan, Takigawa, Keniston, Meadows & Lockwood, 1994).

Treatment

The general principles of treatment of carpal tunnel syndrome, reviewed in Chapters 14 and 15, apply equally to occupational and nonoccupational carpal tunnel syndrome. The prognosis is good for workers undergoing carpal tunnel surgery, but is slightly worse than the prognosis for nonworkers (see Chapter 15, e.g., Tables 15-12 and 15-14). Nonetheless, a small fraction of workers (8% of those undergoing carpal tunnel surgery in Washington State) are disabled longer than 1 year after carpal tunnel surgery (Adams, Franklin & Barnhart, 1994). For musculoskeletal injuries in general, prognosis for return to work is worse once workers have lost 6 months or more of time from work. In some states patients who file workers' compensation claims for carpal tunnel syndrome can face long delays in receiving professional care, claims adjudication, or authorization for treatment (Herbert, Janeway & Schechter, 1999). The Washington State Department of Labor and Industries, as an occupational health pilot project, has developed by expert consensus a schedule of quality indicators for clinical care of workers who have carpal tunnel syndrome. This facilitates proceeding to carpal tunnel surgery, when indicated, within 4 months of presentation for medical care (Table 13-9). As discussed in Chapter 14, many workers have mild carpal tunnel syndrome that does not require surgical care; however, in addition to the usual indications for surgical assessment (see Chapter 14, Table 14-1), any worker who is *missing work* because of hand and arm symptoms needs prompt assessment for possible carpal tunnel syndrome and consideration of timely carpal tunnel surgery if the diagnosis is established as the cause of time loss.

Table 13-9. Schedule of Clinical Process to Improve Quality of Care for Occupational Carpal Tunnel Syndrome

Clinical Care Action	Time Frame
Early screen for presence/absence of carpal tunnel syndrome	First health care visit*
Documented history of physical work and non-work exposures	First or second health care visit
Determination of work-relatedness	First or second health care visit
Activity prescription	Each visit
Communication with employer regarding return to work	First health care visit
Referral to specialist if no RTW or clinical improvement	6 wks
Specialist visit	Within 1–3 wks of referral
Nerve conduction studies	Terminal latency within 2 wks of consideration of surgery
Referral for assessment of RTW impediments	4–6 wks
Surgical decompression	Within 4–6 wks of determination of need for surgery
Ergonomist assessment of work site	Within 2 wks of first health care visit to (1) assist with work modification and (2) determine if physical hazards may put other workers at risk for carpal tunnel syndrome

RTW = return to work.
*The timing column is anchored in time from claim filing or first provider visit related to carpal tunnel syndrome complaints.
Adapted with permission from RB Rosenbaum, G Franklin, DC Clemmons, RT Fraser, M Hennessey, PD Rumrill. Occupational Neurology. Continuum 2001;7:1–136.

Prevention of Occupational Carpal Tunnel Syndrome

The ergonomic method promises an approach to prevention of carpal tunnel syndrome (Armstrong, 1983; Feldman, Goldman & Keyserling, 1983; Cohen, Gjessing, Fine, Bernard & McGlothin, 1997). It starts with a thorough analysis of tasks and tools, looking for those aspects of a job that might contribute to tenosynovial or nerve irritation or lead to increases in carpal canal pressure.

Tichauer and Gage (1977) recommend paying attention to a number of features of hand tool design: optimization of tool forces with good sensory feedback from the tool, distribution of tool contact pressures, use of appropriate work gloves, promotion of optimal postures and motions, and matching tool size to the worker. These principles can translate to some clever adaptations, such as angling the handle of a hammer so that the worker can use the tool with less ulnar wrist deviation (Schoenmarklin & Marras, 1989). Changes in the work task and workstation can also minimize abnormal wrist postures or decrease the need for repetitive movements (Armstrong, 1983). Table 13-10 summarizes some job modifications that might help prevent carpal tunnel syndrome.

The value of ergonomic intervention for prevention of carpal tunnel syndrome has not been rigorously established. Armstrong and colleagues (1982) surveyed a poultry processing plant, using both film and electromyographic data to provide detail on the hand and arm movements required for turkey boning. They then recommended changes in the workers' tools and techniques and in the design of the workstations to minimize hand stresses. They provide no data on the effectiveness of their proposed changes. Feldman and colleagues (1987) proposed ergonomic improvements in an electronics assembly plant to prevent carpal tunnel syndrome but were unable to implement, let alone assess, the changes that they proposed.

Table 13-10. Prevention of Carpal Tunnel Syndrome

Task	Tools
Match worker to job	Keep wrist straight
Improve workstations	Optimize center of gravity
Avoid pinching, wring-	Maximize mechanical advantage
ing, grasping	Avoid palmar pressure
Reduce task frequency	Encourage ambidexterity
Rotate tasks	
Schedule regular breaks	
Use appropriate gloves	
and padding	

Modified from RG Feldman, R Goldman, WM Keyserling. Classical syndromes in occupational medicine. Peripheral nerve entrapment syndromes and ergonomic factors. Am. J. Ind. Med. 1983;4:661–81.

Analysis of a telecommunications manufacturing facility led to modifications in a number of hand tool operations (McKenzie, Storment, Van-Hook & Armstrong, 1985). The following year, the number of workdays lost due to reportable arm-cumulative-trauma disorders dropped precipitously. McKenzie and colleagues did not separate carpal tunnel syndrome from other causes of hand and arm symptoms. They emphasized that their study was not controlled and that the drop in incidence of disorders might not have been attributable to their intervention.

A variety of studies have reported multidisciplinary interventions in industrial settings. For example, a program in an assembly plant included worker education, early diagnosis and job reassignment for symptomatic workers, and ergonomic changes (Chatterjee, 1992). After the program was implemented, the incidence of claims for occupational upper-extremity disorders was decreased. In general, these studies are uncontrolled and either provide no separate data on incidence of carpal tunnel syndrome or fail to show effect of the program on carpal tunnel syndrome (Lincoln, Vernick, Ogaitis, Smith, Mitchell & Agnew, 2000).

A number of variations in mouse or keyboard design have been proposed to decrease risk of development of carpal tunnel syndrome, but they have not been shown to prevent or modify carpal tunnel syndrome in actual occupational settings (Rempel, Tittiranonda, Burastero, Hudes & So, 1999; Lincoln et al., 2000).

Wearing a flexible wrist splint during repetitive hand activity limits wrist range of motion, but has no significant effect on carpal tunnel pressure and no proven value for prevention or treatment of carpal tunnel syndrome (Rempel et al., 1994).

A meat packing company required all employees to perform an arm warm-up exercise program, lasting just over 3 minutes, at the start of each workday. In the year before beginning the program, 40 cases of carpal tunnel syndrome were reported among employees; in the first year of the program, 25 cases of carpal tunnel syndrome were reported (Seradge, Bear & Bithell, 2000). A controlled study of on-the-job strength and flexibility exercises did not find evidence that the exercises prevented carpal tunnel syndrome, but the study was possibly too brief and underpowered (Lincoln et al., 2000).

The Occupational Safety and Health Administration (OSHA) has issued a final Ergonomics Program standard (29 CFR 1910.900) that requires employers to institute ergonomics programs for any job for which an employee has reported developing carpal tunnel syndrome (or other musculoskeletal disorder) and is exposed to risk factors such as vibration and repetitive or forceful activity (OSHA, 2000). The Ergonomics Program standard specifies the severity of the worker's carpal tunnel syndrome and the nature of the risk factors that together mandate institution of the ergonomics program. The program affects over 6 million employers and 102 million employees in the United States. Its effectiveness is debated (Hadler, 2000; Punnett, 2000). OSHA estimates that the standard can prevent 4.6 million work-related musculoskeletal disorders in the next decade. However, the value of ergonomic interventions for primary prevention of occupational carpal tunnel syndrome is unproven.

Medical-Legal Issues

There have been hundreds of court rulings on the causal relationship between numerous occupations and carpal tunnel syndrome. In addition to workers' compensation claims, carpal tunnel syndrome is a potential issue in litigation involving claims of product liability, regulatory violation, disability, unfair labor practices, breach of warranty, misrepresentation, and medical malpractice (Owen, 1994). We shall not review this body of law, but we will mention legal issues that arise for physicians who participate in the care and evaluation of workers who have carpal tunnel syndrome.

When an individual worker develops carpal tunnel syndrome, the workers' compensation system often queries the physician as to the causal relation between the worker's job activities and the development of the syndrome. An informed and well-reasoned medical opinion is essential, because courts, in determining causation, usually rely heavily on medical experts. Analysis of these questions can be challenging; for example, the worker might have had more than one employer, have vigorous avocational hand use, have worked on a job for only a brief period of time, or have personal and anthropometric characteristics or underlying medical conditions that predispose to development of carpal tunnel syndrome. Often, the employers and insurers will offer assistance in these difficult exposure assessments.

Before considering causation, the physician must ascertain that the diagnosis of carpal tunnel syndrome is correct. Epidemics of ill-defined hand complaints can occur in the workplace. Miller and Topliss (1988), studying an epidemic of hand symptoms among Australian workers, found that carpal tunnel syndrome was rarely the cause of their complaints, and many of the workers had no demonstrable pathology.

When rendering an opinion on causation, the physician should assess the worker's vocational and avocational activities with attention to the extent of repetitive hand and wrist use, wrist and grip force, palmar pressure, cold exposure, and vibration exposure. The existence of any medical condition predisposing to carpal tunnel syndrome should be considered. The prevalence of carpal tunnel syndrome in the worker's colleagues is of potential import, but too often this information is anecdotal at best.

The temporal relationship between the suspect activities and symptoms of carpal tunnel syndrome often provides relevant clues to answering the difficult question of causation. The occurrence of symptoms during work, at night, or rest after work is important. Timing of symptoms in relation to changes in job tasks, vacations, days off, and changes in employment can also be relevant.

At times, a careful occupational history establishes that the patient's occupation is the probable, major contributing cause of the carpal tunnel syndrome. In other patients, the carpal tunnel syndrome has nonoccupational causes, or the role of occupation in the genesis of the carpal tunnel syndrome is equivocal.

Summary

Occupational hand use is a common cause of carpal tunnel syndrome. In the last decade, epidemiologic and pathophysiologic evidence for occupational causation of many cases of carpal tunnel syndrome has accumulated. Assessment, treatment, and prevention of occupational carpal tunnel syndrome remains challenging.

References

Abbas MA, Afifi AA, Zhang ZW, Kraus JF. Meta-analysis of published studies of work-related carpal tunnel syndrome. Int. J. Occup. Environ. Health 1998;4:160–67.

Abbas MF, Faris RH, Harber PI, Mishriky AM, El-Shahaly HA, Waheeb YH, Kraus JF. Worksite and personal factors associated with carpal tunnel syndrome in an Egyptian electronics assembly factory. Int. J. Occup. Environ. Health 2001;7:31–36.

Adams ML, Franklin GM, Barnhart S. Outcome of carpal tunnel surgery in Washington State workers' compensation. Am. J. Ind. Med. 1994;25:527–36.

Alaranta H, Seppalainen AM. Neuropathy and the automatic analysis of electromyographic signals from vibration exposed workers. Scand. J. Work Environ. Health 1977;3:128–34.

Aljure J, Eltorai I, Bradley WE, Lin JE, Johnson B. Carpal tunnel syndrome in paraplegic patients. Paraplegia 1985;23:182–86.

Alvarez N, Larkin C, Roxborough J. Carpal tunnel syndrome in athetoid-dystonic cerebral palsy. Arch. Neurol. 1982;39:311–12.

Andersson A. Reaction in the tissues of the carpal tunnel after repeated contractions of the muscles innervated by the median nerve. An experimental investigation on the rabbit. Scand. J. Plast. Reconstr. Surg. 1970;14:3–67.

Armstrong TJ. An Ergonomics Guide to Carpal Tunnel Syndrome. Akron, OH: American Industrial Hygiene Association, 1983.

Armstrong TJ, Castelli WA, Evans FG, Diaz-Perez R. Some histological changes in carpal tunnel contents and their biomechanical implications. J. Occup. Med. 1984;26:197–201.

Armstrong TJ, Chaffin DB. Carpal tunnel syndrome and selected personal attributes. J. Occup. Med. 1979;21:481–86.

Armstrong TJ, Foulke JA, Joseph BS, Goldstein SA. Investigation of cumulative trauma disorders in a poultry processing plant. Am. Ind. Hyg. Assoc. J. 1982;43:103–16.

Armstrong TJ, Silverstein BA. Upper-extremity pain in the workplace—role of usage in causality. In: Hadler NM, ed. Clinical Concepts in Regional Musculoskeletal Illness. Orlando, FL: Grune & Stratton, 1987;333–54.

Barnhart S, Demers PA, Miller M, Longstreth WT, Rosenstock L. Carpal tunnel syndrome among ski manufacturing workers. Scand. J. Work Environ. Health 1991;17:46–52.

Baron S, Milliron M, Habes D, Fidler A. Health Hazard Evaluation Report. HETA 88-344-2092, Shoprite Supermarkets New Jersey–New York, 1991.

Bay BK, Sharkey NA, Szabo RM. Displacement and strain of the median nerve at the wrist. J. Hand Surg. 1997;22A:621–27.

Bernard BP, ed. Musculoskeletal Disorders and Workplace Factors. Cincinnati: National Institute for Occupational Safety and Health, 1997.

Bernard B, Sauter S, Fine L, Petersen M, Hales T. Job task and psychosocial risk factors for work-related musculoskeletal disorders among newspaper employees. Scand. J. Work Environ. Health 1994;20:417–26.

Birkbeck MQ, Beer TC. Occupation in relation to the carpal tunnel syndrome. Rheumatol. Rehabil. 1975;14:218–21.

Bleecker ML, Bohlman M, Moreland R, Tipton A. Carpal tunnel syndrome: role of carpal canal size. Neurology 1985;35:1599–1604.

Bostrom L, Gothe CJ, Hansson S, Lugnegard H, Nilsson BY. Surgical treatment of carpal tunnel syndrome in patients exposed to vibration from handheld tools. Scand. J. Plast. Reconstr. Surg. Hand Surg. 1994;28:147–49.

Bovenzi M, Italian Study Group on Physical Hazards in the Stone Industry. Hand-arm vibration syndrome and dose-response relation for vibration induced white finger among quarry drillers and stonecarvers. Occup. Environ. Med. 1994;51:603–11.

Bovenzi M, Zadini A, Franzinelli A, Borgogni F. Occupational musculoskeletal disorders in the neck and upper limbs of forestry workers exposed to hand-arm vibration. Ergonomics 1991;34:547–62.

Boyle JC, Smith NJ, Burke FD. Vibration white finger. J. Hand Surg. 1988;13B:171–76.

Brain WR, Wright AD, Wilkinson M. Spontaneous compression of both median nerves in the carpal tunnel. Lancet 1947;1:277–82.

Braithwaite IJ. Bilateral median nerve palsy in a cyclist. Br. J. Sports Med. 1992;26:27–28.

Brammer AJ, Pyykko I. Vibration-induced neuropathy. Detection by nerve conduction measurements. Scand. J. Work Environ. Health 1987;13:317–22.

Brammer AJ, Taylor W. Vibration effects on the hand and arm in industry. In: Brammer AJ, Taylor W, eds. Vibration Effects on the Hand and Arm in Industry. New York: John Wiley & Sons, 1988;1–11.

Cannon LJ, Bernacki EJ, Walter SD. Personal and occupational factors associated with carpal tunnel syndrome. J. Occup. Med. 1981;23:255–58.

Charness ME. Unique Upper Extremity Disorders of Musicians. In: Millender LH, Louis DS, Simmons BP, eds. Occupational Disorders of the Upper Extremity. New York: Churchill Livingstone, 1992;227–52.

Chatterjee DS. Workplace upper limb disorders: a prospective study with intervention. Occupational Medicine: State of the Art Reviews 1992;42:129–236.

Chatterjee DS, Barwick DD, Petrie A. Exploratory electromyography in the study of vibration-induced white finger in rock drillers. Br. J. Ind. Med. 1982;39:89–97.

Chell J, Stevens A, Davis TRC. Work practices and histopathological changes in the tenosynovium and flexor retinaculum in carpal tunnel syndrome in women. J. Bone Joint Surg. 1999;81B:868–70.

Chiang HC, Chen SS, Yu HS, Ko YC. The occurrence of carpal tunnel syndrome in frozen food factory employees. Kaohsiung J. Med. Sci. 1990;6:73–80.

Chiang HC, Ko YC, Chen SS, Yu HS, Wu TN, Chang PY. Prevalence of shoulder and upper-limb disorders among workers in the fish-processing industry. Scand. J. Work Environ. Health 1993;19:126–31.

Cobb TK, An KN, Cooney WP. Externally applied forces to the palm increase carpal canal pressure. J. Hand Surg. 1995a;20A:181–85.

Cobb TK, An KN, Cooney WP. Effect of lumbrical muscle incursion within the carpal tunnel on carpal tunnel pressure: a cadaveric study. J. Hand Surg. 1995b;20A:186–92.

Cobb TK, An KN, Cooney WP, Berger RA. Lumbrical muscle incursion into the carpal tunnel during finger flexion. J. Hand Surg. 1994;19B:434–38.

Cobb TK, Cooney WP, An KN. Aetiology of work-related carpal tunnel syndrome: the role of lumbrical muscles and tool size on carpal tunnel pressures. Ergonomics 1996;39:103–7.

Cohen AL, Gjessing CC, Fine LJ, Bernard BP, McGlothin JD. Elements of Ergonomics Programs. A Primer Based on Workplace Evaluations of Musculoskeletal Disorders. Cincinnati: National Institute for Occupational Safety and Health, 1997.

Conrad JC, Conrad KJ, Osborn JB. A short-term epidemiological study of median nerve dysfunction in practicing dental hygienists. J. Dent. Hyg. 1992;66:76–80.

Conrad JC, Conrad KJ, Osborn JB. A short-term, three-year epidemiological study of median nerve sensitivity in practicing dental hygienists. J. Dent. Hyg. 1993;67:268–72.

Daniell WE, Fulton-Kehoe D, Bradley CM, Franklin GM. Occupational carpal tunnel syndrome in Washington State, 1986–1994. Neurology 1998;50:A56–57.

Davidoff G, Werner R, Waring W. Compressive mononeuropathies of the upper extremity in chronic paraplegia. Paraplegia 1991;1:17–24.

Davis L, Wellman H, Punnett L. Surveillance of work-related carpal tunnel syndrome in Massachusetts, 1992-1997: a report from the Massachusetts Sentinel Event Notification System for Occupational Risks (SENSOR). Am. J. Ind. Med. 2001;39:58–71.

De Krom MCTFM, Kester ADM, Knipschild PG, Spaans F. Risk factors for carpal tunnel syndrome. Am. J. Epidemiol. 1990;132:1102–10.

Dent JA, Hadden WA. Not a routine case of carpal tunnel syndrome. J. R. Coll. Surg. Edinb. 1992;37:346–47.

Dozono K, Hachisuka K, Hatada K, Ogata H. Peripheral neuropathies in the upper extremities of paraplegic wheel-chair marathon racers. Paraplegia 1995;33:208–11.

Ekenvall L, Nilsson BY, Gustavsson P. Temperature and vibration thresholds in vibration syndrome. Br. J. Ind. Med. 1986;43:825–29.

English CJ, Maclaren WM, Court-Brown C, Hughes SP, Porter RW, Wallace WA, Graves RJ, Pethick AJ, Soutar CA. Relations between upper limb soft tissue disorders and repetitive movements at work. Am. J. Ind. Med. 1995;27: 75–90.

Faithfull DK, Moir DH, Ireland J. The micropathology of the typical carpal tunnel syndrome. J. Hand Surg. 1986; 11B:131–32.

Falck B, Aarnio P. Left-sided carpal tunnel syndrome in butchers. Scand. J. Work Environ. Health 1983;9:291–97.

Farkkila M, Pyykko I, Jantti V, Aatola S, Starck J, Korhonen O. Forestry workers exposed to vibration: a neurological study. Br. J. Ind. Med. 1988;45:188–92.

Feldman RG, Goldman R, Keyserling WM. Classical syndromes in occupational medicine. Peripheral nerve entrapment syndromes and ergonomic factors. Am. J. Ind. Med. 1983;4:661–81.

Feldman RG, Travers PH, Chirico-Post J, Keyserling WM. Risk assessment in electronic assembly workers: carpal tunnel syndrome. J. Hand Surg. 1987;12A:849–55.

Fletcher RH, Fletcher SW, Wagner EH. Clinical Epidemiology, the Essentials. Baltimore: Williams & Wilkins, 1982.

Franklin GM, Haug J, Heyer N, Checkoway H, Peck N. Occupational carpal tunnel syndrome in Washington State, 1984–1988. Am. J. Public Health 1991;81:741–46.

Franklin GM, Haug JA, Peck NB, Heyer N, Checkoway H. Occupational carpal tunnel syndrome in Washington state, 1984–1987. Neurology 1990;40:420.

Frost P, Andersen JH, Nielsen VK. Occurrence of carpal tunnel syndrome among slaughterhouse workers. Scand. J. Work Environ. Health 1998;24:285–92.

Fuchs PC, Nathan PA, Myers LD. Synovial histology in carpal tunnel syndrome. J. Hand Surg. 1991;16A:753–58.

Fullerton PM, Gilliatt RW. Changes in nerve conduction in caged guinea pigs. J. Physiol. 1965;178:47–48P.

Gelberman RH, Hergenroeder PT, Hargens AR, Lundborg GN, Akeson WH. The carpal tunnel syndrome. A study of carpal canal pressures. J. Bone Joint Surg. 1981;63A:380–83.

Gellman H, Sie I, Waters RL. Late complications of the weight-bearing upper extremity in the paraplegic patient. Clin. Orthop. 1988;132–35.

Gerwatowski LJ, McFall DB, Stach DJ. Carpal tunnel syndrome. Risk factors and preventive strategies for the dental hygienist. Dental Health 1992;31:5–10.

Giersiepen K, Eberle A, Pohlabeln H. Gender differences in carpal tunnel syndrome? Occupational and non-occupational risk factors in a population-based case-control study. Ann. Epidemiol. 2000;10:481.

Gordon C, Bowyer BL, Johnson EW. Electrodiagnostic characteristics of acute carpal tunnel syndrome. Arch. Phys. Med. Rehabil. 1987;68:545–48.

Gordon C, Johnson EW, Gatens PF, Ashton JJ. Wrist ratio correlation with carpal tunnel syndrome in industry. Am. J. Phys. Med. Rehabil. 1988;67:270–72.

Gorsche RG, Wiley JP, Renger RF, Brant RF, Gemer TY, Sasyniuk TM. Prevalence and incidence of carpal tunnel syndrome in a meat packing plant. Occup. Environ. Med. 1999;56:417–22.

Hadler NM. Arm pain in the workplace. A small area analysis. J. Occup. Med. 1992;34:113–19.

Hadler NM. Repetitive upper-extremity motions in the workplace are not hazardous. J. Hand Surg. 1997;22A:19–29.

Hadler NM. Comments on the "Ergonomics Program Standard" proposed by the Occupational Safety and Health Administration. J. Occup. Environ. Med. 2000;42:951–69.

Hagberg M, Morgenstern H, Kelsh M. Impact of occupations and job tasks on the prevalence of carpal tunnel syndrome. Scand. J. Work Environ. Health 1992;18:337–45.

Hagberg M, Nystrom A, Zetterlund B. Recovery from symptoms after carpal tunnel syndrome surgery in males in relation to vibration exposure. J. Hand Surg. 1991;16A: 66–71.

Haines T, Chong JP. Peripheral neurological assessment methods for workers exposed to hand-arm vibration. An appraisal. Scand. J. Work Environ. Health 1987;13:370–74.

Hales TR, Sauter SL, Peterson MR, Fine LJ, Putz-Anderson V, Schleifer LR, Ochs TT, Bernard BP. Musculoskeletal disorders among visual display terminal users in a telecommunications company. Ergonomics 1994;37:1603–21.

Hamanaka I, Okutsu I, Shimizu K, Takatori Y, Ninomiya S. Evaluation of carpal canal pressure in carpal tunnel syndrome. J. Hand Surg. 1995;20A:848–54.

Hamann C, Werner RA, Franzblau A, Rodgers PA, Siew C, Gruninger S. Prevalence of carpal tunnel syndrome and median mononeuropathy among dentists. J. Am. Dent. Assoc. 2001;132:163–70.

Hanrahan LP, Higgins D, Anderson H, Haskins L, Tai S. Project SENSOR: Wisconsin surveillance of occupational carpal tunnel syndrome. Wis. Med. J. 1991;90:80.

Hanrahan LP, Higgins D, Anderson H, Smith M. Wisconsin occupational carpal tunnel syndrome surveillance: the incidence of surgically treated cases. Wis. Med. J. 1993;92:685–89.

Herbert R, Janeway K, Schechter C. Carpal tunnel syndrome and workers' compensation among an occupational clinic population in New York State. Am. J. Ind. Med. 1999; 35:335–42.

Hochberg FH, Leffert RD, Heller MD, Merriman L. Hand difficulties among musicians. JAMA. 1983;249:1869–72.

Hochholzer T, Krause R, Heuk A. Nerve compression syndromes in sports climbers. Sportverletzung Sportschaden 1993;7:84–87.

Hoffman J, Hoffman PL. Staple gun carpal tunnel syndrome. J. Occup. Med. 1985;27:848–49.

Hopkins AP, Morgan-Hughes JA. The effect of local pressure in diphtheritic neuropathy. J. Neurol. Neurosurg. Psychiatry 1969;32:614–23.

Jackson DL, Hynninen BC, Caborn DN, McLean J. Electrodiagnostic study of carpal tunnel syndrome in wheelchair basketball players. Clin. J. Sport Med. 1996;6:27–31.

Jones WA, Scheker LR. Acute carpal tunnel syndrome: a case report. J. Hand Surg. 1988;13B:400–401.

Kasdan ML, Wolens D, Leis VM, Kasdan AS, Stallings SP. Carpal tunnel syndrome not always work related. J. Ky. Med. Assoc. 1994;92:295–97.

Kearns J, Gresch EE, Weichel CY, Eby P, Pallapothu SR. Pre- and post-employment median nerve latency in pork processing employees. J. Occup. Environ. Med. 2000;42:96–100.

Keir PJ, Bach JM, Rempel DM. Effects of finger posture on carpal tunnel pressure during wrist motion. J. Hand Surg. 1998a;23A:1004–9.

Keir PJ, Bach JM, Rempel DM. Fingertip loading and carpal tunnel pressure: differences between a pinching and a pressing task. J. Orthop. Res. 1998b;16:112–15.

Keir PJ, Bach JM, Rempel D. Effects of computer mouse design and task on carpal tunnel pressure. Ergonomics 1999;42:1350–60.

Keir PJ, Wells RP, Ranney DA, Lavery W. The effects of tendon load and posture on carpal tunnel pressure. J. Hand Surg. 1997;22A:628–34.

Kendall D. Non-penetrating injuries of the median nerve at the wrist. Brain 1950;73:84–94.

Kerr CD, Sybert DR, Albarracin NS. An analysis of the flexor synovium in idiopathic carpal tunnel syndrome: report of 625 cases. J. Hand Surg. 1992;17A:1028–30.

Koller RL, Blank NK. Strawberry picker's palsy. Arch. Neurol. 1980;37:320.

Koskimies K, Farkkila M, Pyykko I, Jantti V, Aatola S, Starck J, Inaba R. Carpal tunnel syndrome in vibration disease. Br. J. Ind. Med. 1990;47:411–16.

Kuorinka I, Forcier L, Hagberg M, Silverstein B, Wells R, Smith MJ, Hendrick HW, Carayon P, Pérusse M. Work Related Musculoskeletal Disorders (WMSDs): A Reference Book for Prevention. London: Taylor & Francis, 1995.

Lalumandier JA, McPhee SD, Riddle S, Shulman JD, Daigle WW. Carpal tunnel syndrome: effect on Army dental personnel. Mil. Med. 2000;165:372–78.

Leclerc A, Franchi P, Cristofari MF, Delemotte B, Mereau P, Teyssier-Cotte C, Touranchet A. Carpal tunnel syndrome and work organisation in repetitive work: a cross sectional study in France. Occup. Environ. Med. 1998; 55:180–87.

Lederman RJ. AAEM minimonograph 43: neuromuscular problems in the performing arts. Muscle Nerve 1994;17:569–77.

Lincoln AE, Vernick JS, Ogaitis S, Smith GS, Mitchell CS, Agnew J. Interventions for the primary prevention of work-related carpal tunnel syndrome. Am. J. Prev. Med. 2000;18:37–50.

Liss GM, Jesin E, Kusiak RA, White P. Musculoskeletal problems among Ontario dental hygienists. Am. J. Ind. Med. 1995;28:521–40.

Loslever P, Ranaivosoa A. Biomechanical and epidemiological investigation of carpal tunnel syndrome at workplaces with high risk factors. Ergonomics 1993;36:537–55.

Luchetti R, Schoenhuber R, Nathan P. Correlation of segmental carpal tunnel pressures with changes in hand and wrist positions in patients with carpal tunnel syndrome and controls. J. Hand Surg. 1998;23B:598–602.

Lundborg G, Dahlin LB, Lundstrom R, Necking LE, Stromberg T. Vibrotactile function of the hand in compression and vibration-induced neuropathy. Sensibility index—a new measure. Scand. J. Plast. Reconstr. Surg. Hand Surg. 1992;26:275–79.

Lundborg G, Myers R, Powell H. Nerve compression injury and increased endoneurial fluid pressure: a "miniature compartment syndrome." J. Neurol. Neurosurg. Psychiatry 1983;46:1119–24.

Macfarlane GJ, Hunt IM, Silman AJ. Role of mechanical and psychosocial factors in the onset of forearm pain: prospective population based study. BMJ. 2000;321:676–79.

MacMahon B, Pugh TF. Epidemiology Principles and Methods. Boston: Little, Brown, 1970.

Margolis W, Kraus JF. The prevalence of carpal tunnel syndrome symptoms in female supermarket checkers. J. Occup. Med. 1987;29:953–56.

Marras WS, Schoenmarklin RW. Wrist motions in industry. Ergonomics 1993;36:341–51.

Masear VR, Hayes JM, Hyde AG. An industrial cause of carpal tunnel syndrome. J. Hand Surg. 1986;11A:222–27.

Matias AC, Salvendy G, Kuczek T. Predictive models of carpal tunnel syndrome causation among VDT operators. Ergonomics 1998;41:213–26.

Mausner JS, Kramer K. Mausner and Bahn Epidemiology—An Introductory Text (2nd ed). Philadelphia: WB Saunders, 1985.

McDiarmid M, Oliver M, Ruser J, Gucer P. Male and female rate differences in carpal tunnel syndrome injuries: personal attributes or job tasks? Environ. Res. 2000;83:23–32.

McKenzie F, Storment J, Van-Hook P, Armstrong TJ. A program for control of repetitive trauma disorders associated with hand tool operations in a telecommunications manufacturing facility. Am. Ind. Hyg. Assoc. J. 1985;46:674–78.

McLellan DL, Swash M. Longitudinal sliding of the median nerve during movements of the upper limb. J. Neurol. Neurosurg. Psychiatry 1976;39:566–70.

Mellion MB. Common cycling injuries. Management and prevention. Sports Med. 1991;11:52–70.

Miller MH, Topliss DJ. Chronic upper limb pain syndrome (repetitive strain injury) in the Australian workforce: a systematic cross sectional rheumatological study of 229 patients. J. Rheumatol. 1988;15:1705–12.

Miller RF, Lohman WH, Maldonado G, Mandel JS. An epidemiologic study of carpal tunnel syndrome and hand-arm vibration syndrome in relation to vibration exposure. J. Hand Surg. 1994;19A:99–105.

Moore JS, Garg A. Upper extremity disorders in a pork processing plant: relationships between job risk factors and morbidity. Am. Ind. Hyg. Assoc. J. 1994;55:703–15.

Morgenstern H, Kelsh M, Kraus J, Margolis W. A cross-sectional study of hand/wrist symptoms in female grocery checkers. Am. J. Ind. Med. 1991;20:209–18.

Murata K, Araki S, Okajima F, Saito Y. Subclinical impairment in the median nerve across the carpal tunnel among female VDT operators. Int. Arch. Occup. Environ. Health 1996;68:75–79.

Nakladalova M, Fialova J, Korycanova H, Nakladal Z. State of health in dental technicians with regard to vibration exposure and overload of upper extremities. Cent. Eur. J. Pub. Health 1995;3[Suppl]:129–31.

Nathan PA. Review of ergonomic studies of carpal tunnel syndrome. Am. J. Ind. Med. 1992;21:895–97.

Nathan PA, Keniston RC. Carpal Tunnel Syndrome: Personal Risk Profile and Role of Intrinsic and Behavioral Factors. In: Kasdan ML, ed. Occupational Hand & Upper Extremity Injuries and Diseases (2nd ed). Philadelphia: Hanley & Belfus, 1998;129–39.

Nathan PA, Keniston RC, Myers LD, Meadows KD. Longitudinal study of median nerve sensory conduction in industry: relationship to age, gender, hand dominance, occupational hand use, and clinical diagnosis. J. Hand Surg. 1992; 17A:850–57.

Nathan PA, Keniston RC, Myers LD, Meadows KD, Lockwood RS. Natural history of median nerve sensory conduction in industry: relationship to symptoms and carpal tunnel syndrome in 558 hands over 11 years. Muscle Nerve 1998;21:711–21.

Nathan PA, Meadows KD, Doyle LS. Occupation as a risk factor for impaired sensory conduction of the median nerve at the carpal tunnel. J. Hand Surg. 1988a;13B:167–70.

Nathan PA, Meadows KD, Doyle LS. Sensory segmental latency values of the median nerve for a population of normal individuals. Arch. Phys. Med. Rehabil. 1988b;69: 499–501.

Nathan PA, Takigawa K, Keniston RC, Meadows KD, Lockwood RS. Slowing of sensory conduction of the median nerve and carpal tunnel syndrome in Japanese and American industrial workers. J. Hand Surg. 1994;19B:30–34.

Neal NC, McManners J, Stirling GA. Pathology of the flexor tendon sheath in the spontaneous carpal tunnel syndrome. J. Hand Surg. 1987;12B:229–32.

Neary D, Ochoa J, Gilliatt RW. Sub-clinical entrapment neuropathy in man. J. Neurol. Sci. 1975;24:282–98.

Nemchausky BA, Ubilluz RM. Upper extremity neuropathies in patients with spinal cord injuries. J. Spinal Cord Med. 1995;18:95–97.

Nilsson T, Hagberg M, Burström L, Lundströmj R. Prevalence and Odds Ratios of Numbness and Carpal Tunnel Syndrome in Different Exposure Categories of Platers. In: Okada A, Dupuis WTH, eds. Hand-Arm Vibration. Kanazawa, Japan: Kyoei Press, 1990;235–39.

Nilsson T, Hagberg M, Burstrom L, Kihlberg S. Impaired nerve conduction in the carpal tunnel of platers and truck assemblers exposed to hand-arm vibration. Scand. J. Work Environ. Health 1994;20:189–99.

Noel B. Pathophysiology and classification of the vibration white finger. Int. Arch. Occup. Environ. Health 2000; 73:150–55.

Nordstrom DL, Vierkant RA, DeStefano F, Layde PM. Risk factors for carpal tunnel syndrome in a general population. Occup. Environ. Med. 1997;54:734–40.

Ochoa J, Marotte L. Nature of nerve lesion caused by chronic entrapment in guinea pig. J. Neurol. Sci. 1973; 19:491–95.

Oesterling BR, Morgan RF, Edlich RF, Steers WD. Carpal tunnel syndrome: an occupational hazard for persons with paraplegia. Am. J. Emerg. Med. 1995;13:608–10.

Okutsu I, Ninomiya S, Hamanaka I, Kuroshima N, Inanami H. Measurement of pressure in the carpal canal before and after endoscopic management of carpal tunnel syndrome. J. Bone Joint Surg. 1989;71:679–83.

Oppenheim H. Textbook of Nervous Diseases (5th ed). London: T. N. Foulis, 1911.

Orcutt SA, Kramer WG 3rd, Howard MW, Keenan MA, Stone LR, Waters RL, Gellman H. Carpal tunnel syndrome secondary to wrist and finger flexor spasticity. J. Hand Surg. 1990;15A:940–44.

Oregon Department of Insurance and Finance. Carpal Tunnel Syndrome in Oregon, 1987–1991.

Osborn JB, Newell KJ, Rudney JD, Stoltenberg JL. Carpal tunnel syndrome among Minnesota dental hygienists. J. Dent. Hyg. 1990;64:79–85.

OSHA. Ergonomics Program, Final Rule. Federal Register 2000;65:68261–870.

Osorio AM, Ames RG, Jones J, Castorina J, Rempel D, Estrin W, Thompson D. Carpal tunnel syndrome among grocery store workers. Am. J. Ind. Med. 1994;25:229–45.

Owen RD. Carpal tunnel syndrome: a products liability prospective. Ergonomics 1994;37:449–76.

Park RM, Nelson NA, Silverstein MA, Mirer FE. Use of medical insurance claims for surveillance of occupational disease. An analysis of cumulative trauma in the auto industry. J. Occup. Med. 1992;34:731–37.

Phalen GS. The carpal-tunnel syndrome. Seventeen years' experience in diagnosis and treatment of six hundred fifty-four hands. J. Bone Joint Surg. 1966;48A:211–28.

Phalen GS. The carpal-tunnel syndrome. Clinical evaluation of 598 hands. Clin. Orthop. 1972;83:29–40.

Pocekay D, McCurdy SA, Samuels SJ, Hammond SK, Schenker MB. A cross-sectional study of musculoskeletal symptoms and risk factors in semiconductor workers. Am. J. Ind. Med. 1995;28:861–71.

Podhorodecki AD, Spielholz NI. Electromyographic study of overuse syndromes in sign language interpreters. Arch. Phys. Med. Rehabil. 1993;74:261–62.

Punnett L. Work-Related Musculoskeletal Disorders in Computer Keyboard Operators. In: Gordon SL, Blair SJ, Fine LJ, eds. Repetitive Motion Disorders of the Upper Extremity. Rosemont, IL: American Academy of Orthopedic Surgeons, 1995;43–48.

Punnett L. Commentary on the scientific basis of the proposed Occupational Safety and Health Administration Ergonomics Program Standard. J. Occup. Environ. Med. 2000; 42:970–81.

Punnett L, Robins JM, Wegman DH, Keyserling WM. Soft tissue disorders in the upper limbs of female garment workers. Scand. J. Work Environ. Health 1985;11:417–25.

Radecki P. Variability in the median and ulnar nerve latencies: implications for diagnosing entrapment. J. Occup. Environ. Med. 1995;37:1293–99.

Rempel D. Musculoskeletal Loading and Carpal Tunnel Pressure. In: Gordon SL, Blair SJ, Fine LJ, eds. Repetitive Motion Disorders of the Upper Extremity. Rosemont, IL: American Academy of Orthopedic Surgeons, 1995;123–32.

Rempel D, Bach JM, Gordon L, So Y. Effects of forearm pronation/supination on carpal tunnel pressure. J. Hand Surg. 1998;23A:38–42.

Rempel D, Keir PJ, Smutz WP, Hargens A. Effects of static fingertip loading on carpal tunnel pressure. J. Orthop. Res. 1997;15:422–26.

Rempel D, Manojlovic R, Levinsohn DG, Bloom T, Gordon L. The effect of wearing a flexible wrist splint on carpal tunnel pressure during repetitive hand activity. J. Hand Surg. 1994;19A:106–10.

Rempel D, Tittiranonda P, Burastero S, Hudes M, So Y. Effect of keyboard keyswitch design on hand pain. J. Occup. Environ. Med. 1999;41:111–19.

Rojviroj S, Sirichativapee W, Kowsuwon W, Wongwiwattananon J, Tamnanthong N, Jeeravipoolvarn P. Pressures in the carpal tunnel. A comparison between patients with carpal tunnel syndrome and normal subjects. J. Bone Joint Surg. 1990;72:516–18.

Roquelaure Y, Mechali S, Dano C, Fanello S, Benetti S, Bureau D, Mariel J, Martin YH, Derriennic F, Penneau-Fontbonne D. Occupational and personnel risk factors for carpal tunnel syndrome in industrial workers. Scand. J. Work Environ. Health 1997;23:364–69.

Rosén I, Stromberg T, Lundborg G. Neurophysiological investigation of hands damaged by vibration: comparison with idiopathic carpal tunnel syndrome. Scand. J. Plast. Reconstr. Surg. Hand Surg. 1993;27:209–16.

Rosenbaum RB, Franklin G, Clemmons DC, Fraser RT, Hennessey M, Rumrill PD. Occupational Neurology. Continuum 2001;7:1–136.

Rossignol M, Stock S, Patry L, Armstrong B. Carpal tunnel syndrome: what is attributable to work? The Montreal study. Occup. Environ. Med. 1997;54:519–23.

Rothfleisch S, Sherman D. Carpal tunnel syndrome—biomechanical aspects of occupational occurrence and implications regarding surgical management. Orthop. Rev. 1976;7:107–9.

Sakakibara H, Hirata M, Hashiguchi T, Toibana N, Koshiyama H. Affected segments of the median nerve detected by fractionated nerve conduction measurement in vibration-induced neuropathy. Industrial Health 1998;36:155–59.

Sakakibara H, Hirata M, Hashiguchi T, Toibana N, Koshiyama H, Zhu SK, Kondo T, Miyao M, Yamada S. Digital sensory nerve conduction velocity and vibration perception threshold in peripheral neurological test for hand-arm vibration syndrome. Am. J. Ind. Med. 1996;30:219–24.

Sakakibara H, Hirata M, Hashiguchi T, Toibana N, Koshiyama H, Zhu SK, Yamada S. Digital nerve conduction velocity for evaluation of peripheral nerve impairments in vibration syndrome. Cent. Eur. J. Pub. Health 1995;3[Suppl]: 52–3.

Sakakibara H, Kondo T, Miyao M, Yamada S. Digital nerve conduction velocity as a sensitive indication of peripheral neuropathy in vibration syndrome. Am. J. Ind. Med. 1994;26:359–66.

Scelsi R, Zanlungo M, Tenti P. Carpal tunnel syndrome. Anatomical and clinical correlations and morphological and ultrastructural aspects of the tenosynovial sheath. Ital. J. Orthop. Traumatol. 1989;15:75–80.

Schoenmarklin RW, Marras WS. Effects of handle angle and work orientation on hammering: I. Wrist motion and hammering performance. Hum. Factors 1989;31:397–411.

Schottland JR, Kirschberg GJ, Fillingim R, Davis VP, Hogg F. Median nerve latencies in poultry processing workers: an approach to resolving the role of industrial "cumulative trauma" in the development of carpal tunnel syndrome. J. Occup. Med. 1991;33:627–31.

Schuind F, Ventura M, Pasteels JL. Idiopathic carpal tunnel syndrome: histologic study of flexor tendon synovium. J. Hand Surg. 1990;15A:497–503.

Seradge H, Bear C, Bithell D. Preventing carpal tunnel syndrome and cumulative trauma disorder: effect of carpal tunnel decompression exercises: an Oklahoma experience. J. Okla. State Med. Assoc. 2000;93:150–53.

Seradge H, Jia YC, Owens W. In-vivo measurement of carpal tunnel pressure in the functioning hand. J. Hand Surg. 1995;20A:855–59.

Siegel DB, Kuzma G, Eakins D. Anatomic investigation of the role of the lumbrical muscles in carpal tunnel syndrome. J. Hand Surg. 1995;20A:860–63.

Silverstein BA, Fine LJ, Armstrong TJ. Occupational factors and carpal tunnel syndrome. Am. J. Ind. Med. 1987;11: 343–58.

Silverstein MA, Silverstein BA, Franklin GM. Evidence for work-related musculoskeletal disorders: a scientific counterargument. J. Occup. Environ. Med. 1996;38:477–84.

Smith SM, Kress TA, Hart WM. Hand/wrist disorders among sign language communicators. Am. Ann. Deaf. 2000; 145:22–25.

Stedt JD. Carpal tunnel syndrome: the risk to educational interpreters. Am. Ann. Deaf. 1989;134:223–26.

Stetson DS, Silverstein BA, Keyserling WM, Wolfe RA, Albers JW. Median sensory distal amplitude and latency: comparisons between nonexposed managerial/professional employees and industrial workers. Am. J. Ind. Med. 1993;24:175–89.

Stevens JC, Witt JC, Smith BE, Weaver AL. The frequency of carpal tunnel syndrome in computer users in a medical facility. Neurology 2001;56:1568–70.

Stevens K. The carpal tunnel syndrome in cardiologists. Ann. Intern. Med. 1990;112:796.

Stock SR. Workplace ergonomic factors and the development of musculocutaneous disorders of the neck and upper limbs: a meta-analysis. Am. J. Ind. Med. 1991;19:87–107.

Stockstill JW, Harn SD, Strickland D, Hruska R. Prevalence of upper extremity neuropathy in a clinical dentist population. J. Am. Dent. Assoc. 1993;124:67–72.

Stromberg T, Dahlin LB, Brun A, Lundborg G. Structural nerve changes at wrist level in workers exposed to vibration. Occup. Environ. Med. 1997;54:307–11.

Stromberg T, Dahlin LB, Lundborg G. Hand problems in 100 vibration-exposed symptomatic male workers. J. Hand Surg. 1997;21B:315–19.

Szabo RM. Occupational Carpal Tunnel Syndrome. In: Kasdan ML, ed. Occupational Hand & Upper Extremity Injuries and Diseases (2nd ed). Philadelphia: Hanley & Belfus, 1998;113–27.

Szabo RM, Chidgey LK. Stress carpal tunnel pressures in patients with carpal tunnel syndrome and normal patients. J. Hand Surg. 1989;14A:624–27.

Takeuchi T, Futatsuka M, Imanishi H, Yamada S. Pathological changes observed in the finger biopsy of patients with vibration-induced white finger. Scand. J. Work Environ. Health 1986;12:280–83.

Takeuchi T, Takeya M, Imanishi H. Ultrastructural changes in peripheral nerves of the fingers of three vibration-exposed persons with Raynaud's phenomenon. Scand. J. Work Environ. Health 1988;14:31–35.

Tan M, Tan U. Correlation of carpal tunnel size and conduction velocity of the sensory median and ulnar nerves of male and female controls and carpet weavers. Percept. Mot. Skills 1998;87:1195–1201.

Tanaka S, Wild DK, Cameron LL, Freund E. Association of occupational and non-occupational risk factors with the prevalence of self-reported carpal tunnel syndrome in a national survey of the working population. Am. J. Ind. Med. 1997;32:550–56.

Tanaka S, Wild DK, Seligman PJ, Behrens V, Cameron L, Putz-Anderson V. The US prevalence of self-reported carpal tunnel syndrome: 1988 National Health Interview Survey data. Am. J. Public Health 1994;84:1846–48.

Tanaka S, Wild DK, Seligman PJ, Halperin WE, Behrens VJ, Putz-Anderson V. Prevalence and work-relatedness of self-reported carpal tunnel syndrome among U.S. workers: analysis of the Occupational Health Supplement data of 1988 National Health Interview Survey. Am. J. Ind. Med. 1995;27:451–70.

Tanzer RC. The carpal-tunnel syndrome. J. Bone Joint Surg. 1959;41A:626–34.

Taylor W. Biological effects of the hand-arm vibration syndrome: historical perspective and current research. J. Acoust. Soc. Am. 1988;83:415–22.

Taylor W, Wasserman DE. Occupational Vibration. In: Zenz C, ed. Occupational Medicine (2nd ed). Chicago: Year Book, 1988;324–33.

Tichauer ER, Gage H. Ergonomic principles basic to hand tool design. Am. Ind. Hyg. Assoc. J. 1977;38:622–34.

Tittiranonda P, Burastero S, Rempel D. Risk factors for musculoskeletal disorders among computer users. Occup. Med. 1999;14:17–38.

U.S. Department of Labor, Bureau of Labor Statistics. United States Department of Labor, Lost-Worktime Injuries and Time Away From Work, 1999, released March 28, 2001 via publication USDL 01-71.

Valls-Solé J, Alvarez R, Nuñez M. Limited longitudinal sliding of the median nerve in patients with carpal tunnel syndrome. Muscle Nerve 1995;18:761–67.

Vender MI, Kasdan ML, Truppa KL. Upper extremity disorders: a literature review to determine work-relatedness. J. Hand Surg. 1995;20A:534–41.

Waring WP 3rd, Werner RA. Clinical management of carpal tunnel syndrome in patients with long-term sequelae of poliomyelitis. J. Hand Surg. 1989;14A:865–69.

Werner CO, Elmqvist D, Ohlin P. Pressure and nerve lesion in the carpal tunnel. Acta Orthop. Scand. 1983;54: 312–16.

Werner RA, Armstrong TJ. Carpal tunnel syndrome. Ergonomic risk factors and intracanal pressure. Phys. Med. Rehab. Clin. North Am. 1997;8:555–69.

Werner RA, Franzblau A, Albers JW, Armstrong TJ. Influence of body mass index and work activity on the prevalence of median mononeuropathy at the wrist. Occup. Environ. Med. 1997;54:268–71.

Werner RA, Franzblau A, Albers JW, Buchele H, Armstrong TJ. Use of screening nerve conduction studies for predicting future carpal tunnel syndrome. Occup. Environ. Med. 1997; 54:96–100.

Werner R, Waring W, Davidoff G. Risk factors for median mononeuropathy of the wrist in postpoliomyelitis patients. Arch. Phys. Med. Rehabil. 1989;70:464–67.

Wieslander G, Norback D, Gothe CJ, Juhlin L. Carpal tunnel syndrome (CTS) and exposure to vibration, repetitive wrist movements, and heavy manual work: a case-referent study. Br. J. Ind. Med. 1989;46:43–47.

Wilgis EF, Murphy R. The significance of longitudinal excursion in peripheral nerves. Hand Clin. 1986;2:761–66.

Winn FJ Jr, Habes DJ. Carpal tunnel area as a risk factor for carpal tunnel syndrome. Muscle Nerve 1990;13:254–58.

Wright TW, Glowczewskie F, Wheeler D, Miller G, Cowin D. Excursion and strain of the median nerve. J. Bone Joint Surg. 1996;78A:1897–1903.

Wyles JM, Rodriquez AA. The predictive value of wrist dimension measurement in median sensory latencies in carpal tunnel syndrome. Muscle Nerve 1991;14:902.

Yamaguchi D, Lipscomb P, Soule E. Carpal tunnel syndrome. Minn. Med. 1965;48:22–31.

Chapter 14

Nonsurgical Treatment of Carpal Tunnel Syndrome

Choice of Therapy

Choice of therapy for carpal tunnel syndrome is dependent on the severity of symptoms, underlying cause of the carpal tunnel syndrome, if known, the presence or absence of neurologic deficit, and, of course, on the wishes of the patient (Table 14-1). This chapter reviews nonsurgical treatment, and Chapter 15 reviews surgical treatment. Ergonomic changes and occupational treatment issues are discussed in Chapter 13.

Many carpal tunnel syndrome patients with mild, intermittent symptoms appropriately choose no therapy (Futami, Kobayashi, Wakabayashi, Yonemoto & Nakamura, 1992). These patients should be alerted to watch for progression of symptoms. If pain and paresthesias become more frequent and, particularly if weakness, sensory loss, or atrophy develops, they must seek re-evaluation and reconsider their decision.

Initial therapy for most patients with carpal tunnel syndrome is nonoperative. Phalen (1966) believed that most patients with carpal tunnel syndrome did not require surgical therapy. A survey of hand surgeons showed that they usually begin treatment with a few weeks of nonoperative therapy (Duncan, Lewis, Foreman & Nordyke, 1987). The most common therapies used were splinting (77% of surgeons), steroid injection into the carpal canal (60%), and nonsteroidal anti-inflammatory drugs (NSAIDs) (47%). Oral steroids or diuretics were prescribed less frequently. Many patients can maintain control of their symptoms for years with nonoperative therapies, and some have improvement in abnormal median nerve conduction find-ings after institution of splinting and other nonoperative therapies (Harter, McKiernan, Kirzinger, Archer, Peters & Harter, 1993).

In some patients with acute carpal tunnel syndrome and associated neurologic deficit, surgical therapy should not be delayed.

Patients with established neurologic deficit and neurologic signs of median neuropathy, such as loss of two-point discrimination or thenar atrophy, are unlikely to be cured by nonoperative therapy. Most surgeons operate on these severe cases of carpal tunnel syndrome without delay (Duncan et al., 1987). An alternative approach is a brief trial of conservative modalities: If pain and paresthesias are relieved, and the neurologic deficit is not progressive during careful follow-up, the rare patient with severe carpal tunnel syndrome shows gradual improvement in neurologic deficit with nonoperative therapy.

We are unaware of a randomized trial comparing operative to nonoperative therapy of carpal tunnel syndrome. Indications for surgery are debated (Johnson, 1995; Wilson & Sumner, 1995). The incidence of carpal tunnel surgery varies among communities, partly due to variations in physicians' opinions about the indications for surgery (Keller, Largay, Soule & Katz, 1998). In a prospective, community-based observational study, surgically and nonsurgically treated patients were matched for pretreatment functional status. Most patients treated nonoperatively remained at least partially symptomatic during 30 months of follow-up, but 40% of nonoperatively treated patients (compared with 75% of surgically treated patents) "reported that they would be satisfied to spend the rest of their lives with their current level of carpal

Table 14-1. Treatment of Median Neuropathies at the Carpal Tunnel Based on Severity[a]

Class	Clinical Status	Treatment
0. Asymptomatic	Symptom free	None.
1. Intermittent positive symptoms	1A. Subclinical median nerve irritability	Reassurance.
	1B. Mild carpal tunnel syndrome: symptoms infrequent, linked to specific activities, or specific medical conditions	Modify activities; treat medical condition or await end of pregnancy; nonoperative treatment.
	1C. Moderate intermittent carpal tunnel syndrome: symptoms many times per week	Modify activities; treat medical condition; use nonoperative treatments; consider surgery for (1) unrelieved symptoms that are troublesome to the patient, especially if present for more than 1 year; (2) unrelieved symptoms that are interfering with full work duties, especially if present greater than 3 months[b]; (3) worsening of carpal tunnel syndrome to class 2 or 3.
2. Persistently symptomatic	Deficit absent on neurologic examination	Try nonoperative treatment; consider surgery as for class 1C.
	Deficit present on neurologic examination	Surgery is usually needed, but nonoperative treatment might be tried for a few weeks. Surgery should not be long postponed unless neurologic deficit resolves with nonoperative therapy.
3. Severe	Negative sensory or motor symptoms and neurologic deficit usually present	Surgical therapy is needed unless patient is resigned to endure symptoms and neurologic deficit. Patient should be informed before surgery that neurologic deficit may improve slowly or incompletely after surgery.

[a]For details of classification, see Chapter 3.
[b]See Chapter 13 for a discussion of special occupational issues in treatment of carpal tunnel syndrome, including the importance of timely treatment in preventing long-term disability.

tunnel symptoms" (Katz, Keller, Simmons, Rogers, Bessette, Fossel & Mooney, 1998). Patients with comparable severity at baseline were less likely to be symptomatic at 30-month follow-up if treated surgically.

A prospective longitudinal study of industrial workers has shown that mildly symptomatic carpal tunnel syndrome usually has a benign course (Nathan, Keniston, Myers, Meadows & Lockwood, 1998). Among workers who had mild symptoms and nerve conduction evidence of carpal tunnel syndrome at the onset of the study, only about one-third still had symptomatic carpal tunnel syndrome 11 years later, even though most retained mild median nerve conduction abnormalities. Among workers who had symptoms such as hand numbness, tingling, or nocturnal awakening but did not meet diagnostic criteria for carpal tunnel syndrome, the vast majority did not have the same symptoms 11 years later.

A retrospective follow-up study of a population-based series of patients with carpal tunnel syndrome in the Marshfield, Wisconsin, Epidemiologic Study Area made a number of interesting observations (DeStefano, Nordstrom & Vierkant, 1997). More than one-half of patients with carpal tunnel syndrome who were treated nonoperatively, usually by splinting, NSAIDs, or simple analgesics, had resolution of symptoms within 1 year. Of those who were still symptomatic after 1 year, nearly one-half had subsequent resolution of symptoms without surgery; in other words, approximately three-fourths of patients with carpal tunnel syndrome who did not have carpal tunnel surgery were asymptomatic after 8 years of nonoperative treatment. Patients who had surgery were more likely, by a factor of almost 6, to have resolution of symptoms, but surgery was much less likely to be successful if symptoms had been present longer than 3 years. In contrast, others have found that duration of symptoms was not a predictor of response to carpal tunnel surgery (Cseuz, Thomas, Lambert, Love & Lipscomb, 1966).

A prospective study followed patients who had carpal tunnel syndrome and were not treated with surgery (Padua, Padua, Aprile, Pasqualetti & Tonali, 2001). Over the 10- to 15-month follow-up period after initial evaluation, less than one-fourth of the patients underwent carpal tunnel surgery. Based on a multiperspective evaluation that included patient questionnaires (similar to Tables 15-9 and 15-10), clinical examination, and electrodiagnostic testing, 23% or more of patients improved, and even more patients remained stationary. Positive prognostic factors for improvement included a history of hand stress, shorter duration of symptoms, a negative Phalen's test, unilateral symptoms, and younger age. These patients were not given specific nonoperative therapies, but many of those who reported hand stress were able to modify their hand activities. Our own protocol for choice of therapy is presented in Table 14-1.

Initial Nonoperative Treatment

Treatment should begin with attention to repetitive or strenuous hand activities that are causing or exacerbating symptoms and, whenever possible, with treatment of any medical condition that is contributing to the median nerve compression. In many patients symptoms are closely related to repetitive hand activities. Often, the best treatment for these patients is stopping the offending activity. At times, the activity can be redesigned or modified to protect against carpal tunnel syndrome. The section on Prevention of Occupational Carpal Tunnel Syndrome in Chapter 13 discusses task modification in greater detail.

When carpal tunnel syndrome is caused or exacerbated by a medical condition, carpal tunnel symptoms often resolve with successful treatment of the underlying problem. For example, the response of carpal tunnel syndrome symptoms to treatment of hypothyroidism, acromegaly, or rheumatoid arthritis is discussed in Chapter 6.

When symptoms of carpal tunnel syndrome develop during pregnancy, they usually resolve after delivery (see Chapter 6 for more detailed data). Most pregnant patients with carpal tunnel syndrome need no specific therapy. If symptoms do require therapy, splinting or steroid injection of the carpal tunnel is often successful.

Splinting

Splinting is a mainstay of conservative therapy. It is simple, safe, relatively inexpensive, and often effective, at least initially.

Technique

A wide variety of splints are now available commercially. An example is shown in Figure 14-1. The splint should firmly immobilize the wrist in the neutral position. Pressure in the carpal tunnel is lowest when the wrist is near the neutral position (at 2 ± 9 degrees of extension and 1 ± 9 degrees of ulnar deviation, when measured in patients with carpal tunnel syndrome) (Weiss, Gordon, Bloom, So & Rempel, 1995). In a study comparing neutral splints to 20-degree extension splints, the neutral splints were more likely to relieve the symptoms of carpal tunnel syndrome (Burke, Burke, Stewart & Cambre, 1994). The thumb should be free and able to flex to the index finger, but the splint should prevent thumb opposition to the little finger. Finger movement should be free. The fit, although firm, should not interfere with circulation or cause focal skin irritation (Falkenburg, 1987).

The splint should be worn during sleep and whenever possible during wakefulness. Some carpal tunnel syndrome patients note symptomatic benefit if they can use the splint during their daily activities. This is not always possible because the splint is too restrictive on some hand and finger movements or is too uncomfortable. A study that tried to randomize patients to night-only or full-time splint use found that only one-fourth of patients instructed to wear the splint full-time actually did so, whereas one-fourth of patients instructed on night-only use also used the splints at least part of their waking hours (Walker, Metzler, Cifu & Swartz, 2000).

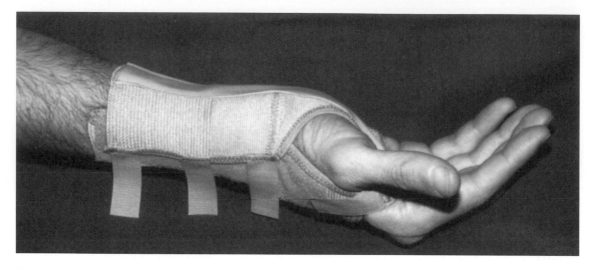

Figure 14-1. The splint used for treatment of carpal tunnel syndrome should maintain the wrist between neutral and 10 degrees or less of extension and 10 degrees or less of ulnar deviation.

Results

In response to the landmark description of carpal tunnel surgery by Brain and colleagues (1947), Roaf (1947) wrote that many patients with carpal tunnel syndrome did not require surgery and suggested 3 to 4 weeks of wrist immobilization as initial treatment of and as a diagnostic test for carpal tunnel syndrome. Heathfield (1957) prescribed wrist splinting in the neutral position for 51 patients with carpal tunnel syndrome. Patients used the splints for 6 to 12 weeks, at night if symptoms were nocturnal, or day and night if symptoms were continual. Forty-eight patients (94%) had excellent relief of symptoms, and only six relapsed.

The success rate in subsequent series has been less impressive. A wrist splint in the neutral position relieved symptoms of carpal tunnel syndrome in 60% to 67% of patients (Quin, 1961; Kruger, Kraft, Deitz, Ameis & Polissar, 1991). The results of Crow (1960) are shown in Figures 14-2 and 14-3. He splinted the wrists of 36 patients in the neutral position at night; approximately one-half of the patients noted immediate relief of nocturnal symptoms and gradual improvement in diurnal symptoms. One-fourth of the patients did not note

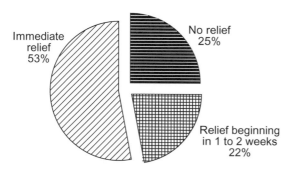

Figure 14-2. Early effects of splinting for treatment of carpal tunnel syndrome. (Data from RS Crow. Treatment of the carpal-tunnel syndrome. BMJ. 1960;1:1611–15.)

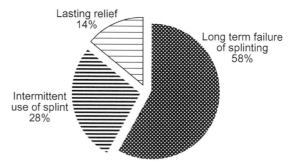

Figure 14-3. Late effects of splinting for treatment of carpal tunnel syndrome. (Data from RS Crow. Treatment of the carpal-tunnel syndrome. BMJ. 1960;1:1611–15.)

benefit until the splints had been in use for a week or two. An occasional patient benefited immediately from splinting and then had a recurrence of symptoms while still using the splint. One-fourth of the patients did not benefit from the splints. Rarely, patients reported an increase in symptoms coincident with splint use.

A randomized controlled trial used a specially designed splint that held the wrist in the neutral position, mildly extended the middle and ring fingers, and slightly approximated the heads to the metacarpals of the index and little fingers (Manente, Torrieri, Di Blasio, Staniscia, Romano & Uncini, 2001). Patients who wore the splint at night for 4 weeks were compared with untreated patients; treated patients had better symptom and function scores (see Tables 15-9 and 15-10) than did untreated patients.

For most patients in Crow's series, symptoms recurred after the splinting was stopped. Only one-seventh of the patients had lasting relief of symptoms after splinting, and usually patients who had sustained improvement after splinting had also changed their hand activities or had been treated for an underlying causal condition.

These mixed clinical responses to wrist splinting correlate with physiologic observations on carpal canal pressure: Wrist splinting can lower intracanal pressure, but sometimes even the lowered pressure is high enough to cause symptomatic nerve compression (Luchetti, Schoenhuber, Alfarano, Deluca, De Cicco & Landi, 1994).

Patients with carpal tunnel syndrome who note symptomatic improvement with splinting can also show improvement of median nerve conduction latencies (Kruger et al., 1991). In a group of patients with carpal tunnel syndrome, Goodman and Gilliatt (1961) performed serial nerve conduction studies during treatment by splinting. In patients with pretreatment median distal motor latencies between 5 and 10 msec, a few showed a 20% or better improvement in distal motor latency, but others showed no improvement or even had slight worsening of median distal motor latency. A study comparing night-only to full-time splint use found better improvement in distal motor and sensory latencies in the full-time splint use group (Walker et al., 2000).

Oral Anti-Inflammatory Drugs, Diuretics, and Anticonvulsants

Many physicians treat carpal tunnel syndrome with NSAIDs. When we do so, we use a 2- to 4-week trial unless limited by side effects such as gastrointestinal intolerance. An occasional patient reports an increase in carpal tunnel syndrome symptoms while on these drugs, possibly because of drug-induced fluid retention. There are no published controlled data that prove the value of NSAIDs for treatment of carpal tunnel syndrome.

Use of a mild diuretic is another common, but poorly studied, treatment of carpal tunnel syndrome. There are a number of letters attesting to the value of diuretics in treatment of carpal tunnel syndrome in pregnancy (Donaldson, 1959; McCallum, 1959; Wood, 1959). The theoretical rationale is to decrease synovial edema or vascular congestion in the carpal tunnel.

Anticonvulsants such as gabapentin and carbamazepine are being used increasingly for treatment of neuropathic pain and dysesthesia. Studies on their use in carpal tunnel syndrome are preliminary (Facchetti, Chiroli, Bascelli & Sasanelli, 1999).

Another preliminary report advocates trials of oral serratiopeptidase for treatment of carpal tunnel syndrome (Panagariya & Sharma, 1999).

The best studies on oral drug treatment of carpal tunnel syndrome show that a brief course of oral steroids can give temporary relief of symptoms of mild to moderate carpal tunnel syndrome (classes 1 or 2). A prospective, randomized, double-blind, placebo-controlled study compared 4 weeks of oral treatment with placebo, NSAID (tenoxicam, 20 mg daily), diuretic (trichlormethiazide, 2 mg daily), or steroids (prednisolone, 20 mg daily for 2 weeks, then 10 mg daily for 2 weeks) in patients with carpal tunnel syndrome confirmed by electrodiagnosis (Chang, Chiang, Lee, Ger & Lo, 1998). None of the treatment groups showed objective improvement at 2 or 4 weeks. The steroid-treated group had a statistically significant improvement in a global symptom scale by which patients subjectively rated pain, numbness, paresthesias, weakness and clumsiness, and nocturnal awakening. The groups treated with diuretic or NSAID did not show improvement in the global symptom score. Another prospective, ran-

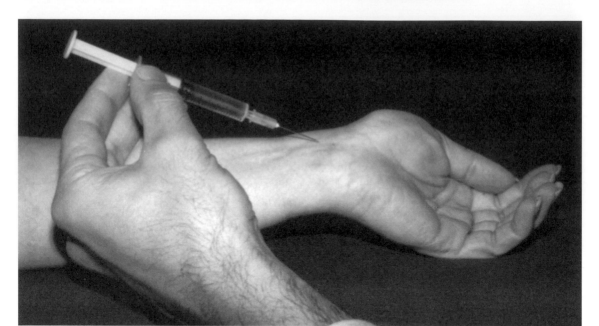

Figure 14-4. One technique for steroid injection into the carpal tunnel: The needle is poised for insertion at an angle of about 30 degrees with the tip 1 cm proximal to the distal wrist crease between the tendons of palmaris longus and flexor carpi radialis.

domized, double-blind, placebo-controlled study compared 2 weeks of oral treatment with placebo or with prednisone (20 mg daily for 1 week, then 10 mg daily for 1 week) (Herskovitz, Berger & Lipton, 1995). The steroid-treated patients reported improvement in the global symptom score after 2 weeks of treatment, but the improvement of symptoms disappeared within 6 weeks of stopping the prednisone.

Steroid Injection into the Carpal Tunnel

Injection of corticosteroids into the carpal tunnel often leads to excellent relief of symptoms. The improvement, however, is rarely permanent. The occasional complication of accidental injection injury to the median nerve can be devastating.

Technique

Steroid injection is typically done with a 25-gauge needle. Various techniques are advocated. The needle can be inserted 1 cm proximal to the distal wrist crease between the palmaris longus

and flexor carpi radialis tendons or on the ulnar side of the palmaris longus tendon (Figure 14-4) (Gelberman, Aronson & Weisman, 1980; Green, 1984). While the needle is advanced about 1 cm to enter the carpal tunnel through the flexor retinaculum, the patient is asked to report any paresthesias. If paresthesias do occur, the needle should be withdrawn and reinserted about 1 cm proximally. If the needle is in the carpal tunnel and not in tendon or the median nerve, there should be no resistance to the injection. When the steroid solution is successfully injected into the carpal tunnel, a slight bulge should be visible or palpable in the proximal palm (Green, 1984). Other approaches to injection into the carpal tunnel have been described (Kay & Marshall, 1992; Kasten & Louis, 1996).

An alternative is to inject proximal to the carpal tunnel, along the flexor tendons 3 cm proximal to the distal wrist crease in line with the third web space with the needle directed distally and about 30 degrees dorsally, inserted to a depth of three-fourths of an inch (Minamikawa, Peimer, Kambe, Wheeler & Sherwin, 1992; Dawson, Hallett & Wilbourn, 1999). Before injection, the patient can be asked to flex his or her fingers slightly; movement of the needle and syringe implies that the needle is in contact with the flexor synovium, in which case slight withdrawal of the needle will ensure injection around, rather than into, the synovial tissue. Even though the steroid is actually injected proximal to the carpal tunnel, it diffuses into the tunnel, perhaps facilitated by tendon sliding during finger flexion and extension. After injection of steroid around the flexor tendons proximal to the tunnel, some recommend massaging the wrist to help move the fluid bolus distally (Dammers, Veering & Vermeulen, 1999).

Results

Phalen and Kendrick (1957) reported treatment of carpal tunnel syndrome by injection of 1 ml of hydrocortisone into the carpal tunnel. Sixteen of 20 patients improved. Kopell (1958) added a case report of treatment by steroid injection into the canal. Van der Bracht (1958) was another early proponent of treatment with injection of hydrocortisone into the canal. Foster (1960) confirmed a similar response rate to this therapy, but noted a high relapse rate at 1-year follow-up. Quin (1961) found that improvement from hydrocortisone injection lasted less than a week in some patients.

Crow (1960) injected 25 to 50 mg of hydrocortisone acetate. He treated 31 hands and noted dramatic improvement in symptoms in 28 hands within 48 hours of injection. Symptomatic relief occurred rapidly, even in patients who had chronic symptoms and objective findings of median nerve dysfunction on examination; however, 80% of patients noted recurrence of symptoms within 1 to 8 months of the injection. On occasion, these patients received a second injection, but most of those who improved after the second injection had recurrence of symptoms within months.

Goodman and Foster (1962) injected 10 mg (1 ml) of prednisolone. They performed repeated median nerve motor conduction studies in their patients before and after injection of steroid into the carpal tunnel. Median distal motor latency often decreased at the initial follow-up, a few weeks after injection, and then again increased in subsequent months, paralleling the clinical observation that symptomatic relief was usually transient.

Gelberman and colleagues (1980) injected 30 mg of triamcinolone (0.75 ml) and an equal volume of 1% lidocaine without epinephrine and then splinted the wrist continuously for 3 weeks in the neutral position. Three-fourths of the patients were asymptomatic 6 weeks after injection, but less than one-fourth remained asymptomatic after months of follow-up. Patients were more likely to have lasting benefit if symptoms were intermittent or had been present less than 1 year before treatment. Some 40% of patients with intermittent symptoms, normal strength, and normal two-point discrimination were asymptomatic 18 months after treatment.

Even an occasional patient with evidence of more severe median neuropathy was cured by the 3-week treatment regimen (Gelberman et al., 1980). Criteria for severe median neuropathy included thenar weakness and atrophy, decreased median two-point discrimination, absent median sensory nerve action potential, median distal motor latency over 6 msec, or fibrillations on thenar electromyography.

Giannini and colleagues (1991) selected patients with mild carpal tunnel syndrome for treatment by canal injection with steroids. They found that 6 months after injection, 93% of their patients had good symptomatic improvement, and many had concomitant improvement in median nerve conduction studies.

One of the most optimistic reports of local steroid injection for carpal tunnel syndrome reported that 84% of injected wrists showed partial or complete symptomatic and electrophysiologic improvement 1 year after injection (Ayhan-Ardic & Erdem, 2000b). Injection therapy was coupled with patient education on avoiding repetitive or symptom-causing wrist activities.

Table 14-2 compares the initial and late response rates to steroid injection into the carpal tunnel in various series. The studies have varied widely in the dose of steroid injected; however, a controlled study of low-dose (25 mg of hydrocortisone) versus high-dose (20 mg of triamcinolone or 100 mg of hydrocortisone) injection found no significant differences in responses at 6 weeks or 6 months (O'Gradaigh & Merry, 2000).

A systematic meta-analysis of randomized controlled studies identified the studies by Dam-

Table 14-2. Efficacy of Steroid Injection in the Carpal Tunnel for Patients with Carpal Tunnel Syndrome

Reference	Number of Hands Treated	Hands with Initial Benefit (%)	Hands with Sustained Benefit (%)
Crow, 1960	81	90	13
Goodman & Foster, 1962	—	88	60
Foster, 1960	25	92	24
Gelberman, Aronson & Weisman, 1980	50	76	22
Phalen, 1972	497	—	13
Wood, 1980	61	90	33
Green, 1984	222	81	37
Ozdogan & Yazici, 1984	37	50*	22
Irwin, Beckett & Suman, 1996	45	51	24
Girlanda, Dattola, Venuto, Mangiapane, Nicolosi & Messina, 1993	27	96*	—
Girlanda, Dattola, Venuto, Mangiapane, Nicolosi & Messina, 1993	91	—	8
Weiss, Sachar & Gendreau, 1994	79	47	13
Babu & Britton, 1994	20	95	35
Ayhan-Ardic & Erdem, 2000	32	—	84
Dammers, Veering & Vermeulen, 1999	30	77*	50*

*Controlled trial with statistically significant benefit compared with control.

mers (1999) and Ozdogan and Yazici (1984) as being of good quality and, based on them, concluded that the trials demonstrate that local corticosteroid injections are more likely than placebo injections to improve symptoms of carpal tunnel syndrome at 1 month after injection (Marshall, Tardif & Ashworth, 2000). Girlanda et al. (1993) came to similar conclusions in a controlled trial but did not report individual patient outcomes. Another controlled trial supporting short-term efficacy of local corticosteroid injections bases its conclusion on electrodiagnostic follow-up rather than clinical assessment (Wu, Chan & Hsu, 1991, available to the English reader only in abstract form).

The value of steroid injection is local rather than systemic. In a controlled series, women with idiopathic carpal tunnel syndrome received 1.5 mg of betamethasone injected into the deltoid or into the carpal tunnel. At follow-up after 1 month, the improvement rate was 50% after carpal tunnel injection, but only 6% after deltoid injection (Ozdogan & Yazici, 1984). In a study that randomized patients who had mild to moderate carpal tunnel syndrome to treatment with prednisolone, 25 mg orally for 10 days, or with methylprednisolone, 15 mg injected once into the

carpal tunnel, the patients who were treated with carpal tunnel injection showed a greater improvement in a global symptom score, and the improvement was still evident 3 months after the injection (Wong, Hui, Tang, Ho, Hung, Wong, Kay & Li, 2001).

Complications

Some patients have transient increase in wrist discomfort at the time of injection. Increased pain may last 1 or 2 days (Phalen, 1966). Experience with injection of other joints suggests that some patients may develop a transient chemical synovitis in response to steroid crystals (Gray & Gottlieb, 1983).

Crow (1960) noted one case of flexor tendon synovial infection introduced in the course of 65 injections. The patient recovered completely from the infection after antibiotic therapy. More severe infection may require acute exploration and drainage of the carpal tunnel (Gottlieb & Riskin, 1980).

Bilateral digital flexor tendon ruptures occurred in a woman treated for idiopathic carpal tunnel syndrome with 29 injections of steroids into the carpal tunnel over 7 years (Gottlieb & Riskin, 1980).

Accidental steroid injection into the median nerve can increase median neuropathy (Linskey & Segal, 1990; McConnell & Bush, 1990; Frederick, Carter & Littler, 1992). The ulnar nerve at the wrist or proximal palm is also vulnerable to injury by misdirected carpal tunnel steroid injection (Frederick et al., 1992; Tavares & Giddins, 1996). When surgery is done after intraneural steroid injection, accumulated material may be visible in the nerve.

Local steroid injections may be complicated on rare occasions by local allergic dermatitis, acne, skin atrophy or depigmentation, or systemic flushing (Gottlieb & Riskin, 1980).

Manipulative Therapy

Case reports described improvement in carpal tunnel syndrome after chiropractic therapy (Ferezy & Norlin, 1989; Valente, 1991; Valente & Gibson, 1994). Subsequently, a variety of manipulative therapies have been proposed for treatment of carpal tunnel syndrome. None of these has proven therapeutic value.

Bonebrake and colleagues (1993) used a variety of manipulative techniques: "variations of ischemic compression, stripping massage, transverse friction massage, skin rolling, tissue stretching, specific muscle exercise and joint manipulation." Hard tissue and soft tissue manipulation were applied on extremities, head, spine, and trunk. Subjects also received a variety of other innovative and unproven therapies. The study was done without a true control group and without objective measures of median nerve recovery. No conclusions about the value of manipulation for treatment of carpal tunnel syndrome can be drawn from this study.

Davis and colleagues (1998) did a single-blind, randomized, controlled trial with two treatment groups: wrist splint plus ibuprofen versus wrist splinting plus "high-velocity low-amplitude manual thrust procedures creating a cavitation response and increased joint motion in the bony joints of the upper extremities including the wrist, elbow, and shoulder as well as in the vertebrae on the cervical and upper thoracic regions." Both treatment groups were improved 1 month after the 9-week treatment

protocol, consistent with the known value of wrist splinting. No deleterious or beneficial effect of manipulation for treatment of carpal tunnel syndrome was shown in this study.

In a series of papers, Sucher (1993a, b, 1994, 1995, 1998) has proposed that specific wrist manipulations designed to stretch the transverse carpal ligament, combined with wrist stretching exercises, can help treat carpal tunnel syndrome. He has demonstrated the distensibility of the transverse carpal ligament by wrist magnetic resonance imaging and in cadaver studies. He has presented case reports of improvement of patients with carpal tunnel syndrome treated with his method, but there are no published controlled studies validating this treatment approach. Furthermore, the relative value of the manipulation versus the stretching exercises is unknown.

A study comparing two different mobilization techniques in patients with carpal tunnel syndrome was inconclusive, perhaps because there were only seven patients in each treatment group (Tal-Akabi & Rushton, 2000). The techniques were carpal bone mobilization and "neurodynamic mobilization," which attempts to mobilize the median nerve by "slight glenohumeral abduction, shoulder girdle depression, elbow extension, lateral rotation of the whole arm, wrist, thumb and finger extension and finally glenohumeral abduction."

New Therapeutic Alternatives

Yoga

A preliminary randomized trial examined yoga as a treatment for carpal tunnel syndrome (Garfinkel, Singhal, Katz, Allan, Reshetar & Schumacher, 1998). The yoga treatment consisted of an 8-week course of twice weekly sessions of yoga instruction. The patients with carpal tunnel syndrome were taught 11 yoga positions (*asanas*) chosen to improve upper body posture, flexibility, and movement, especially of shoulders, arms, wrists, and hands. They held each asana for 30 seconds, then spent 10 to 15 minutes lying in a final relaxation posture. At the end of 8 weeks, they had less hand and wrist pain, more improvement in grip strength, and more remissions of Phalen's sign than did controls who were treated with wrist splints. There were no statistically significant changes in median nerve conduction. The study has been justly criticized for suitability of the control treatment and the subjective nature and relevance of the outcome parameters (Daniell, 1999; Deitchman & Gerr, 1999; Harrast & Kraft, 1999; Mackinnon & Novak, 1999). This study does not establish that yoga is a worthwhile adjunct to treatment of carpal tunnel syndrome.

Nerve and Tendon Gliding Exercises

A study of median nerve and flexor tendon gliding exercises in patients with carpal tunnel syndrome found that patients treated with an exercise program were less likely than historical control patients to have carpal tunnel surgery (Rozmaryn, Dovelle, Rothman, Gorman, Olvey & Bartko, 1998). For tendon gliding exercises, the patient actively moves the fingers through five positions with the wrist neutral: fingers straight, proximal interphalangeal and distal interphalangeal joints flexed, full fist, metacarpophalangeal joints flexed with proximal interphalangeal and distal interphalangeal joints extended, and metacarpophalangeal and proximal interphalangeal joints flexed with distal interphalangeal joints extended. For median nerve gliding, there are six positions: full fist with wrist neutral; wrist neutral with fingers and thumb extended; wrist and fingers extended with thumb neutral; wrist, fingers, and thumb extended; wrist, fingers, and thumb extended with forearm supinated; wrist, fingers, and thumb extended with forearm supinated, then the thumb gently stretched by the other hand. Each position is maintained for 7 seconds, and the sequence is repeated five times. The patient is told to repeat this regimen three to five times each day and to soak hands for 4 minutes in warm water, then 1 minute in cold water twice a day.

Acupuncture

In a small, uncontrolled trial, acupuncture has been reported to relieve pain in patients with carpal tunnel syndrome, including patients who have persistent pain after carpal tunnel surgery (Chen, 1990). The acupuncture points needled include pericardium (PC)-7 over the median nerve at the wrist and PC-6 in the midline of the volar forearm a few centimeters proximal to the wrist. Use of acupressure at the PC-7 and PC-6 points has also been proposed for treatment of symptoms of carpal tunnel syndrome (Chen, 1990).

Percutaneous Laser Stimulation

Low-power percutaneous laser stimulation of the median nerve (so-called "laser acupuncture") reportedly benefits patients with carpal tunnel syndrome (Weintraub, 1997; Padua, Padua, Aprile & Tonali, 1998; Branco & Naeser, 1999). The reports are of small, uncontrolled series. Typical protocols use lasers operating at 670 to 904 nm. For example, one protocol delivered 9 J at each of five different points along the symptomatic median nerve, repeating the treatments for as many as 15 sessions.

Ultrasound

In a small, randomized, controlled trial, ultrasound appeared to benefit patients with carpal tunnel syndrome (Ebenbichler, Resch, Nicolakis, Wiesinger, Uhl, Ghanem & Fialka, 1998). The ultrasound was administered over the wrist, 15 minutes per session, at a frequency of 1 MHz, intensity of 1.0 W/cm^2, pulsed mode 1:4, with a 5 cm^2 transducer. The subjects all had bilateral carpal tunnel syndrome, and the study was controlled by treating one wrist with true ultrasound and one with sham ultrasound for each subject. Treatments were 5 days weekly for the first 2 weeks, then twice weekly for 5 more weeks. The treated wrists showed both symptomatic improvement and improved median distal motor latencies and transcarpal sensory conduction velocities compared with controls. Therapeutic benefit was still evident 6 months after the treatments. However, another small, randomized, controlled trial found no advantage of ultrasound over sham ultrasound (Oztas, Turan, Bora & Karakaya, 1998).

Iontophoresis

In a prospective nonrandomized, nonblinded trial, patients with carpal tunnel syndrome who had not improved using wrist splints and NSAIDs often improved symptomatically after iontophoresis of dexamethasone over the volar wrist (Banta, 1994).

Intravenous Vasodilators

In an uncontrolled series, patients with carpal tunnel syndrome were treated with intravenous infusion of 500 ml of 0.2% procaine with pentoxyphyllin and magnesium sulfuricum, daily for 10 days (Fialova, Bartousek & Nakladalova, 1999). In the majority of patients, median distal motor latency improved following the therapeutic course. No information on symptomatic response or long-term follow-up was reported.

Sternocleidomastoid Exercises

A small group of patients with carpal tunnel syndrome were taught to do sternocleidomastoid exercises aimed at assuring that neck muscle tone was symmetric; over one-half of the patients reported improvement of symptoms of carpal tunnel syndrome after performing the exercises for a number of weeks (Skubick, Clasby, Stuart Donaldson & Marshall, 1993). The authors hypothesized that the exercises corrected abnormalities of forearm flexor muscle tone that had been elicited through a tonic neck reflex.

Pyridoxine (Vitamin B$_6$)

Therapeutic Controversy

Therapy of carpal tunnel syndrome with vitamin B$_6$ (pyridoxine, pyridoxal, pyridoxamine, and their 5'-phosphates) has strong advocates, but proof of its efficacy is still lacking. In a series of papers, Folkers, Ellis, and colleagues have proposed that many cases of carpal tunnel syndrome are caused by vitamin B$_6$ deficiency (Ellis, Kishi, Azuma & Folkers, 1976; Ellis, Azuma, Watanabe, Folkers, Lowell, Hurst, Ho-Ahn & Shuford, 1977; Folkers, Ellis, Watanabe, Saji & Kaji, 1978; Ellis, Folkers, Watanabe, Kaji, Saji, Caldwell, Temple & Wood, 1979; Ellis, Folkers, Levy, Takemura, Shizukuishi, Ulrich & Harrison, 1981;

Fuhr, Farrow & Nelson, 1989; Ellis & Folkers, 1990). They measured erythrocyte glutamic-oxalacetic transaminase (EGOT) activity in vitro before and after addition of pyridoxal phosphate. Patients with carpal tunnel syndrome had lower EGOT activity than controls. Addition of pyridoxal phosphate to the in vitro assay or addition of pyridoxine to the patients' diets led to correction of the EGOT activities of these patients. Two milligrams of oral pyridoxine daily was less effective than 100 mg daily in correcting the results of the assay.

Fuhr and colleagues (1989) found low serum vitamin B$_6$ levels in some patients with carpal tunnel syndrome. Smith and colleagues (1984) found normal pyridoxal and pyridoxal phosphate levels in six patients with carpal tunnel syndrome.

Ellis and colleagues (1982) reported apparent clinical benefit of pyridoxine in seven patients in a crossover, double-blind trial against placebo, but only two of the patients had nerve conduction support for the diagnosis of carpal tunnel syndrome, and the clinical descriptions suggest that all of the patients' symptoms were not those of carpal tunnel syndrome. Wolaniuk and colleagues (1983) reported serial nerve conduction studies in three patients treated with pyridoxine. One of these patients showed statistically significant improvements in right median distal motor latency and left median wrist-to-index finger sensory latency after treatment.

Folkers and colleagues (1984) described a patient in whom they attributed carpal tunnel syndrome to combined pyridoxine and riboflavin deficiency.

Byers and colleagues (1984) criticized the Folkers and Ellis data for poorly separating symptoms of carpal tunnel syndrome from those of other conditions such as peripheral neuropathy. In patients studied by Byers and colleagues, pyridoxine deficiency on the EGOT assay correlated better with evidence of peripheral neuropathy than with evidence of carpal tunnel syndrome.

Others have reported uncontrolled or poorly controlled observations of efficacy of vitamin B$_6$ for treating symptoms of carpal tunnel syndrome (Laso Guzmán, González-Buitrago, de Arriba, Mateos, Moyano & López-Alburquerque, 1989; Bernstein & Dinesen, 1993). In one series, pyridoxine, 100 mg twice daily, was added to a conservative regimen of splinting, anti-inflammatory drugs, job changes, or carpal tunnel steroid injections, and 68% of patients improved without surgery (Kasdan & Janes, 1987). In historical controls given the same conservative regimen without pyridoxine supplements, 14% of patients with carpal tunnel syndrome responded well to conservative therapy. An accompanying discussion emphasized the inadequacy of control data in this paper and called for a well-designed prospective therapeutic trial.

Other small series have reported unimpressive responses to pyridoxine therapy (Amadio, 1985; Scheyer & Haas, 1985). One double-blind study found no benefit of pyridoxine over placebo, but small sample size (six patients treated with pyridoxine) and high response rate in control patients might have masked treatment benefit (Stransky, Rubin, Lava & Lazaro, 1989).

A survey of 125 industrial workers found no relationship between biochemical analysis of individuals' B_6 status and their symptoms of carpal tunnel syndrome or electrodiagnostic evidence of median nerve dysfunction (Franzblau, Rock, Werner, Albers, Kelly & Johnston, 1996). Another study of vitamin B_6 and vitamin C levels in 441 adults found no overall correlation between levels or these vitamins and either carpal tunnel conduction slowing or symptoms of carpal tunnel syndrome (Keniston, Nathan, Leklem & Lockwood, 1997). The authors of the later study did find, however, that low vitamin B_6 levels in men, particularly if the ratio of vitamin C to vitamin B_6 levels was high, correlated with some symptoms of carpal tunnel syndrome.

Pyridoxine Toxicity

Neuropathy is now recognized as a complication of high-dose pyridoxine use (Schaumburg, Kaplan, Windebank, Vick, Rasmus, Pleasure & Brown, 1983; Berger, Schaumburg, Schroeder, Apfel & Reynolds, 1992). A patient receiving 3 g of pyridoxine daily for treatment of carpal tunnel syndrome developed pyridoxine neuropathy (Vasile, Goldberg & Kornberg, 1984). Ellis and Folkers describe use of dose of 200 mg daily in their patients. In patients without carpal tunnel syndrome, pyridoxine toxic neuropathy has been reported in patients on doses as low as 200 mg daily, but most cases of toxicity occur in those taking daily doses of 1 g or more (Parry & Bredesen, 1985).

Synopsis: Pyridoxine in Treatment of Carpal Tunnel Syndrome

There is no convincing proof that vitamin B_6 deficiency causes carpal tunnel syndrome or that pyridoxine supplementation benefits patients with carpal tunnel syndrome. If patients choose to take pyridoxine, they should take care to avoid toxic doses.

Summary

Treatment of patients with carpal tunnel syndrome begins, whenever possible, with efforts to decrease recurrent wrist use and to treat causative medical illnesses. Many patients benefit from a simple wrist splint.

Injection of steroids into the carpal canal often gives impressive relief of symptoms. Some physicians use steroid injections frequently; others are unenthusiastic about injections because benefit is rarely permanent and complications may occur. A brief course of oral steroids can give at least temporary improvement of symptoms of carpal tunnel syndrome. Diuretics or NSAIDs are commonly used, but evidence for their value is only anecdotal. The value of pyridoxine therapy is unproven. If pyridoxine is prescribed, the dose should be kept under 200 mg daily.

Ultrasound therapy of the wrist had some value for treatment of carpal tunnel syndrome when studied in a small controlled trial. Manipulation, yoga, acupuncture, and other new or alternative therapies for carpal tunnel syndrome are innovative but, so far, none has proven value for treatment of carpal tunnel syndrome.

Many patients with carpal tunnel syndrome can be treated successfully without surgery; however, surgical therapy is indicated for most patients with fixed or progressive neurologic deficit and also for those patients without neurologic deficit who have troublesome symptoms that have not been relieved by conservative therapy.

References

Amadio PC. Pyridoxine as an adjunct in the treatment of carpal tunnel syndrome. J. Hand Surg. 1985,10A:237–41.

Ayhan-Ardic FF, Erdem HR. Long-term clinical and electrophysiological results of local steroid injection in patients with carpal tunnel syndrome. Funct. Neurol. 2000b; 15:157–65.

Babu SR, Britton JM. The role of steroid injection in the management of carpal tunnel syndrome. J. Orthop. Rheumatol. 1994;7:59–60.

Banta CA. A prospective, nonrandomized study of iontophoresis, wrist splinting, and antiinflammatory medication in the treatment of early-mild carpal tunnel syndrome. J. Occup. Med. 1994;36:166–68.

Berger AR, Schaumburg HH, Schroeder C, Apfel S, Reynolds R. Dose response, coasting, and differential fiber vulnerability in human toxic neuropathy: a prospective study of pyridoxine neurotoxicity. Neurology 1992;42:1367–70.

Bernstein AL, Dinesen JS. Brief communication: effect of pharmacologic doses of vitamin B_6 on carpal tunnel syndrome, electroencephalographic results, and pain. J. Am. Col. Nutr. 1993;12:73–76.

Bonebrake AR, Fernandez JE, Dahalan JB, Marley RJ. A treatment for carpal tunnel syndrome: results of a follow-up study. J. Manipulative Physiol. Ther. 1993;16:125–39.

Brain WR, Wright AD, Wilkinson M. Spontaneous compression of both median nerves in the carpal tunnel. Lancet 1947;1:277–82.

Branco K, Naeser MA. Carpal tunnel syndrome: clinical outcome after low-level laser acupuncture, microamps transcutaneous electrical nerve stimulation, and other alternative therapies—an open protocol study. J. Altern. Complement. Med. 1999;5:5–26.

Burke DT, Burke MM, Stewart GW, Cambre A. Splinting for carpal tunnel syndrome: in search of the optimal angle. Arch. Phys. Med. Rehabil. 1994;75:1241–44.

Byers CM, DeLisa JA, Frankel DL, Kraft GH. Pyridoxine metabolism in carpal tunnel syndrome with and without peripheral neuropathy. Arch. Phys. Med. Rehabil. 1984;65:712–16.

Chang M-H, Chiang H-T, Lee SS-J, Ger L-P, Lo Y-K. Oral drug of choice in carpal tunnel syndrome. Neurology 1998;51:390–93.

Chen GS. The effect of acupuncture treatment on carpal tunnel syndrome. Am. J. Acupunct. 1990;18:5–9.

Crow RS. Treatment of the carpal-tunnel syndrome. BMJ. 1960;1:1611–15.

Cseuz KA, Thomas JE, Lambert EH, Love JG, Lipscomb PR. Long-term results of operation for carpal tunnel syndrome. Mayo Clin. Proc. 1966;41:232–41.

Dammers JWHH, Veering MM, Vermeulen M. Injection with methylprednisolone proximal to the carpal tunnel: randomised double blind trial. BMJ. 1999;319:884–86.

Daniell HW. Yoga for carpal tunnel syndrome. JAMA. 1999;281: 2087.

Davis P, Hulbert J, Kassak K, Meyer J. Comparative efficacy of conservative medical and chiropractic treatments for carpal tunnel syndrome: a randomized clinical trail. J. Manipulative Physiol. Ther. 1998;21:317–26.

Dawson DM, Hallett M, Wilbourn AJ, eds. Entrapment Neuropathies (3rd ed). Philadelphia: Lippincott–Raven, 1999.

Deitchman S, Gerr F. Yoga for carpal tunnel syndrome. JAMA. 1999;281:2087–88.

DeStefano F, Nordstrom DL, Vierkant RA. Long-term symptom outcomes of carpal tunnel syndrome and its treatment. J. Hand Surg. 1997;22A:200–10.

Donaldson M. Carpal tunnel syndrome. BMJ. 1959;1:1184.

Duncan KH, Lewis RC Jr., Foreman KA, Nordyke MD. Treatment of carpal tunnel syndrome by members of the American Society for Surgery of the Hand: results of a questionnaire. J. Hand Surg. 1987;12A:384–91.

Ebenbichler GR, Resch KL, Nicolakis P, Wiesinger GF, Uhl F, Ghanem AH, Fialka V. Ultrasound treatment for treating the carpal tunnel syndrome: randomised "sham" controlled trial. BMJ. 1998;316:731–35.

Ellis JM, Azuma J, Watanabe T, Folkers K, Lowell JR, Hurst GA, Ho-Ahn C, Shuford EH Jr., Ulrich RF. Survey and new data on treatment with pyridoxine of patients having a clinical syndrome including the carpal tunnel and other defects. Res. Commun. Chem. Pathol. Pharmacol. 1977; 17:165–77.

Ellis JM, Folkers K. Clinical aspects of treatment of carpal tunnel syndrome with vitamin B_6. Ann. NY. Acad. Sci. 1990; 585:302–20.

Ellis JM, Folkers K, Levy M, Shizukuishi S, Lewandowski J, Nishii S, Schubert HA, Ulrich R. Response of vitamin B-6 deficiency and the carpal tunnel syndrome to pyridoxine. Proc. Natl. Acad. Sci. USA. 1982;79: 7494–98.

Ellis J, Folkers K, Levy M, Takemura K, Shizukuishi S, Ulrich R, Harrison P. Therapy with vitamin B_6 with and without surgery for treatment of patients having the idiopathic carpal tunnel syndrome. Res. Commun. Chem. Pathol. Pharmacol. 1981;33:331–44.

Ellis J, Folkers K, Watanabe T, Kaji M, Saji S, Caldwell JW, Temple CA, Wood FS. Clinical results of a cross-over treatment with pyridoxine and placebo of the carpal tunnel syndrome. Am. J. Clin. Nutr. 1979;32:2040–46.

Ellis JM, Kishi T, Azuma J, Folkers K. Vitamin B_6 deficiency in patients with a clinical syndrome including the carpal tunnel defect. Biochemical and clinical response to therapy with pyridoxine. Res. Commun. Chem. Pathol. Pharmacol. 1976;13:743–57.

Facchetti D, Chiroli S, Bascelli C, Sasanelli F. Gabapentin (GBP) vs. carbamazepine (CBZ) in conservative management of carpal tunnel syndrome. Neurology 1999; 52:A203.

Falkenburg SA. Choosing hand splints to aid carpal tunnel syndrome recovery. Occup. Health Saf. 1987;56:60–64.

Ferezy JS, Norlin WT. Carpal tunnel syndrome: a case report. Chiro. Tech. 1989;1:19–22.

Fialova J, Bartousek J, Nakladalova M. Alternative treatment of the carpal tunnel syndrome. Cent. Eur. J. Public. Health 1999;7:168–71.

Folkers K, Ellis J, Watanabe T, Saji S, Kaji M. Biochemical evidence for a deficiency of vitamin B_6 in the carpal tunnel syndrome based on a crossover clinical study. Proc. Natl. Acad. Sci. USA. 1978;75:3410–12.

Folkers K, Wolaniuk A, Vadhanavikit S. Enzymology of the response of the carpal tunnel syndrome to riboflavin and to combined riboflavin and pyridoxine. Proc. Natl. Acad. Sci. USA. 1984;81:7076–78.

Foster JB. Hydrocortisone and the carpal-tunnel syndrome. Lancet 1960;1:454–56.

Franzblau A, Rock CL, Werner RA, Albers JW, Kelly MP, Johnston EC. The relationship of vitamin B$_6$ status to median nerve function and carpal tunnel syndrome among active industrial workers. J. Occup. Environ. Med. 1996; 38:485–91.

Frederick HA, Carter PR, Littler JW. Injection injuries to the median and ulnar nerves at the wrist. J. Hand Surg. 1992;17A:645–47.

Fuhr JE, Farrow A, Nelson HS Jr. Vitamin B$_6$ levels in patients with carpal tunnel syndrome. Arch. Surg. 1989;124:1329–30.

Futami T, Kobayashi A, Wakabayashi N, Yonemoto K, Nakamura K. Natural history of carpal tunnel syndrome. J. Jpn. Soc. Surg. Hand 1992;9:410–12.

Garfinkel MS, Singhal A, Katz WA, Allan DA, Reshetar R, Schumacher HR Jr. Yoga-based intervention for carpal tunnel syndrome: a randomized trial. JAMA. 1998;280: 1601–3.

Gelberman RH, Aronson D, Weisman MH. Carpal-tunnel syndrome. Results of a prospective trial of steroid injection and splinting. J. Bone Joint Surg. 1980;62A:1181–84.

Giannini F, Passero S, Cioni R, Paradiso C, Battistini N, Giordano N, Vaccai D, Marcolongo R. Electrophysiologic evaluation of local steroid injection in carpal tunnel syndrome. Arch. Phys. Med. Rehabil. 1991;72:738–42.

Girlanda P, Dattola R, Venuto C, Mangiapane R, Nicolosi C, Messina C. Local steroid treatment in idiopathic carpal tunnel syndrome: short- and long-term efficacy. J. Neurol. 1993;240:187–90.

Goodman HV, Foster JB. Effect of local corticosteroid injection on median nerve conduction in carpal tunnel syndrome. Ann. Phys. Med. 1962;VI:287–94.

Goodman HV, Gilliatt RW. The effect of treatment on median nerve conduction in patients with the carpal tunnel syndrome. Ann. Phys. Med. 1961;6:137–55.

Gottlieb NL, Riskin WG. Complications of local corticosteroid injections. JAMA. 1980;243:1547–48.

Gray RG, Gottlieb NL. Intra-articular corticosteroids. An updated assessment. Clin. Orthop. 1983;105:235–63.

Green DP. Diagnostic and therapeutic value of carpal tunnel injection. J. Hand Surg. 1984;9A:850–54.

Harrast M, Kraft G. Yoga for carpal tunnel syndrome. JAMA. 1999;281:2088.

Harter BT Jr., McKiernan JE Jr., Kirzinger SS, Archer FW, Peters CK, Harter KC. Carpal tunnel syndrome: surgical and nonsurgical treatment. J. Hand Surg. 1993;18A:734–39.

Heathfield KWG. Acroparaesthesiae and the carpal-tunnel syndrome. Lancet 1957;2:663–66.

Herskovitz S, Berger AR, Lipton RB. Low-dose, short-term oral prednisone in the treatment of carpal tunnel syndrome. Neurology 1995;45:1923–25.

Irwin LR, Beckett R, Suman RK. Steroid injection for carpal tunnel syndrome. J. Hand Surg. 1996;21B:355–57.

Johnson EW. Should immediate surgery be done for carpal tunnel syndrome?—No! Muscle Nerve 1995;18:658–59.

Kasdan ML, Janes C. Carpal tunnel syndrome and vitamin B$_6$. Plast. Reconstr. Surg. 1987;79:456–62.

Kasten SJ, Louis DS. Carpal tunnel syndrome: a case of median nerve injection injury and a safe and effective method for injecting the carpal tunnel. J. Fam. Pract. 1996;43:79–82.

Katz JN, Keller RB, Simmons BP, Rogers WD, Bessette L, Fossel AH, Mooney NA. Maine Carpal Tunnel Study: outcomes of operative and nonoperative therapy for carpal tunnel syndrome in a community-based cohort. J. Hand Surg. 1998;23A:697–710.

Kay NR, Marshall PD. A safe, reliable method of carpal tunnel injection. J. Hand Surg. 1992;17A:1160–61.

Keller RB, Largay AM, Soule DN, Katz JN. Maine Carpal Tunnel Study: small area variations. J. Hand Surg. 1998; 23A:692–96.

Keniston RC, Nathan PA, Leklem JE, Lockwood RS. Vitamin B$_6$, vitamin C, and carpal tunnel syndrome. A cross-sectional study of 441 adults. J. Occup. Environ. Med. 1997;39:949–59.

Kopell HP. Carpal tunnel compression median neuropathy treated nonsurgically. N. Y. State J. Med. 1958;58:744–45.

Kruger VL, Kraft GH, Deitz JC, Ameis A, Polissar L. Carpal tunnel syndrome: objective measures and splint use. Arch. Phys. Med. Rehabil. 1991;72:517–20.

Laso Guzmán FJ, González-Buitrago JM, de Arriba F, Mateos F, Moyano JC, López-Alburquerque T. Carpal tunnel syndrome and vitamin B$_6$. Klin. Wochenschr. 1989;67:38–41.

Linskey ME, Segal R. Median nerve injury from local steroid injection in carpal tunnel syndrome. Neurosurgery 1990;26:512–15.

Luchetti R, Schoenhuber R, Alfarano M, Deluca S, De Cicco G, Landi A. Serial overnight recordings of intracarpal canal pressure in carpal tunnel syndrome patients with and without wrist splinting. J. Hand Surg. 1994;19B:35–37.

Mackinnon SE, Novak CB. Yoga for carpal tunnel syndrome. JAMA. 1999;281:2087.

Manente G, Torrieri F, Di Blasio F, Staniscia T, Romano F, Uncini A. An innovative hand brace for carpal tunnel syndrome: a randomized controlled trial. Muscle Nerve 2001;24:1020–25.

Marshall S, Tardif G, Ashworth N. Local corticosteroid injection for carpal tunnel syndrome (Cochrane Review). The Cochrane Library 2000;4.

McCallum MJ. Acroparaesthesia in pregnancy. BMJ. 1959; 2:1095.

McConnell JR, Bush DC. Intraneural steroid injection as a complication in the management of carpal tunnel syndrome. A report of three cases. Clin. Orthop. 1990;119:181–84.

Minamikawa Y, Peimer CA, Kambe K, Wheeler DR, Sherwin FS. Tenosynovial injection for carpal tunnel syndrome. J. Hand Surg. 1992;17A:178–81.

Nathan PA, Keniston RC, Myers LD, Meadows KD, Lockwood RS. Natural history of median nerve sensory conduction in industry: relationship to symptoms and carpal tunnel syndrome in 558 hands over 11 years. Muscle Nerve 1998;21:711–21.

O'Gradaigh D, Merry P. Corticosteroid injection for the treatment of carpal tunnel syndrome. Ann. Rheum. Dis. 2000;59:918–19.

Ozdogan H, Yazici H. The efficacy of local steroid injections in idiopathic carpal tunnel syndrome: a double-blind study. Br. J. Rheumatol. 1984;23:272–75.

Oztas O, Turan B, Bora I, Karakaya MK. Ultrasound therapy effect in carpal tunnel syndrome. Arch. Phys. Med. Rehabil. 1998;79:1540–44.

Padua L, Padua R, Aprile I, Pasqualetti P, Tonali P. Multiperspective follow-up of untreated carpal tunnel syndrome. A multicenter study. Neurology 2001;56:1459–66.

Padua L, Padua R, Aprile I, Tonali P. Noninvasive laser neurolysis in carpal tunnel syndrome. Muscle Nerve 1998;21:1232–33.

Panagariya A, Sharma AK. A preliminary trial of serratiopeptidase in patients with carpal tunnel syndrome. J. Assoc. Physicians India 1999;47:1170–72.

Parry GJ, Bredesen DE. Sensory neuropathy with low-dose pyridoxine. Neurology 1985;35:1466–68.

Phalen GS. The carpal-tunnel syndrome. Seventeen years' experience in diagnosis and treatment of six hundred fifty-four hands. J. Bone Joint Surg. 1966;48A:211–28.

Phalen GS. The carpal-tunnel syndrome. Clinical evaluation of 598 hands. Clin. Orthop. 1972;83:29–40.

Phalen GS, Kendrick JI. Compression neuropathy of the median nerve in the carpal tunnel. JAMA. 1957;164:524–30.

Quin CE. Carpal tunnel syndrome: treatment by splinting. Ann. Phys. Med. 1961;6:72–75.

Roaf R. Compression of the median nerve in the carpal tunnel. Lancet 1947;1:387.

Rozmaryn LM, Dovelle S, Rothman ER, Gorman K, Olvey KM, Bartko JJ. Nerve and tendon gliding exercises and the conservative management of carpal tunnel syndrome. J. Hand Ther. 1998;11:171–79.

Schaumburg HH, Kaplan A, Windebank A, Vick N, Rasmus S, Pleasure D, Brown MJ. Sensory neuropathy from pyridoxine abuse: a new megavitamin syndrome. N. Engl. J. Med. 1983;309:445–48.

Smith GP, Rudge PJ, Peters TJ. Biochemical studies of pyridoxal and pyridoxal phosphate status and therapeutic trial of pyridoxine in patients with carpal tunnel syndrome. Ann. Neurol. 1984;15:104–7.

Scheyer RD, Haas DC. Pyridoxine in carpal tunnel syndrome. Lancet 1985;2:42.

Skubick DL, Clasby R, Stuart Donaldson CC, Marshall WM. Carpal tunnel syndrome as an expression of muscular dysfunction in the neck. J. Occup. Rehabil. 1993; 3:31–44.

Stransky M, Rubin A, Lava NS, Lazaro RP. Treatment of carpal tunnel syndrome with vitamin B_6: a double-blind study. South. Med. J. 1989;82:841–42.

Sucher BM. Myofascial manipulative release of carpal tunnel syndrome: documentation with magnetic resonance imaging. J. Am. Osteopath. Assoc. 1993a;93:1273–78.

Sucher BM. Myofascial release of carpal tunnel syndrome. J. Am. Osteopath. Assoc. 1993b;93:92–94, 100–101.

Sucher BM. Palpatory diagnosis and manipulative management of carpal tunnel syndrome. J. Am. Osteopath. Assoc. 1994;94:647–63.

Sucher BM. Palpatory diagnosis and manipulative management of carpal tunnel syndrome: Part 2. 'Double crush' and thoracic outlet syndrome. J. Am. Osteopath. Assoc. 1995;95:471–79.

Sucher BM, Hinrichs RN. Manipulative treatment of carpal tunnel syndrome: biomechanical and osteopathic intervention to increase the length of the transverse carpal ligament. J. Am. Osteopath. Assoc. 1998;98:679–86.

Tal-Akabi A, Rushton A. An investigation to compare the effectiveness of carpal bone mobilisation and neurodynamic mobilisation as methods of treatment for carpal tunnel syndrome. Manipulative Ther. 2000;5:214–22.

Tavares SP, Giddins GE. Nerve injury following steroid injection for carpal tunnel syndrome. A report of two cases. J. Hand Surg. 1996;21B:208–9.

Valente R. Chiropractic therapy in carpal tunnel syndrome: a case study. ACA. J. Chiropractic 1991;28:76–78.

Valente R, Gibson H. Chiropractic manipulation in carpal tunnel syndrome. J. Manipulative Physiol. Ther. 1994;17:246–49.

van der Bracht AA. Carpal tunnel syndrome. BMJ. 1958; 1:1180–81.

Vasile A, Goldberg R, Kornberg B. Pyridoxine toxicity: report of a case. J. Am. Osteopath. Assoc. 1984;83:790–91.

Walker WC, Metzler M, Cifu DX, Swartz Z. Neutral wrist splinting in carpal tunnel syndrome: a comparison of night-only versus full-time wear instructions. Arch. Phys. Med. Rehabil. 2000;81:424–29.

Weintraub MI. Noninvasive laser neurolysis in carpal tunnel syndrome. Muscle Nerve 1997;20:1029–31.

Weiss A-P, Sachar K, Gendreau M. Conservative management of carpal tunnel syndrome: a reexamination of steroid injection and splinting. J. Hand Surg. 1994;19A:410–15.

Weiss ND, Gordon L, Bloom T, So Y, Rempel DM. Position of the wrist associated with the lowest carpal-tunnel pressure: implications for splint design. J. Bone Joint Surg. 1995;77A:1695–99.

Wilson JR, Sumner AJ. Immediate surgery is the treatment of choice for carpal tunnel syndrome. Muscle Nerve 1995;18:660–62.

Wolaniuk A, Vadhanavikit S, Folkers K. Electromyographic data differentiate patients with the carpal tunnel syndrome when double blindly treated with pyridoxine and placebo. Res. Commun. Chem. Pathol. Pharmacol. 1983; 41:501–11.

Wong SM, Hui ACF, Tang A, Ho PC, Hung LK, Wong KS, Kay R, Li E. Local vs. systemic corticosteroids in the treatment of carpal tunnel syndrome. Neurology 2001;56: 1565–67.

Wood EC. Acroparaesthesia in pregnancy. BMJ. 1959;2: 1254.

Wood MR. Hydrocortisone injections for carpal tunnel syndrome. Hand 1980;12:62–64.

Wu S, Chan R, Hsu T. Electrodiagnostic evaluation of conservative treatment in carpal tunnel syndrome. Chin. Med. J. (Taipei) 1991;48:125–30.

Chapter 15
Surgical Treatment of Carpal Tunnel Syndrome

Learmonth (1933) first reported the surgical division of the flexor retinaculum to relieve the symptoms of carpal tunnel syndrome. By the late 1940s, Zachary (1945), Cannon and Love (1946), Brain and colleagues (1947), and Phalen et al. (1950) had reported excellent symptomatic relief of carpal tunnel syndrome symptoms after surgery in small series of patients.

The preceding chapter discusses nonsurgical therapy and indications for electing surgical therapy. This chapter covers surgical technique, postoperative care, results of surgery, and complications of surgery.

Technique

The basic concept is simple: complete section of the transverse carpal ligament through an open palmar incision or with an endoscope. A number of variations on the theme are possible regarding particulars such as anesthesia, location of the incisions, care in identifying nerve branches, treatment of the palmaris longus tendon, neurolysis of the median nerve, inspection and débridement of the carpal canal, intraoperative use of steroids, and postoperative care (Hudson, Wissinger, Salazar, Kline, Yarzagaray, Danoff, Fernandez & Field, 1997). Ariyan and Watson (1977), Conolly (1983), Heckler and Jabaley (1986), Birch and colleagues (1998), and Dawson and colleagues (1999) provide descriptions of their personal techniques with photographic illustrations.

Options for Anesthesia and Tourniquet Use

Carpal tunnel surgery can be performed under local or regional anesthesia (Duncan, Lewis, Foreman & Nordyke, 1987; Wilson, 1993; Baguneid, Sochart, Dunlop & Kenny, 1997; Ebskov, Boeckstyns & Sorensen, 1997; Khan & Macey, 2000; Tomaino, Ulizio & Vogt, 2001). When local anesthesia is used, preapplication of topical local anesthetic cream to the palm can decrease the pain caused by the local anesthetic injection (Avramidis, Lewis & Gallagher, 2000). General anesthesia is used for occasional cases. A tourniquet is commonly used to maintain a "bloodless" operative field; however, prolonged application of the tourniquet can be painful and can cause transient nerve block or, even, nerve injury. Tourniquet-induced pain and paresthesias are reduced if the tourniquet is placed on the forearm instead of the upper arm (Hutchinson & McClinton, 1993). Another approach is to eschew use of the tourniquet and maintain hemostasis by using epinephrine with the local anesthetic injected in the hand (Gibson, 1990; Braithwaite, Robinson & Burge, 1993; Tzarnas, 1993).

Open Carpal Tunnel Surgery

Incision

The optimal cutaneous landmarks for the incision are still debated. At issue is the best approach to minimize the possibility of injury to the palmar

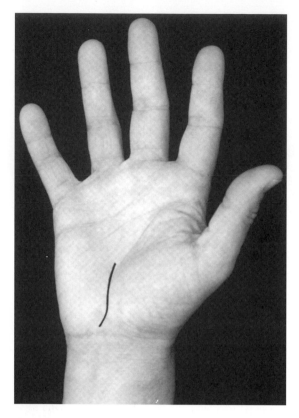

Figure 15-1. Outline of a typical incision for open carpal tunnel surgery.

cutaneous innervation. The palmar cutaneous branch of the median nerve leaves the radial side of the median nerve an average of 4 to 6 cm proximal to the distal wrist crease (range, 27 to 78 mm) (Martin, Seiler & Lesesne, 1996; Watchmaker, Weber & Mackinnon, 1996). The nerve typically crosses the distal wrist crease at the tubercle of the scaphoid bone. Its anatomy and variations are discussed in more detail in Chapter 1. The nerve is vulnerable to transection or to encasement in scar if the surgical incision is carried too far laterally. Figure 1-5 shows some of the unusual, anomalous paths that the nerve can follow; the surgeon must be wary of this even with the recommended longitudinal incision (Das & Brown, 1976).

The ulnar nerve provides cutaneous sensation of the medial palm in various ways. The usual source of medial palmar cutaneous sensation is the nerve of Henle, which also provides the vasa nervorum of the ulnar artery (McCabe & Kleinert, 1990). The cutaneous sensory branches of this nerve often become subcutaneous along the ulnar aspect of the distal wrist crease. Most individuals have additional branches of the ulnar nerve supplying portions of the palm, originating directly from the ulnar nerve or from its hypothenar motor or digital sensory branches; these cutaneous branches typically cross the medial palm transversely, perpendicular to the course of the ulnar nerve. Many of these cutaneous branches are vulnerable to injury with some carpal tunnel surgical incisions (Martin et al., 1996).

A minority of individuals has a distinct palmar cutaneous branch of the ulnar nerve. Engber and Gmeiner (1980) reported two cases of painful neuromas in the hypothenar area after carpal tunnel surgery. They demonstrated that the palmar cutaneous branch of the ulnar nerve could follow a variety of courses in the hypothenar area. This nerve is best avoided if the incision is no more medial than the axis of the ring finger.

Many surgeons have used a curvilinear longitudinal incision in line with the axis of the ring finger (Taleisnik, 1973; Ariyan & Watson, 1977; Heckler & Jabaley, 1986). In the palm, the density of cutaneous nerve branches greater than 75 μm in diameter is lowest along the web space between the ring and middle fingers (Ruch, Marr, Holden, James, Challa & Smith, 1999). An alternative suggestion is a longitudinal incision from the wrist to the palmar point of maximal depression between the thenar and hypothenar eminences; this point is best localized with the wrist fully extended (Watchmaker et al., 1996). Whichever landmarks are used, the surgeon can best protect the cutaneous innervation of the palm by careful identification and preservation of palmar cutaneous nerves (Tomaino & Plakseychuk, 1998).

The operation can be done through a small incision, as outlined in Figure 15-1, but some cases require proximal extension of the incision, and some surgeons routinely use a longer incision (Duncan et al., 1987). The incision is carried down through the palmar aponeurosis to the transverse carpal ligament (Denman, 1981).

In the 1990s, partly in response to the introduction of carpal tunnel endoscopic surgery, there was increased interest in approaching the carpal tunnel through smaller incisions: a 2- to 3-cm mid-palmar incision, a 2-cm transverse incision at the distal wrist crease, or two incisions, one in the distal palm and one at the distal wrist crease (Biyani & Downes, 1993; Bromley, 1994; Wilson, 1994; LoVerme & Saccone, 1995; Shapiro, 1995; Bensimon & Murphy, 1996; Luchetti, Alfarano, Montagna & Soragni, 1996; Jimenez, Gibbs & Clapper, 1998; Avci & Sayli, 2000). Special instruments to guide the knife incising the transverse carpal ligament or to improve visualization have been designed (Carter, 1991; Lee & Jackson, 1996; Serra, Benito & Monner, 1997). An even shorter incision, 1.0 to 1.5 cm, can be used if part of the transverse carpal ligament is sectioned blindly, using a specially designed "carpal tunnel 'tome'" (Lee & Strickland, 1998). A 2-cm incision in the palm can be combined with use of an endoscope to transect the proximal portions of the transverse carpal ligament and extend the transection to the distal antebrachial fascia (Pennino & Tavin, 1996). Small controlled series suggest that compared with traditional open carpal tunnel surgery, small incision open techniques result in less pain and better pinch and grip strength in the early postoperative period (Biyani & Downes, 1993; Wilson, 1994). In a sobering letter, one advocate of combining a small incision and a special instrument to blindly section the transverse carpal ligament reported that he had abandoned the technique after accidentally transecting a median nerve (Murphy, 1997).

Section of the Flexor Retinaculum

The simplest operation is section of the flexor retinaculum without exploration or disturbance of the median nerve or of the contents of the carpal tunnel. Before division of the retinaculum, the recurrent thenar motor branch of the median nerve must be identified and protected. The various possible courses of this branch are illustrated in Chapter 1. The recurrent thenar motor branch is particularly vulnerable to injury when it takes a course through the transverse carpal ligament. If the recurrent thenar motor branch is severed at the time of carpal tunnel surgery, the nerve should be primarily repaired; if the nerve laceration is unrecognized, the patient can require reoperation for secondary repair of the severed nerve (Mannerfelt & Hybbinette, 1972; Lilly & Magnell, 1985; Hybbinette, 1986).

The transverse carpal ligament must be divided from its most proximal to its most distal extent. Distally, care must be taken not to injure the digital nerves and the superficial palmar arterial arch (Semple & Cargill, 1969). Phalen (1966) noted that after complete division, the retinaculum separates by approximately one-fourth of an inch.

A number of idiosyncratic operative techniques have been suggested but have not gained popularity (Pierce, 1976; Fissette, Boucq, Lahaye & Onkelinx, 1981; Paine & Polyzoidis, 1983; Grundberg, 1986; Masear, Hayes & Hyde, 1986; Pearl, 1989; Pagnanelli & Barrer, 1992; Zimmerli, 1992; Hunter, Read & Gray, 1993; Abouzahr, Patsis & Chiu, 1995; Di Giuseppe & Ajmar, 1996; Franzini, Broggi, Servello, Dones & Pluchino, 1996; Loick, Joosten & Lucke, 1997; Nakamichi & Tachibana, 1997; Weber & Sanders, 1997).

Neurolysis

Neurolysis is usually not necessary at the time of carpal tunnel release. Opinion has been divided on its benefits (Phalen, 1966; Curtis & Eversmann, 1973; Hybbinette & Mannerfelt, 1975). One argument for neurolysis is that nerve damage can be assessed and appropriate therapy planned best by inspection of the median nerve through the operating microscope (Palazzi & Palazzi, 1980). Neurolysis starts with longitudinal division of the epineurium. Next, the epineurium is dissected away from the nerve fascicles to obtain an external neurolysis. The dissection typically spares the dorsal epineurium in an effort to preserve microvascular supply to the nerve. The surgeon can proceed with an internal neurolysis to remove fibrosis between the fascicles. A fascicle that is deformed by scarring or neuroma might be resected and grafted. Some surgeons elect internal neurolysis based on the clinical severity of the median nerve deficit; others make a decision on the extent of neurolysis after observing the condition of the nerve at surgery.

Eversmann and Ritsick (1978) recommended internal neurolysis in patients with a preoperative deficit such as thenar atrophy or abnormal median nerve sensory examination. In seven patients undergoing carpal tunnel surgery with internal neurolysis, they measured median distal motor latency before release of the transverse carpal liga-

Table 15-1. Effect of Internal Neurolysis on Intraoperative Median Distal Motor Latency

Patient	Distal Median Motor Latency (msec)		
	Before Surgery	After Ligament Release	After Internal Neurolysis
1	9.7	7.9	6.7
2	8.6	7.1	4.5
3	7.1	6.7	5.1
4	10.1	8.3	5.9
5	4.0	5.1	5.3
6	5.6	5.5	4.6
7	8.3	4.9	5.4
Mean	7.6	6.5	5.4

Data from WW Eversmann Jr, JA Ritsick. Intraoperative changes in motor nerve conduction latency in carpal tunnel syndrome. J. Hand Surg. 1978;3:77–81.

ment, after release, and after internal neurolysis. Five of the seven showed a greater improvement in distal motor latency after internal neurolysis than after release of the transverse carpal ligament but before neurolysis. Table 15-1 shows the values for the seven patients.

Note that in contrast to the impressive improvement in five of the patients after neurolysis, patients number 5 and 7 showed deterioration in median distal motor latency. During surgery in eight patients undergoing carpal tunnel release with neurolysis, Yates and colleagues (1981) measured median distal motor latency and thenar compound muscle action potential amplitude. Three of the patients had a drop in compound muscle potential amplitude after neurolysis, suggesting development of acute partial conduction block.

Even in patients who have intraoperative improvement in nerve conduction after internal neurolysis, the electrical improvement does not guarantee that neurolysis leads to a superior clinical outcome. As discussed in Chapter 8, the correlation between nerve conduction results and symptoms is imperfect. Furthermore, internal neurolysis might lead to delayed fibrosis or nerve ischemia that could negate any of the acute benefits proposed by Eversmann and Ritsick.

A number of clinical studies address the effectiveness of neurolysis in carpal tunnel syndrome. Evrard and Tshiakatumba (1977) reported the

results of carpal tunnel release accompanied by internal neurolysis in 18 hands. Eighty-nine percent of the operations gave excellent or good results; in comparison, they obtained good or excellent results in only 61% of a historical control series. They provide few data on the comparability of the series.

Fissette and Onkelinx (1979) reported a series of 45 carpal tunnel operations in which they inspected the nerve under the microscope and performed an external neurolysis when the nerve was thickened or narrowed. In three cases they found interstitial fibrosis and proceeded with internal neurolysis. They found no definite advantage with this protocol compared with their own experience with division of the transverse carpal ligament without neurolysis.

Lowry and Follender (1988) randomized 50 carpal tunnel operations to transverse carpal ligament release alone or to transverse carpal ligament release followed by internal neurolysis. The patients all had severe carpal tunnel syndrome with thenar atrophy or with a fixed median sensory deficit. Three months after surgery, 67% of the patients who had neurolysis and 65% of the patients who did not have neurolysis reported a good or excellent surgical result. There was no significant difference between the two groups in postoperative median nerve conduction studies or in complication rate.

Holmgran-Larsson and colleagues randomized 48 patients to ligament division either alone or followed by internal neurolysis (Holmgren-Larsson, Leszniewski, Linden, Rabow & Thorling, 1985; Holmgren & Rabow, 1987). At immediate postoperative and 3-year postoperative follow-up, the two groups had no significant differences in improvement after surgery.

Gelberman and colleagues initially favored internal neurolysis in patients with carpal tunnel syndrome that was severe enough to result in objective neurologic deficit (Rhoades, Mowery & Gelberman, 1985). They reported excellent clinical results in 36 hands with this technique. They changed their opinion after evaluating 33 additional hands with equally severe neurologic deficit and obtaining equivalent results after section of the retinaculum without neurolysis (Gelberman, Pfeffer, Galbraith, Szabo, Rydevik & Dimick, 1987).

In 63 carpal tunnel decompressions Mackinnon and colleagues (1991) randomly assigned which patients would undergo internal neurolysis. In this prospective study, neurolysis added no demonstrable benefit to the surgical outcome.

In three prospective trials, patients undergoing carpal tunnel surgery have been randomized to have or not have a linear epineurotomy, incising the epineurium without removing it or attempting more detailed nerve dissection. Surgical outcomes were not significantly different comparing the epineurotomy with the nonepineurotomy groups (Foulkes, Atkinson, Beuchel, Doyle & Singer, 1994; Blair, Goetz, Ross, Steyers & Chang, 1996; Leinberry, Hammond & Siegfried, 1997).

In summary, division of the transverse carpal ligament is extremely effective treatment for most cases of carpal tunnel syndrome. No consistent benefit from neurolysis has been demonstrated.

Flexor Tenosynovectomy

Phalen (1966) advised against routine flexor tenosynovectomy or neurolysis. He performed tenosynovectomy in 4% of his patients, only when the median nerve appeared persistently stretched after section of the ligament. The typical patient who requires tenosynovectomy has carpal tunnel syndrome accompanying rheumatoid arthritis (Straub & Ranawat, 1969; Marmor, 1971; Nalebuff, 1983). Corradi and colleagues (1989) advocate flexor tenosynovectomy in chronic hemodialysis patients who require surgery for carpal tunnel syndrome due to beta-2 microglobulin amyloidosis. In a small, controlled series, Freshwater and Arons (1978) compared 12 patients treated with release of the transverse carpal ligament alone with 14 patients who were treated with transverse carpal ligament release, flexor tenosynovectomy, external neurolysis of the median nerve, and intraoperative instillation of steroids. At follow-up 2 years postoperatively, all 26 patients were asymptomatic. The group with the more extensive surgery had a longer average delay before return to work after surgery.

Palmaris Longus Tendon

Most surgeons do not resect the palmaris longus tendon routinely at the time of carpal tunnel surgery but optionally resect the tendon on those rare occasions when it appears to compress the median nerve (Phalen, 1966; Duncan et al., 1987).

Some surgeons advocate palmaris longus tendon transfer to the thenar muscles as an opponensplasty in selected patients with severe thenar atrophy (Littler & Li, 1967; Braun, 1978; Foucher, Malizos, Sammut, Marin Braun & Michon, 1991; Terrono, Rose, Mulroy & Millender, 1993; Dlabal, 1995; MacDougal, 1995). Other surgeons use various other forearm and hand muscle-tendon units on those rare occasions when opponensplasty is needed (Inglis, Straub & Williams, 1972; Cooney, 1988; Anderson, Lee & Sundararaj, 1992; Brandsma & Ottenhoff-De Jonge, 1992). Planning tendon transfer is more complex when the median nerve injury is proximal to the carpal tunnel or is combined with radial or ulnar neuropathies (Omer, 1992).

Transverse Carpal Ligamentoplasty

A few surgeons reconstruct the transverse carpal ligament after sectioning it. The rationale for this approach is discussed under Analysis of Unsatisfactory Surgical Results, later in this chapter. Techniques include suturing the free radial edge of the transverse carpal ligament to an ulnar edge of the palmar aponeurosis, creating a diagonal flap of the transverse carpal ligament arising from the proximal radial aspect of the ligament and suturing it to the distal ulnar aspect of the ligament, incorporating part of the distal antebrachial fascia into the flap, or a Z-plasty in which the initial incision of the ligament is zigzag, then the cut edges are realigned and resutured to lengthen the ligament (Kapandji, 1990; Jakab, Ganos & Cook, 1991; Schlenker, Koulis & Kho, 1993; Karlsson, Lindau & Hagberg, 1997; Netscher, Mosharrafa, Lee, Polsen, Choi, Steadman & Thornby, 1997). Another surgical variation replaces the traditional linear incision of the transverse carpal ligament with a parabolic incision; although not a ligamentoplasty, this incision offers another approach to preventing herniation or bowstring of canal contents postoperatively (Abdullah, Wolber & Ditto, 1995).

Endoscopic Carpal Tunnel Surgery

Endoscopic section of the transverse carpal ligament with minimal disturbance of the skin or the palmar aponeurosis was introduced by Okutsu and colleagues (1987) and has been studied extensively in the last decade. The risk of complications is highest among surgeons learning the procedure. All surgeons should practice first on cadaver wrists; surgical errors are common during this portion of the training period (Lee, Masear, Meyer, Stevens & Colgin, 1992).

One-Portal Techniques

Okutsu. Okotsu and colleagues (1987) introduced endoscopic carpal tunnel decompression, performed by passing the endoscope through a clear plastic outer sheath, which has been inserted through a small transverse incision proximal to the distal wrist crease, on the ulnar side of the palmaris longus tendon. With the endoscope in place to view the incision, a hook knife is inserted along the ulnar boarder of the sheath, catches the distal edge of the transverse carpal ligament, and incises the ligament as it and the endoscope are withdrawn.

Agee. The most commonly used one-portal endoscopic approach, attributed to Agee (1990), uses a proximal incision at the distal wrist crease between the borders of the flexor carpi radialis and flexor carpi ulnaris tendons (Agee, McCarroll, & North, 1994; Ruch & Poehling, 1996; Rabb & Kernan, 1997). The device is sold commercially by the Orthopedic Products Division of 3M (St. Paul, MN). The endoscope is inserted under the transverse carpal ligament, lateral to the hook of the hamate, in the line of the ring finger. A lateral viewing window at the tip of the endoscope is used to visualize the underside of the transverse carpal ligament, but does not allow further inspection of the contents to the carpal tunnel. The endoscope is passed to the distal border of the transverse carpal ligament, then the cutting blade is elevated, and the endoscope is withdrawn, transecting the retinaculum. A needle, inserted through the palm, can help identify the distal end of the transverse carpal ligament (Wheatley, 1996). The original commercial model was withdrawn from the market in the early 1990s and replaced with a redesigned blade assembly that allowed endoscopic visualization of the point of blade entry into the transverse carpal ligament (Laitt, Jackson & Isherwood, 1996).

Slotted Cannula Techniques. Menon (1993, 1994) described a single-portal endoscopic approach using a D-shaped slotted cannula with a blunt end. The instruments for this approach are sold by Linvatec (Largo, FL) as the Concept Carpal Tunnel Relief Kit. The slotted cannula is inserted through an incision made at the distal wrist crease in line with the radial border of the ring finger. The cannula is advanced under the transverse carpal ligament in line with the ring finger. The underside of the flexor retinaculum is viewed with the endoscope, looking through the slot in the cannula. The ligament is incised by advancing a knife from proximal to distal along the slot of the cannula.

An alternative proximally inserted, single-portal cannula system (Uni-Cut Carpal Tunnel Release Kit; Acufex Microsurgical Inc., Harrogate, UK) uses a dual-slotted cannula, one slot for passage of the hook knife and one for viewing with the endoscope (Worseg, Kuzbari, Korak, Hocker, Wiederer, Tschabitscher & Holle, 1996).

Distal One-Portal Technique. Another endoscopic approach to the carpal tunnel uses a single incision made where the flexed ring finger touches the palm, just lateral to the hypothenar eminence (Tsuruta, Syed & Tsai, 1994; Tsai, Tsuruta, Syed & Kimura, 1995). The palmar fascia is incised at this location and dissected to reveal the distal edge of the transverse carpal ligament. A custom-designed glass tube is inserted under the flexor retinaculum through this portal. The endoscope is passed through the tube, allowing inspection of the transverse carpal ligament and of the carpal canal contents. A special retractor is inserted superficial to the transverse carpal ligament, parallel to the glass tube, so that the two instruments sandwich the retinaculum. Both the tube and the retractor have grooves that allow passage of a knife, guided by the grooves, to divide the retinaculum.

With this technique, the use of the glass tube permits visualization of the carpal tunnel contents that is not possible with the two-portal (Chow) or proximal one-portal (Agee, Menon) techniques. However, the glass tube has been known to chip, adding to the list of possible complications. A similar palmar approach using a slotted cannula rather than a glass tube has also been described (Mirza, King & Tanveer, 1995).

Two-Portal Techniques

Chow (1989) introduced a two-portal endoscopic approach for carpal tunnel surgery (Chow, 1994, 1996). Instruments for this technique are marketed by Smith & Nephew Dyonics, Inc. (Andover, MA) as the Dyonics ECTRA II system. The initial incision is made near the midline of the volar proximal wrist crease, 0.5 cm proximal and 1.5 to 2.0 cm lateral to the proximal pole of the pisiform. An exit portal is created in the proximal, lateral palm. A slotted cannula with a dissecting obturator is placed through the entry incision, under and closely adjacent to the transverse carpal ligament, and out the exit portal. Depending on exact placement of the instrument, the operator can choose a transbursal or extrabursal location of the cannula, defined by whether the instrument enters the ulnar bursa (Resnick & Miller, 1991; Fischer & Hastings, 1996). Chow's original technique used the transbursal approach, so the extrabursal approach is sometimes called the modified Chow technique. Another variation on Chow's techniques uses a dissector and guide tube to develop the path for insertion of the cannula (Lewicky, 1994). Full insertion of the cannula and obturator requires that the wrist be hyperextended, which keeps the canal in contact with the transverse carpal ligament. After the obturator is withdrawn, the slot in the canal permits visualization of the transverse carpal ligament with the endoscope and access to the retinaculum with the knives used to transect it. The operator works with the endoscope inserted through the proximal end of the canal and a knife inserted through the distal end. Once the distal cuts are completed, the positions of the endoscope and knives are reversed to do the proximal cuts. The two-portal endoscope views only the underside of the transverse carpal ligament through the cannula slot, so the technique does not permit visualization of any other anatomic structures or other contents of the carpal tunnel.

Brown et al. (1992) described a modified two-portal technique, using instruments available from Instratek, Inc. (Houston, TX).

Challenges of Endoscopic Surgery

After open carpal tunnel surgery, all layers from the skin to the transverse carpal ligament have been incised. Endoscopic section of the transverse carpal ligament leaves the skin and superficial fascia largely intact. The endoscopist must decide whether to extend the incision volarly into the palmar aponeurosis. In the past, *flexor retinaculum* and *transverse carpal ligament* have been used synonymously. More recent anatomic studies suggest the flexor retinaculum includes both the transverse carpal ligament and the palmar aponeurosis (Cobb, Dalley, Posteraro & Lewis, 1993). The palmar aponeurosis consists of transversely oriented collagen fibers running between the hypothenar and thenar muscles, superficial to the transverse carpal ligament. The palmar aponeurosis has a mean thickness of 1 mm at its lateral and medial edges and ranges from 1.4 to 2.8 mm thick at its center (Cobb et al., 1993). In cadaver studies, even experienced endoscopists often do not completely divide the flexor retinaculum; variations include leaving transverse fibers (probably from the palmar aponeurosis) restraining complete separation of the divided ligament, failing to divide the distal edge of the ligament, or dividing volar but not dorsal fibers of the ligament (Schwartz, Waters & Simmons, 1993; Van Heest, Waters, Simmons & Schwartz, 1995). Division of the transverse carpal ligament without division of the palmar aponeurosis does decrease pressure in the carpal tunnel, but division of both structures drops the pressure further (Okutsu, Hamanaka, Tanabe, Takatori & Ninomiya, 1996a; Nakao, Short, Werner, Fortino & Palmer, 1998).

In most endoscopic techniques, the endoscope is placed in the medial portion of the carpal tunnel, usually in line with the ring finger, just radial to the hook of the hamate. This position is chosen to minimize the risk of injuring the median nerve but increases the risk of injuring the ulnar artery or nerve. These travel as a neurovascular bundle in Guyon's canal, which is bounded medially by the hypothenar muscles, dorsally by the flexor retinaculum, and volarly and laterally by palmar fascia that joins the flexor retinaculum lateral to the hook of the hamate (Cobb, Carmichael & Cooney, 1994). Guyon's canal can be inadvertently opened or entered during endoscopic carpal tunnel surgery (Luallin & Toby, 1993). The pressure in Guyon's canal often drops after open or endoscopic carpal tunnel surgery, and opening

Guyon's canal does not have known adverse consequences unless the neurovascular bundle is traumatized (Ablove, Moy, Peimer, Wheeler & Diao, 1996). However, neurapraxic contusion of the ulnar nerve is reported after many carpal tunnel endoscopies, and more severe ulnar nerve scarring or laceration can occur (Luallin & Toby, 1993).

Anomalies of the hamate such as a "floating," "crooked," or aplastic hook of the hamate can prevent proper placement of the endoscope or lead to inadvertent opening of Guyon's canal while sectioning the transverse carpal ligament (Jebson & Agee, 1996; Richards & Bennett, 1997).

Other structures in the medial palm, including digital nerves, flexor tendons, and arteries such as the superficial palmar arch, are vulnerable to trauma during carpal tunnel endoscopy (Rotman & Manske, 1993). Injuries to these structures are discussed later under Analysis of Unsatisfactory Surgical Results. Training to perform carpal tunnel endoscopy starts with practice on cadaver hands; the trainee often learns of potential complications from personal experience (Lee et al., 1992; Rowland & Kleinert, 1994; Van Heest et al., 1995). Even after cadaver training, endoscopists seem more prone to cause complications in their first 100 cases (Erdmann, 1994; Foucher & Braga Da Silva, 1994).

Postoperative Care

Splinting

Various postoperative regimens are used after carpal tunnel surgery. Four-fifths of hand surgeons apply a compressive dressing after surgery; one-fifth does not (Duncan et al., 1987). Some leave the dressing on only 1 day; others, for more than 10 days. Four-fifths of hand surgeons apply a wrist splint. Surgical opinion is divided on whether the splint should be in extension or neutral position and on duration of splinting. Among those who prescribe a splint, most favor 1 to 3 weeks of splinting.

There are conflicting data on the value of early splinting after carpal tunnel surgery. Whether patients received a bulky soft dressing or a palmar splint immediately after surgery does not affect their postoperative pain in the first 48 hours (Bury, Akelman & Weiss, 1995; Bhatia, Field, Grote & Huma, 2000).

Chaise (1990) randomized 50 patients undergoing carpal tunnel surgery to immediate postoperative active mobilization without splinting or to splinting for 15 to 18 days in 20 degrees of extension. He followed both grip strength and carpal tunnel computed tomographic scanning at 2, 6, and 12 months postoperatively. The patients with active mobilization had weaker grips at follow-up; the grips of these patients were weakest with the wrist flexed. The computed tomographic results suggested that healing without the splint allowed greater anterior bowing of the transverse carpal ligament, resulting in loss of stability and strength of the thenar muscles and of the effective grip of the finger flexors.

In contrast, a randomized study found that grip and pinch strength were the same or better in patients who were not splinted postoperatively compared with patients who were splinted for the first 2 postoperative weeks (Cook, Szabo, Birkholz & King, 1995). Furthermore, the unsplinted patients returned more quickly to activities of daily living, light-duty work, and full-duty work than did splinted patients. No patient in either group developed bowstringing of the flexor tendons, the complication that theoretically might be more common in the unsplinted group.

Postoperative Exercises and Hand Therapy

Early after carpal tunnel surgery, patients are often instructed in tendon gliding exercises to prevent adhesions of the flexor tendons or median nerve within the carpal tunnel (Skirven & Trope, 1994). Active digit exercises with the wrist in the neutral position go through a series of positions: (1) full finger extension, (2) flexion of the proximal and distal interphalangeal joints, (3) flexion of the metacarpal-phalangeal joints while maintaining the proximal and distal interphalangeal joint flexion, (4) extension of the distal interphalangeal joints while maintaining the metacarpal-phalangeal and proximal interphalangeal joint flexion, and (5) reversal of the procedure through steps 3, 2, and 1 (Sailer, 1996). These can be performed even if the wrist is splinted. If the wrist is not splinted, the fingers and wrists should be exercised separately because simultaneous finger and wrist flexion might promote bowstringing of the flexor tendons (Cook et al., 1995). The thumb interphalangeal joints should also be exercised, and range of motion should be maintained at the shoulder, elbow, and forearm.

Median nerve gliding exercises are typically added when the patient can tolerate them, or if a splint is used, when the splint is removed. In the first position, the fingers and thumb are flexed while the wrist and forearm are in a neutral position. Subsequent positions are (2) fingers and thumb extended, (3) wrist extended, (4) forearm supinated, (5) elbow extended, and (6) thumb further extended passively by the contralateral hand (Sailer, 1996). When tolerated, usually about 3 weeks after surgery, hand and wrist strengthening exercises are added to the rehabilitation program.

These exercise and therapy prescriptions are empiric; there are few controlled trials in this area. In a prospective randomized trial, patients were assigned on the twelfth day after carpal tunnel surgery to either a home exercise program or to ten 1-hour therapy sessions over the next 2 weeks (Provinciali, Giattini, Splendiani & Logullo, 2000). The therapy included progressive stretching of the palmar fascia, progressive straightening exercises for abductor pollicis brevis and opponens pollicis, hand massage, motor dexterity exercises, and hand sensory stimulation. The two groups of patients had comparable postoperative symptoms and comparable motor dexterity by 3 months postoperatively. The group that received the hand therapy had earlier return to work and better motor dexterity 1 month after surgery.

In a group of patients after carpal tunnel surgery, Groves and Rider (1989) tried supervised hand therapy with resistive exercises and a work simulator between the third and sixth weeks after surgery. The supervised therapy offered little advantage over unsupervised hand activities such as gentle bending, warm soaks, and pursuit of simple daily tasks.

Return to Work

Many surgeons are now emphasizing early return to work after carpal tunnel surgery. For example, patients can resume a one-hand light duty job as early as the second postoperative day and be back at full duty in 6 to 8 weeks after surgery (Goodman, 1992). Early return to work is facilitated by short incision, early mobilization, and active postoperative hand therapy (Nathan, Meadows & Keniston, 1993). Return to work after endoscopy is discussed in more detail in the following sections.

Results of Carpal Tunnel Surgery

Historical Experience with Carpal Tunnel Surgery

Open Carpal Tunnel Surgery

Once upon a time, assessing the results of carpal tunnel surgery was simple: The surgeon asked the patient's opinion. Patients commonly report dramatic improvement in symptoms after carpal tunnel surgery. Relief of intermittent paresthesias and pain and of nocturnal symptoms is often immediate or evident as soon as incisional pain resolves. Cseuz and colleagues (1966) provided follow-up data on surgical results in 254 hands. The patients were surveyed by questionnaire, months to years after surgery; their assessments of postoperative results are shown in Table 15-2. Numerous surgical series have confirmed patient satisfaction with this operation (Table 15-3).

Table 15-2. Patient's Estimate of Postoperative Improvement

Amount of improvement (%)	100	75	50	25	0	Worse
Number of patients	144	110	23	8	17	11

Data from KA Cseuz, JE Thomas, EH Lambert, JG Love, PR Lipscomb. Long-term results of operation for carpal tunnel syndrome. Mayo Clin. Proc. 1966;41:232–41.

Table 15-3. Results of Open Carpal Tunnel Surgery

Series	No. of Hands	Results
Doyle & Carroll, 1968	100	97% of hands relieved of symptoms or significantly better
Semple & Cargill, 1969	150	75% of hands asymptomatic at follow-up 2 to 7 years after surgery
Farhat, Kahn & Child, 1974	109	65% of hands excellent relief, 30% fair relief
Hybbinette & Mannerfelt, 1975	465	98% of hands relieved of carpal tunnel syndrome pain
Ariyan & Watson, 1977	429	99% of hands improved
Gainer & Nugent, 1977	306	51% of hands cured, 31% greatly improved
Kulick, Gordillo, Javidi, Kilgore & Newmayer, 1986	130	81% of hands free of symptoms at follow-up 2 to 6 years after surgery
Waegeneers, Haentjens & Wylock, 1993	100	93% good to excellent results except that 21% rated strength as fair or poor
Singh, Khoo & Krishnamoorthy, 1994	303	Improvement of symptoms for all patients
Dlabalova, 1995; Nancollas, Peimer, Wheeler & Sherwin, 1995	2,867	Over 96% improved

Endoscopic Carpal Tunnel Surgery

Large uncontrolled clinical series have reported that patients are also generally delighted with the results of endoscopic carpal tunnel surgery (Tables 15-4 and 15-5). However, numerous complications of endoscopic surgery encourage debates about the relative safety and efficacy of open versus endoscopic surgery and about the best way to measure surgical outcomes.

Pathophysiologic Evidence of Efficacy

Both open and endoscopic carpal tunnel surgery effectively lower the pressure in the carpal tunnel

(Okutsu, Ninomiya, Hamanaka, Kuroshima & Inanami, 1989; Brown, Gelberman, Seiler, Abrahamsson, Weiland & Urbaniak, 1993; Hamanaka, Okutsu, Shimizu, Takatori & Ninomiya, 1995; Okutsu et al., 1996a; Hashizume, Nanba, Shigeyama, Hirooka, Yokoi & Inoue, 1997). This change is accompanied by morphologic changes in the canal including widening of the carpal arch, increase in cross-sectional area of the canal, increase in volume of the canal, and volar displacement of the median nerve (Table 15-6).

Measurement of Outcomes

In addition to patient satisfaction and incidence of complications, other measures of treatment of carpal tunnel syndrome include examination for neurologic deficits, such as sensory loss or thenar strength; measurements of hand functions, such as grip or pinch strength, range of motion, or dexterity; median nerve conduction studies; patient reports of functional improvement; generic health assessment measures; or time to return to work or activities (Amadio, Silverstein, Ilstrup, Schleck & Jensen, 1996). A given measure can be more applicable to some patients than to others, and each measure has its own time course of improvement following surgery.

Median Nerve Motor or Sensory Deficits

Most patients who have carpal tunnel syndrome undergo surgery before they develop actual deficits of motor or sensory function. When a deficit is present, it usually improves after surgery, but the improvement can take weeks or months. Because both open and endoscopic surgery effectively decompress the median nerve, the prognosis for recovery of neurologic deficit is not expected to differ between open and endoscopic techniques; initial reports confirm that patients can recover neurologic function after endoscopic surgery (Atroshi, Axelsson, Gummesson & Johnsson, 2000). Patients with preoperative neurologic deficit should be counseled before surgery regarding the uncertainty of neurologic recovery, in contrast to the high probability of surgical relief of pain and dysesthesia. The presence of preoperative neurologic deficit usually does not interfere with other

Table 15-4. Results of One-Portal Endoscopic Carpal Tunnel Surgery

Series	No. of Hands	Good or Excellent (%)	Complications
Agee, Peimer, Pyrek & Walsh, 1995	1,049	—	Conversion to open operation, digital neuropathy, palmar cutaneous neuropathy, mild RSD, palmar sensitivity
Brown, Keyser & Rothenberg, 1992	149	—	6%, including persistent symptoms, RSD, conversion to open operation, and recurrence of carpal tunnel syndrome
Worseg, Kuzbari, Korak, Hocker, Wiederer, Tschabitscher & Holle, 1996 (Uni-Cut)	64	—	11%, including laceration superficial palmar arterial arch, transient digital neuropathy, conversion to open surgery, early RSD
Elmaraghy & Hurst, 1996	86	98	6%, including mild RSD, transient digital neurapraxia, superficial wound infection
Chen, Chen & Wei, 1999	1,214	—	One median nerve laceration; 31% transient new sensory changes, 81% transient scar tenderness
Foucher & Braga Da Silva, 1994	280	100	Conversion to open surgery, paresthesias
Boisrenoult, Desmoineaux & Beaufils, 1998	82	97	Laceration of recurrent thenar motor branch, reoperation, conversion to open operation, pillar pain, ulnar paresthesias
Sturzenegger, 1998	100	—	Median nerve laceration, conversion to open operation, incomplete division of transverse carpal ligament, digital paresthesias
Erhard, Ozalp, Citron & Foucher, 1999	95	94	28% still had some symptoms at 4-year follow-up
Hirooka, Hashizume, Senda, Nagoshi, Inoue & Nagashima, 1999	41	88	—
Benquet, Fabre & Durandeau, 2000	138	98.5	RSD
Feinstein, 1993	61	79	6%, including median nerve lacerations, open operation 1 year later, pillar pain, scan tenderness, pinch and grip weakness, persistent numbness

RSD = reflex sympathetic dystrophy. (See critique of this term in Chapter 16.)

measures of postoperative recovery such as patient satisfaction, upper extremity use, or relief of symptoms such as pain and paresthesias (Katz, Losina, Amick, Fossel, Bessette & Keller, 2001).

Motor Recovery. Phalen (1966) reported results in 112 hands with preoperative thenar atrophy that were examined 5 months or more after surgery (Table 15-7). The rapidity of recovery correlated with the duration of symptoms, but patients could show excellent motor recovery even if atrophy had been present for 3 years or more. Of the hands that failed to improve, seven had had atrophy for more than 20 years, but six had had atrophy for 1 year or less. The single patient with progressive atrophy was re-explored and found to have had incomplete section of the distal transverse carpal ligament at the initial operation. Atrophy is more likely to resolve in younger patients (Nolan, Alkaitis, Glickel & Snow, 1992). Other series have confirmed that atrophy is apt to gradually improve postoperatively (Gelberman et al., 1987; Piaget-Morerod & Chamay, 1991).

Sensory Recovery. Phalen (1966) followed 200 patients who had impaired median cutaneous sensation before surgery. Some 77% had return of normal sensation postoperatively. Prognosis was slightly better in patients without thenar atrophy. Subjective sensory function usually improves within 10 days of surgery and is more likely to improve in patients with intermittent than with persistent preoperative paresthesias (Rosén, Lundborg, Abrahamsson, Hagberg &

Table 15-5. Results of Two-Portal Endoscopic Carpal Tunnel Surgery

Series	No. of Hands	Good or Excellent (%)	Complications
Brown, Keyser & Rothenberg, 1992	152	—	5%, including persistent symptoms, RSD, transient paresthesias
Slattery, 1994a	240	93	2%, including persistent symptoms, RSD, ulnar neurapraxia, median recurrent motor branch neurapraxia, median digital neuropathy, and persistent symptoms
Kelly, Pulisetti & Jamieson, 1994	83	79	27%, including incomplete ligament release, wrong diagnosis, median nerve laceration, digital neuropathy, ulnar neuropathy, persistent symptoms
Atroshi, Johnsson & Ornstein, 1997	255	89	4%, including digital neuropathy, open reoperations for persistent symptoms
Resnick & Miller, 1991	75	92	17%, including ulnar neurapraxia, persistent symptoms, partial median nerve laceration
Payne, Bergman & Ettinger, 1994	20	100	One laceration of the superficial palmar arterial arch
Davies, Pennington & Fritz, 1998	333	98	One transient mild RSD
Chow, 1996	1,299	99	1%, including continued symptoms, recurrent symptoms, transient ulnar palsy
Brief & Brief, 2000	146	86	None
Roth, Richards & MacLeod, 1994	108	94	3.8%, including wound hematoma, cellulitis, flexor tenosynovitis, and incomplete section of the transverse carpal ligament
Papageorgiou, Georgoulis, Makris, Moebius, Varitimidis & Soucacos, 1998	76	100	5%, including transient hypesthesia, palmar hematoma, and scar pain
Kropfl, Gasperschitz & Hertz, 1996	168	84	5%, including laceration of the superficial palmar arch and conversion to open operation
Köstli & Huber, 1998	67	94	7%, including arterial laceration, ulnar neurapraxia and superficial infection
Le Nen, Rizzo, Hu & Brunet, 1998	102	93	4%, including RSD, incomplete section of the transverse carpal ligament, dysesthesia, and superficial palmar arch laceration
Ghaly, Saban, Haley & Ross, 2000	42	86	—
Nagle, Fischer, Harris, Hastings, Osterman, Palmer & Viegas, 1996; Nagle, Harris & Foley, 1994	640	>97	Neurapraxia, RSD, reoperation, palmar tenderness, fewer complications after switch from transbursal to extrabursal technique
Straub, 1999	100	92	3%, including stitch abscesses, palmar hematoma
Brown, MG, Rothenberg, Keyser, Woloszyn & Wolford, 1993	1,236	98	One tendon injury and two recurrences of carpal tunnel syndrome

RSD = reflex sympathetic dystrophy. (See critique of this term in Chapter 16.)

Rosén, 1997). When two-point discrimination is abnormal preoperatively, it can recover as early as the second postoperative week (Rosén et al., 1997). However, recovery of more severe abnormalities of two-point discrimination, are likely to take longer (Table 15-8) (Gelberman et al., 1987).

Quantitative thermotesting (technique discussed in Chapter 9) shows that cold detection, warm detection, and heat pain detection threshold, when abnormal preoperatively, often improve within 6 weeks after surgery. Perception of touch, measured by monofilament testing or by

Table 15-6. Studies Documenting Morphologic Changes in the Carpal Canal after Carpal Tunnel Surgery

Morphologic Change in Carpal Canal	Open Release	Endoscopic Release
Widening of the carpal arch	Gartsman, Kovach, Crouch, Noble & Bennett, 1986; Garcia-Elias, Sanchez-Freijo, Salo & Lluch, 1992; Cobb & Cooney, 1994	Viegas, Pollard & Kaminksi, 1992; Kato, Kuroshima, Okutsu & Ninomiya, 1994; Fuss & Wagner, 1996
Increase in canal cross-sectional area	—	Kato, Kuroshima, Okutsu & Ninomiya, 1994
Increase in canal volume	Ablove, Peimer, Diao, Oliverio & Kuhn, 1994	Richman, Gelberman, Rydevik, Hajek, Braun, Gylys-Morin & Berthoty, 1989; Ablove, Peimer, Diao, Oliverio & Kuhn, 1994
Volar displacement of the median nerve	Ablove, Peimer, Diao, Oliverio & Kuhn, 1994	Richman, Gelberman, Rydevik, Hajek, Braun, Gylys-Morin & Berthoty, 1989; Ablove, Peimer, Diao, Oliverio & Kuhn, 1994

vibrametry, can show some improvement by the third postoperative week but can take 4 to 6 months to reach maximal improvement (Jimenez, Hardy, Horch & Jabaley, 1993; Nygaard, Trumpy & Mellgren, 1996; Rosén et al., 1997). Even 1 year after surgery, sensory recovery is often incomplete if there had been objective preoperative sensory loss (Figure 15-2).

Hand Strength and Dexterity

Hand strength and dexterity can be measured in various ways: dynamometers for grip and pinch strength, and timed activity tests for dexterity. These motor functions are influenced by factors such as pain and tendon gliding and mechanics, rather than just reflecting median-innervated muscle function. Routinely, grip and pinch are weak immediately after carpal tunnel surgery, but for most patients grip and pinch strength return to preoperative levels within about 3 months. Similarly,

hand dexterity for a timed pick-up test improves within 3 months of successful carpal tunnel surgery (Amadio et al., 1996).

For many patients, grip strength was impaired before carpal tunnel surgery, so that by 6 months postoperatively grip and pinch strength are often stronger than they were preoperatively. Gellman and colleagues (1989) measured grip and pinch strength before and after carpal tunnel surgery in 24 hands. Six months after surgery, pinch strength was 126%, and grip strength was 116% of preoperative levels. Another series, with 1 year of postoperative follow-up, found that average grip and pinch strengths were not significantly different from preoperative levels (Leach, Esler & Scott, 1993). The minority of patients who have persistent loss of grip and pinch strength after surgery

Table 15-7. Thenar Motor Status after Surgery in 112 Patients with Thenar Atrophy

Normal or Nearly Normal	Partial Improvement	No Improvement	Progressive Atrophy
76 (68%)	16 (14%)	19 (17%)	1 (1%)

Data from GS Phalen. The carpal-tunnel syndrome. Seventeen years' experience in diagnosis and treatment of six hundred fifty-four hands. J. Bone Joint Surg. 1966;48A:211–28.

Table 15-8. Time to Recovery of Abnormal Two-Point Discrimination after Carpal Tunnel Surgery

Preoperative Median Distribution Two-Point Discrimination (mm)	Mean Time after Surgery until Recovery of Normal (<7 mm) Two-Point Discrimination (mo)
7–10	1.6
11–15	2.0
>15	3.5

Data from RH Gelberman, GB Pfeffer, RT Galbraith, RM Szabo, B Rydevik, M Dimick. Results of treatment of severe carpal-tunnel syndrome without internal neurolysis of the median nerve. J. Bone Joint Surg. 1987;69A:896–903.

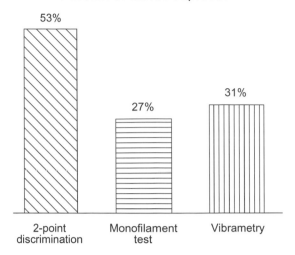

Figure 15-2. Sensory recovery 1 year after carpal tunnel surgery among patients with abnormal preoperative sensory examination. (Data from WB Nolan, D Alkaitis, SZ Glickel, S Snow. Results of treatment of severe carpal tunnel syndrome. J. Hand Surg. 1992;17A:1020–23; B Rosén, G Lundborg, SO Abrahamsson, L Hagberg, I Rosén. Sensory function after median nerve decompression in carpal tunnel syndrome. Preoperative vs postoperative findings. J. Hand Surg. 1997;22B:602–6.)

are discussed in the following section, Analysis of Unsatisfactory Surgical Results.

Nerve Conduction Results

The timing of improvement of median nerve conduction after successful carpal tunnel surgery is discussed in Chapter 8. In general, failure of abnormal median nerve conduction to improve in the months after surgery is indicative of incomplete nerve decompression; otherwise, rapidity or extent of improvement of median nerve conduction is not a useful measure of overall surgical success.

Patient Questionnaires

The self-administered questionnaires of the carpal tunnel symptom severity scale (Table 15-9) and functional status scale (Table 15-10) are reproducible, valid measures of the symptomatic and functional status of patients with carpal tunnel syndrome (Levine, Simmons, Koris, Daltroy, Hohl, Fossel &

Katz, 1993). The symptom severity scale ranges from 11 to 55, and the functional status scales ranges from 8 to 40, with higher scores reflecting more severe symptoms or worse functional status. Other similar hand function questionnaires are available, and at least 13 different patient questionnaires have been published that are intended to assess upper–extremity function (Alderson & McGall, 1999; Davis, Beaton, Hudak, Amadio, Bombardier, Cole, Hawker, Katz & Makela, 1999). Those questionnaires that specifically explore hand symptoms and function reliably document improvement in patients who have had successful open or endoscopic carpal tunnel surgery (Levine et al., 1993; Atroshi, Johnsson & Sprinchorn, 1998). The improvement in these scales is usually evident within 3 months of surgery, and no significant further improvement is present if the patients are questioned 14 months after surgery (Levine et al., 1993). The scales are better than objective assessment of grip or sensation as indicators of patient's postoperative satisfaction (Katz, Gelberman, Wright, Lew & Liang, 1994).

General medical outcome questionnaires have also been studied in patients with carpal tunnel syndrome (Atroshi, Johnsson, Nouhan, Crain & McCabe, 1997). For example, the Medical Outcomes Study 36-Item Short-Form Health Survey queries patients regarding physical function, physical role, body pain, general health perception, vitality, social function, emotional role, and mental health. Although a patient's Medical Outcomes Study 36-Item Short-Form Health Survey score usually improves following successful carpal tunnel surgery, this general scale is less sensitive than the carpal tunnel symptom severity and functional status scales as measures of improvement (Bessette, Sangha, Kuntz, Keller, Lew, Fossel & Katz, 1998; Atroshi, Gummesson, Johnsson & Sprinchorn, 1999; Vaile, Mathers, Ramos-Remus & Russell, 1999).

Resumption of Work or Activity

The interval between carpal tunnel surgery and return to work is an accessible, objective measure. Table 15-11 shows representative data comparing return to work after open and after endoscopic surgery. Time to return to work is influenced by a number of nonphysical factors, such as medical fashion, surgeon enthusiasm, and patient motivation.

Table 15-9. Carpal Tunnel Symptom Severity Scale

The following questions refer to your symptoms for a typical 24-hour period during the past 2 weeks (circle one answer to each question)

How severe is the hand or wrist pain that you have at night?

1. I do not have hand or wrist pain at night
2. Mild pain
3. Moderate pain
4. Severe pain
5. Very severe pain

How often did hand or wrist pain wake you up during a typical night in the past 2 weeks?

1. Never
2. Once
3. Two or three times
4. Four or five times
5. More than five times

Do you typically have pain in your hand or wrist during the daytime?

1. I never have pain during the day
2. I have mild pain during the day
3. I have moderate pain during the day
4. I have severe pain during the day
5. I have very severe pain during the day

How often do you have pain in your hand or wrist during the daytime?

1. Never
2. Once or twice a day
3. Three to five times a day
4. More than five times a day
5. The pain is constant

How long, on average, does an episode of pain last during the daytime?

1. I never get pain during the day
2. Less than 10 minutes
3. 10 to 60 minutes
4. Greater than 60 minutes
5. The pain is constant throughout the day

Do you have numbness (loss of sensation) in your hand?

1. No
2. I have mild numbness
3. I have moderate numbness
4. I have severe numbness
5. I have very severe numbness

Do you have weakness in your hand or wrist?

1. No weakness
2. Mild weakness
3. Moderate weakness
4. Severe weakness
5. Very severe weakness

Do you have tingling sensations in your hand?

1. No tingling
2. Mild tingling
3. Moderate tingling
4. Severe tingling
5. Very severe tingling

How severe is numbness (loss of sensation) or tingling at night?

1. I have no numbness or tingling at night
2. Mild
3. Moderate
4. Severe
5. Very severe

How often did hand numbness or tingling wake you up during a typical night in the past 2 weeks?

1. Never
2. Once
3. Two or three times
4. Four or five times
5. More than five times

Do you have difficulty with grasping and the use of small objects such as keys or pens?

1. No difficulty
2. Mild difficulty
3. Moderate difficulty
4. Severe difficulty
5. Very severe difficulty

Reprinted with permission from DW Levine, BP Simmons, MJ Koris, LII Daltroy, GG Hohl, AH Fossel, JN Katz. A self-administered questionnaire for the assessment of severity of symptoms and functional status in carpal tunnel syndrome. J. Bone Joint Surg. 1993;75A:1585–92.

Table 15-10. Carpal Tunnel Functional Status Scale

On a typical day during the past 2 weeks, have hand and wrist symptoms caused you to have any difficulty doing the activities listed below? Please circle one number that best describes your ability to do the activity.

Activity	No Difficulty	Mild Difficulty	Moderate Difficulty	Severe Difficulty	Cannot Do at All Due to Hand or Wrist Symptoms
Writing	1	2	3	4	5
Buttoning of clothes	1	2	3	4	5
Holding a book while reading	1	2	3	4	5
Gripping of a telephone handle	1	2	3	4	5
Opening of jars	1	2	3	4	5
Household chores	1	2	3	4	5
Carrying of grocery bags	1	2	3	4	5
Bathing and dressing	1	2	3	4	5

Reprinted with permission from DW Levine, BP Simmons, MJ Koris, LH Daltroy, GG Hohl, AH Fossel, JN Katz. A self-administered questionnaire for the assessment of severity of symptoms and functional status in carpal tunnel syndrome. J. Bone Joint Surg. 1993;75A:1585–92.

Long-Term Follow-Up

Follow-up studies of patients after carpal tunnel surgery confirm that 5 years or more after surgery most patients remain satisfied with the operative results (Haupt, Wintzer, Schop, Lottgen & Pawlik, 1993; Nancollas, Peimer, Wheeler & Sherwin, 1995; Lindau & Karlsson, 1999). However, scar discomfort and loss of hand strength persisted in nearly one-fourth to one-third of those available for follow-up; furthermore, one-third or more of patients have some recurrence of hand pain and paresthesias, with average onset 18 to 23 months after surgery (Nancollas et al., 1995). In one series, 10% of patients who had undergone carpal tunnel surgery 6 years previously had recurrent carpal tunnel syndrome at follow-up (Lindau & Karlsson, 1999).

Open versus Endoscopic Carpal Tunnel Surgery

Controlled studies have compared the results of open with the results of endoscopic carpal tunnel surgery (Table 15-12). There is general consensus that the techniques are equally likely to decompress the median nerve and improve the pain and paresthesias of median nerve compression. Any differences in outcomes among the techniques rest with other measures of success such as time to postoperative healing, time to return to work, cost, and nature and incidence of complications.

Many, but not all, studies suggest that patients' average time until return to work after surgery is shorter after endoscopic than after open surgery (see Table 15-11). Usually, neither the surgeon nor the patient is blinded to the type of surgery, so the expectations of both, in addition to physiologic differences, could affect time until return to work. This is particularly important in the series using historical controls, because emphasis on

Table 15-11. Time to Return to Work after Carpal Tunnel Surgery

Type of Surgery	Mean Days to Return to Work		
	Open	Agee	Chow
Data of Agee, McCarroll, Tortosa, Berry, Szabo & Peimer, 1992			
Non-WC	45.5	16.5	—
WC	78	71	—
Data of Kerr, Gittins & Sybert, 1994			
Non-WC	37.9		22.3
WC	49.6		47.0
Data of Palmer, DH, Paulson, Lane-Larsen, Peulen & Olson, 1993			
Non-WC	26.8	10.8	20.3
WC	56.1	29.2	34.6

WC = patients on workers' compensation; Non-WC = patients not on workers' compensation.

Table 15-12. Controlled Studies Comparing Open with Endoscopic Carpal Tunnel Surgery

| Reference | Study Design | Number of Hands | | |
		Open	One-Portal	Two-Portal
Erdmann, 1994	Contralateral simultaneous control	53	—	53
Bande, De Smet & Fabry, 1994	Retrospective contemporary controls	58	44	
Kerr, Gittins & Sybert, 1994	Retrospective, historical matched controls	100	—	100
Agee, McCarroll, Tortosa, Berry, Szabo & Peimer, 1992	Prospective randomized	65	82	—
Brown, Gelberman, Seiler, Abrahamsson, Weiland & Urbaniak, 1993	Prospective randomized (blinded postoperative assessor)	82	—	72
McDonough & Gruenloh, 1993	Retrospective, historical controls	50	5	45
Palmer, Paulson, Lane-Larsen, Peulen & Olson, 1993	Prospective nonrandomized	49	90	72
Skoff & Sklar, 1994	Prospective, historical controls	20	—	20
Futami, 1995	Contralateral control	10	10	—
Hallock & Lutz, 1995	Prospective nonrandomized	71	—	66
Dumontier, Sokolow, Leclercq & Chauvin, 1995	Prospective randomized	40	—	56
Benedetti & Sennwald, 1996	Prospective randomized	22	23	—
Schafer, Sander, Walter & Weitbrecht, 1996	Prospective randomized	54	47	—
Skorpik & Landsiedl, 1996	Prospective nonrandomized	20	—	20
Stark & Engkvist-Lofmark, 1996	Prospective randomized contralateral control	20	20	—
Jacobsen & Rahme, 1996	Prospective randomized (blinded assessment for return to work)	16	—	16
Hoefnagels, van Kleef, Mastenbroek, de Blok, Breukelman & de Krom, 1997	Prospective randomized	91	85	—
Mackenzie, Hainer & Wheatley, 2000	Prospective randomized	14	22	—
Foucher, Buch, Van Overstraeten, Gautherie & Jesel, 1993	Prospective randomized	69	54	—
Sennwald & Benedetti, 1995	Prospective randomized	22	25	—
Frick, Baumeister & Kopp, 1996	Prospective nonrandomized	44	23	—
Worseg, Kuzbari, Korak, Hocker, Wiederer, Tschabitscher & Holle, 1996	Prospective nonrandomized	62	64	—
Mascharka, 1996	Retrospective	250	—	113

early mobilization and return to work has spread in the last decade. An analogous observation is that patients did return to work earlier after short-incision (<2.5 cm) open surgery coupled with early postoperative hand therapy compared with patients who had had longer incision open surgery in earlier years (Nathan et al., 1993). Some dissenting data come from relatively small, European studies. A Swedish prospective randomized study comparing open to two-portal endoscopic surgery that did rely on a blinded observer to determine the date of return to work found no statistical difference in mean time (about 18 days) until return to work between the two treatment groups (Jacobsen & Rahme, 1996). French and Dutch prospective randomized studies found no statistically significant difference in time until return to work comparing open with endoscopic surgery (Foucher et al., 1993; Dumontier, Sokolow, Leclercq & Chauvin, 1995; Hoefnagels, van Kleef, Mastenbroek, de Blok, Breukelman & de Krom, 1997).

Table 15-13. Meta-Analysis of Complication Rates of Carpal Tunnel Surgery Based on Results of 16 Prospective Controlled Studies

	Endoscopic Operations (816)		Open Operations (838)	
	No.	Percent	No.	Percent
Permanent nerve injury	3	0.4	2	0.2
Transient nerve injury	43	5.2	12	1.4
Tendon injury	0	0	1	0.1
Other complications	11	1.3	9	1.1

Adapted from ME Boeckstyns, AI Sorensen. Does endoscopic carpal tunnel release have a higher rate of complications than open carpal tunnel release? An analysis of published series. J. Hand Surg. 1999;24B:9–15.

Early postoperative incisional pain is generally less after endoscopic surgery than after open surgery, but this difference resolves within a few months (Futami, 1995; Hallock & Lutz, 1995; Schafer, Sander, Walter & Weitbrecht, 1996; Stark, & Engkvist-Lofmark, 1996; Hoefnagels et al., 1997). Up to 7 weeks after surgery, 61% of patients who had had open surgery but only 36% of patients who had had two-portal endoscopy had incisional pain (Brown et al., 1993). After one-portal endoscopy, incisional pain resolves sooner than after open surgery, but the differences in pain are undetectable at 3 months after surgery (Agee, McCarroll, Tortosa, Berry, Szabo & Peimer, 1992). Similarly, in a prospective study, both one-portal and two-portal endoscopic surgery led to less scar tenderness than did open surgery, but the difference in scar tenderness was absent 6 months after surgery (Palmer, Paulson, Lane-Larsen, Peulen & Olson, 1993). Although endoscopy may lead to less incisional pain, it does not appear to protect against so-called pillar pain (see Complications, later in this chapter) (Katz, Gelberman, Wright, Abrahamsson & Lew, 1994).

Grip and pinch improve sooner after endoscopic than after open carpal tunnel surgery (Palmer et al., 1993; Erdmann, 1994; Dumontier et al., 1995; Benedetti & Sennwald, 1996; Skorpik & Landsiedl, 1996). This difference is present even if the open operation is done with a short (<2.5 cm) incision (Mackenzie, Hainer & Wheatley, 2000). By 3 to 6 months after surgery, grip and pinch strength is usually at or better than preoperative levels for both endoscopic and open surgical patients (Brownet al., 1993; Palmer et al., 1993; Erdmann, 1994; Skorpik & Landsiedl, 1996).

Complications

Chow reported only three complications after 1,154 operations using the two-portal approach: one incomplete transection of the transverse carpal ligament and two transient ulnar palsies; however, a survey of other surgeons based on 10,640 cases found a complication rate of 2.6% to 5.6% among surgeons who had done less than 25 operations versus less than 1% among surgeons who had done over 100 operations (Chow, 1994).

A meta-analysis of prospective controlled studies comparing open with endoscopic carpal tunnel surgery probably provides the best perspective on the relative safety of the operative methods (Table 15-13) (Boeckstyns & Sorensen, 1999). Endoscopic surgery is more likely than open surgery to be complicated by transient neurapraxias, particularly of the third common digital nerve. Otherwise, well-trained, experienced endoscopists can probably perform the operation as safely as can surgeons who use an open approach.

One comparison of endoscopic with open carpal tunnel surgery uses decision analysis to compare the total theoretical costs of the different approaches (Chung, Walters, Greenfield & Chernew, 1998; Vasen, Kuntz, Simmons & Katz, 1999). The cost differential was particularly affected by the relative risks of complications of the surgical techniques and by differences in return to work time for the two techniques. The decision between endoscopic and open carpal tunnel surgery thus depends on the wishes of the patient, the skills and complication rate of the surgeon, and local economic and occupational factors. Whichever surgical technique is chosen, outcomes are improved by careful patient selection, preoperative patient education, aggressive postoperative mobilization, and emphasis on early return to work.

Contraindications to Carpal Tunnel Endoscopy

Neither one- nor two-portal endoscopy is appropriate for patients who require median nerve neurolysis, flexor synovectomy, inspection of the canal contents, or attention to masses or anomalies within the canal. Endoscopy is contraindicated by hand infection or edema. Patients undergoing repeat carpal tunnel surgery should be explored through an open incision. The two-portal technique cannot be done if the patient's wrist cannot be hyperextended.

Prognostic Factors

Preoperative Symptoms and Signs

Patients who have paresthesias in their index, middle, and ring fingers are more likely than patients with paresthesias or numbness on the arm or dorsal hand to be satisfied with the results of carpal tunnel surgery (Bessette, Keller, Lew, Simmons, Fossel, Mooney & Katz, 1997). Patients whose most troubling preoperative symptoms are nocturnal pain or hand numbness or tingling are more likely to be satisfied with surgical results than are patients whose most troubling symptoms were numbness, hand weakness, or trouble with work tasks (Wintman, Winters, Gelberman & Katz, 1996; Bessette, Keller, Liang, Simmons, Fossel & Katz, 1997). Probability of improvement is independent of duration of symptoms in many series (Cseuz et al., 1966; Harris, Tanner, Goldstein & Pettee, 1979; Yu, Firrell & Tsai, 1992; al-Qattan, Bowen & Manktelow, 1994; Choi & Ahn, 1998; Katz et al., 2001). However, in one series with long-term follow-up, those patients who remained symptomatic yet delayed surgery for 3 years or more after carpal tunnel syndrome was diagnosed had a worse prognosis than those who had earlier surgery (DeStefano, Nordstrom & Vierkant, 1997).

Patients who obtain transient relief of symptoms from steroid injection of the carpal tunnel are more likely to benefit from carpal tunnel surgery than are patients who do not obtain relief from steroid injection (Green, 1984; Kulick, Gordillo, Javidi, Kilgore & Newmayer, 1986).

Preoperative body mass index is not of prognostic import (Yu et al., 1992). Preoperative physical examination findings are not predictive of surgical outcome (Katz et al., 2001).

Preoperative Functional Status

Patients with greater self-reported preoperative limitations of upper extremity use are more likely to have greater symptom severity, functional limitation, and dissatisfaction after surgery (Katz et al., 2001). Similarly, when patients rated their hand use for activities of daily living preoperatively, those with worse preoperative functional status scores (similar to Table 15-10, scoring difficulty on 11 daily activities) were more likely to be dissatisfied with surgical outcomes 6 months after endoscopic carpal tunnel surgery (Atroshi, Johnsson & Ornstein, 1998).

Preoperative Nerve Conduction Results

Preoperative nerve conduction values are not particularly helpful in choosing patients for carpal tunnel surgery, except to the extent that they make the clinician confident or uncertain of the diagnosis of carpal tunnel syndrome and confirm or exclude alternative or additional diagnoses. Patients who have classic clinical presentations of carpal tunnel syndrome and normal nerve conduction results can have excellent relief of symptoms after carpal tunnel surgery and as a group do as well after surgery as do carpal tunnel syndrome patients who have abnormal median nerve conduction (Cseuz et al., 1966; Grundberg, 1983; Yu et al., 1992; Braun & Jackson, 1994; Glowacki, Breen, Sachar & Weiss, 1996; Concannon, Gainor, Petroski & Puckett, 1997; Finsen & Russwurm, 2001).

Higgs and colleagues (1997), who showed that some patients with possible carpal tunnel syndrome and normal median nerve conduction do not improve with surgery, stressed that when median nerve conduction is normal or only slightly abnormal, the clinical diagnosis should be reviewed with care before undertaking carpal tunnel surgery. Harris and colleagues (1979) found that patients who had prolonged median distal motor latency were more likely to have a good surgical response than were patients who had a normal median distal motor latency but prolonged median distal sensory latency. Mendelson and Balla (1973) and Atroshi and colleagues (1998) made similar observations and suggested that this seemingly paradoxical finding might indicate misdiagnoses in some the patients with milder nerve conduction abnormalities. Other studies have not found a relation between the degree of preoperative nerve conduction abnormality and surgical results (Yu et al., 1992; al-Qattan et al., 1994; Choi & Ahn, 1998; Mondclli, Reale, Sicurelli & Padua, 2000). Unfortunately, few of the studies cited in the last two paragraphs combine carefully defined nerve conduction techniques, a range of valid outcome measures, and prospective randomized design.

Co-Existing Neuropathy

Co-existent diffuse peripheral neuropathy does not preclude excellent response of carpal tunnel syndrome to surgery (Clayburgh, Beckenbaugh & Dobyns, 1987; Morgenlander, Lynch & Sanders, 1997). This issue arises most commonly in diabetics. Published studies on this issue are few and imperfectly controlled. Some series suggest that the overall success rate and long-term prognosis may be worse for diabetic carpal tunnel syndrome than for idiopathic carpal tunnel syndrome (Haupt et al., 1993; al-Qattan, Manktelow & Bowen, 1994).

Future studies should carefully distinguish between diabetics who have carpal tunnel syndrome but do not have more diffuse neuropathy and those who have both carpal tunnel syndrome and distal symmetric polyneuropathy (Wilbourn, 1999). The diagnosis of carpal tunnel syndrome in a diabetic must be based on clinical findings, rather than just on electrodiagnostic data (see Chapter 8). Brown and Asbury (1984) state, "When of short duration, these entrapment neuropathies [in diabetics] appear to respond to accepted treatment in a manner similar to that found in patients without polyneuropathy." We suspect that if the diabetic carpal tunnel syndrome has progressed to the stage of objective motor or sensory deficit, postoperative neurologic

recovery will be less likely than in idiopathic carpal tunnel syndrome of similar severity. However, for diabetics who have both distal symmetric polyneuropathy and carpal tunnel syndrome, carpal tunnel surgery can lead to improved hand and arm symptoms and improved two-point discrimination in median-innervated digits (Aszmann, Kress & Dellon, 2000).

Patients on chronic hemodialysis who develop carpal tunnel syndrome can benefit from carpal tunnel surgery (Okutsu, Hamanaka, Ninomiya, Takatori, Shimizu & Ugawa, 1993). However, they continue to deposit amyloid in the flexor retinaculum and, perhaps, are more likely than patients with idiopathic carpal tunnel syndrome to develop postoperative late recurrence (Kim, Shin & Kang, 2000). In hemodialysis patients undergoing carpal tunnel endoscopic surgery, complete division of all portions of the flexor retinaculum is particularly important to optimize nerve decompression (Okutsu, Hamanaka, Tanabe, Takatori & Ninomiya, 1996b).

Social and Psychological Factors

As expected for any medical condition, patients' responses to carpal tunnel surgery are affected by social and psychological factors. In a prospective study, patients' preoperative mental health was assessed using a five-item mental health subscale of the Medical Outcomes Study 36-Item Short-Form Health Survey; worse preoperative mental health scores correlated with greater postoperative symptom severity, functional limitation, and dissatisfaction with surgery (Katz et al., 2001). Drinking more than two alcoholic drinks daily was also an adverse prognostic factor (Katz et al., 2001). Preoperative Minnesota Multiphasic Personality Index scores indicative of depression or somatization decrease the patient's probability of improvement after carpal tunnel surgery (Hamlin, Hitchcock, Hofmeister & Owens, 1996).

Occupation and Workers' Compensation

Most workers who are treated for carpal tunnel syndrome under a workers' compensation claim have good to excellent surgical results (Adams,

Franklin & Barnhart, 1994; Katz et al., 1998). Among workers with carpal tunnel syndrome, those treated surgically are less likely to have disability than those receiving chronic nonoperative therapies (Shin, Perlman, Shin & Garay, 2000). However, the surgical results for these workers are not quite as good as for others with carpal tunnel syndrome (Table 15-14) (Tountas, MacDonald, Meyerhoff & Bihrle, 1983; Glowacki et al., 1996). Whether treated with open or endoscopic surgery, patients on workers' compensation return to work, on average, later than those who are not on workers' compensation (see Table 15-11). Workers are more likely to have difficulty with returning to work and more likely to change jobs, if their occupation before surgery was strenuous or hand-intensive (Yu et al., 1992; Adams et al., 1994; Nancollas et al., 1995; Butterfield, Spencer, Redmond, Rosenbaum & Zirkle, 1997).

Prognostic elements for workers after carpal tunnel surgery include both physical and psychosocial factors. Examples of adverse physical factors are more intense hand work required by the job or need for bilateral carpal tunnel surgery; examples of adverse psychosocial factors include fewer years of education or decreased mental health status (Butterfield et al., 1997). Workers exposed to vibration have a slightly worse prognosis for full postoperative recovery (Hagberg, Nystrom & Zetterlund, 1991; Bostrom, Gothe, Hansson, Lugnegard & Nilsson, 1994). Workers represented by attorneys probably have a worse prognosis (Butterfield et al., 1997; Katz, Lew, Bessette, Punnett, Fossel, Mooney & Keller, 1998; Olney, Quenzer & Makowsky, 1999). However, the mechanisms for this association are complex, and in at least one surgical series, presence or absence of legal representation did not affect rate or extent of postoperative recovery of grip and pinch strength (Braun, Doehr, Mosqueda & Garcia, 1999).

Other Prognostic Factors

In some series, older patients have had a worse prognosis for operative relief of symptoms (Cseuz et al., 1966; Atroshi, Johnsson & Ornstein, 1998). However, in a prospective study there was an inverse correlation between age and symptom

Table 15-14. Results of Carpal Tunnel Surgery and Workers' Compensation Status

Surgical Result	For Patients Covered by Workers' Compensation (%)	For Patients Not Covered by Workers' Compensation (%)
Good	66	85
Fair	23	11
Poor	11	4

Data from CP Tountas, CJ MacDonald, JD Meyerhoff, DM Bihrle. Carpal tunnel syndrome. A review of 507 patients. Minn. Med. 1983;66:479–82.

severity or dissatisfaction with surgery when patients were surveyed 18 months postoperatively (Katz, Losina, Amick, Fossel, Bessette & Keller, 2001), and a retrospective review of patients with occupational carpal tunnel syndrome found that younger patients had less satisfaction with their care (Butterfield et al., 1997). Other series have not found age to be a prognostic indicator (Adams et al., 1994).

The appearance of the median nerve at surgery does not seem to predict the probability of surgical response (Arons, Collins & Arons, 1999).

Analysis of Unsatisfactory Surgical Results

In every series of carpal tunnel operations, a minority of patients has unsatisfactory results. The operation is now done so frequently that treatment and diagnosis of these patients who have not been cured by initial surgery is becoming a common clinical challenge. Patients can be divided into those who have persistent symptoms after surgery, those who have recurrent symptoms of carpal tunnel syndrome after initially successful surgery, and those who have new symptom patterns after surgery. Table 15-15 outlines differential diagnosis for these patients.

Incomplete Relief of Symptoms with Surgery

Patients who have a preoperative neurologic deficit often have slow or incomplete recovery of nerve

Table 15-15. Unsatisfactory Results of Carpal Tunnel Surgery

Incomplete relief of symptoms with surgery
  Preoperative neurologic deficit
  Incorrect or incomplete initial diagnosis
  Incomplete division of the flexor retinaculum
Recurrent carpal tunnel syndrome after initial success
  Perineural fibrosis
  Progressive tenosynovitis
  Unusual canal contents
New symptom patterns after surgery
  Postoperative wrist pain
  Joint stiffness
  Bowstringing of flexor tendons
  Loss of hand strength
  Postoperative wound infection
  Gout
  Arterial injury
  Tendon injury
  Iatrogenic nerve branch injury
  Neurologic complications of axillary nerve block anesthesia
  Postoperative tourniquet palsy
  "Complex regional pain syndrome"

function; however, they usually have excellent postoperative relief of pain and paresthesias if the flexor retinaculum is adequately sectioned (Phalen, 1966). The time course and probability of recovery of neurologic deficit is discussed earlier in this chapter (see Median Nerve Motor or Sensory Deficits). Worsening of neurologic deficit after surgery suggests inadequate decompression of the median nerve, iatrogenic nerve injury, or an alternative neurologic diagnosis.

Sometimes symptoms persist after carpal tunnel surgery because the initial diagnosis was incorrect or the patient has another condition in addition to carpal tunnel syndrome. Crymble (1968) found this pattern in 20% of 140 patients who underwent carpal tunnel surgery. New diagnoses were made postoperatively after the patients had only partial relief of symptoms; diagnoses included de Quervain's tenosynovitis, ulnar nerve compression at the elbow, tenosynovitis of flexor pollicis longus, and lateral epicondylitis. Connolly (1978) reported patients in

whom diagnoses of diffuse peripheral neuropathy or cervical spondylosis became evident after carpal tunnel surgery failed. Eason and colleagues (1985) found that 81% of their patients with suboptimal surgical results had had co-existent neck pain or radiographic evidence of cervical spondylosis, but the authors do not include control data on the incidence of these common findings in a matched population. Chapter 4, on differential diagnosis, documents a number of other conditions that have been confused with, misdiagnosed as, or co-existed with carpal tunnel syndrome.

Patients with multicausal hand symptoms such as carpal tunnel syndrome accompanied by Dupuytren's contracture, flexor tenosynovitis, or arthritis of the basal thumb joint are likely to have hand symptoms after carpal tunnel surgery (Bloem, Pradjarahardja & Vuursteen, 1986). When patients with carpal tunnel syndrome have multifocal areas of musculoskeletal pain and tenderness in the affected arm, even if no specific diagnosis is made, carpal tunnel surgery might relieve their paresthesias and neuropathic pain but not relieve their diffuse musculoskeletal complaints (Lazaro, 1997). Nissenbaum and Kleinert (1980) found that their patients who had had treatment of carpal tunnel syndrome and Dupuytren's contracture in a single operation often had postoperative hand symptoms, but Gonzalez and Watson (1991) reported good results when correcting both conditions at the same operation.

In the past, the most common cause of incomplete relief of symptoms after surgery was incomplete division of the flexor retinaculum (Stark, 1968; Conolly, 1978; MacDonald, Lichtman, Hanlon & Wilson, 1978). Langloh and Linschied (1972) found that among patients who had a second operation because of incomplete section of the transverse carpal ligament, 80% had had incomplete relief of symptoms after the first operation or had had recurrent symptoms within 3 months of the first operation. In another series, 81% of patients who demonstrated incomplete division of the flexor retinaculum at reoperation had 2 weeks or less of symptom relief after their first carpal tunnel surgery (Cobb & Amadio, 1996). Use of a transverse rather than longitudinal incision increases the risk of incomplete visualization of the distal extent of the ligament (Phalen, 1966; Stark, 1968). Incomplete section of the transverse carpal ligament is a particular risk with endoscopic or small-incision carpal tunnel surgery (Shinya, Lanzetta & Conolly, 1995). The endoscopist may fail to divide the distal or central portion of the ligament or decompress Guyon's canal rather than the carpal tunnel (Lee et al., 1992).

Recurrent Carpal Tunnel Syndrome after Initial Surgical Success

An occasional patient reports that symptoms abated shortly after carpal surgery but that typical symptoms of carpal tunnel syndrome recurred months to years later. This timing can occur with incomplete release of the flexor retinaculum, however, it usually signifies an alternative pathologic process, such as fibrosis and reclosure of the flexor retinaculum (Cobb, Amadio, Leatherwood, Schleck & Ilstrup, 1996). Langloh and Linscheid (1972) found that patients with this history often had scar formation in the carpal tunnel or tenosynovial hypertrophy leading to recurrent nerve compression. The same pattern can occur after endoscopic carpal tunnel surgery (Shinya et al., 1995). In 40 wrists re-explored because of recurrent symptoms of carpal tunnel syndrome, Wadstroem and Nigst (1986) found perineural fibrosis in 36 and flexor tenosynovitis in 19. Six patients in a surgical series of 140 experienced excellent initial relief of symptoms postoperatively, but reported recurrent symptoms several months later. At reoperation their retinaculums were thickened and had rejoined. The retinaculums were resectioned and partially removed with lasting relief of symptoms (Magee & Kahn, 1967).

The median nerve can be trapped in the fibrotic retinaculum (Inglis, 1980). Sennwald and Hagen (1990) repeated surgery in 12 patients with recurrent pain after initial carpal tunnel release. At re-exploration, the median nerves of these patients had migrated anteriorly and were fixed in the scar of the transverse carpal ligament. Some patients also had anterior subluxation of the flexor tendons. They suggested that simple section of the transverse carpal ligament should be replaced with reconstruction of the ligament, using tendon from the palmaris brevis or flexor carpi radialis to allow increase in canal volume without the danger of anterior subluxation of the canal contents.

On rare occasion, re-exploration reveals abnormal canal contents that were not recognized at the first operation; reported examples include a ganglion in the canal or chronic granulomatous infection (Kelly, Karlson, Weed & Lipscomb, 1967; Conolly, 1978; Langa, Posner, Hoffman & Steiner, 1986). In an unusual case, recurrent median nerve compression was attributed to a radially inserted palmaris longus tendon that began to compress the median nerve after the antebrachial fascia was divided during a carpal tunnel release (Nakamichi & Tachibana, 2000).

Choice of Patients for Surgical Re-Exploration

Persistent or recurrent carpal tunnel syndrome after carpal tunnel surgery should prompt consideration of surgical re-exploration of the carpal tunnel. Patients with postoperative wrist pain or alternative hand diagnoses are unlikely to benefit from repeated carpal tunnel surgery, so they must be carefully distinguished from those with unrelieved or recurrent median nerve compression. Surgery is definitely indicated in patients with progressive median nerve deficit. However, even with thoughtful patient selection, surgical re-exploration has variable results.

A small series suggested that persistent paresthetic symptoms coupled with a negative Phalen's test was typical of incomplete distal division of the flexor retinaculum (De Smet, 1993). This clinical clue was not confirmed in a larger series (Cobb et al., 1996).

The timing of improvement in median nerve conduction that follows successful carpal tunnel surgery is reviewed in Chapter 8. Failure of nerve conduction to evolve toward normal as expected after surgery is one indicator of incomplete nerve decompression. If patients with persistent or recurrent symptoms after carpal tunnel surgery have normal median nerve conduction studies, they are less likely to benefit from carpal tunnel re-exploration (Cobb et al., 1996). A report to the contrary, that nerve conduction results are not of value in choosing patients for carpal tunnel re-exploration, is difficult to evaluate due to lack of clinical and electrodiagnostic detail (Chang & Dellon, 1993).

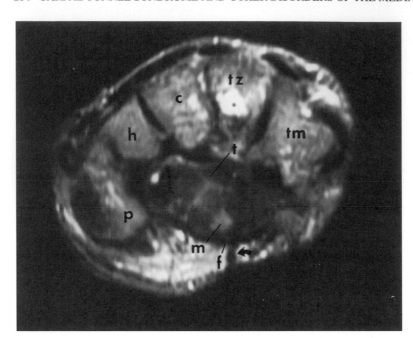

Figure 15-3. Failed carpal tunnel surgery. The axial T2-weighted magnetic resonance image of the wrist shows abnormalities in a patient who had persistent neuropathic symptoms after carpal tunnel surgery. The curved arrow points to postsurgical scarring at the site of the incision. The flexor retinaculum (f) appears continuous and shows thickening and volar bowing. The median nerve (m) is prominent with high signal intensity, suggesting nerve edema or inflammation. There is an incidental interosseous cyst in the trapezoid. (c = capitate; h = hamate; p = pisiform; t = flexor tendons; tm = trapezium; tz = trapezoid.) (Courtesy of Dr. Stephen Quinn.)

Magnetic resonance imaging (MRI) can be particularly helpful for evaluating postoperative symptoms, both to exclude unexpected masses in the carpal canal and to assess the continuity of the transverse carpal ligament (Mesgarzadeh, Schneck, Bonakdarpour, Mitra & Conaway, 1989; Reicher & Kellerhouse, 1990; Buchberger, Judmaier, Birbamer, Hasenohrl & Schmidauer, 1993; Murphy, Chernofsky, Osborne & Wolson, 1993). Ultrasonography has also been used for postoperative assessments but does not visualize canal contents as well as MRI and can be degraded by acoustic shadowing from the surgical scar (Buchberger et al., 1993; Buchberger, 1997).

Postoperative MRIs must be interpreted with caution: After successful carpal tunnel surgery, the median nerve can still look enlarged and abnormally bright on T2-weighted images, and both fat and fibrous tissue can appear proliferated within the carpal tunnel (Buchberger, 1997; Pierre-Jerome, Bekkelund, Mellgren & Nordstrom, 1997). For example, in one series of patients who had undergone clinically successful carpal tunnel surgery, the signal intensity of the median nerve on postoperative MRI had decreased in only two-thirds of the patients. MRI can also show evidence of nerve laceration or neuroma formation (Silbermann-Hoffman, Touam, Mir-

oux, Moysan, Oberlin & Benacerraf, 1998). Figure 15-3 shows an MRI scan of the wrist of a patient who had recurrent symptoms of median nerve compression after carpal tunnel surgery. The MRI finding of an intact or refibrosed transverse carpal ligament was matched by the surgical finding of fibrotic scarring at the site of previous section of the ligament. After the re-exploration, the patient had relief of the symptoms of median nerve compression.

A decision to repeat carpal tunnel surgery requires careful consideration of the differential diagnosis, and most patients with hand symptoms after carpal tunnel surgery do not need re-exploration. When patients for re-exploration are chosen with care, the majority improves after the second surgery (Langloh & Linscheid, 1972; Wadstroem & Nigst, 1986). However, a significant minority have unsatisfactory results of the re-exploration (Table 15-16) (Cobb et al., 1996). Patients whose carpal tunnel syndrome is covered under workers' compensation insurance are less likely than those not under workers' compensation insurance to benefit from recurrent surgery (Cobb et al., 1996; Hulsizer, Staebler, Weiss & Akelman, 1998; Concannon, Brownfield & Puckett, 2000). Patients whose first surgery was endoscopic rather than open are more likely to

Table 15-16. Results of a Second Carpal Tunnel Re-Exploration in 131 Patients with Symptoms of Carpal Tunnel Syndrome after Carpal Tunnel Surgery

Surgical Outcome	Percent of Patients
Complete relief of symptoms	29
Successful but incomplete relief of symptoms	21
Partial relief of symptoms	18
Unsuccessful relief of symptoms	31
Underwent third operation because of unsuccessful relief of symptoms	11

Data from TK Cobb, PC Amadio, DF Leatherwood, CD Schleck, DM Ilstrup. Outcome of reoperation for carpal tunnel syndrome. J. Hand Surg. 1996;21A:347–56.

benefit from open re-operation, perhaps because endoscopic surgery is less likely to fully divide the flexor retinaculum (Forman, Watson, Caulfield, Shenko, Caputo & Ashmead, 1998; Hulsizer et al., 1998).

Operative Techniques

A number of operative techniques are espoused for carpal tunnel re-exploration, but none has been validated in controlled trials (Table 15-17). If re-exploration reveals incomplete division of the flexor retinaculum, simply completing the division is usually sufficient. The more extensive procedures are more likely to be considered in patients whose median nerve is encased in scar tissue (Botte, von Schroeder, Abrams & Gellman, 1996).

New Symptom Patterns after Surgery

Postoperative Wrist and Palm Pain

Following carpal tunnel surgery, pain in the wrist and proximal palm is a problem for a significant minority of patients. Only a few patients have an identifiable infectious, inflammatory, or neuropathic cause of the pain. For most the pain is either *scar pain* or *pillar pain*. Scar pain is persistent sensitivity and discomfort at the site of the incision (Farhat, Kahn & Child, 1974). In a series that found scar sensitivity in 62% of patients after open carpal tunnel release, the maximum

Table 15-17. Surgical Techniques for Recurrent Carpal Tunnel Surgery

Extensive median epineurolysis from distal forearm to palm (Duclos & Sokolow, 1998)

Extensive median epineurolysis from distal forearm to palm, flexor tenosynovectomy, reconstruction of the transverse carpal ligament and the forearm antebrachial fascia (Hunter, 1996)

Wrapping the median nerve with autogenous saphenous vein (Varitimidis, Riano, Vardakas & Sotereanos, 2000)

Re-exploration using a new incision parallel to but more medial than the original operative incision (Dellon & Chang, 1992; Chang & Dellon, 1993)

Median nerve coverage with hypothenar fat pad flap (Plancher, Idler, Lourie & Strickland, 1996; Strickland, Idler, Lourie & Plancher, 1996; Giunta, Frank & Lanz, 1998; Frank, Giunta, Krimmer & Lanz, 1999; Mathoulin, Bahm & Roukoz, 2000)

Median nerve coverage with abductor digiti minimi muscle transposition flap (Reisman & Dellon, 1983; Spokevicius & Kleinert, 1996)

Median nerve coverage with palmaris brevis turnover flap (Rose, Norris, Kowalski, Lucas & Flegler, 1991; Rose, 1996)

Median nerve coverage by transposition of pronator quadratus (Dellon & Mackinnon, 1984)

Median nerve coverage with synovial flap (Wulle, 1993, 1996)

Median nerve coverage with reverse flow radial artery fascial flap (Tham, Ireland, Riccio & Morrison, 1996)

Median nerve coverage with flap from the dorsal forearm supplied by the dorsal ulnar artery (Gilbert & Becker, 1993)

Digital nerve coverage with lumbrical flap (Wilgis, 1984)

Median nerve coverage with dermal fat grafts (McClinton, 1996; Guillemot, Le Nen, Colin, Stindel, Hu & L'Heveder, 1999)

duration of sensitivity was 5 months (Singh, Khoo & Krishnamoorthy, 1994). Cseuz and colleagues (1966) found that 36% of their patients reported scar sensitivity when queried months or years postoperatively. Most patients with scar discomfort reported "minor discomfort which did not interfere with their daily activities"; however, some patients reported scar discomfort for more than 3 years after surgery. Scar pain is more common in the proximal portion of the incision. It cannot be attributed simply to injury of small cutaneous nerve endings because these appear to be equally abundant in the proximal and distal palm (Biyani, Wolfe, Simison & Zakhour, 1996). Shorter incisions, whether as part of open or of

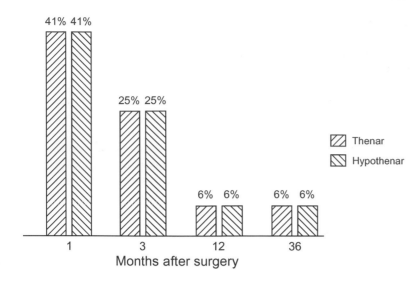

Figure 15-4. Incidence of subjective thenar or hypothenar tenderness after open carpal tunnel surgery. (Data from Povlsen B, Tegnell I. Incidence and natural history of touch allodynia after open carpal tunnel release. Scand. J. Plast. Reconstr. Surg. Hand Surg. 1996;30:221–25.)

endoscopic carpal tunnel surgery, lead to less scar pain (Biyani & Downes, 1993).

Pillar pain is variously defined but refers generally to tenderness over the hypothenar and thenar regions. Its pathophysiology is debated (Ludlow, Merla, Cox & Hurst, 1997). Wilson (1994) suggests examining for it "by applying approximately 2 kg force of pinch to the palm with the thumb on the anterior side and the index finger on the dorsal side of the wrist. Pillar pain was evaluated by thumb palpation immediately radial then ulnar to the long-ring web axis and proximal to Kaplan's cardinal line." Pillar pain is a common experience after carpal tunnel surgery and usually improves in the postoperative months (Figure 15-4). Even patients who are unaware of tenderness in these areas can have abnormal sensitivity to pressure on examination (Povlsen & Tegnell, 1996).

Whether endoscopic carpal tunnel surgery is less likely than open surgery to cause pillar pain is debated. Polvsen and colleagues (1997), measuring tenderness with a pressure gauge, found that 1 month after surgery patients undergoing either procedure were more sensitive than controls to thenar or hypothenar pressure; however, by 3 months after surgery, patients who had had an Agee-endoscopic decompression no longer were hypersensitive to pressure, whereas patients who had had an open carpal tunnel release remained hypersensitive. Pillar pain is less severe after at least some of the small incision techniques of open carpal tunnel surgery, particularly if the incision spares the proximal palm (Wilson, 1994).

Alterations in dynamics of the pisiform bone might be one mechanism of hypothenar pillar pain (Rigoni & Madonia, 1992). Seradge and Seradge (1989) found persistent hypothenar pain 6 months after surgery in 5 patients among 500 who had had carpal tunnel operations. In these five patients, the pain could be induced by ulnar displacement of the pisiform bone. The patients had temporary relief of pain and improvement of grip strength after local anesthetic injection of the piso-triquetrum joint. In all five patients, excision of the pisiform bone relieved the pain.

Decreased median nerve gliding due to postoperative adhesions has been hypothesized as one mechanism of postoperative pain (Hunter, 1996). Various operations that move tissue to protect the median nerve have been suggested to improve median nerve gliding (see Table 15-17). Even their advocates usually reserve these operations for patients who require repeat carpal tunnel operations. In a controlled blinded study of patients requiring bilateral carpal tunnel surgery, the hand in which a hypothenar fat pad was mobilized and placed over the median nerve had no less pain than the hand in which as standard closure was done (Jones, Stuart & Stothard, 1997).

Both scar and pillar pain usually resolve within 6 months of surgery (Das & Brown, 1976). As discussed previously under postoperative splinting and rehabilitation, there are few data on optimal therapy for scar or pillar pain. In one study, pillar pain resolved more quickly in patients who were not splinted after carpal tunnel surgery (Cook et al., 1995). We warn our patients of the risk of these pains preoperatively; reassure them postoperatively that, if these pains occur, they are not evidence of median nerve injury or compression; and encourage them to continue active hand and wrist use as tolerated despite the pain.

An occasional patient develops a hypertrophic wrist scar (MacDonald et al., 1985). This is more likely to occur if the initial incision crosses the distal wrist crease at right angles or extends proximally into the distal forearm.

Joint Stiffness

Rarely, patients describe increased finger stiffness after carpal tunnel surgery (MacDonald et al., 1978). Stiffness can be caused by tendon adhesions or development of trigger digits (Mackinnon, 1991). At the extreme, permanent contractures of interphalangeal joints can develop (Louis et al., 1985). Early active finger use after surgery should minimize the risk of this complication, and hand physical therapy is the treatment of choice if postoperative joint stiffness develops. Trigger digits can be treated with local steroid injections or surgical release.

Bowstringing of Flexor Tendons

After division of the transverse carpal ligament, the flexor tendons, assessed with the wrist in neutral position or in flexion, are more ventral than they had been before surgery (Ferrara & Marcelis, 1997; Netscher et al., 1997). This ventral movement of the tendons can be studied in cadaver models (Kline & Moore, 1992; Kiritsis & Kline, 1995). In some, but not all, cadaver studies, the ventral excursion is less after endoscopic than after open surgery (Brown & Peimer, 2000). Clinically, only a few patients experience postoperative *tendon bowstringing*, movement of the tendons beyond the bounds of the carpal tunnel; when these patients flex their wrists, they can experience pain, a snap-

ping sensation, or paresthesias in a median distribution (MacDonald et al., 1978). The bowstrung tendons are sometimes visible on examination of the flexed wrist.

During surgery, a few surgeons assess the risk of bowstringing after section of the flexor retinaculum by passively moving the fingers with the wrist in the neutral position (Tubiana & Brockman, 1993). The superficial tendon of the small finger is the one most likely to move out of the canal on this intraoperative test; if this occurs, the surgeon can perform a ligamentoplasty after sectioning the transverse carpal ligament.

Loss of Hand Strength

As discussed previously, grip and pinch strength are usually impaired immediately after carpal tunnel surgery but return to preoperative levels within an average of about 3 months. Persistent grip weakness is a problem for some patients after carpal tunnel surgery, particularly for those whose activities require a strong grip. Subjective grip weakness can persist for many months after carpal tunnel surgery (Kluge, Simpson & Nicol, 1996). For example, a survey of employees at a meat processing plant who had undergone carpal tunnel surgery found that 78% of the patients complained that grip strength was persistently decreased after surgery; grip strength was not actually measured in this series (Masear et al., 1986). Gartsman and colleagues (1986) measured grip strength in 46 patients examined 8 months or more after unilateral carpal tunnel surgery. After correcting for hand dominance, they found that the operated hand was a mean of 12% weaker than the nonoperated hand. In a prospective survey with 3 months of postoperative follow-up, 19% of patients had less than 80% of their preoperative grip strength (Young, Logan, Fernando, Grasse, Seaton & Young, 1992).

In some patients, loss of grip strength is due to scar tenderness. Among patients studied 10 months after open carpal tunnel surgery using a 5-cm incision, 19% reported scar tenderness but an even larger fraction were limited by palmar discomfort when they placed pressure on the palm (Kluge et al., 1996).

Loss of grip strength is at least partially related to postoperative changes in configuration of the carpal arch. Gartsman and colleagues (1986) estimated the transverse carpal diameter by measuring the distance between the palmar tips of the ridge of the trapezium and the hook of the hamate on standardized carpal radiographs. They compared the wrist that had surgery to the contralateral unoperated wrist. Some 47 of 50 patients had a postoperative increase in the transverse diameter of the canal. The amount of increase correlated with amount of decrease in the patient's grip strength but not with the presence or absence of postoperative wrist pain. The operated wrists did not lose range of flexion or extension.

Fissette and colleagues (1981) reconstructed the transverse carpal ligament at the time of the initial carpal tunnel surgery using a Dacron and silicone sheet. They compared grip strength after surgery in 26 patients who had the surgery with reconstruction and in 27 patients who had division of the transverse carpal ligament without reconstruction. The group with reconstruction had consistently stronger grips at 3, 6, 9, and 12 months after surgery. There is no preoperative data to see if the groups were truly comparable; however, the groups did not have consistent postoperative differences in strength of pronation or supination. Others have advocated varied techniques for reconstruction of the transverse carpal ligament to improve grip strength (Kapandji, 1990; Jakab et al., 1991; Lluch, 1993; Karlsson et al., 1997; Netscher et al., 1997). In controlled prospective studies patients undergoing transverse carpal ligament reconstruction had better grip and pinch strength 3 months after surgery than did patients undergoing routine open division of the ligament or one-portal endoscopic surgery (Foucher, Buch, Van Overstraeten, Gautherie & Jesel, 1993; Netscher, Steadman, Thornby & Cohen, 1998). A retrospective review, in contrast, found no clear benefit to ligament reconstruction (Karlsson et al., 1997).

These few studies on grip strength after surgery are tantalizing. If grip strength is consistently decreased after surgery, treatment options, particularly for patients who wish to resume vigorous hand use after surgery, need to be reconsidered. More data are needed on the role of transverse carpal ligament reconstruction and of postoperative mobilization or splinting on hand function after surgery.

Postoperative Wound Infection

Minor superficial infections have been reported after as many as 6% of carpal tunnel operations (Gainer & Nugent, 1977). However, the risk of postoperative deep wound infection after carpal tunnel surgery is small. At the Mayo Clinic the incidence of infection was 0.5% in 3,600 operations (Hanssen, Amadio, DeSilva & Ilstrup, 1989). *Staphylococcus aureus* was the most commonly identified organism, but a variety of other organisms can be responsible for postoperative infections. For example, in one case the pathogen was *Prototheca wickerhamii*, an alga-like organism (Moyer, Bush & Dennehy, 1990). Most postoperative infections are easily treated with antibiotics and, where indicated, with surgical drainage. Massive necrosis of the palmar fascia is a rare complication of postoperative infection (Cartotto, McCabe & Mackinnon, 1992; Greco & Curtsinger, 1993). Risk factors for infection include tenosynovectomy, intraoperative steroid installation, use of a surgical drain, and longer operating time. Infections can occur after the newer small incision or endoscopic approaches to the carpal tunnel; no systematic study has demonstrated lower or higher infection risks for these techniques (Rieger, Grunert & Brug, 1996; Shapiro, 1997). Possible sequelae of infection include scar pain, loss of range of motion, tendon rupture, and swan neck deformity. An extraordinary sequence was prior axillary lymph node dissection for breast carcinoma, development of ipsilateral carpal tunnel syndrome years later, postoperative superficial wound infection, then postinfectious lymphedema limited to the operated hand (Smith & Giddins, 1999).

Gout

In susceptible patients, acute gout can be precipitated by surgery. A few case reports document acute gout developing in the operated hand in the first few days after carpal tunnel surgery (Phalen, 1966; Graff, Seiler & Jupiter, 1992; Kalia & Moossy, 1993; Calderon & Chung, 1999).

Arterial Injury

The superficial palmar arterial arch, just distal to the transverse carpal ligament, can be inadvertently lacerated during carpal tunnel surgery and is particularly vulnerable to laceration during carpal tunnel endoscopy (Shinya et al., 1995; Palmer & Toivonen, 1999). The ulnar or, less commonly, the radial artery can also be lacerated, especially during endoscopic surgery (Palmer & Toivonen, 1999). If a laceration is identified when it occurs, it can be repaired without ill effect (Brown et al., 1993; Kropfl, Gasperschitz & Hertz, 1996). Postoperative palmar pain, mass, or discoloration can be caused by hematoma or pseudoaneurysm from superficial arch injury (MacDonald et al., 1978; Murphy, Jennings & Wukich, 1994).

Tendon Injury

In response to a survey on complications of carpal tunnel release, members of the American Society of Hand Surgeons reported a number of incidental tendon lacerations (Palmer & Toivonen, 1999). The risk of tendon laceration is probably higher with endoscopic surgery (Scoggin & Whipple, 1992; McDonough & Gruenloh, 1993). The most commonly affected tendons are those of flexor digitorum profundus to the little finger or of flexor digitorum superficialis to the ring or little fingers. The lacerations are more likely to be partial rather than complete and are usually treated by direct repair without long-term ill effect on the patient.

In an unusual case, a 72-year-old man ruptured his flexor pollicis longus tendon 4 months after ipsilateral carpal tunnel surgery (Christodoulou, Yang & Chamberlain, 2000). His physicians hypothesized that displacement of the tendon resulting from section of the flexor retinaculum contributed to the rupture.

Iatrogenic Nerve Injury

The median nerve proper, the recurrent thenar motor branch, the median palmar cutaneous nerve branch, the ulnar palmar cutaneous nerve branch, the superficial radial nerve, and digital nerve branches are all vulnerable to injury at the time of carpal tunnel surgery. Injury to the median palmar cutaneous branch at the time of carpal tunnel exploration was reported as early as 1924 (Amadio, 1995). When the recurrent thenar motor branch is injured, clinical examination shows the-

nar weakness with preserved lumbrical and median sensory function. Electromyography can confirm the diagnosis and often characterize the nature of the nerve injury. When a sensory branch is injured, local sensory impairment is often accompanied by a painful neuroma and a positive Tinel's sign at the site of nerve injury.

Table 15-18 gives references to examples of iatrogenic nerve injuries from carpal tunnel surgery.

The ulnar nerve is especially at risk during endoscopic procedures in which the endoscope is kept toward the ulnar side of the carpal tunnel. Mechanisms include ulnar nerve contusion, which usually causes transient nerve irritation or neurapraxia, ulnar nerve transection, and delayed onset of ulnar nerve compression due to an anomalous palmaris longus muscle (del Pinal, Cruz-Camara & Jado, 1997; Santoro, Matloub & Gosain, 2000).

Postoperative neuromas of a cutaneous nerve, such as the median or ulnar palmar cutaneous branches, are sometimes treated surgically. Surgical techniques include resection of the neuroma, implantation of the nerve end into tissue such as bone or muscle, or excision of the nerve after stripping it from the median nerve trunk (Evans & Dellon, 1994; Sood & Elliot, 1998; Lanzetta & Nolli, 2000).

Neurologic Complications of Axillary Nerve Block Anesthesia

When axillary nerve block is used for anesthesia for hand surgery, there is a small risk of injury to the brachial plexus or to the proximal median, ulnar, or radial nerves (Regnard, Soichot & Ringuier, 1990; Stark 1996).

Postoperative Tourniquet Palsy

Intraoperative use of an arm tourniquet at pressures above the systolic blood pressure to maintain a bloodless operative field can cause conduction block and axonal injuries to multiple arm nerves (On, Ozdemir & Aksit, 2000). Usually carpal tunnel surgery is completed in less than 1 hour; therefore, clinical postoperative tourniquet palsies should not occur (Flatt, 1972). However, the tourniquet can cause subclinical nerve injury. Nitz and Dobner (1989) performed electromyo-

Table 15-18. Iatrogenic Nerve Injury after Carpal Tunnel Surgery

Nerve	Open Surgery	Endoscopic Surgery
Median	Conolly, 1978; Cartotto, McCabe & Mackinnon, 1992; Slattery, 1994b; Nahabedian, Wittstadt & Wilgis, 1995; Murphy, 1997	Resnick & Miller, 1991; Feinstein, 1993; Herren & Simmen, 1994; Murphy, Jennings & Wukich, 1994; Dheansa & Belcher, 1998; Chen, Chen & Wei, 1999
Digital	Semple & Cargill, 1969; Das & Brown, 1976; Murray, Saccone & Rayan, 1994; Slattery, 1994b	Brown, Gelberman, Seiler, Abrahamsson, Weiland & Urbaniak, 1993; Sennwald & Benedetti, 1995; Jacobsen & Rahme, 1996, radial digital IV; Worseg, Kuzbari, Korak, Hocker, Wiederer, Tschabitscher & Holle, 1996
Median palmar cutaneous	Carroll & Green, 1972; Taleisnik, 1973; Hybbinette & Mannerfelt, 1975; Das & Brown, 1976; Conolly, 1978; MacDonald, Lichtman, Hanlon & Wilson, 1978; Louis, Greene & Noellert, 1985; Murray, Saccone & Rayan, 1994	Herren & Simmen, 1994; Agee, Peimer, Pyrek & Walsh, 1995
Recurrent thenar motor	Mannerfelt & Hybbinette, 1972; Hybbinette & Mannerfelt, 1975; Das & Brown, 1976; Conolly, 1978; Lilly & Magnell, 1985; Hybbinette, 1986	Boisrenoult, Desmoineaux & Beaufils, 1998
Superficial radial	Louis, Greene & Noellert, 1985	—
Ulnar	Favero & Gropper, 1987	Agee, McCarroll, Tortosa, Berry, Szabo & Peimer, 1992; Brown, Gelberman, Seiler, Abrahamsson, Weiland & Urbaniak, 1993; Nath, Mackinnon & Weeks, 1993; Shinya, Lanzetta & Conolly, 1995; del Pinal, Cruz-Camara & Jado, 1997; Müller, Rudig, Blum & Degreif, 1997; Müller, Rudig, Degreif & Rommens, 2000, neurapraxia; Santoro, Matloub & Gosain, 2000
Ulnar deep motor branch	Terrono, Belsky, Feldon & Nalebuff, 1993	De Smet & Fabry, 1995
Ulnar-median digital anastomosis	May & Rosen, 1981	Herren & Simmen, 1994; Agee, Peimer, Pyrek & Walsh, 1995
Ulnar palmar cutaneous	Engber & Gmeiner, 1980	—

graphy in 60 patients 3 weeks before and 3 weeks after carpal tunnel surgery. Patients were randomized in regard to use of a tourniquet during surgery. Tourniquet time was 1 hour or less. After surgery, reportedly 77% of patients in whom a tourniquet was used, but only 3% of patients who did not have a tourniquet, had developed fibrillations, positive sharp waves, or bizarre high-frequency discharges in nonthenar muscles distal to the tourniquet.

Crandall and Weeks (1988) described a 24-year-old woman who developed radial, anterior interosseous, and ulnar neuropathies in an arm that had had carpal surgery with use of a tourniquet. The delayed onset of these neuropathies excluded a classic tourniquet palsy, which is apparent immediately postoperatively. They speculated whether the tourniquet had caused subclinical nerve injury that predisposed to the development of the subsequent neuropathies.

Complex Regional Pain Syndrome

On rare occasion, a patient develops chronic pain and autonomic and vasomotor dysfunction in the operated hand after carpal tunnel surgery (Mac-Donald et al., 1978). The hand can be swollen, warm or cold, and is usually dry. Later, the skin can become cool, pale, or shiny with trophic changes. The patient may describe hyperalgesia and hyperesthesia. The incidence of similar complications was 10 patients in over 7,000 endoscopic surgeries (see Tables 15-4 and 15-5).

This clinical condition is sometime called a *complex regional pain syndrome. Reflex sympathetic dystrophy*, a formerly popular term, is now being abandoned. Chapter 16 discusses the difficulties in definition and diagnosis of complex regional pain syndromes. For example, case 3 in Chapter 16 illustrates how histrionic features complicate evaluation of patients with purported reflex sympathetic dystrophy.

Facile diagnosis of complex regional pain syndrome or reflex sympathetic dystrophy must not prevent careful evaluation for treatable causes of postoperative symptoms. For example, Milward and colleagues (1977) described a patient who developed hand swelling and "scalding" pain after carpal tunnel surgery. Pain did not improve with stellate ganglion block. When the wrist was re-explored, extensive scar formation was found involving both the median and ulnar nerves, and symptoms improved after neurolysis of both nerves.

Early mobilization and physical therapy are important aspects of treatment of patients with complex regional pain syndromes.

Summary

Carpal tunnel surgery is one of the most common and most effective operations in current medical practice. Interest in new developments, such as early mobilization, endoscopy, ligament reconstruction, and better outcome measurement, has led to greater understanding of the pathophysiology of carpal tunnel surgery. The many debates on the best treatment techniques will undoubtedly continue.

References

Abdullah AF, Wolber PH, Ditto EW 3rd. Sequelae of carpal tunnel surgery: rationale for the design of a surgical approach. Neurosurgery 1995;37:931–35; discussion, 935–36.

Ablove RH, Moy OJ, Peimer CA, Wheeler DR, Diao E. Pressure changes in Guyon's canal after carpal tunnel release. J. Hand Surg. 1996;21B:664–65.

Ablove RH, Peimer CA, Diao E, Oliverio R, Kuhn JP. Morphologic changes following endoscopic and two-portal subcutaneous carpal tunnel release. J. Hand Surg. 1994;19A: 821–26.

Abouzahr MK, Patsis MC, Chiu DT. Carpal tunnel release using limited direct vision. Plast. Reconstr. Surg. 1995;95: 534–38.

Adams ML, Franklin GM, Barnhart S. Outcome of carpal tunnel surgery in Washington State workers' compensation. Am. J. Ind. Med. 1994;25:527–36.

Agee JM, McCarroll HR, North ER. Endoscopic carpal tunnel release using the single proximal incision technique. Hand Clin. 1994;10:647–59.

Agee JM, McCarroll HR Jr, Tortosa RD, Berry DA, Szabo RM, Peimer CA. Endoscopic release of the carpal tunnel: a randomized prospective multicenter study. J. Hand Surg. 1992;17A:987–95.

Agee JM, Peimer CA, Pyrek JD, Walsh WE. Endoscopic carpal tunnel release: a prospective study of complications and surgical experience. J. Hand Surg. 1995;20A:165–71.

Agee JM, Tortosa R, Barry D, Peimer CA. Endoscopic release of the carpal tunnel. Transcription of presentation at the American Society for Surgery of the Hand, September 23–27, 1990; Toronto, Canada.

Alderson M, McGall D. The Alderson-McGall hand function questionnaire for patients with carpal tunnel syndrome: a pilot evaluation of a future outcome measure. J. Hand Ther. 1999;12:313–22.

al-Qattan MM, Bowen V, Manktelow RT. Factors associated with poor outcome following primary carpal tunnel release in non-diabetic patients. J. Hand Surg. 1994;19B: 622–25.

al-Qattan MM, Manktelow RT, Bowen CV. Outcome of carpal tunnel release in diabetic patients. J. Hand Surg. 1994; 19B:626–29.

Amadio PC. The first carpal tunnel release? J. Hand Surg. 1995;20B:40–41.

Amadio PC, Silverstein MD, Ilstrup DM, Schleck CD, Jensen LM. Outcome assessment for carpal tunnel surgery: the relative responsiveness of generic, arthritis-specific, disease-specific, and physical examination measures. J. Hand Surg. 1996;21A:338–46.

Anderson GA, Lee V, Sundararaj GD. Opponensplasty by extensor indicis and flexor digitorum superficialis tendon transfer. J. Hand Surg. 1992;17B:611–14.

Ariyan S, Watson HK. The palmar approach for the visualization and release of the carpal tunnel. An analysis of 429 cases. Plast. Reconstr. Surg. 1977;60:539–47.

Arons JA, Collins N, Arons MS. Results of treatment of carpal tunnel syndrome with associated hourglass deformity of the median nerve. J. Hand Surg. 1999;24A:1192–95.

Aszmann OC, Kress KM, Dellon AL. Results of decompression of peripheral nerves in diabetics: a prospective, blinded study. Plast. Reconstr. Surg. 2000;106:816–22.

Atroshi I, Axelsson G, Gummesson C, Johnsson R. Carpal tunnel syndrome with severe sensory deficit: endoscopic release in 18 cases. Acta Orthop. Scand. 2000;71:484–87.

Atroshi I, Gummesson C, Johnsson R, Sprinchorn A. Symptoms, disability, and quality of life in patients with carpal tunnel syndrome. J. Hand Surg. 1999;24A:398–404.

Atroshi I, Johnsson R, Nouhan R, Crain G, McCabe SJ. Use of outcome instruments to compare workers' compensation and non-workers' compensation carpal tunnel syndrome. J. Hand Surg. 1997;22A:882–88.

Atroshi I, Johnsson R, Ornstein E. Endoscopic carpal tunnel release: prospective assessment of 255 consecutive cases. J. Hand Surg. 1997;22B:42–47.

Atroshi I, Johnsson R, Ornstein E. Patient satisfaction and return to work after endoscopic carpal tunnel surgery. J. Hand Surg. 1998;23A:58–65.

Atroshi I, Johnsson R, Sprinchorn A. Self-administered outcome instrument in carpal tunnel syndrome. Reliability, validity and responsiveness evaluated in 102 patients. Acta Orthop. Scand. 1998;69:82–88.

Avci S, Sayli U. Carpal tunnel release using a short palmar incision and a new knife. J. Hand Surg. 2000;25B:357–60.

Avramidis K, Lewis JC, Gallagher P. Reduction in pain associated with open carpal tunnel decompression. J. Hand Surg. 2000;25B:147–49.

Baguneid MS, Sochart DH, Dunlop D, Kenny NW. Carpal tunnel decompression under local anaesthetic and tourniquet control. J. Hand Surg. 1997;22B:322–24.

Bande S, De Smet L, Fabry G. The results of carpal tunnel release: open versus endoscopic technique. J. Hand Surg. 1994;19B:14–17.

Benedetti VR, Sennwald G. Endoskopische Dekompression des N. medianus nach Agee: Prospektive Studie mit Vergleich zur offenen Dekompression Handchir. Mikrochir. Plast. Chir. 1996;28:151–55.

Benquet B, Fabre T, Durandeau A. Neurolysis of the median nerve in the carpal canal using a mini-invasive approach. Apropos of a prospective series of 138 cases. Chir. Main. 2000;19:86–93.

Bensimon RH, Murphy RX Jr. Midpalmar approach to the carpal tunnel: an alternative to endoscopic release. Ann. Plast. Surg. 1996;36:462–65.

Bessette L, Keller RB, Lew RA, Simmons BP, Fossel AH, Mooney N, Katz JN. Prognostic value of a hand symptom diagram in surgery for carpal tunnel syndrome. J. Rheumatol. 1997;24:726–34.

Bessette L, Keller RB, Liang MH, Simmons BP, Fossel AH, Katz JN. Patients' preferences and their relationship with satisfaction following carpal tunnel release. J. Hand Surg. 1997;22A:613–20.

Bessette L, Sangha O, Kuntz KM, Keller RB, Lew RA, Fossel AH, Katz JN. Comparative responsiveness of generic versus disease-specific and weighted versus unweighted health status measures in carpal tunnel syndrome. Medical Care 1998;36:491–502.

Bhatia R, Field J, Grote J, Huma H. Does splintage help pain after carpal tunnel release? J. Hand Surg. 2000;25B:150.

Birch R, Bonney G, Wynn Parry CB. Surgical Disorders of the Peripheral Nerves. Edinburgh, UK: Churchill Livingstone, 1998.

Biyani A, Downes EM. An open twin incision technique of carpal tunnel decompression with reduced incidence of scar tenderness. J. Hand Surg. 1993;18B:331–34.

Biyani A, Wolfe K, Simison AJ, Zakhour HD. Distribution of nerve fibers in the standard incision for carpal tunnel decompression. J. Hand Surg. 1996;21A:855–57.

Blair WF, Goetz DD, Ross MA, Steyers CM, Chang P. Carpal tunnel release with and without epineurotomy: a comparative prospective trial. J. Hand Surg. 1996;21A:655–61.

Bloem JJ, Pradjarahardja MC, Vuursteen PJ. The post-carpal tunnel syndrome. Causes and prevention. Neth. J. Surg. 1986;38:52–55.

Boeckstyns ME, Sorensen AI. Does endoscopic carpal tunnel release have a higher rate of complications than open carpal tunnel release? An analysis of published series. J. Hand Surg. 1999;24B:9–15.

Boisrenoult P, Desmoineaux P, Beaufils P. Single-portal endoscopic treatment of carpal tunnel syndrome. Results of a preliminary series. Rev. Chir. Orthop. Reparatrice Appar. Mot. 1998;84:136–41.

Bostrom L, Gothe CJ, Hansson S, Lugnegard H, Nilsson BY. Surgical treatment of carpal tunnel syndrome in patients exposed to vibration from handheld tools. Scand. J. Plast. Reconstr. Surg. Hand Surg. 1994;28:147–49.

Botte MJ, von Schroeder HP, Abrams RA, Gellman H. Recurrent carpal tunnel syndrome. Hand Clin. 1996;12:731–43.

Brain WR, Wright AD, Wilkinson M. Spontaneous compression of both median nerves in the carpal tunnel. Lancet 1947;1:277–82.

Braithwaite BD, Robinson GJ, Burge PD. Haemostasis during carpal tunnel release under local anaesthesia: a controlled comparison of a tourniquet and adrenaline infiltration. J. Hand Surg. 1993;18B:184–86.

Brandsma JW, Ottenhoff-De Jonge MW. Flexor digitorum superficialis tendon transfer for intrinsic replacement. Long-term results and the effect on donor fingers. J. Hand Surg. 1992;17B:625–28.

Braun RM. Palmaris longus tendon transfer for augmentation of the thenar musculature in low median palsy. J. Hand Surg. 1978;3:488–91.

Braun RM, Doehr S, Mosqueda T, Garcia A. The effect of legal representation on functional recovery of the hand in injured workers following carpal tunnel release. J. Hand Surg. 1999;24A:53–58.

Braun RM, Jackson WJ. Electrical studies as a prognostic factor in the surgical treatment of carpal tunnel syndrome. J. Hand Surg. 1994;19A:893–900.

Brief R, Brief LP. Endoscopic carpal tunnel release: report of 146 cases. Mt. Sinai J. Med. 2000;67:274–77.

Bromley GS. Minimal-incision open carpal tunnel decompression. J. Hand Surg. 1994;19A:119–20.

Brown MG, Keyser B, Rothenberg ES. Endoscopic carpal tunnel release. J. Hand Surg. 1992;17A:1009–11.

Brown MG, Rothenberg ES, Keyser B, Woloszyn TT, Wolford A. Results of 1236 endoscopic carpal tunnel release procedures using the Brown technique. Contemp. Orthop. 1993;27:251–58.

Brown MJ, Asbury AK. Diabetic neuropathy. Ann. Neurol. 1984;15:2–12.

Brown RA, Gelberman RH, Seiler JG 3rd, Abrahamsson SO, Weiland AJ, Urbaniak JR, Schoenfeld DA, Furcolo D. Carpal tunnel release. A prospective, randomized assessment of open and endoscopic methods. J. Bone Joint Surg. 1993;75A:1265–75.

Brown RK, Peimer CA. Changes in digital flexor tendon mechanics after endoscopic and open carpal tunnel releases in cadaver wrists. J. Hand Surg. 2000;25A:112–19.

Buchberger W. Radiologic imaging of the carpal tunnel. Eur. J. Radiol. 1997;25:112–17.

Buchberger W, Judmaier W, Birbamer G, Hasenohrl K, Schmidauer C. The role of sonography and MR tomography in the diagnosis and therapeutic control of the carpal tunnel syndrome. Fortschr. Röntgenstr. 1993;159:138–43.

Bury TF, Akelman E, Weiss AP. Prospective, randomized trial of splinting after carpal tunnel release. Ann. Plast. Surg. 1995;35:19–22.

Butterfield PG, Spencer PS, Redmond N, Rosenbaum R, Zirkle DF. Clinical and employment outcomes of carpal tunnel syndrome in Oregon workers' compensation recipients. J. Occup. Rehabil. 1997;7:61–73.

Calderon MS, Chung KC. Case report. Initial manifestation of gout after carpal tunnel release. Br. J. Plast. Surg. 1999; 52:76–77.

Cannon BW, Love JG. Tardy median palsy; median neuritis; median thenar neuritis amenable to surgery. Surgery 1946; 20:210–16.

Carroll RE, Green DP. The significance of the palmar cutaneous nerve at the wrist. Clin. Orthop. 1972;83:24–28.

Carter SL. A new instrument: a carpal tunnel knife. J. Hand Surg. 1991;16A:178–79.

Cartotto RC, McCabe S, Mackinnon SE. Two devastating complications of carpal tunnel surgery. Ann. Plast. Surg. 1992; 28:472–74.

Chaise F. Immediate active mobilization or rigid postoperative immobilization of the wrist in carpal tunnel syndrome. Comparative analysis of a series of 50 patients. Rev. Rhum. Mal. Osteoartic. 1990;57:435–39.

Chang B, Dellon AL. Surgical management of recurrent carpal tunnel syndrome. J. Hand Surg. 1993;18:467–70.

Chen HT, Chen HC, Wei FC. Endoscopic carpal tunnel release. Chang. Keng. I. Hsueh. Tsa. Chih. 1999;22:386–91.

Choi S-J, Ahn D-S. Correlation of clinical history and electrodiagnostic abnormalities with outcome after surgery for carpal tunnel syndrome. Plast. Reconstr. Surg. 1998;102:2374–80.

Chow JCY. Endoscopic release of the carpal ligament: a new technique for carpal tunnel syndrome. Arthroscopy 1989; 5:19–24.

Chow JC. Endoscopic carpal tunnel release. Two-portal technique. Hand Clin. 1994;10:637–46.

Chow JC. Endoscopic carpal tunnel release. Clin. Sports Med. 1996;15:769–84.

Christodoulou L, Yang XB, Chamberlain ST. Rupture of flexor pollicis longus after carpal tunnel decompression. Injury 2000;31:744–45.

Chung KC, Walters MR, Greenfield ML, Chernew ME. Endoscopic versus open carpal tunnel release: a cost-effectiveness analysis. Plast. Reconstr. Surg. 1998;102: 1089–99.

Clayburgh RH, Beckenbaugh RD, Dobyns JH. Carpal tunnel release in patients with diffuse peripheral neuropathy. J. Hand Surg. 1987;12A:380–83.

Cobb TK, Amadio PC. Reoperation for carpal tunnel syndrome. Hand Clin. 1996;12:313–23.

Cobb TK, Amadio PC, Leatherwood DF, Schleck CD, Ilstrup DM. Outcome of reoperation for carpal tunnel syndrome. J. Hand Surg. 1996;21A:347–56.

Cobb TK, Carmichael SW, Cooney WP. The ulnar neurovascular bundle at the wrist. A technical note on endoscopic carpal tunnel release. J. Hand Surg. 1994;19B:24–26.

Cobb TK, Cooney WP. Significance of incomplete release of the distal portion of the flexor retinaculum. Implications for endoscopic carpal tunnel surgery. J. Hand Surg. 1994;19B: 283–85.

Cobb TK, Dalley BK, Posteraro RH, Lewis RC. Anatomy of the flexor retinaculum. J. Hand Surg. 1993;18A:91–99.

Concannon MJ, Brownfield ML, Puckett CL. The incidence of recurrence after endoscopic carpal tunnel release. Plast. Reconstr. Surg. 2000;105:1662–65.

Concannon MJ, Gainor B, Petroski GF, Puckett CL. The predictive value of electrodiagnostic studies in carpal tunnel syndrome. Plast. Reconstr. Surg. 1997;100:1452–58.

Conolly WB. Pitfalls in carpal tunnel decompression. Aust. N. Z. J. Surg. 1978;48:421–25.

Conolly WB. Color Atlas of Treatment of Carpal Tunnel Syndrome. Oradell, NJ: Medical Economics Books, 1983.

Cook AC, Szabo RM, Birkholz SW, King EF. Early mobilization following carpal tunnel release. A prospective randomized study. J. Hand Surg. 1995;20B:228–30.

Cooney WP. Tendon transfer for median nerve palsy. Hand Clin. 1988;4:155–65.

Corradi M, Paganelli E, Pavesi G. Internal neurolysis and flexor tenosynovectomy: adjuncts in the treatment of chronic median nerve compression at the wrist in hemodialysis patients. Microsurgery 1989;10:248–50.

Crandall RE, Weeks PM. Multiple nerve dysfunction after carpal tunnel release. J. Hand Surg. 1988;13A:584–89.

Crymble B. Brachial neuralgia and the carpal tunnel syndrome. BMJ. 1968;3:470–71.

Cseuz KA, Thomas JE, Lambert EH, Love JG, Lipscomb PR. Long-term results of operation for carpal tunnel syndrome. Mayo Clin. Proc. 1966;41:232–41.

Curtis RM, Eversmann Jr WW. Internal neurolysis as an adjunct to the treatment of the carpal-tunnel syndrome. J. Bone Joint Surg. 1973;55A:733–40.

Das SK, Brown HG. In search of complications in carpal tunnel decompression. Hand 1976;8:243–49.

Davies BW, Pennington GA, Fritz AM. Two-portal endoscopic carpal tunnel release: an outcome analysis of 333 hands. Ann. Plast. Surg. 1998;40:542–48.

Davis AM, Beaton DE, Hudak P, Amadio P, Bombardier C, Cole D, Hawker G, Katz JN, Makela M, Marx RG, Punnett L, Wright JG. Measuring disability of the upper extremity: a rationale supporting the use of a regional outcome measure. J. Hand Ther. 1999;12:269–74.

Dawson DM, Hallett M, Wilbourn AJ. Carpal Tunnel Syndrome. In: Dawson DM, Hallett M, Wilbourn AJ, eds. Entrapment Neuropathies. Philadelphia: Lippincott–Raven, 1999;20–94.

Dellon AL, Chang BW. An alternative incision for approaching recurrent median nerve compression at the wrist. Plast. Reconstr. Surg. 1992;89:576–78.

Dellon AL, Mackinnon SE. The pronator quadratus muscle flap. J. Hand Surg. 1984;9A:423–27.

del Pinal F, Cruz-Camara A, Jado E. Total ulnar nerve transection during endoscopic carpal tunnel release. Arthroscopy 1997;13:235–37.

Denman EE. The anatomy of the incision for carpal tunnel decompression. Hand 1981;13:17–28.

De Smet L. Recurrent carpal tunnel syndrome. Clinical testing indicating incomplete section of the flexor retinaculum. J. Hand Surg. 1993;18B:189.

De Smet L, Fabry G. Transection of the motor branch of the ulnar nerve as a complication of two-portal endoscopic carpal tunnel release: a case report. J. Hand Surg. 1995;20A: 18–19.

DeStefano F, Nordstrom DL, Vierkant RA. Long-term symptom outcomes of carpal tunnel syndrome and its treatment. J. Hand Surg. 1997;22A:200–10.

Dheansa BS, Belcher HJ. Median nerve contusion during endoscopic carpal tunnel release. J. Hand Surg. 1998;23B: 110–11.

Di Giuseppe P, Ajmar R. Carpal tunnel release using minimally invasive technique. Plast. Reconstr. Surg. 1996;97: 1310–11.

Dlabal K. Late results of surgical treatment of opposition of the thumb in peripheral palsy of n. medianus trunk. Acta Chir. Plast. 1995;37:3–6.

Dlabalova V. Our long-term experience and results of surgical management of the carpal tunnel syndrome. Acta Chir. Plast. 1995;37:47–49.

Doyle JR, Carroll RE. The carpal tunnel syndrome. A review of 100 patients treated surgically. Calif. Med. 1968;108: 263–67.

Duclos L, Sokolow C. Management of true recurrent carpal tunnel syndrome: is it worthwhile to bring vascularized tissue? Chir. Main. 1998;17:113–17; discussion, 118.

Dumontier C, Sokolow C, Leclercq C, Chauvin P. Early results of conventional versus two-portal endoscopic carpal tunnel release. A prospective study. J. Hand Surg. 1995; 20B:658–62.

Duncan KH, Lewis RC Jr, Foreman KA, Nordyke MD. Treatment of carpal tunnel syndrome by members of the American Society for Surgery of the Hand: results of a questionnaire. J. Hand Surg. 1987;12A:384–91.

Eason SY, Belsole RJ, Greene TL. Carpal tunnel release: analysis of suboptimal results. J. Hand Surg. 1985;10B:365–69.

Ebskov LB, Boeckstyns ME, Sorensen AI. Operative treatment of carpal tunnel syndrome in Denmark. Results of a questionnaire. J. Hand Surg. 1997;22B:761–63.

Elmaraghy MW, Hurst LN. Single-portal endoscopic carpal tunnel release: Agee carpal tunnel release system. Ann. Plast. Surg. 1996;36:286–91.

Engber WD, Gmeiner JG. Palmar cutaneous branch of the ulnar nerve. J. Hand Surg. 1980;5:26–29.

Erdmann MW. Endoscopic carpal tunnel decompression. J. Hand Surg. 1994;19B:5–13.

Erhard L, Ozalp T, Citron N, Foucher G. Carpal tunnel release by the Agee endoscopic technique. Results at 4 year follow-up. J. Hand Surg. 1999;24B:583–85.

Evans GR, Dellon AL. Implantation of the palmar cutaneous branch of the median nerve into the pronator quadratus for treatment of painful neuroma. J. Hand Surg. 1994;19A: 203–6.

Eversmann WW Jr, Ritsick JA. Intraoperative changes in motor nerve conduction latency in carpal tunnel syndrome. J. Hand Surg. 1978;3:77–81.

Evrard H, Tshiakatumba MB. Intraneural neurolysis. Acta Orthop. Belg. 1977;43:186–90.

Farhat SM, Kahn EA, Child MA. The carpal tunnel syndrome. Surg. Neurol. 1974;2:285–88.

Favero KJ, Gropper PT. Ulnar nerve laceration—a complication of carpal tunnel decompression: case report and review of the literature. J. Hand Surg. 1987;12B:239–41.

Feinstein PA. Endoscopic carpal tunnel release in a community-based series. J. Hand Surg. 1993;18A:451–54.

Ferrara MA, Marcelis S. Ultrasound examination of the wrist. J. Belge Radiol. 1997;80:78–80.

Finsen V, Russwurm H. Neurophysiology not required before surgery for typical carpal tunnel syndrome. J. Hand Surg. 2001;26B:61–64.

Fischer TJ, Hastings H 2nd. Endoscopic carpal tunnel release. Chow technique. Hand Clin. 1996;12:285–97.

Fissette J, Boucq D, Lahaye T, Onkelinx A. Effects of reconstruction of the anterior annular carpal ligament using a silicone sheet in surgery of the carpal tunnel syndrome. Acta Orthop. Belg. 1981;47:375–81.

Fissette J, Onkelinx A. Treatment of carpal tunnel syndrome. Comparative study with and without epineurolysis. Hand 1979;11:206–10.

Flatt AE. Tourniquet time in hand surgery. Arch. Surg. 1972; 104:190–92.

Forman DL, Watson HK, Caulfield KA, Shenko J, Caputo AE, Ashmead D. Persistent or recurrent carpal tunnel syndrome following prior endoscopic carpal tunnel release. J. Hand Surg. 1998;23A:1010–14.

Foucher G, Braga Da Silva J. Ouverture endoscopique du canal carpien. Chirurgie 1994–95;120:100–104.

Foucher G, Buch N, Van Overstraeten L, Gautherie M, Jesel M. Carpal tunnel syndrome. Can it still be a controversial topic? Chirurgie 1993–94;119:80–4.

Foucher G, Malizos C, Sammut D, Marin Braun F, Michon J. Primary palmaris longus transfer as an opponensplasty in carpal tunnel syndrome. J. Hand Surg. 1991;16B:56–60.

Foulkes GD, Atkinson RE, Beuchel C, Doyle JR, Singer DI. Outcome following epineurotomy in carpal tunnel syndrome: a prospective, randomized clinical trial. J. Hand Surg. 1994;19A:539–47.

Frank U, Giunta R, Krimmer H, Lanz U. Relocation of the median nerve after scarring along the carpal tunnel with hypothenar fatty tissue flap-plasty. Handchir. Mikrochir. Plast. Chir. 1999;31:317–22.

Franzini A, Broggi G, Servello D, Dones I, Pluchino MG. Transillumination in minimally invasive surgery for carpal tunnel release. Technical note. J. Neurosurg. 1996;85:1184–86.

Freshwater MF, Arons MS. The effect of various adjuncts on the surgical treatment of carpal tunnel syndrome secondary to chronic tenosynovitis. Plast. Reconstr. Surg. 1978;61:93–96.

Frick A, Baumeister RG, Kopp R. Zur Verfahrenswahl bei der Therapie des distalen N. medianus-Kompressionssyndroms. Handchir. Mikrochir. Plast. Chir. 1996;28:147–50.

Fuss FK, Wagner TF. Biomechanical alterations in the carpal arch and hand muscles after carpal tunnel release: a further approach toward understanding the function of the flexor retinaculum and the cause of postoperative grip weakness. Clin. Anat. 1996;9:100–8.

Futami T. Surgery for bilateral carpal tunnel syndrome. Endoscopic and open release compared in 10 patients. Acta Orthop. Scand. 1995;66:153–55.

Gainer JV Jr, Nugent GR. Carpal tunnel syndrome: report of 430 operations. South. Med. J. 1977;70:325–28.

Garcia-Elias M, Sanchez-Freijo JM, Salo JM, Lluch AL. Dynamic changes of the transverse carpal arch during flexion-extension of the wrist: effects of sectioning the transverse carpal ligament. J. Hand Surg. 1992;17A:1017–19.

Gartsman GM, Kovach JC, Crouch CC, Noble PC, Bennett JB. Carpal arch alteration after carpal tunnel release. J. Hand Surg. 1986;11A:372–74.

Gelberman RH, Pfeffer GB, Galbraith RT, Szabo RM, Rydevik B, Dimick M. Results of treatment of severe carpal-tunnel syndrome without internal neurolysis of the median nerve. J. Bone Joint Surg. 1987;69A:896–903.

Gellman H, Kan D, Gee V, Kuschner SH, Botte MJ. Analysis of pinch and grip strength after carpal tunnel release. J. Hand Surg. 1989;14A:863–64.

Ghaly RF, Saban KL, Haley DA, Ross RE. Endoscopic carpal tunnel release surgery: report of patient satisfaction. Neurol. Res. 2000;22:551–55.

Gibson M. Outpatient carpal tunnel decompression without tourniquet: a simple local anaesthetic technique. Ann. R. Coll. Surg. Engl. 1990;72:408–9.

Gilbert A, Becker C. A Flap Based on Distal Branches of the Ulnar Artery and Its Use in Recurrent Carpal Tunnel Syndrome. In: Tubiana R, ed. The Hand. Philadelphia: Saunders, 1993;499–505.

Giunta R, Frank U, Lanz U. The hypothenar fat-pad flap for reconstructive repair after scarring of the median nerve at the wrist joint. Chir. Main. 1998;17:107–12.

Glowacki KA, Breen CJ, Sachar K, Weiss A-PC. Electrodiagnostic testing and carpal tunnel release outcome. J. Hand Surg. 1996;21A:117–22.

Gonzalez F, Watson HK. Simultaneous carpal tunnel release and Dupuytren's fasciectomy. J. Hand Surg. 1991;16B: 175–78.

Goodman RC. An aggressive return-to-work program in surgical treatment of carpal tunnel syndrome: a comparison of costs. Plast. Reconstr. Surg. 1992;89:715–17.

Graff SN, Seiler JG 3d, Jupiter JB. Acute gout after carpal tunnel release. J. Hand Surg. 1992;17A:1031–32.

Greco RJ, Curtsinger LJ. Carpal tunnel release complicated by necrotizing fasciitis. Ann. Plast. Surg. 1993;30:545–48.

Green DP. Diagnostic and therapeutic value of carpal tunnel injection. J. Hand Surg. 1984;9A:850–54.

Groves EJ, Rider BA. A comparison of treatment approaches used after carpal tunnel release surgery. Am. J. Occup. Ther. 1989;43:398–402.

Grundberg AB. Carpal tunnel decompression in spite of normal electromyography. J. Hand Surg. 1983;8:348–49.

Grundberg AB. Guyon's canal decompression. J. Hand Surg. 1986;11A:454.

Guillemot E, Le Nen D, Colin D, Stindel E, Hu W, L'Heveder G. Perineural fibrosis of the median nerve at the wrist. Treatment by neurolysis and dermal-hypodermal graft. Chir. Main. 1999;18:279–89.

Hagberg M, Nystrom A, Zetterlund B. Recovery from symptoms after carpal tunnel syndrome surgery in males in relation to vibration exposure. J. Hand Surg. 1991;16A: 66–71.

Hallock GG, Lutz DA. Prospective comparison of minimal incision "open" and two-portal endoscopic carpal tunnel release. Plast. Reconstr. Surg. 1995;96:941–47.

Hamanaka I, Okutsu I, Shimizu K, Takatori Y, Ninomiya S. Evaluation of carpal canal pressure in carpal tunnel syndrome. J. Hand Surg. 1995;20A:848–54.

Hamlin C, Hitchcock M, Hofmeister J, Owens R. Predicting surgical outcome for pain relief and return to work [corrected and republished article originally printed in Best Pract. Benchmarking Healthc. 1996;1:258-61]. Best Pract. Benchmarking Healthc. 1996;1: 311–14.

Hanssen AD, Amadio PC, DeSilva SP, Ilstrup DM. Deep postoperative wound infection after carpal tunnel release. J. Hand Surg. 1989;14A:869–73.

Harris CM, Tanner E, Goldstein MN, Pettee DS. The surgical treatment of the carpal-tunnel syndrome correlated with preoperative nerve-conduction studies. J. Bone Joint Surg. 1979;61A:93–98.

Hashizume H, Nanba Y, Shigeyama Y, Hirooka T, Yokoi T, Inoue H. Endoscopic carpal tunnel pressure measurement: a reliable technique for complete release. Acta Medica Okayama 1997;51:105–10.

Haupt WF, Wintzer G, Schop A, Lottgen J, Pawlik G. Longterm results of carpal tunnel decompression. Assessment of 60 cases. J. Hand Surg. 1993;18B:471–74.

Heckler FR, Jabaley ME. Evolving concepts of median nerve decompression in the carpal tunnel. Hand Clin. 1986;2: 723–36.

Herren DB, Simmen BR. Complications after endoscopic carpal tunnel decompression. Z. Unfallchir. Versicherungsmed. 1994; 87:120–27.

Higgs PE, Edwards DF, Martin DS, Weeks PM. Relation of preoperative nerve-conduction values to outcome in workers with surgically treated carpal tunnel syndrome. J. Hand Surg. 1997;22A:216–21.

Hirooka T, Hashizume H, Senda M, Nagoshi M, Inoue H, Nagashima H. Adequacy and long-term prognosis of endoscopic carpal tunnel release. Acta Medica Okayama 1999;53:39–44.

Hoefnagels WA, van Kleef JG, Mastenbroek GG, de Blok JA, Breukelman AJ, de Krom MC. Surgical treatment of carpal tunnel syndrome: endoscopic or classical (open)? A prospective randomized trial. Ned. Tijdschr. Geneeskd. 1997; 141:878–82.

Holmgren H, Rabow L. Internal neurolysis or ligament division only in carpal tunnel syndrome, II. A 3 year follow-up with an evaluation of various neurophysiological parameters for diagnosis. Acta Neurochir. (Wien.) 1987;87:44–47.

Holmgren-Larsson H, Leszniewski W, Linden U, Rabow L, Thorling J. Internal neurolysis or ligament division only in carpal tunnel syndrome—results of a randomized study. Acta Neurochir. (Wien.) 1985;74:118–21.

Hudson AR, Wissinger JP, Salazar JL, Kline DG, Yarzagaray L, Danoff D, Fernandez E, Field EM, Gainsburg DB, Fabi RA, Mackinnon SE. Carpal tunnel syndrome. Surg. Neurol. 1997;47:105–14.

Hulsizer DL, Staebler MP, Weiss AP, Akelman E. The results of revision carpal tunnel release following previous open versus endoscopic surgery. J. Hand Surg. 1998;23A:865–69.

Hunter JM. Reconstruction of the transverse carpal ligament to restore median nerve gliding. The rationale of a new technique for revision of recurrent median nerve neuropathy. Hand Clin. 1996;12:365–78.

Hunter JM, Read RL, Gray R. Carpal tunnel neuropathy caused by injury: reconstruction of the transverse carpal ligament for the complex carpal tunnel syndromes. J. Hand Ther. 1993;6:145–51.

Hutchinson DT, McClinton MA. Upper extremity tourniquet tolerance. J. Hand Surg. 1993;18A:206–10.

Hybbinette CH. Severance of thenar branch. J. Hand Surg. 1986;11A:613.

Hybbinette CH, Mannerfelt L. The carpal tunnel syndrome. A retrospective study of 400 operated patients. Acta Orthop. Scand. 1975;46:610–20.

Inglis AE. Two unusual operative complications in the carpal-tunnel syndrome. A report of two cases. J. Bone Joint Surg. 1980;62A:1208–9.

Inglis AE, Straub LR, Williams CS. Median nerve neuropathy at the wrist. Clin. Orthop. 1972;83:48–54.

Jacobsen MB, Rahme H. A prospective, randomized study with an independent observer comparing open carpal tunnel release with endoscopic carpal tunnel release. J. Hand Surg. 1996;21B:202–4.

Jakab E, Ganos D, Cook FW. Transverse carpal ligament reconstruction in surgery for carpal tunnel syndrome: a new technique. J. Hand Surg. 1991;91A:202–6.

Jebson PJ, Agee JM. Carpal tunnel syndrome: unusual contraindications to endoscopic release. Arthroscopy 1996;12:749–51.

Jimenez DF, Gibbs SR, Clapper AT. Endoscopic treatment of carpal tunnel syndrome: a critical review. J. Neurosurg. 1998;88:817–26.

Jimenez S, Hardy MA, Horch K, Jabaley M. A study of sensory recovery following carpal tunnel release. J. Hand Ther. 1993;6:124–29.

Jones SM, Stuart PR, Stothard J. Open carpal tunnel release. Does a vascularized hypothenar fat pad reduce wound tenderness? J. Hand Surg. 1997;22B:758–60.

Kalia KK, Moossy JJ. Carpal tunnel release complicated by acute gout. Neurosurgery 1993;33:1102–3.

Kapandji AI. Plastic surgical enlargement of the anterior annular carpal ligament in the treatment of carpal tunnel syndrome. Ann. Chir. Main. 1990;9:305–13; discussion 314.

Karlsson MK, Lindau T, Hagberg L. Ligament lengthening compared with simple division of the transverse carpal ligament in the open treatment of carpal tunnel syndrome. Scand. J. Plast. Reconstr. Surg. Hand Surg. 1997;31:65–69.

Kato T, Kuroshima N, Okutsu I, Ninomiya S. Effects of endoscopic release of the transverse carpal ligament on carpal canal volume. J. Hand Surg. 1994;19A:416–19.

Katz JN, Gelberman RH, Wright EA, Abrahamsson SO, Lew RA. A preliminary scoring system for assessing the out-come of carpal tunnel release. J. Hand Surg. 1994; 19A:531–38.

Katz JN, Gelberman RH, Wright EA, Lew RA, Liang MH. Responsiveness of self-reported and objective measures of disease severity in carpal tunnel syndrome. Medical Care 1994;32:1127–33.

Katz JN, Lew RA, Bessette L, Punnett L, Fossel AH, Mooney N, Keller RB. Prevalence and predictors of long-term work disability due to carpal tunnel syndrome. Am. J. Ind. Med. 1998;33:543–50.

Katz JN, Losina E, Amick III BC, Fossel AH, Bessette L, Keller RB. Predictors of outcomes of carpal tunnel release. Arthritis Rheum. 2001;44:1184–93.

Kelly CP, Pulisetti D, Jamieson AM. Early experience with endoscopic carpal tunnel release. J. Hand Surg. 1994; 19B:18–21.

Kelly PJ, Karlson AG, Weed LA, Lipscomb PR. Infection of synovial tissues by mycobacteria other than mycobacterium tuberculosis. J. Bone Joint Surg. 1967;49A:1521–30.

Kerr CD, Gittins ME, Sybert DR. Endoscopic versus open carpal tunnel release: clinical results. Arthroscopy 1994; 10:266–69.

Khan R, Macey A. Open carpal tunnel release under local anaesthesia: a patient satisfaction survey. Ir. Med. J. 2000; 93:19.

Kim SJ, Shin SJ, Kang ES. Endoscopic carpal tunnel release in patients receiving long-term hemodialysis. Clin. Orthop. 2000;376:141–48.

Kiritsis PG, Kline SC. Biomechanical changes after carpal tunnel release: a cadaveric model for comparing open, endoscopic, and step-cut lengthening techniques. J. Hand Surg. 1995;20A:173–80.

Kline SC, Moore JR. The transverse carpal ligament. An important component of the digital flexor pulley system. J. Bone Joint Surg. 1992;74A:1478–85.

Kluge W, Simpson RG, Nicol AC. Late complications after open carpal tunnel decompression. J. Hand Surg. 1996; 21B:205–7.

Köstli A, Huber H. Release of the carpal tunnel by endoscopy. Swiss Surgery 1998;4:311–15.

Kropfl A, Gasperschitz F, Hertz H. Technik, Ergebnisse und Gefahren der endoskopischen Karpaltunnelspaltung. Handchir. Mikrochir. Plast. Chir. 1996;28:120–27.

Kulick MI, Gordillo G, Javidi T, Kilgore ES Jr, Newmayer WL 3d. Long-term analysis of patients having surgical treatment for carpal tunnel syndrome. J. Hand Surg. 1986;11A:59–66.

Langa V, Posner MA, Hoffman S, Steiner GC. Carpal tunnel syndrome secondary to tuberculous tenosynovitis. Bull. Hosp. Joint Dis. 1986;46:137–42.

Langloh ND, Linscheid RL. Recurrent and unrelieved carpal-tunnel syndrome. Clin. Orthop. 1972;83:41–47.

Lanzetta M, Nolli R. Nerve stripping: new treatment for neuromas of the palmar cutaneous branch of the median nerve. J. Hand Surg. 2000;25B:151–53.

Lazaro RP. Neuropathic symptoms and musculoskeletal pain in carpal tunnel syndrome: prognostic and therapeutic implications. Surg. Neurol. 1997;47:115–19.

Leach WJ, Esler C, Scott TD. Grip strength following carpal tunnel decompression. J. Hand Surg. 1993;18B:750–52.

Learmonth JR. Treatment of diseases of peripheral nerves. Surg. Clin. North Am. 1933;13:905–13.

Lee DH, Masear VR, Meyer RD, Stevens DM, Colgin S. Endoscopic carpal tunnel release: a cadaveric study. J. Hand Surg. 1992;17A:1003–8.

Lee H, Jackson TA. Carpal tunnel release through a limited skin incision under direct visualization using a new instrument, the carposcope. Plast. Reconstr. Surg. 1996;98:313–19.

Lee WP, Strickland JW. Safe carpal tunnel release via a limited palmar incision. Plast. Reconstr. Surg. 1998;101:418–24.

Leinberry CF, Hammond 3rd NL, Siegfried JW. The role of epineurotomy in the operative treatment of carpal tunnel syndrome. J. Bone Joint Surg. 1997;79A:555–57.

Le Nen D, Rizzo C, Hu W, Brunet P. Neurolysis of the median nerve at the wrist with 2-portal endoscopic technique. Analysis of 102 consecutive cases. Chir. Main 1998;17: 221–31.

Levine DW, Simmons BP, Koris MJ, Daltroy LH, Hohl GG, Fossel AH, Katz JN. A self-administered questionnaire for the assessment of severity of symptoms and functional status in carpal tunnel syndrome. J. Bone Joint Surg. 1993; 75A:1585–92.

Lewicky RT. Endoscopic carpal tunnel release: the guide tube technique. Arthroscopy 1994;10:39–49.

Lilly CJ, Magnell TD. Severance of the thenar branch of the median nerve as a complication of carpal tunnel release. J. Hand Surg. 1985;10A:399–402.

Lindau T, Karlsson MK. Complications and outcome in open carpal tunnel release. A 6-year follow-up in 92 patients. Chir. Main 1999;18:115–21.

Littler JW, Li CS. Primary restoration of thumb opposition with median nerve decompression. Plast. Reconstr. Surg. 1967; 39:74–75.

Lluch AL. Transverse carpal ligament reconstruction for carpal tunnel syndrome. J. Hand Surg. 1993;18A:170–71.

Loick J, Joosten U, Lucke R. Implantation of oxidized, regenerated cellulose for prevention of recurrence in surgical therapy of carpal tunnel syndrome. Handchir. Mikrochir. Plast. Chir. 1997;29:209–13.

Louis DS, Greene TL, Noellert RC. Complications of carpal tunnel surgery. J. Neurosurg. 1985;62:352–56.

LoVerme PJ, Saccone PG. Limited portal with direct-vision carpal tunnel release. Ann. Plast. Surg. 1995;34:304–8.

Lowry WE Jr, Follender AB. Interfascicular neurolysis in the severe carpal tunnel syndrome. A prospective, randomized, double-blind, controlled study. Clin. Orthop. 1988;227: 251–54.

Luallin SR, Toby EB. Incidental Guyon's canal release during attempted endoscopic carpal tunnel release: an anatomical study and report of two cases. Arthroscopy 1993; 9:382–86.

Luchetti R, Alfarano M, Montagna G, Soragni O. Short palmar incision: a new surgical approach for carpal tunnel syndrome. Chir. Organi Mov. 1996;81: 197–206.

Ludlow KS, Merla JL, Cox JA, Hurst LN. Pillar pain as a postoperative complication of carpal tunnel release: a review of the literature. J. Hand Ther. 1997;10:277–82.

MacDonald RI, Lichtman DM, Hanlon JJ, Wilson JN. Complications of surgical release for carpal tunnel syndrome. J. Hand Surg. 1978;3:70–76.

MacDougal BA. Palmaris longus opponensplasty. Plast. Reconstr. Surg. 1995;96:982–84.

Mackenzie DJ, Hainer R, Wheatley MJ. Early recovery after endoscopic vs. short-incision open carpal tunnel release. Ann. Plast. Surg. 2000;44:601–4.

Mackinnon SE. Secondary carpal tunnel surgery. Neurosurg. Clin. North Am. 1991;2:75–91.

Mackinnon SE, McCabe S, Murray JF, Szalai JP, Kelly L, Novak C, Kin B, Burke GM. Internal neurolysis fails to improve the results of primary carpal tunnel decompression. J. Hand Surg. 1991;16A:211–18.

Magee KR, Kahn EA. The carpal tunnel syndrome. Mich. Med. 1967;66:1424–28.

Mannerfelt L, Hybbinette CH. Important anomaly of the thenar motor branch of the median nerve. A clinical and anatomical report. Bull. Hosp. Joint Dis. 1972;33:15–21.

Marmor L. Surgery of rheumatoid hand and wrist. Semin. Arthritis Rheum. 1971;1:7–24.

Martin CH, Seiler JG 3rd, Lesesne JS. The cutaneous innervation of the palm: an anatomic study of the ulnar and median nerves. J. Hand Surg. 1996;21A:634–38.

Mascharka Z. Zweieinhalbjahrige Erfahrung mit der endoskopischen Karpaltunnelspaltung. Handchir. Mikrochir. Plast. Chir. 1996;28:138–42.

Masear VR, Hayes JM, Hyde AG. An industrial cause of carpal tunnel syndrome. J. Hand Surg. 1986;11A:222–27.

Mathoulin C, Bahm J, Roukoz S. Pedicled hypothenar fat flap for median nerve coverage in recalcitrant carpal tunnel syndrome. Hand Surg. 2000;5:33–40.

May JW Jr, Rosen H. Division of the sensory ramus communicans between the ulnar and median nerves: a complication following carpal tunnel release. A case report. J. Bone Joint Surg. 1981;63A:836–38.

McCabe SJ, Kleinert JM. The nerve of Henle. J. Hand Surg. 1990;15A:784–88.

McClinton M. The use of dermal-fat grafts. Hand Clin. 1996; 12:357–64.

McDonough JW, Gruenloh TJ. A comparison of endoscopic and open carpal tunnel release. Wis. Med. J. 1993;92: 675–77.

Mendelson B, Balla J. Results of surgical treatment of the carpal tunnel syndrome. Proc. Aust. Assoc. Neurol. 1973; 9:129–32.

Menon J. Endoscopic carpal tunnel release: preliminary report. Arthroscopy 1994;10:31–38.

Menon J, Etter C. Endoscopic carpal tunnel release—current status. J. Hand Ther. 1993;6:139–44.

Mesgarzadeh M, Schneck CD, Bonakdarpour A, Mitra A, Conaway D. Carpal tunnel: MR imaging. Part II. Carpal tunnel syndrome. Radiology 1989;171:749–54.

Milward TM, Stott WG, Kleinert HE. The abductor digiti minimi muscle flap. Hand 1977;9:82–85.

Mirza MA, King ET Jr, Tanveer S. Palmar uniportal extrabursal endoscopic carpal tunnel release. Arthroscopy 1995;11: 82–90.

Mondelli M, Reale F, Sicurelli F, Padua L. Relationship between the self-administered Boston questionnaire and electrophysiological findings in follow-up of surgically-treated carpal tunnel syndrome. J. Hand Surg. 2000;25B: 128–34.

Morgenlander JC, Lynch JR, Sanders DB. Surgical treatment of carpal tunnel syndrome in patients with peripheral neuropathy. Neurology 1997;49:1159–63.

Moyer RA, Bush DC, Dennehy JJ. *Prototheca wickerhamii* tenosynovitis. J. Rheumatol. 1990;17:701–4.

Müller LP, Rudig L, Blum J, Degreif J. Komplikationen der endoskopischen Retinakulumspaltung. Handchir. Mikrochir. Plast. Chir. 1997;29:238–42.

Müller LP, Rudig L, Degreif J, Rommens PM. Endoscopic carpal tunnel release: results with special consideration to possible complications. Knee Surg. Sports Traumatol. Arthrosc. 2000;8:166–72.

Murphy RX Jr. Re: Midpalmar approach to the carpal tunnel: an alternative to endoscopic release. Ann. Plast. Surg. 1997; 38:84.

Murphy RX Jr., Chernofsky MA, Osborne MA, Wolson AH. Magnetic resonance imaging in the evaluation of persistent carpal tunnel syndrome. J. Hand Surg. 1993;18A:113–20.

Murphy RX Jr., Jennings JF, Wukich DK. Major neurovascular complications of endoscopic carpal tunnel release. J. Hand Surg. 1994;19A:114–18.

Murray DP, Saccone PG, Rayan GM. Complications after subfascial carpal tunnel release. South. Med. J. 1994;87:416–18.

Nagle DJ, Fischer TJ, Harris GD, Hastings H 2nd, Osterman AL, Palmer AK, Viegas SF, Whipple TL, Foley M. A multicenter prospective review of 640 endoscopic carpal tunnel releases using the transbursal and extrabursal chow techniques. Arthroscopy 1996;12:139–43.

Nagle D, Harris G, Foley M. Prospective review of 278 endoscopic carpal tunnel releases using the modified chow technique. Arthroscopy 1994;10:259–65.

Nahabedian MY, Wittstadt R, Wilgis EF. Median nerve injury following YAG laser carpal tunnel release. J. Hand Surg. 1995;20A:361–62.

Nakamichi K, Tachibana S. Ultrasonographically assisted carpal tunnel release. J. Hand Surg. 1997;22A:853–62.

Nakamichi K, Tachibana S. Median nerve compression by a radially inserted palmaris longus tendon after release of the antebrachial fascia: a complication of carpal tunnel release. J. Hand Surg. 2000;25A:955–58.

Nakao E, Short WH, Werner FW, Fortino MD, Palmer AK. Changes in carpal tunnel pressures following endoscopic carpal tunnel release: a cadaveric study. J. Hand Surg. 1998; 23A:43–47.

Nalebuff EA. Rheumatoid hand surgery—update. J. Hand Surg. 1983;8:678–82.

Nancollas MP, Peimer CA, Wheeler DR, Sherwin FS. Long-term results of carpal tunnel release. J. Hand Surg. 1995; 20B:470–74.

Nath RK, Mackinnon SE, Weeks PM. Ulnar nerve transection as a complication of two-portal endoscopic carpal tunnel release: a case report. J. Hand Surg. 1993;18A:896–98.

Nathan PA, Meadows KD, Keniston RC. Rehabilitation of carpal tunnel surgery patients using a short surgical incision and an early program of physical therapy. J. Hand Surg. 1993;18A:1044–50.

Netscher D, Mosharrafa A, Lee M, Polsen C, Choi H, Steadman AK, Thornby J. Transverse carpal ligament: its effect on flexor tendon excursion, morphologic changes of the carpal canal, and on pinch and grip strengths after open carpal tunnel release. Plast. Reconstr. Surg. 1997;100:636–42.

Netscher D, Steadman AK, Thornby J, Cohen V. Temporal changes in grip and pinch strength after open carpal tunnel release and the effect of ligament reconstruction. J. Hand Surg. 1998;23A:48–54.

Nissenbaum M, Kleinert HE. Treatment considerations in carpal tunnel syndrome with coexistent Dupuytren's disease. J. Hand Surg. 1980;5:544–47.

Nitz AJ, Dobner JJ. Upper extremity tourniquet effects in carpal tunnel release. J. Hand Surg. 1989;14A:499–504.

Nolan WB 3rd, Alkaitis D, Glickel SZ, Snow S. Results of treatment of severe carpal tunnel syndrome. J. Hand Surg. 1992;17A:1020–23.

Nygaard OP, Trumpy JH, Mellgren SI. Recovery of sensory function after surgical decompression in carpal tunnel syndrome. Acta Neurol. Scand. 1996;94:253–57.

Okutsu I, Hamanaka I, Ninomiya S, Takatori Y, Shimizu K, Ugawa Y. Results of endoscopic management of carpal-tunnel syndrome in long-term haemodialysis versus idiopathic patients. Nephrol. Dial. Transplant. 1993;8:1110–14.

Okutsu I, Hamanaka I, Tanabe T, Takatori Y, Ninomiya S. Complete endoscopic carpal canal decompression. Am. J. Orthop. 1996a;25:365–68.

Okutsu I, Hamanaka I, Tanabe T, Takatori Y, Ninomiya S. Complete endoscopic carpal tunnel release in long-term haemodialysis patients. J. Hand Surg. 1996b;21B:668–71.

Okutsu I, Ninomiya S, Hamanaka I, Kuroshima N, Inanami H. Measurement of pressure in the carpal canal before and after endoscopic management of carpal tunnel syndrome. J. Bone Joint Surg. 1989;71:679–83.

Okutsu I, Ninomiya S, Natsuyama M, Takatori Y, Inanami H, Kuroshima N, Hiraki S. Subcutaneous operation and examination under universal endoscope. Nippon Seikeigeka Gakkai Zasshi 1987;61:491–98.

Olney JR, Quenzer DE, Makowsky M. Contested claims in carpal tunnel surgery: outcome study of worker's compensation factors. Iowa Orthop. J. 1999;19:111–21.

Omer GE. Tendon transfers for combined traumatic nerve palsies of the forearm and hand. J. Hand Surg. 1992;17B:603–10.

On AY, Ozdemir O, Aksit R. Tourniquet paralysis after primary nerve repair. Am. J. Phys. Med. Rehabil. 2000;79:298–300.

Pagnanelli DM, Barrer SJ. Bilateral carpal tunnel release at one operation: report of 228 patients. Neurosurgery 1992;31:1030–34.

Paine KW, Polyzoidis KS. Carpal tunnel syndrome. Decompression using the Paine retinaculotome. J. Neurosurg. 1983;59:1031–36.

Palazzi S, Palazzi JL. Neurolsis in compressive neuropathies. Int. Surg. 1980;65:509–14.

Palmer AK, Toivonen DA. Complications of endoscopic and open carpal tunnel release. J. Hand Surg. 1999;24A:561–65.

Palmer DH, Paulson JC, Lane-Larsen CL, Peulen VK, Olson JD. Endoscopic carpal tunnel release: a comparison of two techniques with open release. Arthroscopy 1993; 9:498–508.

Papageorgiou CD, Georgoulis AD, Makris CA, Moebius UG, Varitimidis SE, Soucacos PN. Difficulties and early results of the endoscopic carpal tunnel release using the modified

Chow technique. Knee Surg. Sports Traumatol. Arthrosc. 1998;6:189–93.

Payne JC, Bergman RS, Ettinger DJ. Endoscopic carpal tunnel release. J. Am. Osteopath. Assoc. 1994;94:295–98.

Pearl RM. Use of the laser in treatment of carpal tunnel syndrome. Plast. Reconstr. Surg. 1989;83:577.

Pennino R, Tavin E. Endoscopic-assisted carpal tunnel release: a coupling of endoscopic and open techniques. Ann. Plast. Surg. 1996;36:458–61.

Phalen GS. The carpal-tunnel syndrome. Seventeen years' experience in diagnosis and treatment of six hundred fifty-four hands. J. Bone Joint Surg. 1966;48A:211–28.

Phalen GS, Gardner WJ, La Londe AA. Neuropathy of the median nerve due to compression beneath the transverse carpal ligament. J. Bone Joint Surg. 1950;32A:109–12.

Piaget-Morerod F, Chamay A. Etude d'une série de trente syndromes du tunnel carpien avec atrophie du thénar externe. Helv. Chir. Acta 1991;58:401–5.

Pierce RO. A different surgical approach for carpal tunnel syndrome. J. Natl. Med. Assoc. 1976;68:252.

Pierre-Jerome C, Bekkelund SI, Mellgren SI, Nordstrom R. Bilateral fast magnetic resonance imaging of the operated carpal tunnel. Scand. J. Plast. Reconstr. Surg. Hand Surg. 1997;31:171–77.

Plancher KD, Idler RS, Lourie GM, Strickland JW. Recalcitrant carpal tunnel. The hypothenar fat pad flap. Hand Clin. 1996;12:337–49.

Povlsen B, Tegnell I. Incidence and natural history of touch allodynia after open carpal tunnel release. Scand. J. Plast. Reconstr. Surg. Hand Surg. 1996;30:221–25.

Povlsen B, Tegnell L, Revell M, Adolfsson L. Touch allodynia following endoscopic (single portal) or open decompression for carpal tunnel syndrome. J. Hand Surg. 1997;22B:325–27.

Provinciali L, Giattini A, Splendiani G, Logullo F. The usefulness of hand rehabilitation after carpal tunnel surgery. Muscle Nerve 2000;23:211–16.

Rabb CH, Kernan JC. 3M Agee carpal tunnel release system. Neurosurgery 1997;40:639–41.

Regnard PJ, Soichot P, Ringuier JP. Local complications after axillary block anesthesia. Ann. Chir. Main 1990;9:59–64.

Reicher MA, Kellerhouse LE. Carpal tunnel disease, flexor and extensor tendon disorders. In: Reicher MA, Kellerhouse LE, eds. MRI of the Wrist and Hand. New York: Raven Press, 1990;49–68.

Reisman NR, Dellon AL. The abductor digiti minimi muscle flap: a salvage technique for palmar wrist pain. Plast. Reconstr. Surg. 1983;72:859–65.

Resnick CT, Miller BW. Endoscopic carpal tunnel release using the subligamentous two-portal technique. Contemp. Orthop. 1991;22:269–77.

Rhoades CE, Mowery CA, Gelberman RH. Results of internal neurolysis of the median nerve for severe carpal-tunnel syndrome. J. Bone Joint Surg. 1985;67A:253–56.

Richards RS, Bennett JD. Abnormalities of the hook of the hamate in patients with carpal tunnel syndrome. Ann. Plast. Surg. 1997;39:44–46.

Richman JA, Gelberman RH, Rydevik BL, Hajek PC, Braun RM, Gylys-Morin VM, Berthoty D. Carpal tunnel syndrome: morphologic changes after release of the transverse carpal ligament. J. Hand Surg. 1989;14A:852–57.

Rieger H, Grunert J, Brug E. A severe infection following endoscopic carpal tunnel release. J. Hand Surg. 1996;21B:672–74.

Rigoni G, Madonia F. Piso-triquetral syndrome following incision of the retinaculum flexorum. Helv. Chir. Acta 1992; 58:413–17.

Rose EH. The use of the palmaris brevis flap in recurrent carpal tunnel syndrome. Hand Clin. 1996;12:389–95.

Rose EH, Norris MS, Kowalski TA, Lucas A, Flegler EJ. Palmaris brevis turnover flap as an adjunct to internal neurolysis of the chronically scarred median nerve in recurrent carpal tunnel syndrome. J. Hand Surg. 1991;16A:191–201.

Rosén B, Lundborg G, Abrahamsson SO, Hagberg L, Rosén I. Sensory function after median nerve decompression in carpal tunnel syndrome. Preoperative vs postoperative findings. J. Hand Surg. 1997;22B:602–6.

Roth JH, Richards RS, MacLeod MD. Endoscopic carpal tunnel release. Can. J. Surg. 1994;37:189–93.

Rotman MB, Manske PR. Anatomic relationships of an endoscopic carpal tunnel device to surrounding structures. J. Hand Surg. 1993;18A:442–50.

Rowland EB, Kleinert JM. Endoscopic carpal-tunnel release in cadavers. An investigation of the results of twelve surgeons with this training model. J. Bone Joint Surg. 1994;76A:266–68.

Ruch DS, Marr A, Holden M, James P, Challa V, Smith BP. Innervation density of the base of the palm. J. Hand Surg. 1999;24A:392–97.

Ruch DS, Poehling GG. Endoscopic carpal tunnel release. The Agee technique. Hand Clin. 1996;12:299–303.

Sailer SM. The role of splinting and rehabilitation in the treatment of carpal and cubital tunnel syndromes. Hand Clin. 1996;12:223–41.

Santoro TD, Matloub HS, Gosain AK. Ulnar nerve compression by an anomalous muscle following carpal tunnel release: a case report. J. Hand Surg. 2000;25A:740–44.

Schafer W, Sander KE, Walter A, Weitbrecht WU. Endoskopische Operation des Karpaltunnelsyndroms nach Agee im Vergleich mit der offenen Operationstechnik. Handchir. Mikrochir. Plast. Chir. 1996;28:143–46.

Schlenker JD, Koulis CP, Kho LK. Synovialectomy and reconstruction of the retinaculum flexorum in median nerve decompression: technique and early results. Handchir. Mikrochir. Plast. Chir. 1993;25:66–71.

Schwartz JT, Waters PM, Simmons BP. Endoscopic carpal tunnel release: a cadaveric study. Arthroscopy 1993;9:209–13.

Scoggin JF, Whipple TL. A potential complication of endoscopic carpal tunnel release. Arthroscopy 1992;8:363–65.

Semple JC, Cargill AO. Carpal-tunnel syndrome. Results of surgical decompression. Lancet 1969;1:918–19.

Sennwald GR, Benedetti R. The value of one-portal endoscopic carpal tunnel release: a prospective randomized study. Knee Surg. Sports Traumatol. Arthrosc. 1995; 3:113–16.

Sennwald G, Hagen K. Decompression of the carpal tunnel. Apropos of 16 reoperated cases. Schweiz. Med. Wochenschr. 1990;120:931–35.

Seradge H, Seradge E. Piso-triquetral pain syndrome after carpal tunnel release. J. Hand Surg. 1989;14A:858–62.

Serra JM, Benito JR, Monner J. Carpal tunnel release with short incision. Plast. Reconstr. Surg. 1997;99:129–35.

Shapiro S. Microsurgical carpal tunnel release. Neurosurgery 1995;37:66–70.

Shapiro S. Microsurgical carpal tunnel release. Neurosurgery Focus 1997;3:1–8.

Shin AY, Perlman M, Shin PA, Garay AA. Disability outcomes in a worker's compensation population: surgical versus non-surgical treatment of carpal tunnel syndrome. Am. J. Orthop. 2000;29:179–84.

Shinya K, Lanzetta M, Conolly WB. Risk and complications in endoscopic carpal tunnel release. J. Hand Surg. 1995; 20B:222–27.

Silbermann-Hoffman O, Touam C, Miroux F, Moysan P, Oberlin C, Benacerraf R. Contribution of magnetic resonance imaging for the diagnosis of median nerve lesion after endoscopic carpal tunnel release. Chir. Main 1998; 17: 291–99.

Singh I, Khoo KM, Krishnamoorthy S. The carpal tunnel syndrome: clinical evaluation and results of surgical decompression. Ann. Acad. Med. Singapore 1994;23:94–97.

Skirven T, Trope J. Complications of immobilization. Hand Clin. 1994;10:53–61.

Skoff HD, Sklar R. Endoscopic median nerve decompression: early experience. Plast. Reconstr. Surg. 1994;94:691–94.

Skorpik G, Landsiedl F. Das Karpaltunnelsyndrom. Ein Vergleich der endoskopischen und offenen operativen Behandlung. Handchir. Mikrochir. Plast. Chir. 1996;28:133–37.

Slattery PG. Endoscopic carpal tunnel release. Use of the modified Chow technique in 215 cases. Med. J. Aust. 1994a; 160:104–7.

Slattery PG. Median nerve injury and the transverse wrist crease incision in open carpal tunnel release. Aust. N. Z. J. Surg. 1994b;64:768–70.

Smith WK, Giddins GE. Lymphoedema and hand surgery. J. Hand Surg. 1999;24B:138.

Sood MK, Elliot D. Treatment of painful neuromas of the hand and wrist by relocation into the pronator quadratus muscle. J. Hand Surg. 1998;23B:214–19.

Spokevicius S, Kleinert HE. The abductor digiti minimi flap: its use in revision carpal tunnel surgery. Hand Clin. 1996; 12:351–55.

Stark B, Engkvist-Lofmark C. Endoskopische Operation oder konventionelle offene Operationstechnik bei Karpaltunnelsyndrom: Eine prospektive, vergleichende Studie. Handchir. Mikrochir. Plast. Chir. 1996;28:128–32.

Stark RH. Neurologic injury from axillary block anesthesia. J. Hand Surg. 1996;21A:391–96.

Stark WA. Carpal tunnel syndrome, failure of surgery. J. Indiana State Med. Assoc. 1968;61:1547–50.

Straub LR, Ranawat CS. The wrist in rheumatoid arthritis. Surgical treatment and results. J. Bone Joint Surg. 1969;51:1–20.

Straub TA. Endoscopic carpal tunnel release: a prospective analysis of factors associated with unsatisfactory results. Arthroscopy 1999;15:269–74.

Strickland JW, Idler RS, Lourie GM, Plancher KD. The hypothenar fat pad flap for management of recalcitrant carpal tunnel syndrome. J. Hand Surg. 1996;21A:840–48.

Sturzenegger M. Carpal tunnel treated with endoscopic decompression. Rev. Med. Suisse Romande 1998;118: 451–55.

Taleisnik J. The palmar cutaneous branch of the median nerve and the approach to the carpal tunnel. An anatomical study. J. Bone Joint Surg. 1973;55:1212–17.

Terrono AL, Belsky MR, Feldon PG, Nalebuff EA. Injury to the deep motor branch of the ulnar nerve during carpal tunnel release. J. Hand Surg. 1993;18A:1038–40.

Terrono AL, Rose JH, Mulroy J, Millender LH. Camitz palmaris longus abductorplasty for severe thenar atrophy secondary to carpal tunnel syndrome. J. Hand Surg. 1993; 18A:204–6.

Tham SK, Ireland DC, Riccio M, Morrison WA. Reverse radial artery fascial flap: a treatment for the chronically scarred median nerve in recurrent carpal tunnel syndrome. J. Hand Surg. 1996;21A:849–54.

Tomaino MM, Plakseychuk A. Identification and preservation of palmar cutaneous nerves during open carpal tunnel release. J. Hand Surg. 1998;23B:607–8.

Tomaino MM, Ulizio D, Vogt MT. Carpal tunnel release under intravenous regional or local infiltration anaesthesia. J. Hand Surg. 2001;26B:67–68.

Tountas CP, MacDonald CJ, Meyerhoff JD, Bihrle DM. Carpal tunnel syndrome. A review of 507 patients. Minn. Med. 1983;66:479–82.

Tsai TM, Tsuruta T, Syed SA, Kimura H. A new technique for endoscopic carpal tunnel decompression. J. Hand Surg. 1995;20B:465–69.

Tsuruta T, Syed SA, Tsai T. Comparison of proximal and distal one portal entry techniques for endoscopic carpal tunnel release. A cadaver study. J. Hand Surg. 1994;19B:618–21.

Tubiana R, Brockman R. General Considerations in Carpal Tunnel Syndrome. In: Tubiana R, ed. The Hand. Philadelphia: Saunders, 1993;441–49.

Tzarnas CD. Carpal tunnel release without a tourniquet. J. Hand Surg. 1993;18A:1041–43.

Vaile JH, Mathers DM, Ramos-Remus C, Russell AS. Generic health instruments do not comprehensively capture patient perceived improvement in patients with carpal tunnel syndrome. J. Rheumatol. 1999;26:1163–66.

Van Heest A, Waters P, Simmons B, Schwartz JT. A cadaveric study of the single-portal endoscopic carpal tunnel release. J. Hand Surg. 1995;20A:363–66.

Varitimidis SE, Riano F, Vardakas DG, Sotereanos DG. Recurrent compressive neuropathy of the median nerve at the wrist: treatment with autogenous saphenous vein wrapping. J. Hand Surg. 2000;25B:271–75.

Vasen AP, Kuntz KM, Simmons BP, Katz JN. Open versus endoscopic carpal tunnel release: a decision analysis. J. Hand Surg. 1999;24A:1109–17.

Viegas SF, Pollard A, Kaminksi K. Carpal arch alteration and related clinical status after endoscopic carpal tunnel release. J. Hand Surg. 1992;17A:1012–16.

Wadstroem J, Nigst H. Reoperation for carpal tunnel syndrome. A retrospective analysis of forty cases. Ann. Chir. Main. 1986;5:54–58.

Waegeneers S, Haentjens P, Wylock P. Operative treatment of carpal tunnel syndrome. Acta Orthop. Belg. 1993;59:367–70.

Watchmaker GP, Weber D, Mackinnon SE. Avoidance of transection of the palmar cutaneous branch of the median nerve in carpal tunnel release. J. Hand Surg. 1996;21A: 644–50.

Weber RA, Sanders WE. Flexor carpi radialis approach for carpal tunnel release [published erratum appears in J. Hand Surg. 1997;22:950–51]. J. Hand Surg. 1997;22A:120–26.

Wheatley MJ. A simple technique for identification of the distal extent of the transverse carpal ligament during single-portal endoscopic carpal tunnel release. J. Hand Surg. 1996; 21A:1109–10.

Wilbourn AJ. Diabetic Entrapment and Compression Neuropathies. In: Dyck PJ, Thomas PK, eds. Diabetic Neuropathy (2nd ed). Philadelphia: Saunders, 1999;480–508.

Wilgis EF. Local muscle flaps in the hand. Anatomy as related to reconstructive surgery. Bull. Hosp. Joint Dis. 1984; 44:552–57.

Wilson KM. Distal forearm regional block anesthesia for carpal tunnel release. J. Hand Surg. 1993;18A:438–40.

Wilson KM. Double incision open technique for carpal tunnel release: an alternative to endoscopic release. J. Hand Surg. 1994;19A:907–12.

Wintman BI, Winters SC, Gelberman RH, Katz JN. Carpal tunnel release. Correlations with preoperative symptomatology. Clin. Orthop. 1996;326:135–45.

Worseg AP, Kuzbari R, Korak K, Hocker K, Wiederer C, Tschabitscher M, Holle J. Endoscopic carpal tunnel release using a single-portal system. Br. J. Plast. Surg. 1996;49:1–10.

Wulle C. Synovial flap repair in treating recurrent carpal tunnel syndrome. Handchir. Mikrochir. Plast. Chir. 1993;25:236–40.

Wulle C. The synovial flap as treatment of the recurrent carpal tunnel syndrome. Hand Clin. 1996;12:379–88.

Yates SK, Hurst LN, Brown WF. Physiological observations in the median nerve during carpal tunnel surgery. Ann. Neurol. 1981;10:227–29.

Young VL, Logan SE, Fernando B, Grasse P, Seaton M, Young AE. Grip strength before and after carpal tunnel decompression. South. Med. J. 1992;85:896–900.

Yu GZ, Firrell JC, Tsai TM. Pre-operative factors and treatment outcome following carpal tunnel release. J. Hand Surg. 1992;17B:646–50.

Zachary RB. Thenar palsy due to compression of the median nerve. Surg. Gynecol. Obstet. 1945;81:213–17.

Zimmerli W. Double incision for operation of carpal tunnel syndrome—14 years experience. Helv. Chir. Acta 1992;58: 395–400.

Chapter 16

Median Nerve "Causalgia," "Reflex Sympathetic Dystrophy," and "Complex Regional Pain Syndrome"

Clinicians assessing the hand and its innervation are routinely confronted by cases of chronic hand pain, commonly associated with positive or negative motor, sensory, or autonomic manifestations, that strongly suggest "neuropathic" dysfunction. In these patients, the clinical challenge is to determine

1. The presence or absence of detectable peripheral nerve dysfunction
2. The relationship of the positive and negative clinical phenomena to nerve dysfunction, when present
3. The role, if any, of the sympathetic system as a cause of pain
4. The possible origin of the syndrome in the psychoneurologic brain

This diagnostic exercise calls for special zeal because

1. Most nerve injuries do not lead to chronic pain.
2. Refined electrophysiologic methods can detect subtle subclinical local nerve dysfunction, which may be wrongly construed as the authentic basis for the clinical symptoms (Gilliatt, 1978).
3. Accumulating research data refute the role of the sympathetic system as a determinant of the sensory, motor, and pain phenomena.
4. In many patients with a picture of presumed nerve injury, the absence of nerve pathology and the presence of high cortical dysfunction can be convincingly demonstrated (pseudoneurologic dysfunction; Shorter, 1995).

Historical Concepts and Terminology

Causalgia

The term *causalgia* (from the Greek *kausos*, "burning" and *algos*, "pain") is currently obsolete. It was used by Weir Mitchell (1872) in his descriptions of painful limbs that he investigated in Civil War veterans. He described a number of cases of causalgia after median nerve injury.

After Weir Mitchell, the term was also used by Leriche (1916), Doupe et al. (1944), Livingston (1947), Nathan (1947), Loh and Nathan (1978), and then many others to describe patients with chronic pains and sensorimotor manifestations, usually associated with vasomotor changes. Some of the patients seemed responsive to sympathetic blocks or sympathectomy. Eventually, causalgia was defined in different ways by different authors [International Association for the Study of Pain (IASP) 1986; Abram, Blumberg, Boas, Haddox, Jänig, Kruescher, Racz, Raj, Roberts, Stanton-Hicks, et al., 1990; Bonica, 1990; Ochoa & Verdugo, 1992]. Common features of several definitions of causalgia included chronic pains and hyperalgesias, often associated with sensory, motor, and autonomic signs, resulting from nerve trauma (or disease).

Reflex Sympathetic Dystrophy

Convictions on the supposed role of the sympathetic nervous system in some patients with chronic limb pain led to introduction of the diagnostic term *reflex sympathetic dystrophy* (RSD) (Bonica, 1990). Attempts to define RSD took varied approaches:

1. Emphasizing chronic pain in the absence of nerve injury. A multi-author attempt published by the IASP (1986; emphasis added) defined RSD as "continuous pain in a portion of an extremity after trauma which may include fracture but *does not involve a major nerve*, associated with *sympathetic hyperactivity*. . . . The pain is described as burning, continuous, exacerbated by movement, cutaneous stimulation, or stress." This definition did not mention a motor component (other than disuse atrophy) or significant sensory components (other than pain exacerbated by "cutaneous stimulation").

2. Including overt motor and sensory nerve dysfunction among the diagnostic criteria (Abram, Blumberg, Boas, Haddox, Jänig, Kruescher, Racz, Raj, Roberts & Stanton-Hicks, 1990; Jänig, Blumberg, Boas & Campbell, 1991). If motor and sensory neurologic dysfunction were necessary components of RSD, the definition of RSD was so similar to classic definitions of causalgia that the terminology became redundant (Ochoa & Verdugo, 1992).

3. Offering a compromise definition to include patients with and without nerve injury and to avoid the debate on the importance of the sympathetic nervous system in the pathogenesis of the clinical phenomena. The Consensus Statement on RSD Definition by Jänig et al. (1991; emphasis added) stated that "RSD is a descriptive term meaning a *complex disorder or a group of disorders* that may develop *as a consequence of trauma* affecting the limbs, *with or without an obvious nerve lesion* . . . it consists of *pain and related sensory abnormalities*, *abnormal blood flow* and sweating, *abnormalities in the motor system* and changes in structure of both superficial and deep tissues . . . it is agreed that the name reflex sympathetic dystrophy is used in a descriptive sense and *does not imply specific underlying mechanisms*." This definition logically abandoned the therapeutic connotations in RSD and specific pathophysiologic assumptions regarding the role of the sympathetic system in pain. However, by retaining the term *sympathetic*, it invited indiscriminate

assault to that system in seeking pain relief for any of a broad variety of conditions. In the early 1990s, we recommended abandoning the term RSD because the meanings and roles of *reflex*, *sympathetic*, and *dystrophy* in the clinical syndrome were all unestablished (Verdugo & Ochoa, 1992; Ochoa, 1995).

Sympathetically Maintained Pain and Placebo Effect

Roberts (1986) introduced the term *sympathetically maintained pain* (SMP) to describe patients with "a) a history of physical trauma on the painful areas; b) the presence of a continuous burning pain together with mechanical hyperalgesia-allodynia (painful sensation to touch); and c) relief from the pain during sympathetic block." In his original paper, Roberts summarized SMP as "pain relieved during sympathetic block." Subsequently, others have defined SMP as "that aspect of pain that is dependent on sympathetic efferent activity in the painful part" (Raja, Treede, Davis & Campbell, 1991, p. 691) or as "all pain syndromes that can be relieved by sympathetic blockade" (Treede, Raja, Davis, Meyer & Campbell, 1991).

The proposed pathophysiologic basis for SMP assumed that sympathetic efferent activity supplying a symptomatic limb naturally activates receptors of low-threshold (tactile) mechanoreceptors (Roberts, 1986; Roberts & Kramis, 1991). Such afferent input would impinge on previously sensitized *wide dynamic range* neurons in the spinal dorsal horn assumed to be capable of evoking pain. Spontaneous pain would be a consequence of natural, tonic sympathetic efferent activity that through low-threshold mechanoreceptors would excite the secondarily abnormal, pain-evoking, wide dynamic range neurons. Mechanical hyperalgesia-allodynia would be the consequence of natural activation by external stimuli of normally responsive low-threshold mechanoreceptor tactile units, again impinging on the same hypothetically sensitized central neurons.

The concept of SMP can be fairly criticized on two fronts: First, it heavily relies on the volunteered testimony of an individual concerning a subjective experience in response to a medical intervention that combines pharmacologic and placebo effects. These two effects are traditionally not separated by those who perform sympathetic blocks. This flaw is magnified by the inordinately high incidence of placebo responders among these patients (Verdugo & Ochoa, 1991). The incidence of placebo response in patients with chronic causalgiform syndromes is twice as high (Verdugo & Ochoa, 1991) as the placebo response in the general population (Evans, 1974). Sympathetic blocks are typically not controlled for placebo pain response (Ochoa, 1991a, 1991b, 1992; Verdugo & Ochoa, 1994; Verdugo, Campero & Ochoa, 1994). When controlled, efficacy of the active drug is found to be no better than placebo (Glynn & Jones, 1990; Glynn, 1992; Verdugo, Rosenblum & Ochoa, 1991; Verdugo & Ochoa, 1994; Verdugo et al., 1994; Ramamurthy, Hoffman & Guanethidine study group, 1995; Jadad, Carroll, Glynn & McQuay, 1995). These observations reemphasize the importance of psychological mechanisms in patients with causalgiform pain syndromes. They also call for re-evaluation of theories on the pathogenesis of the syndrome that assume that these pain patients are specifically responsive to sympathetic blockade. Thus, the strongest clinical support for the idea of SMP, the patients' subjective report of pain improvement after a ritualistic intervention that may remove pain by nonspecific mechanisms, has little current scientific weight. Clinical evidence against the existence of SMP is that sympathectomy and sympathetic blocks do not cure patients with causalgia, RSD, or SMP (Ochoa, 1991a, 1991b, 1992; Ochoa & Verdugo, 1992; Tanelian, 1996).

Second, there is no demonstrable activation of low-threshold mechanoreceptor units in symptomatic parts of patients when the sympathetic system has been effectively recruited by reflex maneuvers (Dotson, Ochoa, Cline, Roberts, Yarnitsky, Simone & Marchettini, 1990). Moreover, whereas one subtype of mechanical hyperalgesia in patients is undoubtedly mediated by large-caliber afferents, there are several alternative hypotheses to explain this observation, and in many patients, the hyperalgesia is definitely mediated by sensitized peripheral nociceptors, rather than by normal low-threshold tactile units (Ochoa, Roberts, Cline, Dotson, & Yarnitsky, 1989).

In summary, for causalgia as defined by the IASP (1986), that is, for the painful syndrome after organic nerve injury, multiple different pathophysiologic processes may be operant throughout the length of sick primary sensory units and also in second-order or higher-order neurons in the sensory pathway. Clearly, more than one mechanism can contribute to the complex painful syndrome in any one case. The idea of a critical role of the sympathetic system in maintaining the pains after nerve injury in humans is not supported by rigorous evidence.

Complex Regional Pain Syndrome

Today's taxonomy subclassifies chronic neuropathic pain patients into two major descriptive categories that imply different pathophysiologic backgrounds: those carrying sufficient primary nerve pathology (the old *causalgia*, today's CRPS II), and the atypical ones not carrying sufficient peripheral pathology, but instead, hypothetical secondary pathology in the spinal cord, caused by past, resolved, peripheral injury (CRPS I). These atypical patients display

1. Nondermatomal and nonmyotomal sensory and motor dysfunction
2. Paradoxical expansion and worsening of symptoms with time
3. Normal reflexes
4. Normality of neurophysiologic tests, both for peripheral and central motor and sensory conduction

The mere existence of the atypical neuropathic pain patients was a fundamental reason for extrapolation of the experimental concept of secondary central neuronal sensitization into the clinics. Indeed, the concept of secondary neuronal sensitization was originated by default when the clinical features of an atypical subgroup of "neuropathic" pain patients was found not to be explainable by the laws of neurology and neuropathology. There was nonanatomic expansion of sensory and motor symptoms, and touch now caused pain: "In the painful states associated with hyperesthesia and hyperpathia, the lesion in the periphery induced abnormal functioning in the central nervous system, presumably at spinal level. This statement is based on the fact that tactile stimulation causes pain and on the fact of spread of pain and hypersensitivity beyond the territory of the lesion" (Loh & Nathan, 1978).

Experimentally, cellular "wind up" and sensitization of dorsal horn neurons are unquestionable as transient events in animals with nerve injury or peripheral inflammation and continue to be invoked as key abnormalities: "Continual input to the dorsal horn as a result of spontaneous firing in C fibre sensory neurons causes sensitization of dorsal horn neurons, which increases their excitability such as they respond to normal (A-beta fibre) input in an exaggerated and extended way. Thus, stimuli that would normally be innocuous are now painful" (Woolf & Mannion, 1999).

"Neuropathic pains" in patients not subjected to stringent differential diagnosis were attributed to this hypothetical dorsal horn dysfunction while ignoring the observation that the experimental hyperexcitable central state is self-limited, whereas symptoms in patients are chronic (Gracely, Lynch & Bennett, 1992). There is no cellular neurophysiologic data in atypical chronic (CRPS I) patients to support the secondary central hypothesis. Moreover, animals and patients with sizable nerve injury do not develop the atypical clinical profiles that are blamed on hypothetical secondary central changes.

When Verdugo first showed in the early 1990s that SMP is a placebo artifact, these atypical patients could no longer be explained as reflecting SMP. When the SMP theory was discredited, it carried with it the concept of RSD. CRPS then came out of the ashes. The official definition from the IASP specifies that in CRPS I there is no nerve injury. Regarding the system affected, it states, "peripheral nervous system, possibly central nervous system." About the usual cause, the IASP states, "variable." About pathology, it states, "unknown." Criteria number four is intriguing: "This diagnosis is excluded by the existence of conditions that would otherwise account for the degree of pain and dysfunction" (Merskey & Bogduk, 1994). Thus, CRPS I holds as a tentative diagnostic term only as long as the physician is perplexed. Others have regarded the current criteria for CRPS as having inadequate specificity and, therefore, likely to lead to overdiagnosis (Bruehl, Harden, Galer, Saltz, Bertram, Backonja, Gayles, Rudin, Bhugra & Stanton-Hicks, 1999).

We emphasize that causalgia, RSD, SMP, and CRPS are purely descriptive terms. To the extent that they are given different meanings by different authors and practitioners, they cause confusion. Moreover, they perpetuate the illusion of understanding causes, mechanisms, and cures for these chronic painful syndromes (Ochoa, 1990, 1991a, 1991b, 1992, 1995, 1999; Ochoa & Verdugo, 1992). These terms should be updated. At this point, keeping in mind the urgent need to formulate solid concepts to effectively assess and treat patients with causalgia-RSD-SMP-CRPS, one of Dr. Samuel Johnson's (1773) lighthearted quotes may be applicable to our currently biased notions: "A cucumber should be well sliced, and dressed with pepper and vinegar, and then thrown out, as good for nothing."

Sensory Pathophysiology in Neuropathy

Most patients with nerve injury develop sensory dysfunction. A minority of patients develops chronic spontaneous pains after nerve injury. For some, gentle stimulation of the symptomatic area also induces pain with abnormal ease (hyperalgesia; allodynia). In both the peripheral and the central nervous systems, a number of hypothetical or proven pathophysiologic phenomena may be responsible for these positive, spontaneous or stimulus-induced, sensory symptoms:

1. *Sensitization of nerve endings* of high-threshold sensory units that normally respond specifically to potentially damaging stimuli (nociceptors) can lead to pain, spontaneously or in response to normally nonpainful stimulus energy. This mechanism was envisioned more than half a century ago by Sir Thomas Lewis to explain certain clinical observations. He proposed that the vasomotor phenomena and "tenderness of the skin in causalgia are all due to the release of substances peripherally; the release is supposed to bring the corresponding skin into a condition similar to what has been called erythralgic skin" (Lewis, 1942).

He further hypothesized that the mechanism of the pain is release into the skin of a substance that lowers the threshold of the pain nerve endings to various forms of stimulation (Lewis, 1936). Others subsequently supported Lewis's hypothesis on the grounds of experience with

Figure l6-1. (A) Within the hatched area of hyperalgesia, the receptive field of an identified C nociceptor is marked (*cross*). **(B)** Intradermal electrical stimulation in the receptive field evoked a slowly conducted unitary response recorded with a microelectrode in the superficial radial nerve (conduction velocity of 1.25 m/sec). **(C)** Intraneural recording of C-unit response to nine consecutive gentle mechanical stimuli applied to the receptive field. Such low-threshold response of a human polymodal nociceptor to innocuous energy implies sensitization. (Reproduced with permission from M Cline, JL Ochoa, HE Torebjörk. Chronic hyperalgesia and skin warming caused by sensitized C-nociceptors. Brain 1989;112: 621–47.)

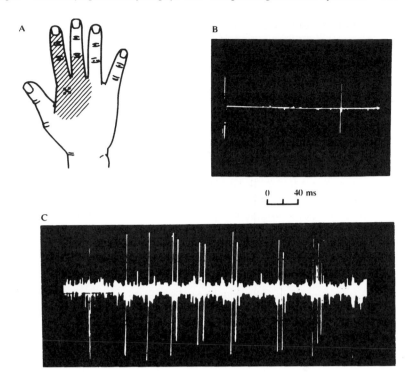

their own patients (Jung, 1941). Note that the term *causalgia* was being applied loosely by Lewis to signify the presence of a burning pain associated with vasodilatation; associated hyperalgesia improved if the temperature of the skin was lowered. Lewis (1936) stated that the condition does not reflect abnormality of the vasomotor system. Rather, the neurosecretory process that lowered the threshold of the pain nerve endings and changed the vasomotor tone would be an affair of sensory nerves, which he termed *nocifensor*. Basic research on antidromic vasodilation and neurogenic inflammation now supports many of Lewis's ideas (Chahl, Szolcsanyi & Lembeck, 1984; Serra, Campero & Ochoa, 1998). Furthermore, rigorous research methods have demonstrated that in a subset of "causalgic" patients, sensitization of nociceptors and antidromic nociceptor-dependent vasodilatation are the basis for the painful and vasomotor phenomena (Figure 16-1) (Ochoa, 1986a, 1986b; Cline, Ochoa & Torebjörk, 1989).

However, this specific pathophysiologic basis for causalgia applies only to a subset of chronic pain patients who have the variant termed *erythralgia* (Lewis, 1936) or *ABC syndrome* (Ochoa,

1986a). Although animal or human models of erythralgia or ABC syndrome are readily reproduced in the laboratory by application to tissues of substances that "irritate" nociceptor nerve fibers (Culp, Ochoa, Cline & Dotson, 1989), and repetitive experimental excitation of nociceptor peripheral nerve fibers in humans does cause antidromic vasodilation and pain (see Color Plates 10-1C and D), there is not yet a self-perpetuating animal model of erythralgia or ABC syndrome that can be generated by experimentally disturbing peripheral nerve trunks. Certain features of Bennett's model of painful nerve injury, however, suggest elements of ABC syndrome (Bennett & Ochoa, 1991).

2. *Ectopic impulse generation* from pathologic axons within locally injured nerve trunks definitely contributes to the generation of pain induced by mechanical challenge of the abnormal nerve (Tinel's sign, and so forth) and may even contribute to spontaneous pain in patients (Ochoa, Torebjörk, Culp & Schady, 1982; Nordin, Nystrom, Wallin & Hagbarth, 1984; Campero, Serra & Ochoa, 1998). Whether abnormal foci of increased axonal excitability within locally injured nerve trunks contribute spontane-

ous pains through electrical or chemical ephaptic cross excitation from sympathetic efferents was a favorite question in the past. After initial popularity (Doupe et al., 1944; Nathan, 1947; Devor & Jänig, 1981), this theory has received decreasing support (Ochoa & Verdugo, 1992), because the sympathetic pathophysiology is purely hypothetical, and the sympathetic blocks consistently relieve pain through placebo effect, whether or not the pain is associated with nerve injury. Experience with placebo-controlled sympathetic block reveals that suppression of sympathetic function does not relieve pain in patients with chronic pain associated with bona fide nerve pathology (Verdugo et al., 1994; Ramamuthy & Hoffman, 1994; Jadad, Carroll, Glynn & McQuay, 1995).

3. There has been rigorous experimental research since the mid 1980s on *secondary central nervous system derangements following nerve injury.* Morphologic, histochemical, neurophysiologic, cellular, and molecular biological studies have shown that a host of changes can occur in the dorsal horns and more rostrally that might contribute to the pathogenesis of some components of the painful syndrome (Devor & Wall, 1981; Simone, Baumann, Collins & LaMotte, 1989; and many others now). However, although such secondary changes are found consistently after experimental nerve injury, patients and animals with nerve injury infrequently develop chronic painful syndromes (Ochoa, 1999).

4. *Pseudoneuropathy* often masquerades as painful neuropathy. This condition, which is usually underdiagnosed, causes much confusion among treating physicians and almost invariably leads to iatrogenesis and litigation. Pseudoneuropathy is treated separately (see Pseudoneuropathy, later in this chapter).

Role of the Sympathetic Nervous System

Many patients with chronic painful limb syndromes have changes in limb temperature, skin color, texture, and, to a lesser extent, sweat pattern of the symptomatic area. These vasomotor and sudomotor abnormalities have traditionally focused attention on the sympathetic nervous system in patients with "causalgia" and continue to

invite dedicated clinical investigation (Wasner, Schattschneider, Heckmann, Maier & Baron, 2001).

The autonomic phenomena, particularly the vasomotor deviations, may indeed be a consequence of changes in sympathetic nervous system activity. However,

1. The sympathetic activity may be a physiologic reflex response to pain rather than a primary pathologic state.
2. Excessive activity of sympathetic effector organs may be the consequence of sympathetic denervation supersensitivity rather than of hyperactivity of sympathetic nerves.
3. The vasomotor phenomena may be entirely unrelated to the sympathetic system; they may reflect antidromic vasodilatation mediated by sensory nociceptive fibers (see Color Plates 10-1 C and D).
4. The vasomotor phenomena may be entirely due to disuse.
5. Regardless of the physiology of the vasomotor phenomena, the assumption that sympathetic actions determine the pain is not rigorously founded (Ochoa, 1986a, 1990, 1991a, 1991b; Ochoa & Verdugo, 1992; Ochoa, 1999).

In sum, vasomotor changes are not always of sympathetic origin, and sympathetic function need not be the cause of pain.

Observations of vasomotor and sudomotor abnormalities in chronic pain patients led to trials of sympatholytic therapies. Reports that sympathetic blocks or sympathectomy transiently improved pain in some "causalgic" patients were followed by a century of treatment of patients by sympatholysis. Neither the pathophysiology of the transient responses to blocks nor the long-term value of this therapy was ever rigorously assessed (Ochoa, 1991a, 1992, 1991c, 1991d; Ochoa & Verdugo, 1991; Tanelian, 1996).

Another important source of mystification of the idea of sympathetic participation in chronic painful syndromes has been the progressive misunderstanding of the writings by classic authors. For example, Weir Mitchell (1872) actually wrote that "causalgia" was an affair of somatic nerves, foreign to the sympathetic system. Livingston (1947) explicitly stated, "In seeking for a clue as to what this unknown alternative might be, one might start by abandoning, for the time being, the assumption that the activities of the sympathetic nerves represent the essential factor in either the cause or the cure of the causalgic syndrome." Leriche's (1916) Corporal G., who had a severe neurovascular lesion at left retroclavicular level, did not have RSD or CRPS by current IASP criteria: What Leriche severed for therapy was his patient's humeral perivascular sympathetic innervation, and what he cured were probably ischemic ulcers, not neuropathic pain (Ochoa & Verdugo, 1992).

Animal Models

At times, the science behind the concepts of causalgia, RSD, SMP, and CRPS have been absurdly extrapolated. There are excellent animal models of nerve injury (Bennett & Xie, 1988; Seltzer, Dubner & Shir, 1990; and so forth). However, it is questionable that they provide legitimate models of human RSD, SMP, or CRPS. In humans, persistent chronic pain after nerve injury is not common, so the multiple primary peripheral and secondary central nervous system abnormalities consistently demonstrated after experimental nerve injury in animals must include idiosyncrasies inadequate to explain the uncommon and multifaceted human pain syndromes. The specific pathology and pathophysiology of the animal nerve injury models (Jänig, 1991) are unlikely to represent the universal pathology and pathophysiology of human RSD-CRPS and related syndromes. Observations on *normal* animal physiology have shown activation of tactile sensory receptors by sympathetic efferent discharge (Roberts, 1986). However, in humans the sympathetic system does not activate low-threshold mechanoreceptors (Dotson et al., 1990), so this animal model does not establish the validity of the concept of SMP for humans. Currently, there are no authentic animal models for these descriptive conditions with absence of nerve injury. Given the all-embracing consensus definition of RSD by Jänig et al. (1991), and of CRPS by the IASP (Merskey & Bogduck, 1994), it would be surprising if a unitary animal model could be found for that diffuse complex. Moreover, to the extent that psychological mechanisms are so

intrinsic to some of the human conditions it is hard to conceive an appropriate animal model for them.

Psychological Factors

The psyche always participates in the human experience of pain. Older methods of investigation of neurologic function frequently did not allow determination of the relative roles of nerve injury and psychological mechanisms in chronic posttraumatic syndromes that were associated with pains and motor and sensory phenomena. The French master neuropsychiatrists attributed the clinical presentation of a subset of such patients to hysteria (Charcot, 1877, 1889; Déjérine, 1901). In 1944, Doupe et al. reemphasized that chronic posttraumatic "causalgic" syndromes might be caused by either organic or psychogenic dysfunction. By present standards, an unmeasurable percentage of previously described "causalgic" patients must have had no nerve injury at all. However, debate on proportions of organic versus psychogenic causalgia remains current (Merskey, 1988; Weintraub, 1988; Ochoa, 1991b, 1997). The limbic system (emotional brain) becomes abnormally activated in atypical chronic pains (Derbyshire, Jones, Devani, Friston, Feinmann, Harris, Pearce, Watson & Frackowiak, 1994).

Pseudoneuropathy

There is urgent need to upgrade the differential diagnosis of painful neuropathy to incorporate the concept of painful pseudoneuropathy. Such diagnostic consideration is mandatory and yet, is commonly neglected. This omission predictably breeds iatrogenesis, both by omission and by commission (Ochoa, 2001).

Neglecting differentiation between painful neuropathy and painful pseudoneuropathy is the norm when these patients go under the exclusive care of pain management experts. The typical outcome is implementation of invasive or dangerous therapeutic interventions before pursuit of evidence-based diagnosis. Pain is a nonspecific symptom that may affect any system of the body. The mechanisms of pain from different systems are distinct and fall within the expertise of the specialists in those systems. An across-the-board pain specialist does not have expertise in a specific system. Pain specialists develop the skills to palliate the symptom pain but not to identify or treat the disorder that underlies it. Pain specialists commonly fail to understand patients who display pains associated with neurologic sensory, motor, or autonomic symptomatology. Pseudomononeuropathy is highly prevalent. In those cases, the sensory numbness or hyperalgesia, muscle weakness and spasms or dystonia, which appear to be neuropathic, in reality result from conversion somatization, or malingering (Weintraub, 1995).

Chronic pain from median pseudoneuropathy is not rare. Typically in those patients there is no physiologic dysfunction of peripheral sensory or motor pathways underlying the sensorimotor positive and negative psychophysical phenomena. Moreover, the central sensory and motor pathways serving areas of hypoesthesia or paresis are also normal. The clinical profile is characteristic enough. Diagnosis is not by default: It is not just based on absence of evidence of physiologic impairment. These patients commonly display psychophysical motor or sensory findings that, by their nature, can be traced to the interface between the emotional brain and the sensorimotor cortex (Derbyshire et al., 1994; Vuilleumier, Chicherio, Assal, Schwartz, Slosman & Landis, 2001). Explicit examples of pseudoneurologic dysfunction include, on the motor side, give-way weakness with electromyographic evidence of interruption of an otherwise intact upper motor neuron drive of abundant peripheral motor units. On the sensory side, a dramatic example is the disappearance of sensory loss with placebo, as is the disappearance of paresis with placebo (Verdugo & Ochoa, 1998). Neurologists readily understand that sensory or motor losses that disappear through a phenomenon mediated through the psyche cannot be based on structural pathology of the system. Of course, organically based *pain* may clearly disappear with placebo, but this is quite different from abolition of a sensory or motor deficit, which implies axonal loss, demyelinating block, or synaptic block.

A strong clue suggesting pseudoneuropathic identity for chronic pains associated with motor, sensory, or vasomotor phenomena is progressive worsening with time and expansion in the body space of the symptomatology after a discrete acute physical injury. Another strong argument for psychogenicity is the cure of the painful sensory and motor phenomenon through psychotherapy (Color Plate 16-2 illustrates one such case of psychogenic pseudoneuropathy).

Patient Evaluation

With or without nerve injury, patients can develop a chronic posttraumatic syndrome of pains and sensory, motor, and autonomic dysfunctions. The neurologic assessment should document the level of function of each category of nerve fiber systems. This must rely not just on conventional nerve conduction studies, which only detect normality versus deficit and only for large-caliber fibers. Documentation of the physiologic status of nerve fibers must include quantitative somatosensory thermotest (see Chapter 9) and quantitative autonomic testing (see Chapter 10) to evaluate small-caliber nerve fiber function and to differentiate normal from deficient or excessive function. Where available, microneurographic recording may prove the critical test (see Figure 16-1) (Cline et al., 1989; Serra, Campero, Ochoa & Bostock, 1999).

Differentiating between an organic basis and a psychologic basis for the patient's symptoms and signs starts with routine physical and neurologic history and examination. At times, further studies are needed to explicitly demonstrate that muscle weakness, spasms, sensory loss, hyperalgesia, and pains are of cerebral, rather than of neuromuscular, origin. Strategies for this involve refined subspecialty testing. Again, criteria do not just rely on absence of organic neuromuscular dysfunction or on presence of psychological dysfunction. Nor do they rely on a menu of traditional but controverted clinical phenomena (Gould, Miller, Goldberg & Benson, 1986). In "weak" muscles, electromyographic evidence of unimpaired volitional drive of upper motor neurons, with recruitment of full interference pattern interrupted by pauses of decruitment, in absence of pain, is strongly suggestive of psychogenic origin. So is the disappearance of neuromuscular motor or sensory *deficit* after diagnostic block (Verdugo & Ochoa, 1992, 1998; Ochoa, 1997) (Color Plate 16-2).

A traditional handicap in our ability to assess the real nature of many patients with the picture of CRPS, whether in the absence or presence of nerve injury, is that these patients are usually not evaluated by neurologists for what is essentially a neurologic picture of pain, motor phenomena, sensory phenomena, and apparent neurovascular phenomena involving the peripheral nervous system. Pain management experts and anesthesiologists usually care for these patients, bypassing the necessary and complex specialized neurologic evaluation. When patients who display "CRPS" but no specific nerve trauma are evaluated thoroughly to assess function in subpopulations of nerve fibers, they often have no *pertinent* peripheral nerve dysfunction; express subjective responses to medical interventions that are, in some two-thirds, voided by placebo effect (Verdugo & Ochoa, 1991, 1994; Verdugo et al., 1994); and display psychologically mediated numbness or hyperalgesia and psychologically mediated weakness or "dystonic" muscle spasms (Verdugo & Ochoa, 2000).

Three Clinical Cases of "Causalgia–Reflex Sympathetic Dystrophy–Complex Regional Pain Syndrome"

Case 1: Rapid Development of ABC Syndrome after Nerve Trauma

The young man in Figure 16-3 was seen in the summer of 1989. Symptoms started 5 months earlier, immediately after a gunshot wound to the right upper arm, with the bullet exiting in the medial upper arm. "I heard the shot coming from the car that fled. I felt burning and pins and needles in the hand and some of my fingers. When I rubbed the skin, I felt pain and tingling in the area which was numb and burning. My hand was weak. I thought the shot hit me in the hand, but there was nothing there; there was blood pouring down my elbow." In the emergency room, 2 hours after injury, "the right hand became swollen and hot; it was just those parts [of the skin] which were tingling and burning that became hot and red." The initial pain was severe enough for him to require narcotics. The hand remained "definitely tender to touch and, at the same time, numb." He described the sensory symptoms as confined to the median nerve territory

of palm and fingers, splitting the ring finger. A few days after the injury, he started noticing a Tinel's sign at the site of bullet exit.

A few weeks after the injury, he first noticed thinning of the muscles in the forearm. Early after injury, he had become aware of thermal dependence of his painful syndrome when he discovered that while in bed his pain would lessen if the arm was kept outside of the covers. Subsequently, he realized that in a sauna his pains would be much worse, but in a cold pool, they would significantly improve. The spontaneous burning pain was the most temperature-dependent symptom; the touch-induced tingling and pain seemed to be less influenced by cold immersion. Tinel's sign was not influenced by temperature.

From clinical, electrodiagnostic, and thermographic assessment, the referring doctor from Florida established the diagnosis of local nerve injury to median nerve, with axonal involvement and hypothesized development of an ABC syndrome. As shown in Figure 16-3B, with time the affected fingers, particularly the index, became tapered and moderately "dystrophic."

When seen in our clinic, months after the injury, the sign of Tinel remained close to the scar of bullet exit (see Figure 16-3A). The area of abnormal cutaneous sensation was strictly confined to textbook median nerve territory and included hypoesthesia to all submodalities and mechanical hyperalgesia of both dynamic and static subtypes (see Figure 16-3A, C, and D) (Ochoa et al., 1989). The symptomatic burning hand was hypothermic to touch and to thermography, particularly the skin of the most symptomatic index and middle fingers. Residual ability to vasodilate in response to reflex sympathetic maneuvers revealed a degree of autonomic control on the cold skin. Therefore, the switch from a "hot" to a "cold" symptomatic state meant interjection of vasoconstriction, either as a consequence of partial sympathetic denervation supersensitivity or engagement of exaggerated sympathetic vasoconstrictor neural outflow, or a combination of both.

Perhaps the most remarkable feature in this patient, who might have been one of Weir Mitchell's soldiers with "causalgia," and who by modern criteria have "RSD" (CRPS II) with clear dystrophic features in the symptomatic parts, is the development almost immediately after injury

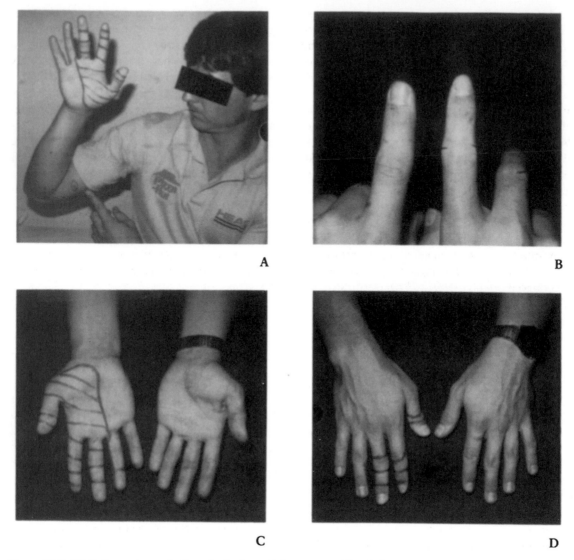

Figure 16-3. (A) Patient points to bullet exit site in medial upper arm. The circle enclosing the scar defines the point of Tinel's sign. **(B)** Dystrophic features of right index finger. **(C–D)** The hatched areas of skin on volar and dorsal aspects of hands and digits delineate well-defined sensory dysfunction combining hyperalgesia and hypoesthesia to all modalities. The area corresponds to usual median nerve territory.

of an erythralgic or ABC syndrome, characterized by vasodilatation, heat and mechanical hyperalgesia, and significant improvement by passive cooling. The locally irritated polymodal nociceptors-in-continuity probably discharged ectopically, orthodromically evoking spontaneous burning pain, while antidromically evoking vasodilatation and perhaps sensitization of peripheral receptors.

Another striking feature is the unsurprising similarity between this case and many features of Bennett's animal model of nerve injury (Bennett & Xie, 1988). Indeed, vasodilatation leading eventually to vasoconstriction, spontaneous pain behavior, mechanical hyperalgesia, thermal hyperalgesia, and even dystrophic features are shared by the experimental animal state. The mechanical hyperalgesia in the particular animal model of Bennett (and in the ABC syndrome) is probably explained on the grounds of nociceptor sensitization, since myelinated fibers are practically devastated and therefore A fiber-mediated hyperalgesia (allodynia) could not apply (Ochoa, 1990). In this patient, however, the mechanical hyperalgesia was dichotomized into two phenomenologic types, one (dynamic) mediated by myelinated fibers, the other (static) by unmyelinated (Ochoa & Yarnitsky, 1993). The striking dynamic mechanical hyperalgesia was rapidly abolished by A-fiber blocks. In retrospect, it was abolished too rapidly. The effect may well have been a placebo response. Because this dynamic mechanical hyperalgesia developed immediately after injury, we suspect that rather than reflecting instantaneous development of secondary dorsal horn pathophysiologic changes, the hyperalgesia simply reflects echo and amplification and reverberations at the site of injury as a result of ephapses (Rasminsky, 1982).

Unfortunately, the patient could not tolerate microneurography intended to explore (1) the basis for the Tinel's sign, (2) the kind of afferent activity recorded during elicitation of mechanical hyperalgesia, (3) whether any of such activity was reflected antidromically after elicitation, and (4) possible presence of ectopic discharge in C nociceptors.

Case 2: Painful Digital Nerve Injury with Distal Neuropathic Pain Mechanism

This worker suffered a deep cut by broken glass on the radial border of the right palm in May 1991 (Color Plate 16-4A). He immediately felt painful tingling in the index finger, associated with a combination of diminution of sensory acuity and painful hypersensitivity to gentle mechanical skin stimulation. Shortly after the injury, a plastic surgeon microscopically repaired a digital nerve in the palm. When seen 6 months after the injury, the patient still complained of constant local pain in the region of the scar, associated with a local Tinel's sign. Lightly touching the lateral aspect of the right index finger continued to induce a weird unpleasant sensation, and pressure in the same area induced a sharp pain, "like someone is sticking a needle." Color Plate 16-4A shows the patient puzzled by concurrence of painful exaggeration (red)

next to diminution (black) of sensitivity to touching the symptomatic skin. Cold temperature would increase the painful symptoms, and the hand always felt cold to the patient and was diffusely cold thermographically (Color Plate 16-4B).

A sham "block" of the right median nerve at wrist level revealed no placebo response. In contrast, lidocaine block caused multimodality sensory loss in "classic" median nerve territory, while abolishing Tinel's sign, hyperalgesia, and spontaneous pain (Color Plate 16-4C). The corresponding territory of skin warmed up considerably, as shown in the thermogram (Color Plate 16-4D). Note remarkable matching between anesthetic and vasodilated areas.

In this case, the positive and negative sensory phenomena, including multimodality hypoesthesia, mechanical hyperalgesia, Tinel's sign, and spontaneous pain, were all in complete harmony with the anatomically proven local nerve injury. The positive sensory phenomena were erased by anesthetic nerve block proximal to the injury but not by inert placebo block. The locally abnormal nerve physiology therefore must explain the whole of the sensory syndrome. Indeed, the spontaneous and the stimulus-induced pains must be sustained by activity coming from below the site of nerve block. The diffuse hypothermia affecting the whole of the symptomatic hand, rather than just the territory of the affected nerve, is consistent with recruitment of somatosympathetic vasoconstrictor reflex; the vasodilatation in response to blockade of sympathetic vasoconstrictor efferent outflow at wrist level indicates its abolition. This case is to be contrasted with the next.

Case 3: Histrionic Pain Syndrome after Carpal Tunnel Surgery

There are numerous reports in the surgical literature of RSD developing as a complication of carpal tunnel surgery, but none is reported with sufficient neurologic detail to give insight into the neuropathophysiology or possible psychopathology of the painful condition.

The patient shown in Color Plate 16-2 developed classical carpal tunnel syndrome on the left side. Clinical and electrodiagnostic testing were clearly abnormal. She underwent surgical decom-

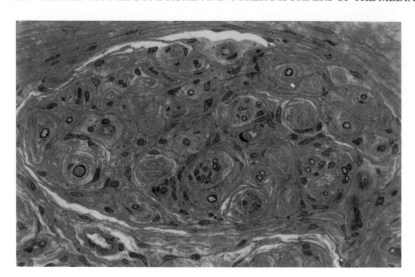

Figure 16-5. Light micrograph of cross section of median nerve fascicle obtained from patient shown in Color Plate 16-4 during carpal tunnel surgery on the affected left hand. Severe dropout of myelinated fibers is obvious.

pression of the median nerve at carpal tunnel in the spring of 1989. The surgeon was sufficiently impressed with the gigantic median nerve to biopsy a nerve fascicle. As shown in Figure 16-5, the nerve specimen was profoundly abnormal, with marked depopulation of myelinated fibers.

After surgery, she complained of a new, extremely severe pain (grade 10 on the 10-point scale) in the whole hand. There was also mechanical hyperalgesia, both of the static and dynamic subtypes. She reported that cooling might abolish the pain but not the mechanical hyperalgesia, and that the hand tended to become "red or pink." In addition, she claimed profound sensory loss all the way up to elbow level (see Color Plate 16-2A, hatched area). A hypothetical organic explanation for the new pain syndrome was that it might be caused by surgical trauma to an anomalous nerve that supplied the whole hand or, alternatively, that it might be a nerve injury that became complicated by secondary "centralization," as has been proposed for RSD-SMP.

Local anesthetic diagnostic block of the median nerve, supplemented by thermography, clarified the issue. As compared with a normal symmetric baseline thermogram (see Color Plate 16-2B), the post-lidocaine block thermogram (see Color Plate 16-2D) showed objective warming (paralytic vasodilatation) confined to the typical normal left median nerve territory. This correlated with deep, legitimate anesthesia in the same territory (see Color Plate 16-2C). But the

blocked nerve did not supply sympathetic fibers to the nonmedian areas of the hand that she had described as extremely painful and hyperalgesic. At the same time, the hypothesis of centralization was not supported, but rather dismissed, because the diagnostic block intriguingly abolished the long glove of deep anesthesia. In other words, this medical intervention took away the deficit. This miraculous recovery is not explicable in terms of organic dysfunction (Verdugo & Ochoa, 1992; 1998). Furthermore, the glove of anesthesia was of psychological nature: On multiple occasions, while blindfolded, the patient punctually announced with a "no" every stimulus to an anesthetic part.

In summary, this RSD case is complex. Of course, the patient did have histologically proven nerve pathology, but beyond doubt, she also had a psychogenic sensory syndrome. Without thorough investigation, the bizarre sensory profile might have erroneously been attributed to hypothetical secondary spinal cord changes.

References

Abram SE, Blumberg H, Boas RA, Haddox JD, Jänig W, Kruescher H, Racz GB, Raj PP, Roberts WJ, Stanton-Hicks M, et al. Proposed definition of reflex sympathetic dystrophy. In: Stanton-Hicks M, Wilfrid J, Boas RA, eds. Reflex Sympathetic Dystrophy. Boston: Kluwer, 1990;207–10.

Bennett GJ, Ochoa JL. Thermographic observations on rats with experimental neuropathic pain. Pain 1991;45:61–67.

Bennett GJ, Xie Y-K. A peripheral mononeuropathy in rat that produces disorders of pain sensation like those seen in man. Pain 1988;33:87–107.

Bonica JJ. The Management of Pain. Vol 1. Philadelphia: Lea & Febiger, 1990.

Bruehl S, Harden RN, Galer BS, Saltz S, Bertram M, Backonja M, Gayles R, Rudin N, Bhugra MK, Stanton-Hicks M. External validation of IASP diagnostic criteria for complex regional pain syndrome and proposed research diagnostic criteria. International Association for the Study of Pain. Pain 1999;81:147–54.

Chahl LA, Szolcsanyi J, Lembeck F, eds. Antidromic Vasodilatation and Neurogenic Inflammation. Budapest: Akademiai Kiado, 1984.

Campero M, Serra J, Ochoa J. Ectopic impulse generation and autoexcitation in single myelinated afferent fibers in patients with peripheral neuropathy and positive sensory symptoms. Muscle Nerve 1998;21:1661–67.

Charcot JM. (Clinical) lectures on the diseases of the nervous system. Vols. 1, 3. New Sydenham Society, London, Special Edition (1985), Critchley M, ed. The Classics of Neurology and Neurosurgery Library. Birmingham, AL: Gryphon Editions, 1877, 1889.

Cline M, Ochoa JL, Torebjörk HE. Chronic hyperalgesia and skin warming caused by sensitized C nociceptors. Brain 1989;112:621–47.

Culp WJ, Ochoa JL, Cline M, Dotson R. Heat and mechanical hyperalgesia induced by capsaicin: cross modality threshold modulation in human C-nociceptors. Brain 1989; 112: 1317–31.

Déjérine PJ. Sémiologíe du systeme nerveux. In: Traité de Pathologie Generale. Paris: Masson et Cie, 1901;559–1168.

Derbyshire SWG, Jones AKP, Devani P, Friston KJ, Feinmann C, Harris M, Pearce S, Watson JDG, Frackowiak RSJ. Cerebral responses to pain in patients with atypical facial pain measured by positron emission tomography. J. Neurol. Neurosurg. Psychiatry 1994;57:1166–72.

Devor M, Jänig W. Activation of myelinated afferents ending in a neuroma by stimulation of the sympathetic supply in the rat. Neurosci. Lett. 1981;24:43–47.

Devor M, Wall PD. Plasticity in the spinal cord sensory map following peripheral nerve injury in rats. J. Neurosci. 1981;148:679–84.

Dotson R, Ochoa JL, Cline M, Roberts W, Yarnitsky D, Simone D, Marchettini P. Sympathetic effects on human low threshold mechanoreceptors (abstr). Soc. Neurosci. 1990; 16:1280.

Doupe J, Cullen CH, Chance GQ. Post-traumatic pain and the causalgic syndrome. J. Neurol. Neurosurg. Psychiatry 1944;7:33–48.

Evans FJ. The placebo response in pain reduction. Adv. Neurol. 1974;4:289–96.

Gilliatt RW. Sensory conduction studies in the early recognition of nerve disorders. Muscle Nerve 1978;1:352–59.

Glynn CJ. (1991) in Ochoa JL. Controversies on chronic somatic pain and the sympathetic system. A five-year chronicle. In: Hamann W, Wedley JR, eds. Physiological Mechanisms of Pain and Pharmacology of Analgesia. London: Gordon and Breach, 1992.

Glynn CJ, Jones PC. An investigation of the role of clonidine in the treatment of reflex sympathetic dystrophy. In: Stanton-Hicks M, Wilfrid J, Boas RA, eds. Reflex Sympathetic Dystrophy. Boston: Kluwer, 1990;187–96.

Gracely RH, Lynch SA, Bennett GJ. Painful neuropathy: altered central processing maintained dynamically by peripheral input. Pain 1992;51:175–94.

Gould R, Miller BL, Goldberg MA, Benson DF. The validity of hysterical signs and symptoms. J. Nerv. Ment. Dis. 1986;174:593–97.

International Association for the Study of Pain (IASP). Classification of chronic pain. Descriptions of chronic pain syndromes and definitions of pain terms. Prepared by the Subcommittee on Taxonomy. Pain Suppl 3;1986.

Jadad AR, Carroll D, Glynn CJ, McQuay HJ. Intravenous regional sympathetic blockade for paint relief in reflex sympathetic dystrophy: a systematic review and a randomized, double-blind crossover study. J. Pain Symp. Manage. 1995;10:13–20.

Jänig W. Experimental approach to reflex sympathetic dystrophy and related syndromes. Pain 1991;46:241–45.

Jänig W, Blumberg H, Boas RA, Campbell JN. The reflex sympathetic dystrophy syndrome: consensus statement and general recommendations for diagnosis and clinical research. In: Bond MR, Charlton JE, Woolf CJ, eds. Proceedings of the VIth World Congress on Pain. Amsterdam: Elsevier, 1991;373–76.

Johnson SJ. Quoted by James Boswell in Life of Johnson. (L. F. Powell's revision of G. B. Hill's edition.) 1773, Oxford Dictionary of Quotations. Oxford: Oxford University Press, 1979;280.

Jung R. Die allgemeine Symptomatologle der Nervenverletzungen und ihre Physiologischen grundlagen. Nervenarzt 1941;14:493–516.

Leriche R. De la causalgie, envisagée comme une nevrite du sympathique et de son traltement par la dénudation et l'excision des plexus nerveux péri-arteriels. Presse Med. 1916;24:178–80.

Lewis T. Vascular Disorders of the Limbs, Described for Practitioners and Students. London: Macmillan, 1936;93.

Lewis T. Pain. London: Macmillan, 1942.

Livingston WK. Pain Mechanisms. New York: Macmillan, 1947;209–23.

Loh L, Nathan PW. Painful peripheral states and sympathetic blocks. J. Neurol. Neurosurg. Psychiatry 1978;41:664–71.

Merskey H. Regional pain is rarely hysterical. Arch. Neurol. 1988;45:915–18.

Merskey H, Bogduk N, eds. Classification of Chronic Pain. Descriptions of Chronic Pain Syndromes and Definitions of Pain Terms (2nd ed). Prepared by the task force on taxonomy of the International Association for the Study of Pain. Seattle, IASP Press, 1994.

Mitchell SW. Injuries of Nerves and Their Consequences. 1872; Reprinted, New York: Dover Publications, 1965.

Nathan PW. On the pathogenesis of causalgia in peripheral nerve injuries. Brain 1947;70:145–70.

Nordin M, Nystrom B, Wallin U, Hagbarth K-E. Ectopic sensory discharges and paresthesiae in patients with disorders of peripheral nerves, dorsal roots and dorsal columns. Pain 1984;20:231–45.

Ochoa JL. The newly recognized painful ABC syndrome: thermographic aspects. Thermology 1986a;2:65–107.

Ochoa JL. Unmyelinated fibers, microneurography, thermography and pain. (abstr). Ninth annual continuing education course B, American Association of Electromyography and Electrodiagnosis, Rochester, 1986b;29–34.

Ochoa JL. Neuropathic pains, from within: personal experiences, experiments, and reflections on mythology. In: Dimitrijevic MR, ed. Recent Achievements in Restorative Neurology. Altered Sensation and Pain. Basel, Switzerland: Karger, 1990;100–11.

Ochoa JL. Afferent and sympathetic roles in chronic "neuropathic" pains: confessions on misconceptions. In: Besson JM, Guilbaud G, eds. Lesions of Primary Afferent Fibers as a Tool for the Study of Clinical Pain. Amsterdam: Elsevier, 1991a.

Ochoa JL. A dangerous diagnosis to be given. Eur. J. Pain 1991b;12:63–64.

Ochoa J. Editorial: Reflex? Sympathetic? Dystrophy? Triple Questioned Again. Mayo Clin. Proc. 1995;70:1124–26.

Ochoa J. Chronic pain associated with positive and negative sensory, motor, and vasomotor manifestations: CPSMV (RSD; CRPS?). Heterogeneous somatic versus psychopathological origins. J. Contemp. Neurol. 1997;2:21–23.

Ochoa JL. Truths, errors and lies around "reflex sympathetic dystrophy " and "CRPS." J. Neurol. (Eur.) 1999;246:870–75.

Ochoa J. Neuropathic pain and iatrogenesis. Continuum, iatrogenic neurology. A program of the American Academy of Neurology. 2001;7:91–104.

Ochoa JL, Roberts WJ, Cline MA, Dotson R, Yarnitsky D. Two mechanical hyperalgesias in human neuropathy Soc. Neurosci. (abst). 1989;15:472.

Ochoa JL, Torebjörk HE, Culp WJ, Schady W. Abnormal spontaneous activity in single sensory nerve fibers in humans. Muscle Nerve 1982;5:S74–77.

Ochoa JL, Verdugo R. Reflex sympathetic dystrophy. Definitions and history of the ideas. A critical review of human studies. In: Low PA, ed. The Evaluation and Management of Clinical Autonomic Disorders. Boston: Little, Brown, 1992.

Ochoa J, Yarnitsky D. Mechanical hyperalgesias in neuropathic pain patients: dynamic and static subtypes. Ann. Neurol. 1993;33:465–72.

Raja SN, Treede R-D, Davis K, Campbell J. Systemic alpha-adrenergic blockade with phentolamine: a diagnostic test for sympathetically maintained pain. Anesthesiology 1991;74:691–98.

Ramamurthy S, Hoffman J, Guanethidine study group. Intravenous regional guanethidine in the treatment of reflex sympathetic dystrophy/causalgia: a randomized, double-blind study. Anesth. Analg. 1995;81:718–23.

Rasminsky M. Ectopic excitation, emphatic excitation and autoexcitation in peripheral nerve fibers of mutant mice. In: Culp WJ, Ochoa J, eds. Abnormal Nerves and Muscles as Impulse Generators. New York: Oxford University Press, 1982.

Roberts WJ. A hypothesis on the physiological basis for causalgia and related pains. Pain 1986;24:297–311.

Roberts WJ, Kramis RC. Sympathetically dependent pain: physiology and clinical expression. In: Wynn-Parry CB, ed. Management of Pain in the Hand and Wrist. London: Churchill Livingstone, 1991;14–27.

Seltzer Z, Dubner R, Shir Y. A novel behavioral model of neuropathic pain disorders produced by partial sciatic nerve injury in rats. Pain 1990;43:205–18.

Serra J, Campero M, Ochoa J. Flare and hyperalgesia following intradermal capsaicin injection in human skin. J. Neurophysiol. 1998;80:2801–10.

Serra J, Campero M, Ochoa J, Bostock H. Activity-dependent slowing of conduction differentiates functional subtypes of C fibres innervating human skin. J. Physiol. 1999; 15:799–811.

Shorter E. The borderland between neurology and history: conversion reactions. Neurol. Clin. 1995;10:229–39.

Simone DA, Baumann TK, Collins JG, LaMotte RH. Sensitization of cat dorsal horn neurons to innocuous mechanical stimulation after intradermal injection of capsaicin. Brain 1989;486:185–89.

Tanelian DL. Reflex sympathetic dystrophy. A reevaluation of the literature. Pain Forum 1996;5:247–56.

Treede RD, Raja SN, Davis KD, Meyer RA, Campbell JN. Evidence that peripheral α-adrenergic receptors mediate sympathetically maintained pain. In: Bond MR, Charlton JE, Woolf CJ, eds. Proceedings of the VIth World Congress on Pain. Amsterdam: Elsevier, 1991;377–82.

Verdugo R, Ochoa JL. High incidence of placebo responders among chronic neuropathic pain patients (abstr). Ann. Neurol. 1991;30:294.

Verdugo R, Rosenblum S, Ochoa J. Phentolamine sympathetic blocks mislead diagnosis (abstr). Soc. Neurosci. 1991; 17:107.

Verdugo RJ, Ochoa J. Hypoesthesia erased by somatic nerve block, or placebo: a pseudoneuropathic, psychogenic sign, in causalgia/RSD (abstr). Soc. Neurosci. 1992;16:235.

Verdugo RJ, Ochoa JL. Reversal of hypoesthesia by nerve block, or placebo: a psychologically mediated sign in chronic pseudoneuropathic pain patients. J. Neurol. Neurosurg. Psychiatry 1998;65:196–203.

Verdugo R, Campero M, Ochoa J. Phentolamine sympathetic block in painful polyneuropathies. II. Further questioning of the concept of 'sympathetically maintained pain.' Neurology 1994;44:1010–14.

Verdugo R, Ochoa J. Sympathetically maintained pain. I. Phentolamine block questions the concept. Neurology 1994; 44:1003–10.

Verdugo RJ, Ochoa JL. Abnormal movements in complex regional pain syndrome: assessment of their nature. Muscle Nerve 2000;23:198–205.

Vuilleumier P, Chicherio C, Assal F, Schwartz S, Slosman D, Landis T. Functional neuroanatomical correlates of hysterical sensorimotor loss. Brain 2001;124:1077–90.

Wasner G, Schattschneider J, Heckmann K, Maier C, Baron R. Vascular abnormalities in reflex sympathetic dystrophy (CRPS 1): mechanisms and diagnostic value. Brain 2001;124:587–99.

Weintraub MI. Malingering and conversion reactions. Neurol. Clin. 1995;139:2.

Weintraub MI. Regional pain is usually hysterical. Arch. Neurol. 1988;4S:914–15.

Woolf CJ, Mannion RJ. Neuropathic pain: etiology, symptoms, mechanisms, and management. Lancet 1999;353: 1959–64.

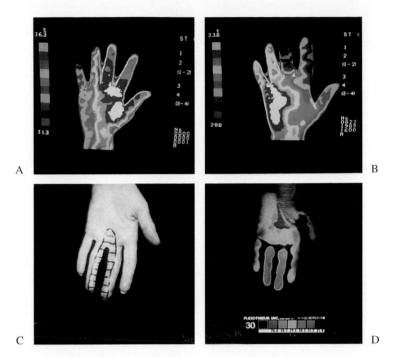

Color Plate 10.1. Thermograms displaying three typical patterns determined by different kinds of abnormal nerve function (see text pp. 11,177–178,307–308).

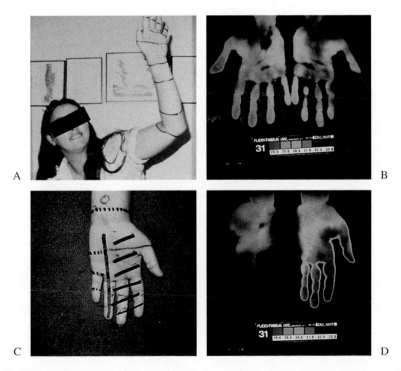

Color Plate 16.2. Usefulness of combined local anesthetic block and thermography in assessing abnormal neurophysiology of cold painful limb (see text pp. 11,177,310,313–314).

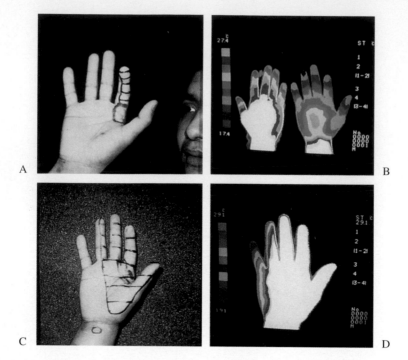

Color Plate 16.4. Usefulness of combined local anesthetic block and thermography in differentiating organic versus psychogenic sensory profiles (see text pp. 11,177–179,313–314).

Chapter 17

Median Neuropathy Proximal to the Carpal Tunnel

From its formation by the medial and lateral cords of the brachial plexus to its entrance into the carpal tunnel, the median nerve runs a gauntlet of potential injuries and compressions. Nonetheless, the total prevalence of proximal median neuropathies is only a small fraction of the prevalence of carpal tunnel syndrome. Figure 17-1 shows the sites and Table 17-1 shows the relative prevalences of median nerve compression at these sites reported in one series; most clinicians find that this overestimates the incidence of median neuropathies proximal to the carpal tunnel (Gessini, Jandolo, Pietrangeli & Senese, 1983).

Laceration and repair of the median nerve is amply covered in textbooks of peripheral nerve surgery (Seddon, 1972; Mackinnon & Dellon, 1988; Birch, Bonney & Wynn Parry, 1998; Omer, Spinner & Van Beek, 1998). We shall discuss other proximal median neuropathies starting in the distal forearm and tracing the nerve to the brachial plexus.

Median Neuropathy in the Distal Forearm

Median nerve compression in the distal forearm has been called *pseudocarpal tunnel syndrome*. It is usually discovered on those rare occasions when a patient presents with features indicative of carpal tunnel syndrome, but the contents of the carpal tunnel are found to be normal at the time of flexor retinaculum release. In these patients, the surgeon should trace the course of the median nerve over its first few centimeters into the distal forearm in search of an unusual site of nerve compression.

The possibility of compression of the median nerve by the palmaris longus muscle-tendon unit, just proximal to the carpal tunnel, has been discussed in Chapter 6. For example, median nerve compression has been reported to occur from a bifid palmaris longus tendon, some 5 cm proximal to the tunnel, or by an anomalously bifid median nerve entangled in the muscle belly or tendon of flexor digitorum sublimis (Baruch & Hass, 1977; Dorin & Mann, 1984; Fernandez-Garcia, Pi-Folguera & Estallo-Matino, 1994). A lipoma on the anterior wrist, proximal to the carpal tunnel and superficial to the median nerve, or a tendon sheath fibroma in the distal forearm can cause symptoms of median nerve compression (Phalen, Kendrick & Rodriguez, 1971; Bertolotto, Rosenberg, Parodi, Perrone, Gentile, Rollandi & Succi, 1996). An unsuspected foreign body penetrating the median nerve from prior injury has been found at the time of surgical exploration (Rainer, Schoeller, Wechselberger, Bauer & Hussl, 2000).

Pseudocarpal tunnel syndrome may develop acutely after trauma. For example, marked median neuropathy developed over 36 hours after a tire fell on the dorsum of a patient's hand and forearm. At surgery the median nerve was compressed against the forearm fascia by flexor digitorum superficialis muscle (Dansereau & Cianciulli, 1968).

With distal forearm injuries, there are many potential mechanisms for median nerve injury, including nerve contusion or stretch at the time of injury or the time of fracture reduction, compression or stretch of the nerve over a hematoma or displaced fracture, or compression in a compartment syndrome of the carpal tunnel or volar forearm. For

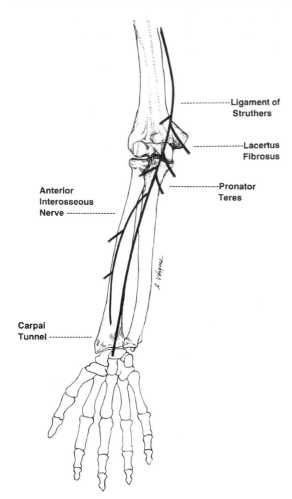

Ligament of Struthers

Lacertus Fibrosus

Pronator Teres

Anterior Interosseous Nerve

Carpal Tunnel

Figure 17-1. Potential sites of compression of the median nerve. The relative prevalence of compression at these sites is shown in Table 17-1.

Table 17-1. Sites of Median Nerve Compression in 238 Cases of Median Neuropathy

Site of Compression	No. of Cases
Carpal tunnel	201
Pronator teres	21
Anterior interosseous nerve	3
Lacertus fibrosus	2
Struthers' ligament	1

Data from L Gessini, B Jandolo, A Pietrangeli. Entrapment neuropathies of the median nerve at and above the elbow. Surg. Neurol. 1983;19:112–16.

(Lewis, 1978). The relationship between Colles' fracture and carpal tunnel syndrome is discussed further in Chapter 6. In some instances, median nerve deficit resolves when a wrist or forearm fracture is reduced (Binfield, Sott-Miknas & Good, 1998). If a patient has median nerve deficit after reduction of the fracture, measuring compartment pressures in the carpal tunnel and distal forearm can clarify the mechanism of nerve injury.

Median Palmar Cutaneous Neuropathy

Isolated compression or injury of the palmar cutaneous branch of the median nerve is very unusual. There are case reports of its compression by ganglion, palmaris longus tendon, atypical palmaris longus muscle, antebrachial fascia, or fascia of flexor digitorum superficialis (Stellbrink, 1972; Gessini et al., 1983; Buckmiller & Rickard, 1987; Shimizu, Iwasaki, Hoshikawa & Yamamuro, 1988; Haskin, 1994; Duncan, Yospur, Gomez-Garcia & Lesavoy, 1995; Semer, Crimmins & Jones, 1996; De Smet, 1998). Mechanisms of compression vary along the course of the nerve, described in Chapter 1 (al-Qattan, 1997). For example, the nerve is briefly adjacent to the flexor carpi radialis tendon and theoretically could be compressed in this area by focal tenosynovitis (Naff, Dellon & Mackinnon, 1993). In the proximal hand, the palmar cutaneous branch runs briefly (9 to 16 mm) in a tunnel within the flexor retinaculum, where a ganglion as small as few millimeters in diameter may compress it (al-Qattan & Robertson, 1993). It may be injured with surgery of the volar wrist,

instance, Sumner and Khuri (1984) reported a case of median nerve entrapment in an epiphyseal fracture-dislocation of the distal radioulnar joint. In this case the entrapment was corrected acutely, and clinical nerve injury was prevented. Another example is a displaced distal radial epiphyseal fracture (Salter-Harris type II) (Waters, Kolettis & Schwend, 1994). Evaluation of nerve function is more complex if a flexor tendon of a median innervated muscle is also entrapped in the fracture. In some patients who acutely develop symptoms of median nerve compression after Colles' fracture, the median nerve may be compressed by a hematoma beneath the fascia of the distal forearm particularly with surgery for carpal tunnel release (see Table 15-18).

There is no well-established method to study nerve conduction in the median palmar cutaneous nerve. In most of the case reports of median palmar cutaneous neuropathy, the diagnosis has been made on clinical grounds without electrodiagnostic confirmation. However, Lum and Kanakamedala (1986) proposed studying nerve conduction of the median palmar cutaneous nerve using a pair of surface recording electrodes over the thenar eminence while stimulating the nerve antidromically. With stimulation 10 cm proximal to the recording electrode, mean latency to the negative peak of the nerve action potential was 2.6 msec. Mean amplitude of the evoked response was 12 mV. However, Dumitru and colleagues (1989) showed that the nerve action potential recorded by this method did not reliably originate from the palmar cutaneous nerve. They found that this nerve action potential persisted after the median palmar cutaneous nerve was blocked by local anesthetic but disappeared after the median nerve was blocked by local anesthetic injection in the palm.

Alternatively, median palmar cutaneous nerve conduction can be tested orthodromically by stimulating over the thenar eminence and recording over the median nerve 10 cm proximally (Chang & Lien, 1991). Upper limit of normal latency to negative peak was 2.56 msec for 40 controls and 3.04 msec for 43 patients with suspected carpal tunnel syndrome. The sensory nerve action potential amplitude may be low, requiring averaging of multiple stimuli to record accurately, and the absence of a reproducible sensory nerve action potential may represent technical failure rather than be evidence of an abnormality of the median palmar cutaneous nerve.

Anterior Interosseous Neuropathy

Anterior interosseous nerve palsy is of interest for its distinctive clinical presentation and varied etiologies. The anatomy of the anterior interosseous nerve is discussed in Chapter 1. Palsy limited to the distribution of this nerve was described by Kiloh and Nevin (1952), hence the eponym *Kiloh-Nevin syndrome*. They reported two cases of sudden onset of focal weakness without preceding trauma. A 52-year-old man presented with painless weakness of flexor pollicis longus and of flexor digitorum profundus to index and middle fingers. A 28-year-old man awoke with pain along the lateral forearm and weakness of flexor pollicis longus. Within months both patients recovered spontaneously. Kiloh and Nevin postulated that these patients had a variant of acute brachial plexitis.

Anterior interosseous nerve palsies account for much less than 1% of median neuropathies. In 7 years, physicians at the Mayo Clinic saw two cases of anterior interosseous palsy while seeing 39 cases of pronator syndrome (Hartz, Linscheid, Gramse & Daube, 1981).

Clinical Presentation

The hallmark of anterior interosseous nerve palsy is weakness limited to flexor pollicis longus, flexor digitorum profundus to the index finger, and pronator quadratus. Occasionally, flexor digitorum profundus to the middle finger is weak. In the classic posture the patient extends the distal interphalangeal joint of the thumb and index finger when trying to pinch these two fingers together (Figure 17-2). The normal hand can form a circle with this pinch. Patients with isolated anterior interosseous nerve palsy have no associated sensory loss. Pain in the wrist or forearm is a variable symptom.

The palsy may be partial with clinical weakness limited to flexor pollicis longus or to flexor digitorum profundus to the index finger (Hill, Howard & Huffer, 1985; Conway & Thomas, 1990). To test pronator quadratus while minimizing the action of pronator teres, pronation is tested with the elbow flexed; even with this technique, mild to moderate weakness of pronator quadratus can be difficult to detect.

Anomalous neuroanatomy can lead to unusual clinical presentations. In the most common form of Martin-Gruber anastomosis, motor axons travel with the median nerve into the forearm, accompany the anterior interosseous nerve, cross to join the ulnar nerve proximal to the wrist, and innervate ulnar intrinsic hand muscles, particularly adductor pollicis and first dorsal interosseous (Mannerfelt, 1966). The diagnostically puzzling combination of weakness of ulnar-innervated hand muscles and of the muscles classically innervated by the anterior

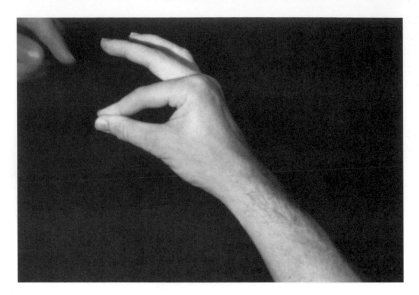

Figure 17-2. The classic hand posture of the patient with anterior interosseous nerve palsy results from paresis of flexor pollicis longus and of flexor digitorum profundus to the index finger.

interosseous nerve occurs if anterior interosseous nerve palsy affects a patient with Martin-Gruber anastomosis (Spinner, 1970).

At times, both the main trunk of the median nerve and the anterior interosseous nerve supply flexor digitorum superficialis. When this occurs, this muscle of a patient who has anterior interosseous neuropathy might show some neuropathic changes on needle electromyography (EMG), even when it is not clinically weak (Wertsch, 1992).

In another variation, a patient presented with features of anterior interosseous palsy but with an unusual degree of pronator weakness. EMG showed fibrillations in both pronator teres and pronator quadratus. Surgical exploration of the forearm showed compression of the anterior interosseous nerve, which arose anomalously, proximal to the heads of pronator teres, and gave off an anomalous branch to pronator teres (Ashworth, Marshall & Classen, 1997).

Causes

Anterior Interosseous Nerve Compression. Anterior interosseous nerve palsy may be caused by chronic isolated compression of the anterior interosseous nerve (Fearn & Goodfellow, 1965) (Table 17-2). Symptoms of compression may develop gradually or, in relation to a forearm strain or injury, more abruptly. Patients typically have deep, aching elbow and forearm pain associated with forearm tenderness to deep pressure. Paresthesias, such as "pins and needles," should be absent. Weakness confined to muscles supplied by the anterior interosseous nerve develops gradually and may lag behind the painful symptoms in appearance.

Clinical clues to anterior interosseous nerve compression, in addition to the characteristic pattern of weakness, can include a positive Tinel's sign over the nerve in the forearm or an increase in elbow pain elicited by pronating the forearm against resistance, then extending the elbow while keeping the fingers and wrists hyperflexed ("modified Mill's test") (Rask, 1979). A rare patient notes that muscles innervated by the anterior interosseous nerve develop weakness after excessive forearm use and recover within days of stopping the excessive activity (Hill et al., 1985).

A number of structures in the forearm are potential compressors of the anterior interosseous nerve. At times the *deep head of pronator teres* forms a tough arch of fibrous tissue that can compress the anterior interosseous nerve as it passes between the two heads of this muscle (Spinner & Schreiber, 1969; Wiens & Lau, 1978; Hill et al., 1985; Megele, 1988). The *origin of flexor digitorum superficialis* crosses the anterior interosseous nerve approximately 4 cm distal to the origin of the nerve. At this point, the muscle origin is sometimes tendinous and can appear to compress the nerve (Stern,

Rosner & Blinderman, 1967; Vichare, 1968; Schmidt & Eiken, 1971; Wiens & Lau, 1978). Fearn and Goodfellow (1965) described compression of the nerve by a crescentic fibrous band ("the arcuate ligament of Fearn and Goodfellow") distally continuous with the aponeurosis attached to the deep surface of the humeral head of pronator teres and fanned out proximally to blend with the insertion of the brachialis; various *other fibrous structures* seem to compress the nerve in some individuals (Rask, 1979; Hill et al., 1985). In a patient with isolated paresis of flexor pollicis longus, the fibrous band crossed the branch of the anterior interosseous nerve that innervated this muscle (Stern & Kutz, 1980). An *accessory head of flexor pollicis longus* ("Gantzer's muscle"), when present, can compress the nerve (Figure 17-3) (Nelson & Currier, 1980). The *anterior interosseous artery* can thrombose after trauma and perhaps contributes to nerve compression in some cases (Spinner, 1970).

Complicating interpretation of the reports mentioned previously, structures often cross the anterior interosseus nerve as asymptomatic anatomic variants. Sixteen of 31 cadaver arms had a fibrous arch crossing the anterior interosseous nerve (Dellon, 1986). The arch may originate from the flexor digitorum superficialis or from either head of pronator teres. In 10% of cadavers, the anterior interosseous nerve branches from the median nerve proximal to the distal edge of the pronator teres

Table 17-2. Causes of Anterior Interosseous Neuropathy

Compression
    Arcuate ligament of Fearn and Goodfellow
    Other fibrous bands
    Heads of pronator teres
    Tendinous origin of flexor digitorum superficialis
    Accessory head of flexor pollicis longus (Gantzer's muscle)
    Anterior interosseous artery
Acute trauma
    Nerve laceration
    Supracondylar humeral fracture in children
    Proximal humeral fracture
    Distal humeral or olecranon fracture
    Posterior elbow dislocation
    Monteggia fracture of the ulna
    Internal fixation of proximal radius
    Closed fracture of proximal ulna
    Closed fracture of radius and ulna
    Volkmann's contracture
    Closed forearm compression or soft tissue trauma
Antecubital mischief ("pseudoanterior interosseus palsy")
    Antecubital cardiac catheterization
    Elbow arthroscopy
    Antecubital venipuncture
    Brachial artery blood gas collection
Neuralgic amyotrophy
Miscellaneous
    Metastatic tumor in forearm

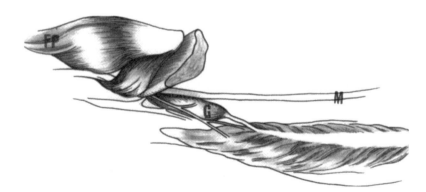

Figure 17-3. Forearm; distal is toward the right. Gantzer's muscle (G), an accessory head of flexor pollicis longus, sometimes compresses the anterior interosseous nerve (unlabeled). (M = median nerve; FP = flexor and pronator muscles.) (Reproduced with permission from AL Dellon, SE Mackinnon. Musculoaponeurotic variations along the course of the median nerve in the proximal forearm. J. Hand Surg. 1987;12B:359–63.)

(Johnson, Spinner & Shrewsbury, 1979). An accessory head of flexor pollicis longus originates from the medial humeral epicondyle and crosses to the lateral forearm between the median nerve and the anterior interosseous nerve in more than one-half of arms (Mangini, 1960; al-Qattan, 1996; Shirali, Hanson, Branovacki & Gonzalez, 1998). The mere presence of one of these structures crossing the anterior interosseous nerve does not prove pathologic compression.

For years, the site of nerve compression could be confirmed only with surgery. More recent case reports suggest that modern imaging can elucidate the cause of some cases of anterior interosseous palsy. A man developed anterior interosseous palsy acutely while weight lifting; ultrasound of the forearm showed a fluid collection in the vicinity of the volar forearm muscles (Internullo, Marcuzzi, Busa, Cordella & Caroli, 1995). In another case, magnetic resonance imaging of the forearm showed selective edema of involved muscles (Duteille, Amara, Dautel & Merle, 2000).

Peters and Todd (1983) described an unusual occurrence: compression of the anterior interosseous nerve by a metastasis from bronchogenic carcinoma.

Anterior Interosseous Nerve Trauma. Trauma can cause isolated anterior interosseous nerve injury. Spinner and Schreiber (1969) described six cases of anterior interosseous nerve palsy occurring after *supracondylar humeral fractures* in children. In each case neuropathic weakness was limited to flexor pollicis longus and flexor digitorum profundus, and recovery occurred within 8 weeks. Occasionally, the weakness is not detected until a few days after the fracture (Geutjens, 1995).

Spinner and Schreiber investigated the mechanism of the nerve injury. At the level of the fracture, median nerve fascicles destined for the anterior interosseous nerve are situated posteriorly and in close proximity to motor fascicles for pronator teres and flexor digitorum superficialis and to sensory fascicles. Therefore, partial direct contusion of the median nerve would be unlikely to selectively paralyze flexor pollicis longus and flexor digitorum profundus. In cadavers, they found that supracondylar fracture with posterior displacement placed tension on the anterior interosseous nerve at the level of the proximal third of the forearm and suggested that nerve stretching at this point in the forearm was the probable mechanism of nerve injury. A case of documented anterior interosseous nerve avulsion at its origin from the median nerve that occurred in association with an open humeral fracture gives credence to this hypothesized mechanism (Collins & Weber, 1983). However, other cases might be due to selective fascicular trauma: Shortly after a *fracture of the proximal third of the humerus*, a patient had weakness limited to the anterior interosseous distribution, but EMG a number of weeks later showed that axons to pronator teres had also been interrupted (Apergis, Aktipis, Giota, Kastanis, Nteimentes & Papanikolaou, 1998). Anterior interosseous palsy can also accompany *olecranon fracture* (Galbraith & McCullough, 1979).

Anterior interosseous nerve palsy can also occur as a delayed effect after *posterior dislocation of the elbow* (Beverly & Fearn, 1984; Katirji, 1986). The anterior interosseous nerve may also be injured in association with *forearm fractures*, such as ulnar fracture with ipsilateral dislocation of the radial head ("Monteggia fracture") and, more rarely, with less severe fractures of the proximal ulna or of the radius and ulna (Warren, 1963; Engber & Keene, 1983; Mirovsky, Hendel & Halperin, 1988; Geissler, Fernandez & Graca, 1990). The Monteggia fracture is more commonly accompanied by posterior interosseous nerve injury. Hope (1988) reported an anterior interosseous nerve palsy appearing within the first 3 weeks after open reduction and internal fixation of a radial fracture. A bone-holding forceps was used at surgery, and cadaver studies suggested that the forceps might have temporarily compressed the anterior interosseous nerve during surgery.

Penetrating *injuries of the forearm* may lacerate the anterior interosseous nerve directly. Closed forearm injury can lead to anterior interosseous neuropathy as a delayed effect of the injury due to secondary scarring and nerve compression (Spinner, 1970).

Anterior interosseous nerve palsy has also been reported secondary to *thrombosis of the anterior interosseous artery* or as a sequel of *Volkmann's contracture* of the forearm. *External pressure on the forearm* can cause anterior interosseous nerve palsy; examples include pressure on the forearm during surgery with the patient prone, compression by an arm sling applied for treatment of acromioclavicular joint dislocation, compression by the strap of a heavy purse carried across the forearm, and constriction by a tight band wrapped around the forearm to treat "tennis elbow" (Spinner, 1970; Albanese, Buterbaugh, Palmer, Lubicky & Yuan, 1986; O'Neill, Zarins, Gelberman, Keating & Louis, 1990; Enzenauer & Nordstrom, 1991). In an instance of anterior interosseous palsy following forearm casting placed after hand surgery, an anomalous median artery penetrating the anterior interosseous nerve perhaps increased nerve vulnerability (Proudman & Menz, 1992).

Neuralgic Amyotrophy. In the syndrome of neuralgic amyotrophy, patients present with acute arm pain and focal weakness. In some patients weakness may be limited to the distribution of the anterior interosseous nerve. In their series of 136 patients with neuralgic amyotrophy or acute brachial plexitis, Parsonage and Turner (1948) noted that flexor pollicis longus and flexor digitorum profundus were at times preferentially weakened in patients with the syndrome. They described a single case in which the motor abnormality was limited to flexor pollicis longus and flexor digitorum profundus to the index finger and assumed that this presentation was part of the spectrum of neuralgic amyotrophy. Kiloh and Nevin (1952) considered their two cases of isolated anterior interosseous nerve palsy as a "neuritis" analogous to the cases of Parsonage and Turner. Features linking Kiloh and Nevin's cases to neuralgic amyotrophy were sudden, often painful, onset and spontaneous, but delayed, motor recovery beginning more than 1 year after onset of symptoms. Other patients may have sudden onset of pain and focal anterior interosseous nerve weakness and recover more rapidly (Smith & Herbst, 1974; Verhagen & Dalman, 1995). Rarely, the neuralgic amyotrophy causes bilateral weakness limited to the anterior interosseous distribution (Verhagen & Dalman, 1995). The following cases, which bridge the gap between neuralgic amyotrophy and isolated anterior interosseous nerve neuritis, are instructive.

A 31-year-old man developed right antecubital pain and weakness of flexor digitorum profundus to the right index finger 11 days after an illness characterized by headache, fever, and malaise (Dunne, Prentice & Stewart-Wynne, 1987). Five days later he developed similar pain on the left with weakness in left flexor digitorum profundus and flexor pollicis longus. Tenderness adjacent to the biceps tendon interfered with elbow extension. Clues to disease beyond the territory of the anterior interosseous nerves were slight tingling of the thumbs, decreased sensation reported at the tip of the left thumb, and decreased appreciation of pin prick over the upper lateral right arm. Using a needle recording electrode in the pronator quadratus and stimulating in the antecubital fossa, the distal motor latency of the anterior interosseous nerve was prolonged at 6.8 msec over 24 cm on the left and was unobtainable on the right.

EMG examination with a needle electrode showed increased insertional activity, fibrillations, and reduced interference pattern bilaterally in pronator quadratus, flexor pollicis longus, and flexor digitorum profundus. The left pronator teres and flexor carpi radialis showed similar abnormalities.

Cytomegalovirus infection was diagnosed based on cytomegalovirus-specific serology and cytomegalovirus isolation from the urine. After 5 months, he had partially recovered strength.

The second case is that of a 20-year-old man who presented with a left anterior interosseous nerve palsy coincident with a myalgic flulike illness (Rennels & Ochoa, 1980). Motor abnormalities were initially limited to the anterior interosseous nerve distribution, but hyperesthesia in both arms and asymmetrically depressed deep tendon reflexes hinted at more diffuse neurologic involvement. Light taping in the antecubital fossa elicited intense forearm pain. Sixteen days later he developed weakness in the right serratus anterior. Recovery of left hand strength was first noted 19 months after onset of symptoms and was nearly complete by 23 months after onset.

These cases match the cases of isolated anterior interosseous neuritis in sudden onset and prominent pain and indicate that in some instances, although the anterior interosseous nerve may be preferentially involved, the neuropathy is actually more widespread. In these two cases there was EMG evidence of axonal degeneration, and the delayed recovery is consistent with axonal regeneration over a distance similar to the distance from brachial plexus to forearm using the approximation of 1 mm of axonal regrowth daily. However, the hypothesis that the pathology is a patchy process in the brachial plexus rather than in the anterior interosseous nerve itself is unproven.

In fact, other cases compatible with neuralgic amyotrophy show axonopathy of multiple arm nerves, suggesting a mononeuritis multiplex rather than a brachial plexitis (England & Sumner, 1987). Cases may show isolated denervation in pronator teres, sensory change in a palmar cutaneous pattern, or more complete median neuropathy proximal to the branch to pronator teres. In some cases time to reinnervation favors lesions in the arm or forearm rather than the brachial plexus. The anatomically noncommittal label, *neuralgic amyotrophy*, rather than *brachial plexitis*, is appropriate to this condition because of the varied sites of nerve pathology.

The differentiation between anterior interosseous nerve compression and anterior interosseous neuralgic amyotrophy is challenging at times. Sudden onset of proximal pain, rapid evolution of weakness, subtle neuropathy beyond the innervation of the anterior interosseous nerve, and EMG evidence of axonal interruption favor the diagnosis of neuralgic amyotrophy. Note that in the previously mentioned cases nerve sensitivity to percussion in the forearm (Tinel's sign) can be prominent in neuralgic amyotrophy and is not a reliable indicator of focal nerve compression. In problematic cases a meticulous search, both by neurologic examination and EMG, for evidence of neuropathy beyond the distribution of the anterior interosseous nerve may resolve the issue. When neuropathy is clearly restricted to the anterior interosseous nerve, clinical judgment becomes especially important. Retrospective reading of case reports of anterior interosseous nerve compression suggests that some patients are unnecessarily explored for compressive lesions (Wong & Dellon, 1997). For example, Miller-Breslow and colleagues (1990) describe two cases of anterior interosseous nerve palsy in which they found no pathology on surgical exploration of the forearm; they warn other surgeons of the danger of overhasty surgical exploration when neuralgic amyotrophy is a likely diagnosis.

A provocative Japanese report concerns patients who developed spontaneous, usually painful, anterior interosseous nerve palsy and underwent nerve exploration when no motor recovery was evident 3 months after onset of weakness (Nagano, Shibata, Tokimura, Yamamoto & Tajiri, 1996). In eight of nine operations, an hourglass-like constriction limited to fascicles destined for the anterior interosseous nerve was found within the median nerve 2.0 to 7.5 cm proximal to the medial epicondyle. The authors performed fascicular neurolysis and recommended this surgical approach to any spontaneous anterior interosseous palsy that does not begin to recover within 3 months. However, they have acknowledged that at least some of their patients had neuralgic amyotrophy (Yamamoto, Nagano, Mikami, Tajiri, Kawano & Itaka, 1999). Others have also reported constriction of individual nerve fascicles in patients presenting with dysfunction of the anterior interosseous or proximal median nerves (Haussmann & Patel, 1996). An operative approach is unnecessary in patients who have had an episode of neuralgic amyotrophy and are apt to recover spontaneously.

Differential Diagnosis

The importance of a careful clinical and EMG evaluation is highlighted by the *pseudo-anterior interosseus nerve syndrome*. At times a partial median neuropathy with injury in the vicinity of the antecubital space, proximal to the takeoff of the anterior interosseous nerve, may masquerade as an anterior interosseus nerve syndrome. Phlebotomy, brachial artery blood gas collection, cutdown for catheterization, and elbow arthroscopy are typical causes of this type of injury (Schneck, 1960; Finelli, 1977; Saeed & Gatens, 1983; Ruch & Poehling, 1997). Only subtle findings may document more widespread median nerve involvement. For example, a 55-year-old man presented 2 days after right antecubital cardiac catheterization with forearm and hand discomfort and weakness restricted to the right flexor pollicis longus and flexor digitorum profundus (Wertsch, Sanger & Matloub, 1985). The clues to more widespread median nerve involvement were a 4-mm diameter area of sensory loss at the tips of the right index finger and thumb and mild asymmetries of nerve conduction comparing right and left median nerves. EMG needle examination of median-innervated muscles showed sharp waves and fibrillations in flexor pollicis longus and pronator quadratus but was otherwise normal. At exploration, dense fibrosis was noted around the median nerve in the antecubital space at the site of previous cutdown for catheterization, whereas the anterior interosseous nerve itself was normal.

Katirji (1986) reported a similar case in a 30-year-old man who sustained a posterior elbow dislocation that was reduced without surgery. Weakness limited to flexor pollicis longus and flexor digitorum profundus developed a few weeks later, and sensory examination was normal. Median motor and sensory conduction studies to the hand were normal and symmetric, except that the thenar compound muscle action potential was 6.6 mV on the symptomatic side compared with 16.0 mV contralaterally. The most convincing evidence of more extensive median nerve injury was neuropathic abnormalities on needle EMG involving not only flexor pollicis longus, pronator quadratus, and flexor digitorum profundus, but also to a lesser extent, abductor pollicis brevis, pronator teres, and flexor digitorum sublimis. At antecubital exploration, scarring was found around the median nerve.

These cases of pseudo-anterior interosseous nerve syndrome are consistent with the fascicular organization of the median nerve (Figure 17-4); the fibers intended for the anterior interosseous nerve are grouped discretely in the posterior portion of the median nerve (Jabaley, Wallace & Heckler, 1980). For more than 93 mm above the medial epicondyle, the anterior interosseous nerve can be microdissected free from the main median nerve because the epineurium divides the two nerve bundles.

Rupture of flexor pollicis longus or flexor digitorum profundus tendons, or rare congenital absence of one of these muscles can easily be confused with anterior interosseous nerve palsy (Stern & Kutz, 1980; Hill et al., 1985; Mahring, Semple & Gray, 1985). Tendon rupture can occur traumatically or spontaneously, particularly in patients with rheumatoid arthritis (Boyes, Wilson & Smith, 1960; Moberg, 1965; Mannerfelt & Norman, 1969). The confusion is heightened because a partial anterior interosseous nerve palsy can present with weakness clinically evident in only a single muscle. The tenodesis effect can be used as part of the physical examination to distinguish anterior interosseous palsy from flexor pollicis longus tendon rupture (Mody, 1992; Schantz & Riegels-Nielsen, 1992). The patient's wrist is held in full dorsiflexion. The examiner hyperextends the patient's thumb at the carpal-metacarpal and metacarpal-phalangeal joints. If the flexor

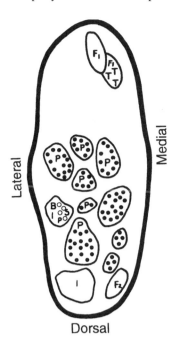

Figure 17-4. Fascicular anatomy of median nerve at the antecubital level. The fibers destined for the anterior interosseous nerve (I) are predominantly dorsal so that partial nerve injury of the posterior aspect of the nerve can cause a "pseudo-interosseous nerve syndrome." (Other fibers: B = cutaneous fibers from the second interspace; F_1 = proximal common flexors, F_2 = distal common flexors; round dots = mixed fibers; P = palmar cutaneous; T = pronator teres; S = flexor digitorum superficialis.) (Reproduced with permission from S Sunderland. The intraneural topography of the radial, median and ulnar nerves. Brain 1945;68:243–98; and S Sunderland. The Median Nerve. Anatomical and Physiological Considerations. In: Nerves and Nerve Injuries [2nd ed]. Edinburgh, UK: Churchill Livingstone, 1978;674.)

pollicis longus muscle-tendon unit is continuous, the interphalangeal joint of the thumb flexes spontaneously or at least resists passive extension. Electrodiagnosis can also be helpful in making the distinction.

Electrodiagnosis

Nerve conduction studies of the anterior interosseous nerve are limited to assessment of motor conduction. A number of different techniques have been proposed.

The compound muscle action potential of pronator quadratus can be recorded with surface elec-

Table 17-3. Normal Values for Anterior Interosseous Nerve Conduction

	Mean	Range	Standard Deviation	Maximum Side to Side Variation
Distal motor latency (msec)	3.6	2.8–4.4	0.4	0.4
Compound muscle action potential amplitude	3.1 mV	2.0–5.5 mV	0.8 mV	25%
Compound muscle action potential duration (msec)	7.8	5.6–10.5	1.3	—

Data from WJ Mysiw, SC Colachis 3rd. Electrophysiologic study of the anterior interosseous nerve. Am. J. Phys. Med. Rehabil. 1988;67:50–54.

trodes while the median nerve is stimulated at the antecubital space with the forearm pronated and the elbow flexed 90 degrees (Mysiw & Colachis, 1988). The active recording electrode is placed on the dorsum of the forearm 3 cm proximal to the ulnar styloid with the reference electrode at the ulnar styloid. The distance from stimulus site in the antecubital space to the recording electrode varies from 17 to 28 cm. Table 17-3 shows the normal values for this technique based on Mysiw and Colachis' study of 26 healthy individuals.

Nakano and colleagues (1977) reported normative data on latency obtained by recording in pronator quadratus with a needle electrode. With stimulation in the ventromedial arm adjacent to the biceps tendon, mean latency was 5.1 msec with a 95% confidence upper limit of 6.0 msec. With stimulation in the forearm 10 cm distal to the lateral epicondyle, mean latency was 3.6 msec with a 95% confidence upper limit of 4.4 msec. Nakano and colleagues studied seven patients with anterior interosseous nerve palsy; all had prolonged duration of the muscle action potential, and five had prolonged motor latency.

Rosenberg (1990) proposed recording the muscle action potential from pronator quadratus with a monopolar active intramuscular electrode using a surface reference electrode. With stimulation of the median nerve proximal to the antecubital fossa, the latencies to the pronator quadratus and abductor pollicis brevis are measured, and the ratio of these latencies is used to compare anterior interosseous nerve and median nerve conductions.

The compound muscle action potential of the flexor pollicis longus can be recorded using an active surface electrode over the lateral distal third of the anterior forearm (Craft, Currier & Nelson, 1977). The active electrode should be placed three-eighths of the distance between the distal wrist crease and the antecubital crease with the reference electrode placed distally over the flexor pollicis longus tendon. Ideally, the body of flexor pollicis longus should be palpated to confirm electrode placement, but this is not always possible if flexor pollicis longus is severely paretic. With stimulation of the median nerve just proximal to the elbow, the amplitude of the compound muscle action potential ranged from 3.8 to 7.5 mV, and the latency ranged from 1.8 to 3.6 msec in 25 healthy women.

Electrodiagnostic study of patients with suspected anterior interosseous nerve palsy should include motor and sensory studies of the main trunk of the median nerve, which should be normal (O'Brien & Upton, 1972). EMG needle electrode examination should be performed to confirm localization of the abnormality to the muscles supplied by the anterior interosseous nerve. Accurate needle electrode placement in pronator quadratus can be technically challenging (Wertsch, 1992). If neuropathic abnormalities are noted in ulnar-innervated hand intrinsic muscles, nerve stimulation can check for a Martin-Gruber anastomosis. EMG needle electrode examination is also helpful in characterizing the degree of axonal interruption contributing to the anterior interosseous nerve dysfunction.

Treatment

Appropriate treatment, of course, varies with cause. Some patients with compressive neuropathy improve with decreased forearm use. In some cases this is imposed by casting the arm in supination (Rask, 1979). If no improvement occurs in 4 to 8 weeks, many surgeons favor forearm exploration for correction of entrapment (Mills, Mukherjee & Bassett, 1969; Spinner, 1970; Stern, 1984). If the clinical presentation suggests gradual development of compressive symptoms and if the EMG shows evidence of axonal interruption, surgical exploration should not be delayed. Postoperative worsening of a partial anterior interosseous palsy is a rare complication of surgery (al-Qattan, Manktelow & Murray, 1994). In patients who have had axonal interruption, recovery of strength is usually successful but can take a year (Schantz & Riegels-Nielsen, 1992).

If the clinical presentation favors neuralgic amyotrophy, decompressive surgery is obviously without value, and improvement may take 2 years or more.

In patients who have persistent weakness in flexor pollicis longus or flexor digitorum profundus after the predicted recovery time, tendon transfer surgery may be of value. Spinner (1970) suggested releasing the flexor digitorum superficialis tendon of the ring finger and attaching it to the flexor pollicis longus tendon. The tendon of the brachioradialis or the flexor digitorum profundus of ring or middle finger can be transferred to the flexor digitorum profundus tendon of the index finger.

Terminal Branch of Anterior Interosseous Nerve

Dellon and colleagues (1984) reported a series of 12 patients whom they believed had had focal injury to the terminal branch of the anterior interosseous nerve. This branch of the nerve provides sensory innervation of the anterior radiocarpal and intercarpal joints. The patients complained of dull, aching volar wrist pain, exacerbated by some wrist movements, particularly hyperextension. The symptoms developed and became chronic after hyperextension wrist injuries. No neurologic or electrophysiologic testing can confirm the diagnosis. Dellon and colleagues suggest a diagnostic test of terminal anterior interosseous nerve block with injection of local anaesthetic at the interosseous membrane after piercing the pronator quadratus; a positive test includes pain relief and normal grip testing after the block. This report, however, did not include control blocks with placebo injection or block of other nerves. Dellon and colleagues proposed treatment by resection of the terminal anterior interosseous nerve. Their patients reportedly had long-standing good to excellent response to surgery. Evaluation of the diagnosis and of results of treatment is complicated because many of the patients had concomitant treatment of other problems, including carpal tunnel surgery and ganglionectomy, and because many of the patients had unresolved litigation or worker's compensation claims.

Median Neuropathy in the Antecubital Space and Proximal Forearm

Compression by Normal or Anomalous Anatomic Structures

The pronator syndrome, defined as median nerve compression by the pronator teres muscle, was described by Seyffarth (1951). We now recognize that the median nerve is vulnerable to compression at a variety of sites as it enters the forearm. The pronator teres is the most common of these sites. Other possible points of nerve compression include a tendinous origin of flexor digitorum superficialis, the lacertus fibrosus, or the ligament of Struthers (Figures 17-5 through 17-7). The anatomy of the course of the median nerve through the antecubital space and into the forearm is reviewed in Chapter 1.

Clinical Presentation

Pronator syndrome presents with aching forearm distress and muscle fatigability, often related to repetitive forearm pronation. Intermittent, but vaguely localized, numbness in the hand, especially in the thumb and index finger, sometimes accompanies use-induced distress.

Nocturnal awakening with pain or paresthesias is *not* characteristic of pronator syndrome. Symptoms typically develop insidiously and are often present for months before diagnosis. Occasionally symptoms appear more abruptly after a specific sprain or episode of heavy forearm use or focal trauma (Hartz, Linscheid, Gramse & Daube, 1981). Examples include development of the syndrome after rock climbing or tuning a harp (Hochholzer, Krause & Heuk, 1993; Lederman, 1994). Pronator syndrome is much rarer than carpal tunnel syndrome. Reported clinical series are relatively small (Morris & Peters, 1976; Johnson et al., 1979; Hartz et al., 1981; Gross & Jones, 1992). Male subjects are more commonly affected in some

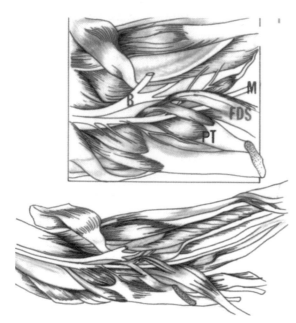

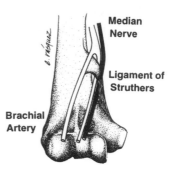

Figure 17-7. The supracondylar spur of Struthers and its associated ligament are anomalies that, when present, sometimes compress the median nerve.

Figure 17-5. In this patient, the median nerve (M) is crossed by two arches, one formed by the flexor digitorum superficialis (FDS) and the other formed by the superficial head of pronator teres (PT). B labels the brachial artery. Left arm; distal is toward the right. Other patients have no crossing arch or a single arch. (Reproduced with permission from AL Dellon, SE Mackinnon. Musculoaponeurotic variations along the course of the median nerve in the proximal forearm. J. Hand Surg. 1987;12B:359–63.)

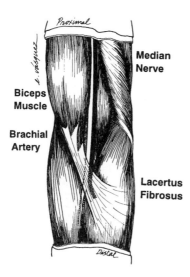

Figure 17-6. The lacertus fibrosus, a fascial band that stretches between the biceps tendon and the proximal ulna, potentially compresses the median nerve.

series, whereas female subjects predominate in others. Typically the dominant arm is symptomatic, but bilateral cases occur. At times, anomalous configuration of pronator teres or anomalous course of the median nerve appears to contribute to development of compression (Lacey & Soldatis, 1993; Tulwa, Limb & Brown, 1994).

Most reports of pronator syndrome are of sporadic cases. In contrast, a survey of Swedish women who worked at milking machines diagnosed pronator syndrome in 23 cases (Stål, Hagert & Moritz, 1998). The diagnoses were based on clinical findings of forearm tenderness and muscle weakness, but electrodiagnostic tests were not done on these patients.

Instances of median nerve compression by lacertus fibrosus seem to be quite rare (Laha, Lunsford & Dujovny, 1978; Gessini, Jandolo, Pietrangeli & Bove, 1980; Gessini, Jandolo & Pietrangeli, 1983; Swiggett & Ruby, 1986). In one case, the role of the lacertus fibrosus in compressing the nerve was supported by intraoperative short segment nerve conduction studies (Nelson, Goodheart, Salotto & Tibbs, 1994).

Median nerve entrapment by the ligament of Struthers or by the supracondylar process of the humerus is much rarer than entrapment by the pronator muscle (Barnard & McCoy, 1946; Winkelman, 1980; Rofes-Capo, Ramirez-Ruiz, Bordas-Sales, Gomez-Bonfills & Lopez-de-Vega, 1981; Gessini et al., 1983; Suranyi, 1983; Ivins, 1996; Sener, Takka & Cila, 1998). Case reports show that compression by Struthers' ligament can occur in children, bilaterally, or in the absence of a supracondylar process (Smith & Fisher, 1973; al-Qattan & Husband, 1991; Schrader & Reina, 1994; Murali, Ashcroft & Scotland, 1995; Straub, 1997; Aydinlioglu, Cirak, Akpinar, Tosun & Dogan, 2000). The entrapment may first become symptomatic after fracture of the supracondylar process (al-Naib, 1994; Sener et al., 1998). These entrapments along the distal humerus may be clinically suspected and distinguished from entrapments in the antecubital space or proximal forearm if there is concomitant arterial compression, if symptoms are increased with elbow flexion or extension with the arm supinated, or if a supracondylar process is palpable or is visible on humeral radiographs (Symeonides, 1972; Bilge, Yalaman, Bilge, Çokneseli & Barut, 1990; Aydinlioglu et al., 2000). The process is best visualized with oblique radiographs of the humerus (Ivins, 1996). Rarely, the ulnar nerve may also be compressed by the supracondylar process (Thomsen, 1977; Mittal & Gupta, 1978). In many cases, a clinical localization of the site of median nerve compression is impossible until the course of the nerve is surgically explored.

Physical Examination Findings

The clue to the diagnosis of pronator syndrome on physical examination is abnormal findings on palpation of the ventral forearm over the pronator teres. This muscle originates at or proximal to the medial epicondyle and crosses to the proximal forearm at about a 45-degree angle to insert on the radius 7 to 10 cm distal to the lateral epicondyle. The muscle may feel firm, tender, or enlarged. Hartz and colleagues (1981) found tenderness at this point in 37 of 39 patients. The proximal forearm at the level of the pronator teres may be visibly enlarged. If the lacertus fibrosus is responsible for the compression, it may create a depressed contour in the antecubital space. Some patients also note tenderness over the thenar eminence (Seyffarth, 1951). A Tinel's sign is elicited over the median nerve in the proximal forearm in approximately one-half of the cases (Hartz et al., 1981; Werner, Rosén & Thorngren, 1985). A positive Phalen's wrist flexion test can be a misleading finding (Hartz et al., 1981).

In the larger series of pronator syndrome collected by orthopedists and hand surgeons, objective sensory loss is usually absent and motor impairment in the median distribution is subtle or absent (Johnson et al., 1979; Hartz et al., 1981). A smaller series from a neurology group found muscle weakness and sensory loss in most patients with the diagnosis (Morris & Peters, 1976). Did the neurologist do a more thorough neurologic examination? Did the orthopedists overdiagnose the syndrome? Did the neurologists not make the diagnosis until the syndrome was more advanced? The third hypothesis could explain at least part of the discrepancy; In chronic compressive neuropathies, the expected pattern is for intermittent pain and paresthesias to precede objective neurologic deficit. The second hypothesis also merits consideration; there is no standard test to prove the diagnosis, and distinguishing mild cases of pronator syndrome from other causes of forearm pain is challenging.

On rare occasions, *focal dystonia*, manifest as involuntary hand posturing, induced or increased by action, has been reported in patients with purported proximal median neuropathy (Scherokman, Husain, Cuetter, Jabbari & Maniglia, 1986).

Provocative Tests

A number of provocative tests are proposed to localize median compression in the forearm (Figure 17-8) (Spinner, 1980):

1. When forearm pain and hand paresthesias are increased with resisted pronation or with elbow extension with the forearm pronated, the entrapment is probably at the level of the pronator teres.
2. When forearm pain and hand paresthesias are increased by resisted flexion of the proximal interphalangeal joint of the middle finger, entrapment at the arch formed by flexor digitorum superficialis is the favored diagnosis.
3. When forearm pain and hand paresthesias are increased by maintaining elbow flexion against resistance with the forearm supinated, the expected level of entrapment is at the lacertus fibrosus or at Struthers' ligament.
4. When forearm pain and hand paresthesias are increased by maintaining elbow extension against resistance with the forearm supinated, the level of entrapment can be anywhere from Struthers' ligament to the arch of flexor digito-

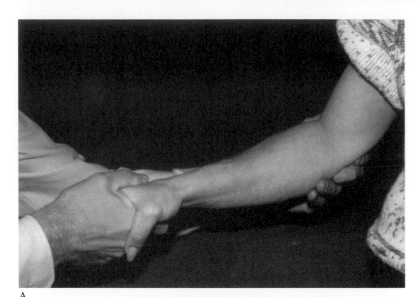

A

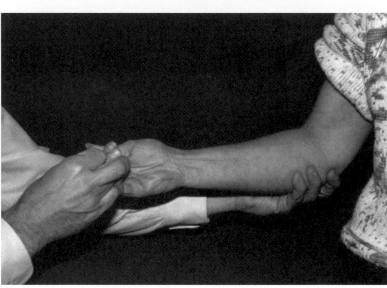

B

Figure 17-8. Spinner (1980) recommended three provocative tests for median nerve entrapment in the forearm: resisted pronation (**A**), resisted flexion of the proximal interphalangeal joint of the middle finger (**B**), and sustained elbow flexion with forearm supinated (**C**).

rum superficialis (Goldner, 1984; Aydinlioglu et al., 2000).

5. For the pronator compression test, the examiner's thumb presses firmly on the patient's volar forearm just proximal and lateral to the edge of pronator teres (Gainor, 1990; Olehnik, Manske & Szerzinski, 1994). The test is positive if the patient describes pain and paresthesias in the median nerve distribution after 30 seconds or less of compression. Falsely localizing positive responses can occur in patients with carpal tunnel syndrome (Rayhack, 1989).

6. In some patients, symptoms are reproduced by full passive supination of the forearm (Olehnik et al., 1994).

These are nerve compression postures and should be maintained for a standardized length of time, such as 1 minute. The specificity and sensitivity of the test vary depending on the test duration. The specificity of each test is improved if elicitation of paresthesias in the median cutaneous distribution, rather than pain alone, is used as the criterion for a positive test. In 39 patients reported

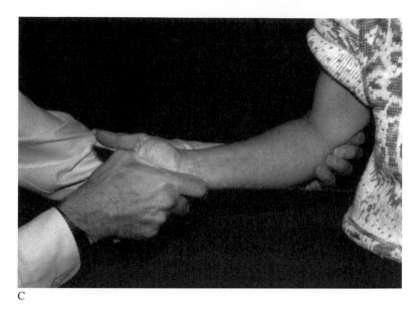

C

by Hartz and colleagues (1981), 30 had paresthesias provoked by test 1 in the previous list and 14 had paresthesias provoked by test 2. The correlation between which test was positive and the surgically identified site of entrapment was imperfect. There are few data available on the false-positive rates for these provocative tests. Extrapolating from the false-positive incidence of Phalen's wrist flexion test in carpal tunnel syndrome, from the high incidence of potential sites of median nerve compression in the asymptomatic forearm, and from the possibility that unrelated musculoskeletal pains can confuse the results, abundant false-positive results on these forearm provocative tests should be anticipated (Dellon, 1986; Gellman, Gelberman, Tan & Botte, 1986).

Electrodiagnosis

Median nerve conduction studies are sometimes abnormal in patients with median nerve entrapment in the forearm. Median motor conduction velocity to the abductor pollicis brevis may be slowed in the forearm with a normal distal motor latency (Morris & Peters, 1976). Median motor latency between the antecubital space and flexor digitorum profundus or flexor digitorum superficialis may be prolonged, or median sensory conduction may be slowed across the site of entrapment (Buchthal, Rosenfalck & Trojaborg,

1974). All 18 patients reported by Buchthal and colleagues and Morris and Peters had deteriorated to the stage of clinical weakness in median-innervated muscles; two-thirds of the patients showed an abnormality in motor or sensory median nerve conduction, but each test was not done in every patient. In comparison, the incidence of median nerve conduction abnormalities in the larger clinical series was quite low, and abnormalities, when present, were usually not of value in localizing the site of compression; even intraoperative median nerve conduction studies usually failed to demonstrate localized slowing of nerve conduction (Johnson et al., 1979; Hartz et al., 1981). Among 14 patients who had proximal median neuropathy confirmed by EMG needle examination, only five had abnormal median motor or sensory conduction (Gross & Jones, 1992).

The sensitivity of nerve conduction tests perhaps improves by combining them with provocative maneuvers (Werner et al., 1985). In nine patients with a clinical diagnosis of pronator syndrome, routine median motor nerve conduction to the thenar eminence was normal, but three of the patients showed abnormalities when nerve conduction was repeated during isometric forearm pronation. In one patient the abnormality was a 40% drop in the compound muscle action potential amplitude and a 0.5-msec increase in the motor latency with antecubital median nerve stimulation.

In two patients the change was a 20% drop in the compound muscle action potential amplitude. In these three patients the abnormalities were reversed after surgical decompression.

In a minority of patients, EMG needle examination shows neuropathic changes in median-innervated hand or forearm muscles (Buchthal et al., 1974; Hartz et al., 1981; Werner et al., 1985). Although the median nerve branches to pronator teres usually leave the nerve before its site of entrapment by the pronator, some branching to pronator teres may occur distal to the entrapment, and neuropathic changes on EMG of pronator teres are seen on rare occasions in pronator syndrome (Aiken & Moritz, 1987). On occasion, nerve branches to flexor carpi radialis and flexor digitorum superficialis leave the median nerve proximal to the site of entrapment, in which case these muscles are normal on EMG even though other median-innervated muscles are abnormal (Gessini, Jandolo & Pietrangeli, 1987).

Treatment

Initial nonsurgical therapy traditionally includes avoiding those arm activities that induce symptoms, anti-inflammatory medication, physical therapy, or forearm immobilization. Local steroid infiltration of the pronator teres might relieve symptoms even if objective neurologic abnormalities are present (Morris & Peters, 1976).

If surgery is undertaken, the course of the median nerve through the antecubital space from Struthers' ligament to the flexor digitorum superficialis must be explored. To minimize the risk of hypertrophic postoperative scarring in the antecubital fossa, varied skin incisions are advocated (Mackinnon & Dellon, 1988; Eversmann, 1992; Gainor, 1993; Tsai & Syed, 1994). Clinical findings do not reliably localize the exact site of entrapment, and multiple sites of entrapment may be present. The most optimistic view of surgery is provided by Johnson and colleagues (1979), who claim only four failures in 51 operations. They, however, do not precisely describe their follow-up criteria.

In the Mayo Clinic series of 36 operations, eight patients had complete relief of symptoms; 20 patients had good relief of symptoms to the extent that they could return to previous activities;

five patients had some relief of symptoms but persistence of some residual disability; and three patients did not improve (Hartz et al., 1981). Another experience after 39 operations for presumed pronator syndrome reported 10 patients cured, 20 patients improved, and nine patients unimproved (Olehnik et al., 1994). Postoperative immobilization for 2 to 3 weeks followed by gradual mobilization and strengthening exercises with 6 weeks of avoidance of strenuous arm use probably contributed to the improvement. These surgical series are uncontrolled; the therapeutic value of the postoperative protocol alone without surgery is unknown.

The course of recovery after nerve decompression depends on the severity of median nerve injury. If there has been no axonal interruption, both positive and negative sensorimotor symptoms should resolve quickly, and neurologic function should recover within a few weeks (Eversmann, 1986). Persistent forearm pain should prompt reconsideration of the differential diagnosis. Incomplete exploration and decompression of the nerve should be considered; for example, if the surgical scar does not extend above the elbow flexion crease, inadequate evaluation for Struthers' ligament would be suspected. An alternative or additional site of nerve entrapment must be considered; for example, carpal tunnel syndrome may co-exist with pronator syndrome. Persistent forearm pain associated with forearm paresthesias or sensory loss raises the possibility of injury to the lateral antebrachial cutaneous nerve at the time of surgery.

Differential Diagnosis

In addition to median nerve compression, the differential diagnosis of median neuropathies in the arm, antecubital space, and forearm can be subdivided as follows.

Traumatic Median Neuropathies

Acute *median nerve traumatic transection* may occur anywhere along the course of the nerve. In the upper arm, trauma that transects the median nerve usually injures the ulnar nerve as well. In the distal few centimeters of the upper arm, the median and ulnar nerves are separated as the ulnar nerve courses posteriorly and medially to run behind the medial epicondyle while the median nerve pursues its antecubital course. Isolated median nerve laceration has been reported 6 cm or less above the medial epicondyle (Boswick & Stromberg, 1967). The brachial artery is often transected with the same injury. Primary nerve repair is advisable where possible (Birch & Raji, 1991). Recovery of protective hand sensation may take 18 to 26 months. Motor recovery in median forearm muscles may begin within 6 to 12 months. Thenar motor recovery is less likely to occur and may require tendon transfer surgery to reconstitute thumb opposition.

An acute median injury in the antecubital area can occur, particularly in children, after *elbow dislocations* or their reduction (Linscheid & Wheeler, 1965). The ulnar nerve is injured more frequently than the median; occasionally, both are injured (Linscheid & Wheeler, 1965). Rarely, the median nerve is transected (Rana, Kenwright, Taylor & Rushworth, 1974). Distinguishing between nerve entrapment and traction injury is challenging. There are at least four different mechanisms of entrapment (Figure 17-9) (Hallett, 1981; al-Qattan, Zuker & Weinberg, 1994). Peripheral nerve function of patients being treated for elbow dislocation should be assessed before and after reduction. If median nerve function deteriorates after reduction, acute surgical nerve release is indicated (Floyd, Gebhardt & Emans, 1987; Rao & Crawford, 1995). When patients present with persistent median nerve dysfunction weeks or months after elbow dislocation, clues to nerve entrapment include loss of elbow range of motion and a history of accompanying fracture of the medial epicondyle. When the nerve is entrapped in the medial epicondylar fracture, anteroposterior elbow radiographs taken months after the injury sometimes show a depression in the cortical bone on the ulnar side of the distal humeral metaphysis (Matev, 1976). If diagnosis and surgical decompression are delayed, the median nerve deficit can become irreversible (Holmes, Skolnick & Hall, 1979; Boe & Holst-Nielsen, 1987; al-Qattan et al., 1994).

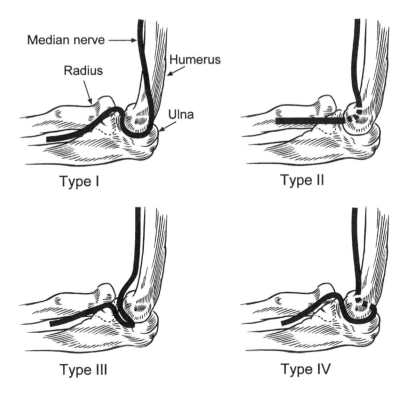

Figure 17-9. Mechanism of median nerve entrapment after elbow dislocations. The dotted lines indicate areas where the median nerve is running through healed epicondylar fracture. (Reprinted with permission from MM al-Qattan, RM Zuker, MJ Weinberg. Type 4 median nerve entrapment after elbow dislocation. J. Hand Surg. 1994;19B: 613–15.)

Injury to the anterior interosseous nerve, the most common nerve injury accompanying *supracondylar humeral fractures*, has been mentioned previously. More extensive median nerve injuries can also occur with this fracture (Lipscomb & Burleson, 1955; Jones & Louis, 1980; McGraw, Akbarnia, Hanel, Keppler & Burdge, 1986; Culp, Osterman, Davidson, Skirven & Bora, 1990). Of 210 children who had supracondylar humeral fractures, 34 sustained median nerve injuries, usually limited to the anterior interosseous branch; however, median sensory neuropathy or even complete median neuropathy can occur (Lyons, Quinn & Stanitski, 2000). One partial anterior interosseous nerve palsy and four median nerve palsies, all in children, were noted in a series of 465 supracondylar fractures of the humerus (Galbraith & McCullough, 1979). In other series, the incidence of any nerve injury with this fracture has been 10% to 15% (Cramer, Green & Devito, 1993; Dormans, Squillante & Sharf, 1995). The radial or ulnar nerves and the brachial artery can be injured concomitantly. The risk of nerve injury is highest when there is lack of cortical contact between the distal and proximal fragments (type III fractures), especially after an extension injury with posterolateral displacement of the distal humerus (Campbell, Waters, Emans, Kasser & Millis, 1995). For example, in one series of children, all those who had median nerve injuries experienced displacement exceeding 90% of the diameter of the humeral shaft, and the probability of nerve injury was high if the displacement was 150% of the diameter (Kiyoshige, 1999). If the brachial artery is compromised by the injury, emergent surgical exploration of the neurovascular bundle is often necessary (Karlsson, Thorsteinsson, Thorleifsson & Arnason, 1986). If circulation is intact but the median nerve is injured, some patients show gradual recovery from neurapraxic injury, and others require delayed nerve exploration for neurolysis or secondary nerve repair.

The median nerve can be injured at the time of *fracture of the humeral supracondylar process* (Spinner, Lins, Jacobson & Nunley, 1994). Delayed effects of this fracture have been discussed previously in regard to compression at Struthers' ligament. Median nerve injury after more proximal humeral fractures is unusual

(Blom & Dahlback, 1970; Apergis et al., 2000). A rare site of traumatic median neuropathy is at the level of mid-humerus associated with greenstick humeral fracture. The median neuropathy may worsen as the fracture heals, reflecting nerve entrapment in fracture callus (Macnicol, 1978).

After forearm injury of various types, patients may develop a *compartment syndrome* characterized by increased pressure in the fascial compartment of the volar forearm (Mubarak & Hargens, 1981). If left untreated, Volkmann's contracture may develop with dysfunction arising both from direct muscle necrosis and from nerve damage. The median, ulnar, and radial nerves may be injured in forearm compartment syndromes, but the median nerve is the most vulnerable. The nerve can be injured through direct nerve trauma, from focal compression or perineural scarring, or from nerve ischemia secondary to the high compartment pressure (Holmes, Highet & Seddon, 1944; Moberg, 1960). If the patient is treated with prompt decompressive fasciotomy and fracture stabilization, the prognosis for median nerve recovery is good (Brostrom, Stark & Svartengren, 1990).

A few case reports describe median nerve injury after *greenstick fracture of the proximal ulna or radius*. The median nerve can be progressively entrapped at the fracture site as callus develops or even partially transected (Nunley & Urbaniak, 1980; Huang, Pun & Coleman, 1998; Proubasta, De Sena & Caceres, 1999). Forearm radiographs sometimes show a bone spur or bone canal at the site of nerve entrapment (al-Qattan, Clarke & Zimmer, 1994). Median neuropathy can also be entrapped in Monteggia ulnar fractures (Watson & Singer, 1994).

Rarer Median Neuropathies of the Forearm

Case reports document a variety of unusual causes of median nerve compression in the forearm or antecubital space. A persistent median artery might compress the median nerve in the forearm (Gainor & Jeffries, 1987; Jones & Ming, 1988). A partial tear of the distal biceps brachii tendon resulted in a swollen synovial bursa that compressed the median nerve in the proximal forearm (Foxworthy & Kinninmonth, 1992). A child born with congenital ring constrictions can suffer nerve entrapments from the remnants of the constricting rings (Marlow, Jarratt & Hosking, 1981; Uchida & Sugioka, 1991). The median and ulnar nerves were compressed by synovial osteochondromatosis of the elbow; pure ulnar neuropathy is more common with this condition (Nogueira, Alcelay, Pena, Sarasua & Madrigal, 1999).

Patients may develop median neuropathy after placement of forearm vascular shunts for hemodialysis; in some patients the neuropathy appears to be on an ischemic basis as demonstrated by resolution of symptoms when the shunt remains in place but is closed (Matolo, Kastagir, Stevens, Chrysanthakopolulos, Weaver & Klinkman, 1971). Other patients develop scarring around the shunt that compresses the median nerve (Zamora, Rose, Rosario & Noon, 1986). A brachial pseudoaneurysm may develop at the antecubital end of the shunt and cause nerve compression (Ergungor, Kars & Yalin, 1989).

In anticoagulated patients, acute median neuropathy can develop from antecubital hematomas after brachial arterial puncture for blood gas testing or even after repeated venipuncture (Macon & Futrell, 1973; Luce, Futrell, Wilgis & Hoopes, 1976; Blankenship, 1991). These patients often require urgent surgical decompression. Another potential mechanism for median nerve compression in anticoagulated patients is an acute syndrome of the biceps brachii compartment after rupture of the biceps tendon (McHale, Geissele & Perlik, 1991). Patients with hemophilia can develop median neuropathy from intraneural hematomas, from external compression by hematomas, or from compartment syndrome due to soft tissue or intramuscular bleeding (Ehrmann, Lechner, Mamoli, Novotny & Kow, 1981; Dumontier, Sautet, Man, Bennani & Apoil, 1994).

The median nerve is the nerve most commonly injured by electric burns of the arm (DiVincenti, Moncrief & Pruitt, 1969; Solem, Fischer & Strate, 1977). Onset of the neuropathy is sometimes delayed until weeks after the electric shock (Parano, Uncini, Incorpora, Pavone & Trifiletti, 1996).

The median basilic vein in the antecubital space crosses just anterior to the median nerve (Pask & Robson, 1954). Thrombophlebitis in this vein can cause a secondary median neuropathy (Oh & Kim, 1967). A venous varix in the antecubital space can compress the nerve (Zikel, Davis, Auger & Cherry, 1997). The median nerve can be damaged if medication that is intended for intravenous administration through this vein is inadvertently injected into the nerve (Seddon, 1972; Hudson, Kline & Gentili, 1980). Even a misdirected venipuncture can injure the median nerve as it crosses the antecubital region (Pradhan & Gupta, 1995).

Median neuropathy is a rare complication of elbow arthroscopy (Andrews & Carson, 1985; Lynch, Meyers, Whipple & Caspari, 1986). The cases reported have been transient palsies, one attributed to extravasation of local anesthetic and one attributed to nerve compression by the joint capsule when it was inflated for the procedure.

A report of an unusual case describes median nerve compression by non-Hodgkin's lymphoma in supratrochlear lymph nodes near the medial epicondyle (Desta, O'Shaughnessy & Milling, 1994). Proximal median mononeuropathy can develop acutely in sickle cell crisis (Shields, Harris & Clark, 1991). Bilateral median neuropathy has been reported complicating sarcoidosis (Kömpf, Neundörfer, Kayser-Gatchalian, Meyer-Wahl & Ranft, 1976).

Median nerve compression neuropathy may result from improper body positioning during anesthesia or from prolonged arm constriction by a tourniquet (Parks, 1973; Bolton & McFarlane, 1978; Munin, Balu, & Sotereanos, 1995). The pathology of tourniquet paralysis is discussed in Chapter 12.

Median Neuropathy with Multiple Mononeuropathies

Vasculitis and other causes of focal nerve ischemia can cause median mononeuropathy, either in isolation or as part of mononeuritis multiplex (Figure 17-10). These ischemic neuropathies should be particularly suspected when focal lesions develop suddenly at sites other than common areas of nerve compression. In mononeuritis multiplex the first nerve affected is more likely to be in the legs than in the arms; nonetheless, eventual median nerve involvement is common. For example, among 12 patients with nonsystemic vasculitic mononeuritis multiplex, six had median neuropathies (Dyck, Benstead, Conn, Stevens, Windebank & Low, 1987). In another series, 26%

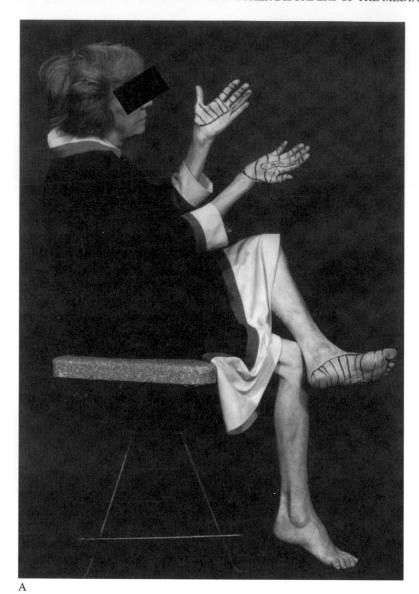

Figure 17-10. (A) Areas of sensory deficit in one patient with mononeuritis multiplex, including the median, ulnar, and posterior tibial nerves. (B) Electron micrograph of this patient's biopsied nerve. Note the cellular exudate adjacent to epineurial blood vessel and eosinophils at the corner. The clinical diagnosis was asthma and allergic granulomatosis and angiitis (Churg-Strauss syndrome).

A

of patients with mononeuritis multiplex had sensory or motor deficits in the median nerve distribution (Hellmann, Laing, Petri, Whiting-O'Keefe & Parry, 1988). The mechanism of median neuropathy is usually nerve ischemia due to inflammation of epineurial arterioles. However, in an unusual case, a patient who had vasculitis and median and ulnar neuropathies, pronator teres biopsy evidence of intramuscular vasculitis and magnetic resonance imaging showed that the pronator teres was swollen, probably compressing the median nerve (Asami, Takayama & Hotokebuchi, 1999).

A patient with idiopathic thrombocytopenic purpura developed mononeuropathies of multiple nerves, including the median; at autopsy multiple intraneural hemorrhages were found (Greenberg & Sonoda, 1991). Some other causes of multiple mononeuropathies such as diabetes, leprosy, and hereditary liability to pressure palsies are discussed in Chapter 5 and 6.

Median Neuropathies at Other Sites

Carpal tunnel syndrome is a much more common cause of forearm pain than is pronator syndrome.

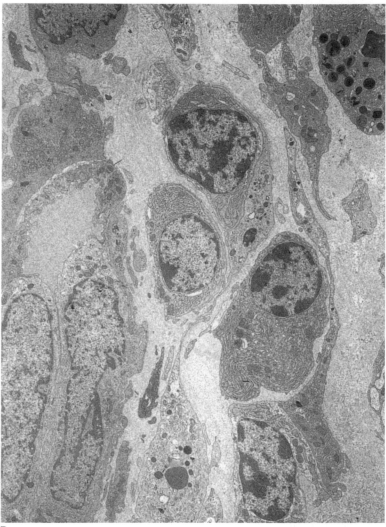

B

Criteria favoring pronator syndrome are focal tenderness over the pronator muscle, weakness of forearm muscles, and diurnal persistence of pain. In theory, proximal median neuropathies should have sensory changes not only in the fingers, but also over the thenar eminence, because the recurrent palmar sensory branch leaves the median nerve proximal to the carpal tunnel; in practice this sensory distinction is rarely reliable. Criteria favoring carpal tunnel syndrome are a typical nocturnal or rest-induced pattern of sensory symptoms; motor findings, when present, limited to thenar muscles and lumbricals; and sensory changes, when present, limited to digital nerves. In patients with pronator syndrome, an initial erroneous diagnosis of carpal tunnel syndrome is common; at times both conditions co-exist. The rare median neuropathies originating in the axilla or upper arm are discussed later in this chapter.

Other Neuropathic Syndromes of the Forearm

Compression of the lateral antebrachial cutaneous nerve in the antecubital space presents with forearm pain and antecubital tenderness (Nunley & Howson, 1989). The tenderness in a typical case is located lateral to the biceps tendon in the antecubital space rather than over the pronator muscle. Paresthesias and sensory signs on examination are localized to the lateral forearm, rather than to the hand, but the sensory territory of the anterior branch of the nerve can overlap the territory of the median palmar cutaneous nerve. Motor deficit is absent. Elbow extension can be limited by pain when the forearm is pronated, a finding potentially confused with a positive provocative test for pronator syndrome.

Other neuropathic processes that merit consideration include ulnar neuropathy, radial or posterior interosseous neuropathy, brachial plexopathies, and cervical radiculopathy. Ulnar or radial neuropathies should be distinguishable by their specific patterns of motor and sensory impairment. Tinel's sign may be localized over the course of the appropriate nerve. Brachial plexopathies, when predominantly affecting the lateral cord of the brachial plexus, may lead to diagnostic difficulty. Isolated disease of this part of the plexus is rare.

The problem of distinguishing neuralgic amyotrophy from median neuropathy is discussed previously in regard to the anterior interosseous nerve. A 36-year-old woman described by Swiggett and Ruby (1986) exemplifies the difficulty of making this distinction. She had sudden onset of pain followed over 10 days by weakness in both median and ulnar muscles and no sensory changes. The authors present this patient as an example of median nerve compression by the lacertus fibrosus, but neuralgic amyotrophy should be considered in the differential diagnosis based on the timing of symptoms and the involvement of more than one nerve.

Cervical radiculopathy presents at times with forearm pain, particularly when the sixth or seventh cervical roots are implicated. Clues favoring cervical radiculopathy include neck pain, reproduction of forearm pain with neck movements ("Spurling's sign"), sensory signs on the dorsum of the hand beyond the distribution of the median nerve, and appropriate changes in tendon reflexes. When muscle weakness is present, the distinction should be relatively easy: Radiculopathic weakness of median-innervated forearm muscles is almost invariably accompanied by triceps weakness because these muscles receive innervation from both the sixth and seventh cervical roots.

Nonneuropathic Syndromes of the Forearm

Focal tenderness in the forearm without focal neurologic dysfunction introduces a differential diagnosis of a variety of localized soft tissue problems. The localization of tenderness should allow separation of lateral epicondylitis from focal sprain or strain of the pronator teres or forearm flexor muscles. A greater diagnostic challenge is separating pronator syndrome from ventral forearm musculoligamentous pains. If *pronator syndrome* is defined as median neuropathy caused by compression of the nerve at the level of the pronator teres, the diagnosis must require some evidence of median nerve dysfunction such as weakness, sensory change, or reproduction of cutaneous parenthetic symptoms by provocative tests.

Median Neuropathy in the Axilla

Infraclavicular nerve compression isolated to the median nerve is extremely rare. Reported causes include nerve compression by aberrant axillary arch muscles, vascular anomalies, thickening of the deltopectoral fascia, or a single case of a large infraclavicular lipoma (Mayfield, 1970; Spinner, 1976, 1980; Weinzweig & Browne, 1988). The clinical picture includes weakness or sensory changes in the median distribution and exacerbation of neurologic findings by shoulder abduction or external rotation. Spinner (1980) has emphasized that sensation may be spared and paralysis may be partial, involving particularly forearm muscles. This pattern reflects preferential damage of nerve fibers from the lateral cord of the brachial plexus.

Cases of median nerve compression in the axilla are so unusual that reported cases deserve critical reading. For example, Spinner (1976) describes a case in which paralysis was isolated to the right flexor pollicis longus. The patient was a 25-year-old woman who presented with acute onset of severe right shoulder pain 10 days preceding the weakness. She had tenderness and a Tinel's sign over the neurovascular bundle at the level of the coracoid process, distinguishing the case from an anterior interosseous nerve palsy. When her axilla was surgically explored, the median nerve was penetrated by an anomalous posterior circumflex artery and vein. These vessels were ligated. Postoperatively, pain was quickly relieved, but weakness took 4 months to resolve. The case was interpreted as an unusual entrapment of the median nerve in the axilla caused by the vascular anomaly. We present an alternative pathogenic hypothesis: The sudden onset, prominence of pain, and rapid development of severe weakness are strongly suggestive of neuralgic amyotrophy. The course of clinical recovery, with pain clearing relatively quickly, but motor recovery taking many months, is also a feature of neuralgic amyotrophy. Neurovascular anomalies of the median nerve in relation to brachial vessels occur asymptomatically in 8% of the population (Miller, 1939).

Acute median neuropathy can evolve over hours or a few days after axillary or brachial arteriography or axillary block anesthesia (Stall, van Voorthuisen & van Dijk, 1966; Carroll & Wilkins, 1970; Molnar & Paul, 1972; Westcott & Taylor, 1972; Lyon, Hansen & Mygind, 1975; O'Keefe, 1980; Groh, Gainor, Jeffries, Brown & Eggers, 1990; Regnard, Soichot & Ringuier, 1990; Stark, 1996; Kennedy, Grocott, Schwartz, Modarres, Scott & Schon, 1997; Colville & Colin, 1998; Busono & Wilbourn, 1999). Possible mechanisms include direct nerve trauma or injection, ischemia, or hematoma or pseudoaneurysm formation in the neurovascular bundle that includes the axillary or brachial artery and median nerve. The neuropathy can be limited to the median nerve, or the radial, ulnar, or musculocutaneous nerves, in close proximity to the median nerve at this level, and can also be injured.

An acute compressive neuropathy, isolated to the proximal median nerve, can occur as a "sleep" palsy, but it is much rarer than the well-known radial nerve "Saturday night" palsy. In Marinacci's (1967) report of 67 patients with "pressure neuropathy from 'hanging arm,'" only nine patients had neuropathy limited to the median nerve. The typical patients awaken from sleep with paralysis including all median-innervated muscles and with sensory changes in the median distribution (Roth, Ludy & Egloff-Baer, 1982). There is often a history of heavy alcohol use the previous night. Recovery occurs either quickly or over the course of many months. Nerve conduction studies sometimes show conduction block in the median nerve just distal to the anterior border of the axilla formed by the pectoralis muscle. The ulnar nerve may be clinically spared, and ulnar motor nerve conduction may confirm no conduction block with stimulation at Erb's point. The

median nerve compression occurs in the proximal arm, after the median and ulnar nerves separate, while the median nerve is in the brachial canal of the arm.

On rare occasion the median nerve may be injured by dislocations of the shoulder or fractures of the proximal humerus (Blom & Dahlback, 1970). Joint and bone injuries at this level are much more likely to affect the axillary rather than the median nerve.

The median nerve may be injured by inadvertent injection of local anesthetic into the nerve during attempted nerve block in the axilla (Hudson, 1987).

Summary

Familiarity with the proximal median neuropathies, uncommon though they are, is important. They are included in the differential diagnosis of cases presenting with arm pain, weakness, or sensory change. Their diagnosis and management requires knowledge of median nerve anatomy and careful attention to details of clinical presentation.

References

Aiken BM, Moritz MJ. A typical electromyographic findings in pronator teres syndrome. Arch. Phys. Med. Rehabil. 1987; 68:173–75.

Albanese S, Buterbaugh G, Palmer AK, Lubicky JP, Yuan HA. Incomplete anterior interosseous nerve palsy following spinal surgery. A report of two cases. Spine 1986;11: 1037–38.

al-Naib I. Humeral supracondylar spur and Struthers' ligament. A rare cause of neurovascular entrapment in the upper limb. Int. Orthop. 1994;18:393–94.

al-Qattan MM. Gantzer's muscle. J. Hand Surg. 1996;21B:269–70.

al-Qattan MM. Anatomical classification of sites of compression of the palmar cutaneous branch of the median nerve. J. Hand Surg. 1997;22B:48–49.

al-Qattan MM, Clarke HM, Zimmer P. Radiological signs of entrapment of the median nerve in forearm shaft fractures. J. Hand Surg. 1994;19B:713–19.

al-Qattan MM, Husband JB. Median nerve compression by the supracondylar process: a case report. J. Hand Surg. 1991; 16B:101–3.

al-Qattan MM, Manktelow RT, Murray KA. An unusual complication of surgical decompression of partial anterior interosseous nerve syndrome. Can. J. Plast. Surg. 1994; 2:93–94.

al-Qattan MM, Robertson GA. Entrapment neuropathy of the palmar cutaneous nerve within its tunnel. J. Hand Surg. 1993;18B:465–66.

al-Qattan MM, Zuker RM, Weinberg MJ. Type 4 median nerve entrapment after elbow dislocation. J. Hand Surg. 1994; 19B:613–15.

Andrews JR, Carson WG. Arthroscopy of the elbow. Arthroscopy 1985;1:97–107.

Apergis E, Aktipis D, Giota A, Kastanis G, Nteimentes G, Papanikolaou A. Median nerve palsy after humeral shaft fracture: case report. J. Trauma 1998;45:825–26.

Asami A, Takayama G, Hotokebuchi T. Pronator teres syndrome associated with mononeuritis multiplex in polyarteritis nodosa. Hand Surg. 1999;4:189–92.

Ashworth NL, Marshall SC, Classen DA. Anterior interosseous nerve syndrome presenting with pronator teres weakness: a case report. Muscle Nerve 1997;20:1591–94.

Aydinlioglu A, Cirak B, Akpinar F, Tosun N, Dogan A. Bilateral median nerve compression at the level of Struthers' ligament. Case report. J. Neurosurg. 2000;92:693–96.

Barnard LB, McCoy SM. The supracondyloid process of the humerus. J. Bone Joint Surg. 1946;28:845–50.

Baruch A, Hass A. Anomaly of the median nerve. J. Hand Surg. 1977;2:331–32.

Bertolotto M, Rosenberg I, Parodi RC, Perrone R, Gentile S, Rollandi GA, Succi S. Case report: fibroma of tendon sheath in the distal forearm with associated median nerve neuropathy: US, CT and MR appearances. Clin. Radiol. 1996;51:370–72.

Beverly MC, Fearn CB. Anterior interosseous nerve palsy and dislocation of the elbow. Injury 1984;16:126–28.

Bilge T, Yalaman O, Bilge S, Çokneseli B, Barut S. Entrapment neuropathy of the median nerve at the level of the ligament of Struthers. Neurosurgery 1990;27:787–89.

Binfield PM, Sott-Miknas A, Good CJ. Median nerve compression associated with displaced Salter-Harris type II distal radial epiphyseal fracture. Injury 1998;29:93–94.

Birch R, Bonney G, Wynn Parry CB. Surgical Disorders of the Peripheral Nerves. Edinburgh, UK: Churchill Livingstone, 1998.

Birch R, Raji ARM. Repair of median and ulnar nerves. J. Bone Joint Surg. 1991;73B:154–57.

Blankenship JC. Median and ulnar neuropathy after streptokinase infusion. Heart Lung 1991;20:221–23.

Blom S, Dahlback LO. Nerve injuries in dislocations of the shoulder joint and fractures of the neck of the humerus: a clinical and electromyographic study. Acta Chir. Scand. 1970;136:461–66.

Boe S, Holst-Nielsen F. Intra-articular entrapment of the median nerve after dislocation of the elbow. J. Hand Surg. 1987;12B:356–58.

Bolton FB, McFarlane RM. Human pneumatic tourniquet paralysis. Neurology 1978;28:787–93.

Boswick JA, Stromberg Jr. WB. Isolated injury of the median nerve above the elbow. J. Bone Joint Surg. 1967;49A:653–58.

Boyes JH, Wilson JN, Smith JW. Flexor tendon ruptures of the forearm and hand. J. Bone Joint Surg. 1960;42A:637–46.

Brostrom LA, Stark A, Svartengren G. Acute compartment syndrome in forearm fractures. Acta Orthop. Scand. 1990; 61:50–53.

Buchthal F, Rosenfalck A, Trojaborg W. Electrophysiological findings in entrapment of the median nerve at wrist and elbow. J. Neurol. Neurosurg. Psychiatry 1974;37:340–60.

Buckmiller JF, Rickard TA. Isolated compression neuropathy of the palmar cutaneous branch of the median nerve. J. Hand Surg. 1987;12A:97–99.

Busono SJ, Wilbourn AJ. Iatrogenic proximal median neuropathy due to cardiac catheterization: clinical and electrodiagnostic aspects. Neurology 1999;52[Suppl 2]: A310.

Campbell CC, Waters PM, Emans JB, Kasser JR, Millis MB. Neurovascular injury and displacement in type III supracondylar humerus fractures. J. Pediatr. Orthop. 1995;15: 47–52.

Carroll SE, Wilkins WW. Two cases of brachial plexus injury following percutaneous arteriograms. Can. Med. Assoc. J. 1970;102:861–62.

Chang C-W, Lien I-N. Comparison of sensory nerve conduction in the palmar cutaneous branch and first digital branch of the median nerve: a new diagnostic method for carpal tunnel syndrome. Muscle Nerve 1991;14:1173–76.

Collins DN, Weber ER. Anterior interosseous nerve avulsion. Clin. Orthop. 1983;181:175–78.

Colville RJ, Colin JF. Median nerve palsy after high brachial angiography. J. R. Soc. Med. 1998;91:387.

Conway RR, Thomas R. Isolated complete denervation of the flexor pollicis longus. Arch. Phys. Med. Rehabil. 1990; 71:406–7.

Craft S, Currier DP, Nelson RM. Motor conduction of the anterior interosseous nerve. Phys. Ther. 1977;57:1143–47.

Cramer KE, Green NE, Devito DP. Incidence of anterior interosseous nerve palsy in supracondylar humerus fractures in children. J. Pediatr. Orthop. 1993;13:502–5.

Culp RW, Osterman AL, Davidson RS, Skirven T, Bora Jr. FW. Neural injuries associated with supracondylar fractures of the humerus in children. J. Bone Joint Surg. 1990; 72A:1211–14.

Dansereau JG, Cianciulli R. Carpal tunnel syndrome. Union Med. Can. 1968;97:326–31.

Dellon AL. Musculotendinous variations about the medial humeral epicondyle. J. Hand Surg. 1986;11B:175–81.

Dellon AL, Mackinnon SE, Daneshvar A. Terminal branch of anterior interosseous nerve as source of wrist pain. J. Hand Surg. 1984;9B:316–22.

De Smet L. Entrapment of the palmar cutaneous branch of the median nerve. J. Hand Surg. 1998;23B:115–16.

Desta K, O'Shaughnessy M, Milling MA. Non-Hodgkin's lymphoma presenting as median nerve compression in the arm. J. Hand Surg. 1994;19B:289–91.

DiVincenti FC, Moncrief JA, Pruitt Jr. BA. Electrical injuries: a review of 65 cases. J. Trauma 1969;9:497–507.

Dorin D, Mann RJ. Carpal tunnel syndrome associated with abnormal palmaris longus muscle. South. Med. J. 1984;77: 1210–11.

Dormans JP, Squillante R, Sharf H. Acute neurovascular complications with supracondylar humerus fractures in children. J. Hand Surg. 1995;20A:1–4.

Dumitru D, Walsh NE, Ramamurthy S. The premotor potential. Arch. Phys. Med. Rehabil. 1989;70:537–40.

Dumontier C, Sautet A, Man M, Bennani M, Apoil A. Entrapment and compartment syndromes of the upper limb in haemophilia. J. Hand Surg. 1994;19B:427–29.

Duncan GJ, Yospur G, Gomez-Garcia A, Lesavoy MA. Entrapment of the palmar cutaneous branch of the median nerve by a normal palmaris longus tendon. Ann. Plast. Surg. 1995;35:534–36.

Dunne JW, Prentice DA, Stewart-Wynne EG. Bilateral anterior interosseous nerve syndromes associated with cytomegalovirus infection. Muscle Nerve 1987;10:446–48.

Duteille F, Amara B, Dautel G, Merle M. Isolated palsy of the flexor pollicis longus in anterior interosseous nerve syndrome. Rev. Chir. Orthop. Reparatrice. Appar. Mot. 2000; 86:306–9.

Dyck PJ, Benstead TJ, Conn DL, Stevens JC, Windebank AJ, Low PA. Nonsystemic vasculitic neuropathy. Brain 1987; 110:843–54.

Ehrmann L, Lechner K, Mamoli B, Novotny C, Kow K. Peripheral nerve lesions in hemophilia. J. Neurol. 1981;225:175–82.

Engber WD, Keene JS. Anterior interosseous nerve palsy associated with a Monteggia fracture. A case report. Clin. Orthop. 1983;156:133–37.

England JD, Sumner AJ. Neuralgic amyotrophy: an increasingly diverse entity. Muscle Nerve 1987;10:60–68.

Enzenauer RJ, Nordstrom DM. Anterior interosseous nerve syndrome associated with forearm band treatment of lateral epicondylitis. Orthopedics 1991;14:788–90.

Ergungor MF, Kars HZ, Yalin R. Median neuralgia caused by brachial pseudoaneurysm. Neurosurg. 1989;24:924–25.

Eversmann WW Jr. Complications of Compression or Entrapment Neuropathies. In: Boswick Jr. JA, ed. Complications in Hand Surgery. Philadelphia: Saunders, 1986;99–115.

Eversmann Jr. WW. Proximal median nerve compression. Hand Clin. 1992;8:307–15.

Fearn CBd'A, Goodfellow JW. Anterior interosseous nerve palsy. J. Bone Joint Surg. 1965;47B:91–93.

Fernandez-Garcia S, Pi-Folguera J, Estallo-Matino F. Bifid median nerve compression due to a musculotendinous anomaly of FDS to the middle finger. J. Hand Surg. 1994; 19B:616–17.

Finelli PF. Anterior interosseous nerve syndrome following cutdown catheterization. Ann. Neurol. 1977;1:205–6.

Floyd WE, Gebhardt MC, Emans JB. Intra-articular entrapment of the median nerve after elbow dislocation in children. J. Hand Surg. 1987;12A:704–7.

Foxworthy M, Kinninmonth AW. Median nerve compression in the proximal forearm as a complication of partial rupture of the distal biceps brachii tendon. J. Hand Surg. 1992;17B:515–17.

Gainor BJ. The pronator compression test revisited. A forgotten physical sign. Ortho. Rev. 1990;19:888–92.

Gainor BJ. Modified exposure for pronator syndrome decompression: a preliminary experience. Orthopedics 1993;16: 1329–31.

Gainor BJ, Jeffries JT. Pronator syndrome associated with a persistent median artery. A case report. J. Bone Joint Surg. 1987;69:303–4.

Galbraith KA, McCullough CJ. Acute nerve injury as a complication of closed fractures or dislocations of the elbow. Injury 1979;11:159–64.

Geissler WB, Fernandez DL, Graca R. Anterior interosseous nerve palsy complicating a forearm fracture in a child. J. Hand Surg. 1990;15A:44–47.

Gellman H, Gelberman RH, Tan AM, Botte MJ. Carpal tunnel syndrome. An evaluation of the provocative diagnostic tests. J. Bone Joint Surg. 1986;68A:735–37.

Gessini L, Jandolo B, Pietrangeli A. Entrapment neuropathies of the median nerve at and above the elbow. Surg. Neurol. 1983;19:112–16.

Gessini L, Jandolo B, Pietrangeli A. The pronator teres syndrome. Clinical and electrophysiological features in six surgically verified cases. J. Neurosurg. Sci. 1987;31:1–5.

Gessini L, Jandolo B, Pietrangeli A, Bove L. The Seyffarth syndrome (round pronator syndrome). Considerations on 19 cases. Chir. Organi. Mov. 1980;66:481–89.

Gessini L, Jandolo B, Pietrangeli A, Senese A. Compression of the palmar cutaneous nerve by ganglions of the wrist. J. Neurosurg. Sci. 1983;27:241–43.

Geutjens GG. Ischaemic anterior interosseus nerve injuries following supracondylar fractures of the humerus in children. Injury 1995;26:343–44.

Goldner JL. Median nerve compressions lesions: anatomical and clinical analysis. Bull. Hosp. Joint Dis. 1984;44:199–223.

Greenberg MK, Sonoda T. Mononeuropathy multiplex complicating idiopathic thrombocytopenic purpura. Neurology 1991;41:1517–18.

Groh GI, Gainor BJ, Jeffries JT, Brown M, Eggers Jr. GWN. Pseudoaneurysm of the axillary artery with median-nerve deficit after axillary block anesthesia. J. Bone Joint Surg. 1990;72A:1407–8.

Gross PT, Jones Jr. HR. Proximal median neuropathies: electromyographic and clinical correlation. Muscle Nerve 1992;15:390–95.

Hallett J. Entrapment of the median nerve after dislocation of the elbow. J. Bone Joint Surg. 1981;63B:408–12.

Hartz CR, Linscheid RL, Gramse RR, Daube JR. The pronator teres syndrome: compressive neuropathy of the median nerve. J. Bone Joint Surg. 1981;63A:885–90.

Haskin Jr. JS. Ganglion-related compression neuropathy of the palmar cutaneous branch of the median nerve: a report of two cases. J. Hand Surg. 1994;19A:827–28.

Haussmann P, Patel MR. Intraepineurial constriction of nerve fascicles in pronator syndrome and anterior interosseous nerve syndrome. Orthop. Clin. North Am. 1996;27:339–44.

Hellmann DB, Laing TJ, Petri M, Whiting-O'Keefe Q, Parry GJ. Mononeuritis multiplex: the yield of evaluations for occult rheumatic diseases. Medicine 1988;67:145–53.

Hill NA, Howard FM, Huffer BR. The incomplete anterior interosseous nerve syndrome. J. Hand Surg. 1985;10A:4–16.

Hochholzer T, Krause R, Heuk A. Nerve compression syndromes in sports climbers. Sportverletzung Sportschaden 1993;7:84–87.

Holmes JC, Skolnick MD, Hall JE. Untreated median-nerve entrapment in bone after fracture of the distal end of the humerus: postmortem findings after forty-seven years. J. Bone Joint Surg. 1979;61A:309–10.

Holmes W, Highet WE, Seddon HJ. Ischaemic nerve lesions occurring in Volkmann's contracture. Br. J. Surg. 1944; 32:259–75.

Hope PG. Anterior interosseous nerve palsy following internal fixation of the proximal radius. J. Bone Joint Surg. 1988;70B:280–82.

Huang K, Pun WK, Coleman S. Entrapment and transection of the median nerve associated with greenstick fractures of the forearm: case report and review of the literature. J. Trauma 1998;44:1101–2.

Hudson AR. Nerve injection injuries. In: Terzis JK, ed. Microreconstruction of Nerve Injuries. Philadelphia: Saunders, 1987;173–79.

Hudson A, Kline D, Gentili F. Peripheral Nerve Injection Injury. In: Omer JR GE, Spinner M, eds. Management of Peripheral Nerve Problems. Philadelphia: Saunders, 1980; 639–53.

Internullo G, Marcuzzi A, Busa R, Cordella C, Caroli A. Kiloh-Nevin syndrome: a clinical case of compression of the anterior interosseous nerve. Chir. Organi Mov. 1995;80: 345–48.

Ivins GK. Supracondylar process syndrome: a case report. J. Hand Surg. 1996;21A:279–81.

Jabaley ME, Wallace WH, Heckler FR. Internal topography of major nerves of the forearm and hand: a current view. J. Hand Surg. 1980;5:1–18.

Johnson RK, Spinner M, Shrewsbury MM. Median nerve entrapment syndrome in the proximal forearm. J. Hand Surg. 1979;4:48–51.

Jones ET, Louis DS. Median nerve injuries associated with supracondylar fractures of the humerus in children. Clin. Orthop. 1980;150:181–86.

Jones NF, Ming NL. Persistent median artery as a cause of pronator syndrome. J. Hand Surg. 1988;13A:728–32.

Karlsson J, Thorsteinsson T, Thorleifsson R, Arnason H. Entrapment of the median nerve and brachial artery after supracondylar fractures of the humerus in children. Arch. Orthop. Trauma Surg. 1986;104:389–91.

Katirji MB. Pseudo-anterior interosseous nerve syndrome. Muscle Nerve 1986;9:266–67.

Kennedy AM, Grocott M, Schwartz MS, Modarres H, Scott M, Schon F. Median nerve injury: an underrecognised complication of brachial artery cardiac catheterisation? J. Neurol. Neurosurg. Psychiatry 1997;63:542–46.

Kiloh LG, Nevin S. Isolated neuritis of the anterior interosseous nerve. BMJ. 1952;1:850–51.

Kiyoshige Y. Critical displacement of neural injuries in supracondylar humeral fractures in children. J. Pediatr. Orthop. 1999;19:816–17.

Kömpf D, Neundörfer B, Kayser-Gatchalian C, Meyer-Wahl L, Ranft K. Mononeuritis multiplex bei Boeckscher Sarkoidose. Nervenarzt 1976;47:687–89.

Lacey SH, Soldatis JJ. Bilateral pronator syndrome associated with anomalous heads of the pronator teres muscle: a case report. J. Hand Surg. 1993;18A:349–51.

Laha RK, Lunsford LD, Dujovny M. Lacertus fibrosus compression of the median nerve. Case report. J. Neurosurg. 1978;48:838–41.

Lederman RJ. AAEM minimonograph #43: neuromuscular problems in the performing arts. Muscle Nerve 1994;17: 569–77.

Lewis MH. Median nerve decompression after Colles's fracture. J. Bone Joint Surg. 1978;60-B:195–96.

Linscheid RL, Wheeler DK. Elbow dislocations. JAMA. 1965;194:1171–76.

Lipscomb PR, Burleson RJ. Vascular and neural complications in supracondylar fractures of the humerus in children. J. Bone Joint Surg. 1955;37A:487–92.

Luce EA, Futrell JW, Wilgis EFS, Hoopes JE. Compression neuropathy following brachial arterial puncture in anticoagulated patients. J. Trauma 1976;16:717–21.

Lum PB, Kanakamedala R. Conduction of the palmar cutaneous branch of the median nerve. Arch. Phys. Med. Rehabil. 1986;67:805–6.

Lynch GJ, Meyers JF, Whipple TL, Caspari RB. Neurovascular anatomy and elbow arthroscopy: inherent risks. Arthroscopy 1986;2:190–97.

Lyon BB, Hansen BA, Mygind T. Peripheral nerve injury as a complication of axillary arteriography. Acta. Neurol. Scand. 1975;51:29–36.

Lyons ST, Quinn M, Stanitski CL. Neurovascular injuries in type III humeral supracondylar fractures in children. Clin. Orthop. 2000;376:62–67.

Mackinnon SE, Dellon AL. Surgery of the Peripheral Nerves. New York: Thieme Medical, 1988.

Macnicol MF. Roentgenographic evidence of median nerve entrapment in a Greenstick humeral fracture. A case report. J. Bone Joint Surg. 1978;60A:998–1000.

Macon WL, Futrell JW. Median-nerve neuropathy after percutaneous puncture of the brachial artery in patients receiving anticoagulants. N. Engl. J. Med. 1973;288:1396.

Mahring M, Semple C, Gray IC. Attritional flexor tendon rupture due to a scaphoid non union imitating an anterior interosseous nerve syndrome: a case report. J. Hand Surg. 1985;10B:62–64.

Mangini U. Flexor pollicis longus muscle—its morphology and clinical significance. J. Bone Joint Surg. 1960;42a: 467–70.

Mannerfelt L. Studies on the hand in ulnar nerve paralysis. Acta. Orthop. Scand. 1966;S87:1–176.

Mannerfelt L, Norman O. Attrition ruptures of flexor tendons in rheumatoid arthritis caused by bony spurs in the carpal tunnel: clinical and radiological study. J. Bone Joint Surg. 1969;51B:270–77.

Marinacci AA. The value of electromyogram in the diagnosis of pressure neuropathy from "hanging arm." Electromyogr. Clin. Neurophysiol. 1967;7:5–10.

Marlow N, Jarratt J, Hosking G. Congenital ring constrictions with entrapment neuropathies. J. Neurol. Neurosurg. Psychiatry 1981;44:247–49.

Matev I. A radiological sign of entrapment of the median nerve in the elbow joint after posterior dislocation. J. Bone Joint Surg. 1976;58B:353–55.

Matolo N, Kastagir B, Stevens LE, Chrysanthakopolulos S, Weaver DH, Klinkman H. Neurovascular complications of brachial arteriovenous fistula. Am. J. Surg. 1971;121:716–19.

Mayfield FH. Compression. In: Vinken PJ, Bruyn GW, eds. Handbook of Clinical Neurology. Diseases of the Nerves. New York: American Elsevier, 1970.

McGraw JJ, Akbarnia BA, Hanel DP, Keppler L, Burdge RE. Neurological complications resulting from supracondylar fractures of the humerus in children. J. Pediatr. Orthop. 1986;6:647–50.

McHale KA, Geissele A, Perlik PD. Compartment syndrome of the biceps brachii compartment following rupture of the long head of the biceps. Orthopedics 1991;14:787–88.

Megele R. Anterior interosseous nerve syndrome with atypical nerve course in relation to the pronator teres. Acta Neurochir. (Wien.) 1988;91:144–46.

Miller RA. Observations upon the arrangement of the axillary artery and brachial plexus. Am. J. Anat. 1939;64:143–63.

Miller-Breslow A, Terrono A, Millender LH. Nonoperative treatment of anterior interosseous nerve paralysis. J. Hand Surg. 1990;15A:493–96.

Mills RH, Mukherjee K, Bassett IB. Anterior interosseous nerve palsy. BMJ. 1969;2:555.

Mirovsky Y, Hendel D, Halperin N. Anterior interosseous nerve palsy following closed fracture of the proximal ulna. A case report and review of the literature. Arch. Orthop. Trauma Surg. 1988;107:61–64.

Mittal RL, Gupta BR. Median and ulnar-nerve palsy: an unusual presentation of the supracondylar process. J. Bone Joint Surg. 1978;60A:557–58.

Moberg E. Examination of sensory loss by the ninhydrin printing test in Volkmann's contracture. Bull. Hosp. Joint Dis. 1960;21:296–303.

Moberg E. Tendon grafting and tendon suture in rheumatoid arthritis. Am. J. Surg. 1965;109:375–76.

Mody BS. A simple clinical test to differentiate rupture of flexor pollicis longus and incomplete anterior interosseous paralysis. J. Hand Surg. 1992;17B:513–14.

Molnar W, Paul DJ. Complications of axillary arteriotomies. Radiology 1972;104:269–76.

Morris HH, Peters BH. Pronator syndrome: clinical and electrophysiological features in seven cases. J. Neurol. Neurosurg. Psychiatry 1976;39:461–64.

Mubarak SJ, Hargens AR. Compartment Syndromes and Volkmann's Contracture. Philadelphia: Saunders, 1981.

Munin MC, Balu G, Sotereanos DG. Elbow complications after organ transplantation. Case report. Am. J. Phys. Med Rehabil. 1995;74:67–72.

Murali SR, Ashcroft P, Scotland T. Bilateral compression of the median nerve by supracondylar spurs. J. Pediatr. Orthop. 1995;4B:118–20.

Mysiw WJ, Colachis SC 3d. Electrophysiologic study of the anterior interosseous nerve. Am. J. Phys. Med. Rehabil. 1988;67:50–54.

Naff N, Dellon AL, Mackinnon SE. The anatomical course of the palmar cutaneous branch of the median nerve, including a description of its own unique tunnel. J. Hand Surg. 1993;18B:316–17.

Nagano A, Shibata K, Tokimura H, Yamamoto S, Tajiri Y. Spontaneous anterior interosseous nerve palsy with hourglasslike fascicular constriction within the main trunk of the median nerve. J. Hand Surg. 1996;21A:266–70.

Nakano KK, Lundergran C, Okihiro MM. Anterior interosseous nerve syndromes. Diagnostic methods and alternative treatments. Arch. Neurol. 1977;34:477–80.

Nelson KR, Goodheart R, Salotto A, Tibbs P. Median nerve entrapment beneath the bicipital aponeurosis: investigation with intraoperative short segment stimulation. Muscle Nerve 1994;17:1221–23.

Nelson RM, Currier DP. Anterior interosseous syndrome: a case report. Phys. Ther. 1980;60:194.

Nogueira A, Alcelay O, Pena C, Sarasua JG, Madrigal B. Synovial osteochondromatosis at the elbow producing ulnar and median nerve palsy. Case report and review of the literature. Chir. Main. 1999;18:108–14.

Nunley JA, Urbaniak JR. Partial bony entrapment of the median nerve in a greenstick fracture of the ulna. J. Hand Surg. 1980;5:557–59.

Nunley II JA, Howson P. Lateral Antebrachial Nerve Compression. In: Szabo RM, ed. Nerve Compression Syndromes. Thorofare, NJ: SLACK Inc., 1989;201–08.

O'Brien MD, Upton AR. Anterior interosseous nerve syndrome. A case report with neurophysiological investigation. J. Neurol. Neurosurg. Psychiatry 1972;35:531–36.

Oh SJ, Kim KW. Thrombophlebitis-induced median neuropathy. South. Med. J. 1967;67:1041–42.

O'Keefe DM. Brachial plexus injury following axillary arteriography. Case report and review of the literature. J. Neurosurg. 1980;53:853–57.

Olehnik WK, Manske PR, Szerzinski J. Median nerve compression in the proximal forearm. J. Hand Surg. 1994;19A:121–26.

Omer Jr. GE, Spinner M, Van Beek AL, eds. Management of Peripheral Nerve Problems (2nd ed). Philadelphia: Saunders, 1998.

On AY, Ozdemir O, Aksit R. Tourniquet paralysis after primary nerve repair. Am. J. Phys. Med. Rehabil. 2000;79:298–300.

O'Neill DB, Zarins B, Gelberman RH, Keating TM, Louis D. Compression of the anterior interosseous nerve after use of a sling for dislocation of the acromioclavicular joint. A report of two cases. J. Bone Joint Surg. 1990;72A:1100–2.

Parano E, Uncini A, Incorpora G, Pavone V, Trifiletti RR. Delayed bilateral median nerve injury due to low-tension electric current. Neuropediatrics 1996;27:105–7.

Parks BJ. Postoperative peripheral neuropathies. Surgery 1973;74:348–57.

Parsonage MJ, Turner JWA. Neuralgic amyotrophy: the shoulder-girdle syndrome. Lancet 1948;1:973–78.

Pask EA, Robson JG. Injury to the median nerve. Anaesthesia 1954;9:94–95.

Peters WJ, Todd TR. Anterior interosseous nerve compression syndrome: from metastatic bronchogenic carcinoma to the forearm. Plast. Reconstr. Surg. 1983;72:706–7.

Phalen GS, Kendrick JI, Rodriguez JM. Lipomas of the upper extremity. Am. J. Surg. 1971;121:298–306.

Pradhan S, Gupta A. Iatrogenic median and femoral neuropathy. J. Assoc. Physicians India 1995;43:141.

Proubasta IR, De Sena L, Caceres EP. Entrapment of the median nerve in a greenstick forearm fracture. A case report and review of the literature. Bull. Hosp. Joint Dis. 1999;58:220–23.

Proudman TW, Menz PJ. An anomaly of the median artery associated with the anterior interosseous nerve syndrome. J. Hand Surg. 1992;17B:507–9.

Rainer C, Schoeller T, Wechselberger G, Bauer T, Hussl H. Median nerve injury caused by missed foreign body. Case report. Scand. J. Plast. Reconstr. Surg. Hand Surg. 2000; 34:401–3.

Rana NA, Kenwright J, Taylor RG, Rushworth G. Complete lesion of the median nerve associated with dislocation of the elbow joint. Acta. Orthop. Scand. 1974;45:365–69.

Rao SB, Crawford AH. Median nerve entrapment after dislocation of the elbow in children. A report of 2 cases and review of literature. Clin. Orthop. 1995;312:232–37.

Rask MR. Anterior interosseous nerve entrapment: (Kiloh-Nevin syndrome) report of seven cases. Clin. Orthop. 1979; 176–81.

Rayhack JM. Pronator compression test: a new sign of carpal tunnel syndrome. FL Ortho. Soc. J. 1989;7:21.

Regnard PJ, Soichot P, Ringuier JP. Local complications after axillary block anesthesia. Ann. Chir. Main. 1990;9:59–64.

Rennels GD, Ochoa J. Neuralgic amyotrophy manifesting as anterior interosseous nerve palsy. Muscle Nerve 1980;3: 160–64.

Rofes-Capo S, Ramirez-Ruiz G, Bordas-Sales JL, Gomez-Bonfills J, Lopez-de-Vega J. Median nerve compression on the level of the ligament of Struthers. Case report. Acta Orthop. Belg. 1981;47:884–89.

Rosenberg JN. Anterior interosseous/median nerve latency ratio. Arch. Phys. Med. Rehabil. 1990;71:228–30.

Roth G, Ludy J-P, Egloff-Baer S. Isolated proximal median neuropathy. Muscle Nerve 1982;5:247–49.

Ruch DS, Poehling GG. Anterior interosseus nerve injury following elbow arthroscopy. Arthroscopy 1997;13:756–58.

Saeed MA, Gatens PF. Anterior interosseous nerve syndrome: unusual etiologies. Arch. Phys. Med. Rehabil. 1983;64:182.

Schantz K, Riegels-Nielsen P. The anterior interosseous nerve syndrome. J. Hand Surg. 1992;17B:510–12.

Scherokman B, Husain F, Cuetter A, Jabbari B, Maniglia E. Peripheral dystonia. Arch. Neurol. 1986;43:830–32.

Schmidt H, Eiken O. The anterior interosseous nerve syndrome. Case reports. Scand. J. Plast. Reconstr. Surg. 1971; 5:53–56.

Schneck SA. Peripheral and cranial nerve injuries resulting from general surgical procedures. Arch. Surg. 1960;81: 855–59.

Schrader PA, Reina CR. Struthers' ligament neuropathy in a juvenile. Orthopedics 1994;17:723–25.

Seddon H. Surgical Disorders of the Peripheral Nerves. Baltimore: Williams & Wilkins, 1972.

Semer N, Crimmins C, Jones NF. Compression neuropathy of the palmar cutaneous branch of the median nerve by the antebrachial fascia. J. Hand Surg. 1996;21B:666–67.

Sener E, Takka S, Cila E. Supracondylar process syndrome. Arch. Orthop. Trauma Surg. 1998;117:418–19.

Seyffarth H. Primary myosis in the m. pronator teres as cause of lesion of the n. medianus (The pronator syndrome). Acta Psychiatr. Scand. 1951;251–54.

Shields Jr. RW, Harris JW, Clark M. Mononeuropathy in sickle cell anemia: anatomical and pathophysiological basis for its rarity. Muscle Nerve 1991;14:370–74.

Shimizu K, Iwasaki R, Hoshikawa H, Yamamuro T. Entrapment neuropathy of the palmar cutaneous branch of the median nerve by the fascia of flexor digitorum superficialis. J. Hand Surg. 1988;13A:581–83.

Shirali S, Hanson M, Branovacki G, Gonzalez M. The flexor pollicis longus and its relation to the anterior and posterior interosseous nerves. J. Hand Surg. 1998;23B:17072.

Smith BH, Herbst BA. Anterior interosseous nerve palsy. Arch. Neurol. 1974;30:330–31.

Smith RV, Fisher RG. Struthers ligament: a source of median nerve compression above the elbow. Case report. J. Neurosurg. 1973;38:778–79.

Solem L, Fischer RP, Strate RG. The natural history of electrical injury. J. Trauma 1977;17:487–92.

Spinner M. The anterior interosseous-nerve syndrome, with special attention to its variations. J. Bone Joint Surg. 1970;52A:84–94.

Spinner M. Cryptogenic infraclavicular brachial plexus neuritis (preliminary report). Bull. Hosp. Joint Dis. 1976;37:98–104.

Spinner M. Management of Nerve Compression Lesions of the Upper Extremity. In: Omer Jr. GE, Spinner M, eds. Management of Peripheral Nerve Problems. Philadelphia: Saunders, 1980;569.

Spinner M, Schreiber SN. Anterior interosseous-nerve paralysis as a complication of supracondylar fractures of the humerus in children. J. Bone Joint Surg. 1969;51A:1 584–90.

Spinner RJ, Lins RE, Jacobson SR, Nunley JA. Fractures of the supracondylar process of the humerus. J. Hand Surg. 1994;19A:1038–41.

Stål M, Hagert CG, Moritz U. Upper extremity nerve involvement in Swedish female machine milkers. Am. J. Ind. Med. 1998;33:551–59.

Stall A, van Voorthuisen AE, van Dijk LM. Neurological complications following arterial catheterisation by the axillary approach. Br. J. Radiol. 1966;39:115–16.

Stark RH. Neurologic injury from axillary block anesthesia. J. Hand Surg. 1996;21A:391–96.

Stellbrink G. Compression of the palmar branch of the median nerve by atypical palmaris longus muscle. Handchirurgie 1972;4:155–57.

Stern MB. The anterior interosseous nerve syndrome (the Kiloh-Nevin syndrome). Report and follow-up study of three cases. Clin. Orthop. 1984;157:223–27.

Stern MB, Rosner LJ, Blinderman EE. Kiloh-Nevin syndrome. Report of a case and review of the literature. Clin. Orthop. 1967;53:95–98.

Stern PJ, Kutz JE. An unusual variant of the anterior interosseous nerve syndrome: a case report and review of the literature. J. Hand Surg. 1980;5:32–34.

Straub R. Bilateral supracondylar process of the humeri with unilateral median nerve compression in an 8-year-old child. A case report. Handchir. Mikrochir. Plast. Chir. 1997;29: 314–15.

Sumner JM, Khuri MD. Entrapment of the median nerve and flexor pollicis longus tendon in an epiphyseal fracture-dislocation of the distal radioulnar joint: a case report. J. Hand Surg. 1984;9A:711–14.

Sunderland S. The intraneural topography of the radial, median and ulnar nerves. Brain 1945;68:243–98;

Sunderland S. The Median Nerve. Anatomical and Physiological Considerations. In: Nerves and Nerve Injuries, (2nd ed). Edinburgh, UK: Churchill Livingstone, 1978;674.

Suranyi L. Median nerve compression by Struther's ligament. J. Neurol. Neurosurg. Psychiatry 1983;46:1047–49.

Swiggett R, Ruby LK. Median nerve compression neuropathy by the lacertus fibrosis: report of three cases. J. Hand Surg. 1986;11A:700–3.

Symeonides PP. The humerus supracondylar process syndrome. Clin. Orthop. 1972;82:141–43.

Thomsen PB. Processus supracondyloidea humeri with concomitant compression of the median nerve and ulnar nerve. Acta. Orthop. Scand. 1977;48:391–93.

Tsai TM, Syed SA. A transverse skin incision approach for decompression of pronator teres syndrome. J. Hand Surg. 1994;19B:40–42.

Tulwa N, Limb D, Brown RF. Median nerve compression within the humeral head of pronator teres. J. Hand Surg. 1994;19B:709–10.

Uchida Y, Sugioka Y. Peripheral nerve palsy associated with congenital band constriction. J. Hand Surg. 1991;16B:109–12.

Veilleux M, Richardson P. Proximal median neuropathy secondary to humeral neck fracture. Muscle Nerve 2000;23:426–29.

Verhagen WIM, Dalman JE. Bilateral anterior interosseus nerve syndrome. Muscle Nerve 1995;18:1352.

Vichare NA. Spontaneous paralysis of the anterior interosseous nerve. J. Bone Joint Surg. 1968;50:806–8.

Warren JD. Anterior interosseous nerve palsy as a complication of forearm fractures. J. Bone Joint Surg. 1963;45B:511–12.

Waters PM, Kolettis GJ, Schwend R. Acute median neuropathy following physeal fractures of the distal radius. J. Pediatr. Orthop. 1994;14:173–77.

Watson JA, Singer GC. Irreducible Monteggia fracture: beware nerve entrapment. Injury 1994;25:325–27.

Weinzweig N, Browne EZ Jr. Infraclavicular median nerve compression caused by a lipoma. Orthopedics 1988;11:1077–78.

Werner CO, Rosén I, Thorngren KG. Clinical and neurophysiologic characteristics of the pronator syndrome. Clin. Orthop. 1985;231–36.

Wertsch JJ. AAEM case report #25: anterior interosseous nerve syndrome. Muscle Nerve 1992;15:977–83.

Wertsch JJ, Sanger JR, Matloub HS. Pseudo-anterior interosseous nerve syndrome. Muscle Nerve 1985;8:68–70.

Westcott JL, Taylor PT. Transaxillary selective four-vessel arteriography. Radiology 1972;104:277–81.

Wiens E, Lau SC. The anterior interosseous nerve syndrome. Can. J. Surg. 1978;21:354–57.

Winkelman NZ. Aberrant sensory branch of the median nerve to the third web space—case report. J. Hand Surg. 1980;5:566–67.

Wong L, Dellon AL. Brachial neuritis presenting as anterior interosseous nerve compression—implications for diagnosis and treatment: a case report. J. Hand Surg. 1997;22A:536–39.

Yamamoto S, Nagano A, Mikami Y, Tajiri Y, Kawano K, Itaka K. Fascicular constriction in the anterior interosseous nerve and other motor branches of the median nerve. Muscle Nerve 1999;22:547–48.

Zamora JL, Rose JE, Rosario V, Noon GP. Double entrapment of the median nerve in association with PTFE hemodialysis loop grafts. South. Med. J. 1986;79:638–40.

Zikel OM, Davis DH, Auger RG, Cherry KJ Jr. Venous varix causing median neuropathy. Case illustration. J. Neurosurg. 1997;87:130.

Chapter 18
Median Neuropathy
Distal to the Carpal Tunnel

Digital Nerves

The digital nerves are the most commonly injured peripheral nerves, both because of the vulnerability of the hand to injuries and because of the location of the proper digital nerves approximately 3 mm below the skin. For example, of 100 orthopedists who were surveyed, 15 had injured their own digital nerves severely enough to cause at least transient focal sensory loss (Roberts & Allan, 1988). Extensive discussion of the treatment and prognosis of digital nerve lacerations and of treatment of posttraumatic neuromas is available in hand surgery or peripheral nerve surgery texts (Birch, Bonney & Wynn Parry, 1998; Omer, Spinner & Van Beek, 1998).

Clinical Presentation

Digital nerve injury that is severe enough to interrupt nerve function causes sensory disturbance in the distribution of the injured nerve. For a proper digital nerve, this disturbance is typically along the volar surface of the ipsilateral half of the finger. The extent of sensory disturbance at the finger pulp depends on the degree of overlap at the pulp of fibers from the contralateral proper digital nerve. Sensation on the dorsal fingertip is affected unless the injury is distal to the take-off of the dorsal branch of the proper digital nerve.

Digital nerve injury is often accompanied by disturbance of blood flow to the finger both because the digital nerve supplies sympathetic fibers to the finger and because the digital artery accompanies the digital nerve so that the nerve and artery can be damaged by the same injury.

Injury to a common digital nerve causes sensory disturbance in two adjoining half-fingers and in the web space between them. A proximal partial median nerve injury that selectively damages the fascicles that carry fibers to a common digital nerve can cause the same pattern of sensory dysfunction (Figure 18-1).

Causes

The proper digital nerves, because of their location between skin and bone, are frequently compressed by objects held in the hand. Repeated compression can lead to development of a "neuroma" in continuity. Pathologically, these are not truly neuromas because there is proliferation of perineural fibrous tissue rather than of a knot of regenerating nerve fibers (Dobyns, O'Brien, Linscheid & Farrow, 1972). Symptoms include focal thickening of the nerve and surrounding connective tissue. Tinel's sign is often elicitable over the neuroma. The patient can have paresthesias or sensory loss distal to the neuroma.

The ulnar digital nerve of the thumb is the most common site of a compression neuroma. A typical cause is nerve irritation by the thumbhole of a bowling ball, hence the diagnosis of "bowler's thumb" (Siegel, 1965; Marmor, 1966; Howell & Leach, 1970; Dobyns et al., 1972; Minkow & Bassett, 1972). Similar injury occurs from use of a variety of objects including scissors, baseball bats, staple guns, tennis rackets,

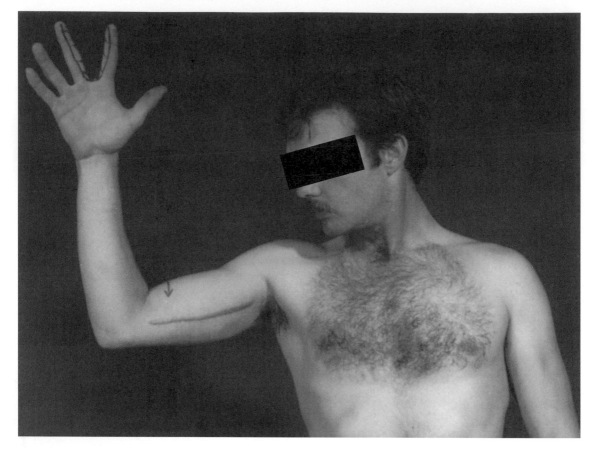

Figure 18-1. Pattern of sensory loss in a patient with a partial median nerve injury in the upper arm. The arrow points to the site of penetrating trauma. The sensory loss was confined to the territory of a single common digital nerve, suggesting injury to a single nerve fascicle.

and axes (Howell & Leach, 1970; Dawson, Hallett & Wilbourn, 1999). Instruments as diverse as piano, flute, violin, viola, cello, oboe, trombone, and marimba have been credited as causes of digital neuropathies in musicians (Cynamon, 1981; Charness, 1992; Lederman, 1994). The ulnar digital nerve of the thumb can be compressed by a hand splint (Rayan & O'Donoghue, 1983).

Cessation of repeated compression is often sufficient treatment of a compression neuroma; occasionally patients are treated surgically with external neurolysis or by constructing a protective muscle flap over the neuroma (Howell & Leach, 1970; Dawson et al., 1999).

Digital nerves can also be compressed by abnormal masses in the hand or by external trauma. Kopell and Thompson (1976) describe patients who developed digital neuropathies after

forced finger hyperextension, after blunt repeat hand trauma with the palm extended, with arthritis of a metacarpal-phalangeal joint, with abnormalities of the tendons near a proximal interphalangeal joint, or even after a particularly crushing handshake. Table 18-1 gives additional examples.

Digital neuropathy is a rare complication in patients with rheumatoid arthritis. The patients usually have a co-existent distal sensory neuropathy in the feet and, at times, more than one digit nerve in the hands is affected (Pallis & Scott, 1965).

As discussed in Chapter 15, digital neuropathy is a well-described complication of carpal tunnel surgery (Semple & Cargill, 1969; Das & Brown, 1976; Brown, Gelberman, Seiler, Abrahamsson, Weiland & Urbaniak, 1993; Murray, Saccone &

Rayan, 1994; Slattery, 1994; Sennwald & Benedetti, 1995; Jacobsen & Rahme, 1996; Worseg, Kuzbari, Korak, Hocker, Wiederer, Tschabitscher & Holle, 1996). Nerve tumors of the digital nerves are discussed in Chapter 19.

Both nerves and sensory receptors in the fingers can be injured by prolonged finger exposure to high-frequency vibration (Hjortsberg, Rosén, Orbaek, Lundborg & Balogh, 1989). The typical patients are dentists and dental technicians who work with tools vibrating at 15,000 to 30,000 Hz. The patients develop numb fingers with increased thresholds to quantitative sensory testing of vibratory function and to heat and cold on quantitative thermotest. Digital nerve conduction studies are normal. The results suggest that the vibration damages small myelinated and unmyelinated fibers. The abnormalities on vibratory testing might be explained by damage to mechanoreceptor end organs or by subtle damage to larger myelinated fibers. This response to high-frequency vibration is distinct from the effect of low-frequency vibration discussed in Chapter 13 under Vibration Exposure and Carpal Tunnel Syndrome.

Digital Nerve Conduction Studies

Median sensory nerve conduction studies between a finger and the wrist are discussed in Chapter 7. Whether done orthodromically, stimulating the finger, or antidromically, recording from the finger, the studies combine the conduction of both digital nerves of the finger. If conduction is impaired in one proper digital nerve, the sensory nerve action potential amplitude sometimes is decreased (Shields & Jacobs, 1986). Slowed conduction in one proper digital nerve can result in a bifid appearance of the sensory nerve action potential recorded at the wrist after finger stimulation (Jablecki & Nazemi, 1982). A technique has been proposed to study conduction in both branches of a common digital nerve: two-sided disc electrodes, with recording gel on both sides, are placed between a pair of fingers and held in place by tapping the fingers together; an antidromic sensory nerve action potential can be recorded from these electrodes after wrist stimulation (Chiou-Tan, Vennix, Dinh & Robinson, 1996).

Table 18-1. Case Reports: Digital Nerve Compression

Cause	Reference
Cysts of the flexor tendon sheath	Dawson, Hallett & Wilbourn, 1999
Digital osteophytes	Dawson, Hallett & Wilbourn, 1999
Dupuytren's contracture	Dawson, Hallett & Wilbourn, 1999
Hand clapping	Shields & Jacobs, 1986
Osteochondroma, third metacarpal	Richmond, 1973
Pacinian corpuscle	Zweig & Burns, 1968; Hart, Thompson, Hildreth & Abell, 1971; Cameron, 1976; Gama & Franca, 1980; Jones & Eadie, 1991; Calder, Holten, Terenghi & Smith, 1995
Palmar lipoma	Schmitz & Keeley, 1957; Paarlberg, Linscheid & Soule, 1972; Oster, Blair & Steyers, 1989
Posttraumatic palmar aneurysm	O'Connor, 1972; Tyler & Stein, 1988
Sandblasting injury	Belsole, Nolan & Eichberg, 1982
Calcinosis in CREST syndrome	Polio & Stern, 1989

CREST = calcinosis, Raynaud's phenomenon, esophageal dysfunction, sclerodactyly, telangiectasia.

Terminal Motor Branches

When the median nerve is injured distal to the departure of the recurrent thenar motor branch, the patient can lose motor function of the median-innervated lumbricals and sensation from the digital branches of the median nerve while retaining function of the thenar muscles (Busis, Logigian & Shahani, 1986).

The recurrent thenar motor branch can be selectively injured in the palm. Typical case reports are listed in Table 18-2.

Widder and Shons (1988) described a patient who had bilateral carpal tunnel syndrome but with unilateral thenar atrophy. At the time of carpal tunnel surgery, the recurrent thenar motor branch on the side with thenar atrophy was compressed between the flexor retinaculum and a prominent superficial palmar branch of the radial artery.

The median nerve fascicles that form the recurrent thenar motor branch are usually located on the

Table 18-2. Causes of Thenar Motor
Branch Neuropathy

Cause	Reference
Puncture wound	Yates, Yaworski & Brown, 1981
Complication of open carpal tunnel surgery	Mannerfelt & Hybbinette, 1972; Conolly, 1978; Lilly & Magnell, 1985; Hybbinette, 1986; Hybbinette & Mannerfelt, 1975; Das & Brown, 1976
Complication of endoscopic carpal tunnel surgery	Boisrenoult, Desmoineaux & Beaufils, 1998
Repeated blunt palmar trauma	Lemmi, Amick & Canale, 1966
Compression by a palmar ganglion	Kato, Ogino, Nanbu & Nakamura, 1991; Crowley, Gschwind & Storey, 1998
Compression by anomalous thenar muscle	Yamanaka, Horiuchi & Yabe, 1994
Compression by a palmar artery	Widder & Shons, 1988

anterior surface of the median nerve. The differential diagnosis of thenar motor branch injury includes more proximal partial median nerve injury of these anterior fascicles (Perotto & Delagi, 1979; Yates, Yaworski & Brown, 1981). Atrophy due to recurrent thenar branch neuropathy must be distinguished from congenital thenar hypoplasia, discussed in Chapter 4 (Cavanagh, Yates & Sutcliffe, 1979).

References

Belsole RJ, Nolan M, Eichberg RD. Sandblasting injury of the hand. J. Hand Surg. 1982;7:523–25.

Birch R, Bonney G, Wynn Parry CB. Surgical Disorders of the Peripheral Nerves. Edinburgh, U.K.: Churchill Livingstone, 1998.

Boisrenoult P, Desmoineaux P, Beaufils P. Single-portal endoscopic treatment of carpal tunnel syndrome. Results of a preliminary series. Rev. Chir. Orthop. Reparatrice Appar. Mot. 1998;84:136–41.

Brown RA, Gelberman RH, Seiler JG 3rd, Abrahamsson SO, Weiland AJ, Urbaniak JR, Schoenfeld DA, Furcolo D. Carpal tunnel release. A prospective, randomized assessment of open and endoscopic methods. J. Bone Joint Surg. 1993; 75A:1265–75.

Busis NA, Logigian EL, Shahani BT. Electrophysiologic assessment of a median nerve injury in the palm. Muscle Nerve 1986;9:208–10.

Calder JS, Holten I, Terenghi G, Smith RW. Digital nerve compression by hyperplastic pacinian corpuscles. A case report and immunohistochemical study. J. Hand Surg. 1995;20B: 218–21.

Cameron S. Two rare cases of nerve entrapment. J. Bone Joint Surg. 1976;58B:266.

Cavanagh NP, Yates DA, Sutcliffe J. Thenar hypoplasia with associated radiologic abnormalities. Muscle Nerve 1979; 2:431–36.

Charness ME. Unique upper extremity disorders of musicians. In: Millender LH, Louis DS, Simmons BP, eds. Occupational Disorders of the Upper Extremity. New York: Churchill Livingstone, 1992;227–52.

Chiou-Tan FY, Vennix MJ, Dinh TI, Robinson LR. Comparison of techniques for detecting digital neuropathy. Am. J. Phys. Med. Rehabil. 1996;75:278–82.

Conolly WB. Pitfalls in carpal tunnel decompression. Aust. N. Z. J. Surg. 1978;48:421–25.

Crowley B, Gschwind CR, Storey C. Selective motor neuropathy of the median nerve caused by a ganglion in the carpal tunnel. J. Hand Surg. 1998;23B:611–12.

Cynamon KB. Flutist's neuropathy. N. Engl. J. Med. 1981; 305:961.

Das SK, Brown HG. In search of complications in carpal tunnel decompression. Hand 1976;8:243–49.

Dawson DM, Hallett M, Wilbourn AJ. Digital nerve entrapment in the hand. In: Dawson DM, Hallett M, Wilbourn AJ, eds. Entrapment Neuropathies (3rd ed). Philadelphia: Lippincott–Raven, 1999;251–63.

Dobyns JH, O'Brien ET, Linscheid RL, Farrow GM. Bowler's thumb: diagnosis and treatment. J. Bone Joint Surg. 1972; 54A:751–55.

Gama C, Franca LCM. Nerve compression by pacinian corpuscles. J. Hand Surg. 1980;5:208–10.

Hart WR, Thompson NW, Hildreth DH, Abell MR. Hyperplastic pacinian corpuscles: a cause of digital pain. Surgery 1971;70:730–35.

Hjortsberg U, Rosén I, Orbaek P, Lundborg G, Balogh I. Finger receptor dysfunction in dental technicians exposed to high-frequency vibration. Scand. J. Work Environ. Health 1989; 15:339–44.

Howell AE, Leach RE. Bowler's thumb. J. Bone Joint Surg. 1970;52A:379–81.

Hybbinette CH. Severance of thenar branch. J. Hand Surg. 1986;11A:613.

Hybbinette CH, Mannerfelt L. The carpal tunnel syndrome. A retrospective study of 400 operated patients. Acta Orthop. Scand. 1975;46:610–20.

Jablecki C, Nazemi R. Unsuspected digital nerve lesions responsible for abnormal median sensory responses. Arch. Phys. Med. Rehabil. 1982;63:135–38.

Jacobsen MB, Rahme H. A prospective, randomized study with an independent observer comparing open carpal tunnel release with endoscopic carpal tunnel release. J. Hand Surg. 1996;21B:202–4.

Jones NF, Eadie P. Pacinian corpuscle hyperplasia in the hand. J. Hand Surg. 1991;16A:865–69.

Kato H, Ogino T, Nanbu T, Nakamura K. Compression neuropathy of the motor branch of the median nerve caused by palmar ganglion. J. Hand Surg. 1991;16A:751–52.

Kopell HP, Thompson WAL. Peripheral Entrapment Neuropathies (2nd ed). Malabar, FL: Robert E. Krieger Publishing Company, 1976.

Lederman RJ. AAEM minimonograph #43: neuromuscular problems in the performing arts. Muscle Nerve 1994;17: 569–77.

Lemmi H, Amick LD, Canale DJ. Median acromotor neuropathy (pseudo carpal tunnel syndrome): report of a case. Arch. Phys. Med. Rehabil. 1966;47:306–9.

Lilly CJ, Magnell TD. Severance of the thenar branch of the median nerve as a complication of carpal tunnel release. J. Hand Surg. 1985;10A:399–402.

Mannerfelt L, Hybbinette CH. Important anomaly of the thenar motor branch of the median nerve. A clinical and anatomical report. Bull. Hosp. Joint Dis. 1972;33:15–21.

Marmor L. Bowler's thumb. J. Trauma 1966;6:282–84.

Minkow FV, Bassett FH 3rd. Bowler's thumb. Clin. Orthop. 1972;83:115–17.

Murray DP, Saccone PG, Rayan GM. Complications after subfascial carpal tunnel release. South. Med. J. 1994;87:416–18.

O'Connor RL. Digital nerve compression secondary to palmar aneurysm. Clin. Orthop. 1972;83:149–50.

Omer Jr. GE, Spinner M, Van Beek AL, eds. Management of Peripheral Nerve Problems (2nd ed). Philadelphia: Saunders, 1998.

Oster LH, Blair WF, Steyers CM. Large lipomas in the deep palmar space. J. Hand Surg. 1989;14A:700–704.

Paarlberg D, Linscheid RL, Soule EH. Lipomas of the hand. Including a case of lipoblastomatosis in a child. Mayo Clin. Proc. 1972;47:121–24.

Pallis CA, Scott JT. Peripheral neuropathy in rheumatoid arthritis. BMJ. 1965;1:1141–47.

Perotto AO, Delagi EF. Funicular localization in partial median nerve injury at the wrists. Arch. Phys. Med. Rehabil. 1979;60:165–69.

Polio JL, Stern PJ. Digital nerve calcification in CREST syndrome. J. Hand Surg. 1989;14A:201–3.

Rayan GM, O'Donoghue DH. Ulnar digital compression neuropathy of the thumb caused by splinting. Clin. Orthop. 1983;175:170–72.

Richmond DA. Uncommon causes of nerve compression with hand symptoms. Hand 1973;5:209–13.

Roberts AP, Allan DB. Digital nerve injuries in orthopaedic surgeons. Injury 1988;19:233–34.

Schmitz RL, Keeley JL. Lipomas of the hand. Surgery 1957; 42:696–700.

Semple JC, Cargill AO. Carpal-tunnel syndrome. Results of surgical decompression. Lancet 1969;1:918–19.

Sennwald GR, Benedetti R. The value of one-portal endoscopic carpal tunnel release: a prospective randomized study. Knee Surg. Sports Traumatol. Arthrosc. 1995;3:113–16.

Shields RW, Jacobs IB. Median palmar digital neuropathy in a cheerleader. Arch. Phys. Med. Rehabil. 1986;67:824–26.

Siegel IM. Bowling-thumb neuroma. JAMA. 1965;192:163.

Slattery PG. Median nerve injury and the transverse wrist crease incision in open carpal tunnel release. Aust. N. Z. J. Surg. 1994;64:768–70.

Tyler G, Stein A. Aneurysm of a common digital artery: resection and vein graft. J. Hand Surg. 1988;13B:348–49.

Widder S, Shons AR. Carpal tunnel syndrome associated with extra tunnel vascular compression of the median nerve motor branch. J. Hand Surg. 1988;13A:926–27.

Worseg AP, Kuzbari R, Korak K, Hocker K, Wiederer C, Tschabitscher M, Holle J. Endoscopic carpal tunnel release using a single-portal system. Br. J. Plast. Surg. 1996;49:1–10.

Yamanaka K, Horiuchi Y, Yabe Y. Compression neuropathy of the motor branch of the median nerve due to an anomalous thenar muscle. J. Hand Surg. 1994;19B:711–12.

Yates SK, Yaworski R, Brown WF. Relative preservation of lumbrical versus thenar motor fibres in neurogenic disorders. J. Neurol. Neurosurg. Psychiatry 1981;44:768–74.

Zweig J, Burns H. Compression of digital nerves by pacinian corpuscles. A report of two cases. J. Bone Joint Surg. 1968;50A:999–1001.

Chapter 19
Tumors of the Median Nerve

"The trouble about these tumors is that they are just common enough to come within the experience of almost all surgeons and rare enough to cause embarrassment in diagnosis and treatment" (Seddon, 1972). Peripheral nerve tumors of any nerve of the arm account for less than 5% of all hand and arm tumors. Strickland and Steichen (1977) found only six nerve tumors in their series of 689 tumors of the hand and arm. Study of median nerve tumors is complicated both by their rarity and by the variety of synonyms that are used for related histologic types. Harkin and Reed (1969, 1983) provide a detailed pathologic review and discussion of the nomenclature. Nonneurogenic masses in the carpal tunnel are listed in Table 6-4.

Neurilemmoma

Neurilemmomas, or schwannomas, are the most common solitary nerve tumors. They are benign tumors that originate from Schwann cells, typically present as masses, and infrequently cause neurologic deficit or sensory symptoms (Birch, 1993). The tumor is usually discovered by palpation. In consistency and mobility the neurilemmoma may be mistaken for a ganglion: The neurilemmoma is more likely to be tender; however, nerve tumors are so much rarer than ganglions that tender subcutaneous masses are usually not nerve tumors. A classic but not invariable finding that favors the diagnosis of neurilemmoma is a mass that is movable laterally but not longitudinally. In some cases, percussion of the tumor elicits distal paresthesias.

Neurilemmomas of the median nerve may be found in the volar forearm, in the palm, or in a branch such as a digital nerve or the recurrent thenar motor branch (Phalen, 1976; Rinaldi, 1983; Mintz & Carneiro, 1989; Ritt & Bos, 1991; Squarzina, Adani, Cerofolini, Bagni & Caroli, 1993). Among 50 patients with neurilemmomas, Stout (1935) found seven arising from the palm, digital nerves, or median nerve. When the tumor occurs within the carpal tunnel, it may cause symptoms of carpal tunnel syndrome (Barre, Shaffer, Carter & Lacey, 1987). In an extraordinary case, a median neurilemmoma in the carpal tunnel stretched the recurrent thenar branch of the nerve causing thenar weakness (Josty & Sykes, 2001). Rarely, a patient has multiple neurilemmomas (Lewis, Nannini & Cocke, 1981; Barre et al., 1987; Birch, 1993).

Neurilemmomas are encapsulated and arise from a single nerve fascicle. They usually can be completely removed surgically without disturbing nerve continuity or function (Phalen, 1976).

Neurofibroma

Neurofibromas are benign tumors that arise from the perineurium and the endoneurium. They grow slowly and interdigitate with nerve fibers, so they are more likely than neurilemmomas to cause pain, other sensory symptoms, or neurologic deficit. When a neurofibroma involves the median nerve in the carpal tunnel, the symptoms may be those of an asymptomatic mass or of a progressive median neuropathy.

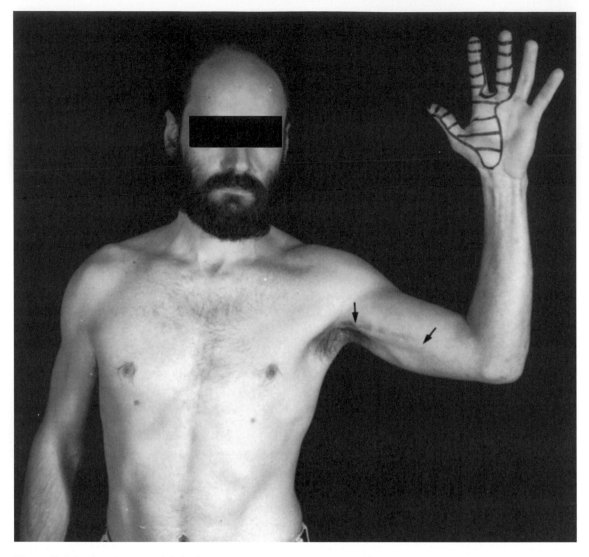

Figure 19-1. Pattern of sensory deficit after resection of a median nerve neurofibroma in the upper arm. The patient also had a profound postoperative median motor deficit.

Neurofibromas are usually cutaneous, rather than on main nerve trunks, and present either as an isolated finding or as part of von Reckling-hausen's neurofibromatosis. Whether as isolated tumors or as part of neurofibromatosis, neurofibromas in the median or digital nerves are even rarer than neurilemmomas (Nagey, McCabe & Wolff, 1990; Bahm, von Saldern & Pallua, 1999; Pascual-Castroviejo, Pascual-Pascual, Viano & Martinez, 2000).

Surgical resection of neurofibromas usually requires nerve transection, often followed by nerve grafting to re-establish nerve continuity (Figure 19-1) (Rinaldi, 1983). Successful microscopic excision of neurofibromas while maintaining nerve continuity is rare (Strickland & Steichen, 1977).

Neurofibromatosis

Median nerve tumors may occur in patients with either type 1 or type 2 neurofibromatosis (von Recklinghausen's disease). Tumors include median nerve neurofibromas, plexiform neurofibromas, and malignant peripheral nerve sheath tumors. The semantics are sometimes confusing, because the most common neurofibromas in patients with neurofibromatosis are small tumors that arise from cutaneous nerves in the dermis. In patients who have median nerve neurofibromas, the characteristics of the tumor are the same whether or not the patient has neurofibromatosis. The diagnosis of neurofibromatosis rests on cutaneous manifestations of the disease, on the genetic history, and on the presence of other nervous system tumors.

Plexiform neurofibromas are distinctive nerve tumors that are seen only in patients with neurofibromatosis (Harkin, 1980). Multiple nerve fascicles are swollen and contain accumulations of Schwann cells, endoneurial cells, and undifferentiated cells. The fascicular swelling creates a macroscopic "tangle-of-worms" appearance. For example, Brooks (1984) described plexiform median nerve fibromas localized to the carpal tunnel in a 5-year-old boy, and extending along the nerve from axilla to elbow in a 17-year-old girl.

Both neurofibromas and plexiform neurofibromas may undergo malignant transformation. Neurofibromatosis is the most common setting for development of malignant peripheral nerve sheath tumors.

Malignant Peripheral Nerve Tumors

The vast majority of peripheral nerve sheath tumors are benign. Clinical clues to malignancy are spontaneous pain, swelling, and associated neurologic deficit. However, most malignant peripheral nerve tumors present as painless masses (Das Gupta & Brasfield, 1970). Malignant nerve sheath tumors arise as solitary lesions or by malignant transformation of neurofibromas in patients with neurofibromatosis (Ducatman, Scheithauer, Piepgras, Reiman & Ilstrup, 1986). Malignant transformation should be suspected when a nerve tumor shows accelerated growth. Malignancy is even rarer for neurilemmomas than for neurofibromas (Nayler, Leiman, Omar & Cooper, 1996). In a series of 31 malignant tumors of peripheral nerve, Vieta and Pack (1951) encountered five arising from the median nerve. Malignant median nerve tumor in the hand can masquerade as carpal tunnel syndrome (Wood, Erdmann & Davies, 1993).

Primitive neuroectodermal tumors are rare nerve tumors that can spread aggressively. In a few instances these tumors arise in the median nerve (Cohn, 1928; Mennel & Zulch, 1971; Akeyson, McCutcheon, Pershouse, Steck & Fuller, 1996).

Treatment of malignant nerve tumors is by total excision. Even after excision, patients are at high risk for local recurrence or development of metastases (Rogalski & Louis, 1991). Association with neurofibromatosis or tumor diameter greater than 5 cm are adverse prognostic signs (Ducatman et al., 1986).

Fatty Nerve Tumors

Fatty tumors of the median nerve include isolated lipomas encapsulated within the nerve, infiltrative lipofibromatous hamartomas of the nerve, or macrodystrophia lipomatosa in which there is fatty infiltration of both the median nerve and of subcutaneous tissue of the hand. These all have clinical and histologic features distinct from median nerve compression by a lipoma external to the nerve (see Table 6-4).

Encapsulated lipomas are rarely found within the median nerve. They have been reported to occur in the nerve within the carpal tunnel or in the forearm (Morley, 1964; Watson-Jones, 1964; Rusko & Larsen, 1981). The soft, subcutaneous mass may be palpable for years before it causes paresthesias. The encapsulated tumor can be surgically completely removed without damaging nerve fascicles, and microscopic examination shows no nerve fibers within the tumor capsule. Some cases, initially reported as median nerve lipomas, did not have the typical histologic encapsulation and excisability of a lipoma and were probably lipofibromatous hamartomas (Mikhail, 1964; Friedlander, Rosenberg & Graubard, 1969).

Lipofibromatous hamartomas of the median nerve are known by a number of synonyms: fibrolipoma, fibrolipomatous hamartoma, fibrofatty proliferation, fatty infiltration of nerve, reactive perineural fibroblastic proliferation of nerve, and intraneural lipofibroma (Pulvertaft, 1964; Yeoman, 1964; Callison, Thoms & White, 1968; Johnson & Bonfiglio, 1969; Abu Jamra & Rebeiz, 1979; Kalisman & Dolich, 1982; Louis, Hankin, Greene & Dick, 1985; Bodne, Quinn, Kloss, Bolton, Murray,

Roberts & Cochran, 1988; Houpt, Storm van Leeuwen & van den Bergen, 1989; Berry, Mallucci, Banwell & Heywood, 1999). This tumor has been the subject of numerous more recent case reports, prompted by its distinctive imaging characteristics and pathology (Guthikonda, Rengachary, Balko & van Loveren, 1994; Evans, Donnelly, Johnson, Blebea & Stern, 1997; Canga, Abascal, Cerezal, Bustamante, Perez-Carro & Vazquez-Barquero, 1998; Sagtas, Orguc, Elcin, Memis & Menzilcioglu, 1999; Kameh, Perez-Berenguer & Pearl, 2000; Lowenstein, Chandnani & Tomaino, 2000). The median nerve is much more likely than other nerves to develop a hamartoma (Silverman & Enzinger, 1985). The tumors have a predilection for the carpal tunnel, spreading distally into the palm and proximally into the forearm. The symptoms are those of a slowly growing palmar or forearm mass, often accompanied by symptoms of carpal tunnel syndrome. Symptoms usually start in childhood, but some patients do not develop symptoms until their seventh decade (Guthikonda et al., 1994). Extraordinary instances of bilateral lipofibromatous hamartomas or of hamartomas of both median and ulnar nerves can occur (Salon, Guero & Glicenstein, 1995; Meyer, Roricht & Schmitt, 1998).

Radiographs occasionally show calcification within the hamartoma (Louis et al., 1985). When the tumor mass is within the carpal tunnel, it occupies the usual location of the median nerve with the flexor tendons dorsal to it and the transverse carpal ligament volar to it. On computed tomographic (CT) scan the tumor appears as an inhomogeneous mass with fatty components (Declercq, De Man, Van Herck, Tanghe & Lateur, 1993). On ultrasound the appearance has been called "cablelike," composed of longitudinally oriented bands that are alternately hypoechogenic and hyperechogenic (Carson, Gumpert & Jefferson, 1971). The magnetic resonance imaging (MRI) appearance is most characteristic, showing longitudinally oriented serpiginous cylinders that are low intensity on T1- and T2-weighted sequences and are separated by fibrous and fatty elements (Figure 19-2) (Bodne et al., 1988; Walker, Adams, Barnes, Roloson & FitzRandolph, 1991; Cavallaro, Taylor, Gorman, Haghighi & Resnick, 1993; Giuliano, Outwater, Mitchell & Burke, 1997; De Maeseneer, Jaovisidha, Lenchick, Witte, Schweitzer, Sartoris & Resnick, 1997). The tumor is usually fusiform or of variable width, extends 5 to 30 cm, and can follow the branching pattern of the nerve.

At surgery a lipofibromatous hamartoma typically appears as a fusiform enlargement of nerve within the epineurium. If the epineurium is divided, the tumor is seen closely intertwined with nerve fascicles so that microdissection of the tumor is usually impossible. Release of the flexor retinaculum, usually accompanied by fascicular biopsy, is often sufficient treatment, at least for the symptoms of median neuropathy. Rowland

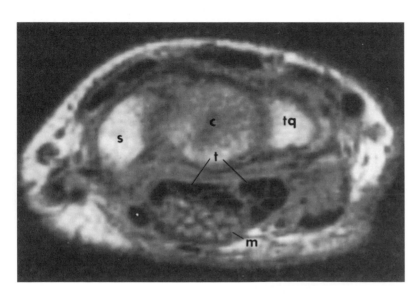

Figure 19-2. Lipofibromatous hamartoma of the median nerve. The axial magnetic resonance imaging of the wrist shows marked enlargement of the median nerve (m). The perineural fibroblastic proliferation is so prominent that individual nerve fascicles can be identified. Sagittal images (not shown) confirmed fatty infiltration of the nerve. (c = capitate; s = scaphoid; t = flexor tendons; tq = triquetrum.) (Reproduced with permission from D Bodne, SF Quinn, J Kloss, et al. Reactive perineural fibroblastic proliferation of the median nerve: MR characteristics. J. Comput. Assist. Tomogr. 1988;12:532–34.)

(1977) followed a patient for 10 years after initial biopsy of a lipofibromatous hamartoma and noted regression of the tumor, but other patients have progressive or recurrent symptoms of median nerve compromise despite carpal tunnel release (Louis et al., 1985). For most patients, even those with progressive symptoms, the value of tumor debulking or resection with nerve grafting is debatable (Camilleri & Milner, 1998; Berry et al., 1999).

Rarely, a lipofibromatous hamartoma is limited to a single digital nerve (Steentoft & Sollerman, 1990). These tumors present as focal swelling of the finger or distal palm with or without sensory disturbance. When only a digital nerve is involved, the tumor can occasionally be dissected free of the nerve with aid of the microscope (Kalisman & Dolich, 1982).

Macrodactyly of one or more digits often accompanies lipofibromatous hamartoma of the corresponding digital nerve or of the median nerve (Hueston & Millroy, 1968; Paletta & Rybka, 1972; Frykman & Wood, 1978; Silverman & Enzinger, 1985; Boren, Henry & Wintch, 1995; Mirza, King & Reinhart, 1998; Nogueira, Pena, Martinez, Sarasua & Madrigal, 1999; Brodwater, Major, Goldner & Layfield, 2000; Sone, Ehara, Tamakawa, Nishida & Honjoh, 2000). The combination is sometimes called *macrodystrophia lipomatosa*. At times, fibrous rather than lipomatous change is the predominant histologic finding in nerve (Moore, 1942; Allende, 1967). The macrodactyly is often congenital (Barsky, 1967). In extraordinary cases, lipofibromatous hamartoma of the median nerve accompanies more widespread congenital disorders such as Proteus syndrome, port-wine stains, or angio-osteohypertrophy (Klippel-Trenaunay-Weber syndrome) (Amadio, Reiman & Dobyns, 1988; Ban, Kamiya, Sato & Kitajima, 1998; Choi, Wey & Borah, 1998).

Vascular Tumors

Hemangiomas of the median nerve are extremely rare; it is hard to find more than a handful of reported cases (Kojima, Ide, Marumo, Ishikawa & Yamashita, 1976; Peled, Iosipovich, Rousso & Wexler, 1980; Kon & Vuursteen, 1981; Patel, Tsai & Kleinert, 1986; Prosser & Burke, 1987; Coes-sens, De Mey, Lacotte & Vandenbroeck, 1991; Louis & Fortin, 1992; Ergin, Druckmiller & Cohen, 1998). These tumors may present in childhood or adolescence with a visible, compressible soft tissue tumor or, when the hemangioma is within the carpal tunnel, with symptoms of carpal tunnel syndrome. Angiomyoma (vascular leiomyoma) of the median nerve and hemangioendothelioma adjacent to the nerve are even more unusual vascular tumors; the later has the potential to metastasize (Zingale, Bruno, Giuffre, Carpinteri & Albanese, 1993; Piers, Terrono, Hayek & Millender, 1996).

MRI is probably the best imaging technique for vascular tumors (Ergin, Druckmiller & Cohen, 1998). CT scan of the tumor with contrast can confirm the vascular nature of the tumor (Feyerabend, Schmitt, Lanz & Warmuth-Metz, 1990). Angiography is positive for only some of the tumors (Ergin et al., 1998).

Intraneural Mucoid Cysts

Resection of an intraneural median nerve cyst containing clear viscous fluid was described over a century ago (Hartwell, 1901). These benign mucoid cysts can cause symptoms of nerve compression or local pain. They are more common in the legs than in the arms and more common in the ulnar nerve than in the median nerve (Giele & Le Viet, 1997). Some appear to be ganglions, originating from tenosynovium and growing into the nerve (Jaradeh, Sanger & Maas, 1995). Others appear to arise among the nerve fibers or in the epineurium (Allieu & Cenac, 1989; Patel, Naik, Mody & Pollack, 1997). Depending on the relation of nerve fibers to the cyst capsule, surgical treatment is complete or partial excision.

Digital Nerve Tumors

Two nerve tumors specifically involve the digital nerves. *Dermal nerve sheath myxoma* is a rare benign tumor that probably originates from Schwann cells (Webb, 1979; Blumberg, Kay & Adelaar, 1989). It presents as a small digital mass. It can become painful or manifest Tinel's sign.

Hyperplastic pacinian corpuscles may also cause small painful subcutaneous digital masses. Normal pacinian corpuscles are sensory end organs for mechanical stimuli that are formed by concentrically arranged squamous epithelium derived from perineurium. On rare occasions, they may become tender and hyperplastic, particularly after hand trauma, and present either as a single mass or as a string of masses (Sandzen & Baksic, 1974; Bas, Oztek & Numanoglu, 1993; Reznik, Thiry & Fridman, 1998). At times, a hyperplastic pacinian corpuscle can cause digital nerve compression with resulting pain and paresthesias (Zweig & Burns, 1968; Hart, Thompson, Hildreth & Abell, 1971; Cameron, 1976; Gama & Franca, 1980; Jones & Eadie, 1991; Calder, Holten, Terenghi & Smith, 1995). Surgical excision of the corpuscles often succeeds in relieving symptoms.

Glomus tumors rarely involve a digital nerve, causing digital paresthesias (Kline, Moore & deMente, 1990). Glomus tumors are small painful benign tumors that are more commonly found under the nail bed or in the fingertip pulp (Van Geertruyden, Lorea, Goldschmidt, de Fontaine, Schuind, Kinnen & Ledoux, 1996; Abou Jaoude, Roula Farah, Sargi, Khairallah & Fakih, 2000). Symptoms of glomus tumor include sensitivity of the tip of the digit to gentle mechanical or cold stimulation, relief of pain by warm stimulation, an evident nodule, or a spot of bluish discoloration (Ochoa, Marchettini & Cline, 1991). MRI can often visualize these tumors (Drape, Idy-Peretti, Goettmann, Wolfram-Gabel, Dion, Grossin & Benacerraf, 1995).

Granular cell tumor is a benign tumor that appears to arise from Schwann cells. It occurs most frequently in tongue, skin, or subcutaneous tissue but has been found arising from a digital nerve (Enghardt & Jordan, 1991).

Localized Hypertrophic Neuropathy (Intraneural Perineurioma)

Localized hypertrophic neuropathy (intraneural perineurioma) is an exceedingly rare cause of focal mononeuropathy (Mitsumoto, Wilbourn & Goren, 1980; Phillips, Persing & Vandenberg, 1991). The clinical presentation is usually insidious evolution of painless motor deficit and little sensory change.

Macroscopic nerve hypertrophy often spans a few inches of nerve, and nerve biopsy shows focal onion bulb formation; it is unclear whether to class this as a benign neoplasm. A few instances of localized hypertrophy of the median nerve have been reported (Peckham, O'Boynick, Meneses & Kepes, 1982; Bilbao, Khoury, Hudson & Briggs, 1984; Jazayeri, Robinson & Legolvan, 2000). One case involved the recurrent thenar motor branch of the median nerve (Mitsumoto, Estes, Wilbourn & Culver, 1992). In another case, a patient with macrodactyly had onion bulb formation noted on biopsy of the localized hypertrophy of the median nerve in the carpal tunnel (Appenzeller & Kornfeld, 1974).

Metastatic Tumor

Tumor metastases specifically to the median nerve are very rare. Squamous cell carcinoma of the finger, especially of the nail bed, can spread up the median nerve, causing a palmar mass or carpal tunnel syndrome (Mackay & Barua, 1990; Canovas, Dereure & Bonnel, 1998). Subungual neurotropic melanoma can spread proximally along the median nerve; histologically, the tumor in nerve can be difficult to distinguish from a malignant peripheral nerve sheath tumor (Iyadomi, Ohtsubo, Gotoh, Kohda & Narisawa, 1998; Ogose, Emura, Iwabuchi, Hotta, Inoue & Saito, 1998). Another metastatic example is spread of bronchogenic carcinoma to the anterior interosseous nerve (Peters & Todd, 1983).

Infection Mistaken for Tumor

Two case reports illustrate an oddity: A mass lesion attached to nerve may be infectious rather than neoplastic. A painful, 2-cm diameter, mobile nodule attached to the median nerve in the upper arm was thought to be a neurilemmoma until pathologic examination showed that it was a cysticercus cyst (Nosanchuk, Agostini, Georgi & Posso, 1980). A 55-year-old woman, who presented with a forearm mass and a distal median neuropathy, was found at surgery to have a calcified mass adherent to the median nerve. A calcified guineaworm (*Dracunculus medinensis*) was identified under the nerve sheath (Balasubramanian & Ramamurthi, 1965).

Tumor Imaging

MRI scanning, CT scanning, and ultrasound can aid in the diagnosis of median nerve tumors. The first characteristic of a nerve sheath tumor is localization of the tumor in or contiguous with a nerve. On MRI the tumors typically are intermediately or moderately bright on T1-weighted images, moderately bright on proton-density weighted images, and bright on T2-weighted images (Stull, Moser, Kransdorf, Bogumill & Nelson, 1991; Hems, Burge & Wilson, 1997). The signal is usually heterogeneous. This combination of findings is seen with neurilemmomas, neurofibromas, and malignant nerve sheath tumors. Tumor margins are usually well defined; an irregular or indistinct margin may occur with malignant tumors, plexiform neurofibromas, or after nerve biopsy.

CT scanning can also be used to confirm the location of a soft tissue tumor in relation to peripheral nerve (Powers, Norman & Edwards, 1983). At times CT appearance gives clues to tumor histology (Feyerabend, Schmitt, Lanz & Warmuth-Metz, 1990). Neurilemmomas appear as well-defined, hypodense masses; after administration of intravenous contrast, the tumor mass may appear unenhanced, inhomogeneously enhanced, or ring-enhanced (Levine, Huntrakoon & Wetzel, 1987; Zingale, Consoli, Tigano, Pero & Albanese, 1993). Neurofibromas are similar in appearance but may be less well defined and occasionally contain areas of calcification. Lipomas and lipofibromatous hamartomas are distinguished by low CT numbers because of their fat content. Hemangiomas show rapid transient enhancement.

On high-resolution real-time ultrasound, the normal median nerve can be identified with an echogenic fibrillar texture (Fornage, 1988). Relative immobility with joint movement helps distinguish it from flexor tendons, which have similar echogenicity. Nerve tumors, like other soft tissue tumors, appear as hypoechoic masses; usually their attachment to nerve is the only clue to their origin. Neurilemmomas usually have more well-defined contours than neurofibromas. Neurilemmomas

may also show distal sound enhancement (Fornage, 1988).

With the possible exception of lipomas and hemangiomas, CT and MRI findings rarely are specific to tumor pathology. For example, they do not reliably distinguish neurofibromas and neurilemmomas from malignant peripheral nerve sheath tumors.

Conclusion

Median nerve tumors should be considered whenever a patient presents with a mass along the course of the median nerve. The diagnosis should be particularly suspected in patients with neurofibromatosis or when the mass is accompanied by symptoms of median neuropathy. Even with modern imaging techniques, the final diagnosis is often not established before biopsy of the mass. Appropriate surgical management is determined by the tumor type and location and by the extent of associated neurologic deficit.

References

Abou Jaoude JF, Roula Farah A, Sargi Z, Khairallah S, Fakih C. Glomus tumors: report on eleven cases and a review of the literature. Chir. Main. 2000;19:243–52.

Abu Jamra FN, Rebeiz JJ. Lipofibroma of the median nerve. J. Hand Surg. 1979;4:160–63.

Akeyson EW, McCutcheon IE, Pershouse MA, Steck PA, Fuller GN. Primitive neuroectodermal tumor of the median nerve. Case report with cytogenetic analysis. J. Neurosurg. 1996;85:163–69.

Allende BT. Macrodactyly with enlarged median nerve associated with carpal tunnel syndrome. Plast. Reconstr. Surg. 1967;39:578–82.

Allieu PY, Cenac PE. Peripheral nerve mucoid degeneration of the upper extremity. J. Hand Surg. 1989;14A:189–94.

Amadio PC, Reiman HM, Dobyns JH. Lipofibromatous hamartoma of nerve. J. Hand Surg. 1988;13A:67–75.

Appenzeller O, Kornfeld M. Macrodactyly and localized hypertrophic neuropathy. Neurology 1974;24:767–71.

Bahm J, von Saldern S, Pallua N. Neurofibroma of the palm of the hand in Recklinghausen disease. A case report. Handchir. Mikrochir. Plast. Chir. 1999;31:282–84.

Balasubramanian V, Ramamurthi B. An unusual location of guineaworm infestation. J. Neurosurg. 1965;23:537–38.

Ban M, Kamiya H, Sato M, Kitajima Y. Lipofibromatous hamartoma of the median nerve associated with macrodactyly and port-wine stains. Pediatr. Dermatol. 1998;15:378–80.

Barre PS, Shaffer JW, Carter JR, Lacey SH. Multiplicity of neurilemomas in the upper extremity. J. Hand Surg. 1987; 12A:307–11.

Barsky AJ. Macrodactyly. J. Bone Joint Surg. 1967;49A:1255–66.

Bas L, Oztek I, Numanoglu A. Subepineural hyperplastic pacinian corpuscle: an unusual cause of digital pain. Plast. Reconstr. Surg. 1993;92:151–53.

Berry MG, Mallucci P, Banwell PE, Heywood AJ. Fibrolipoma of the median. J. R. Soc. Med. 1999;92:408–9.

Bilbao JM, Khoury NJ, Hudson AR, Briggs SJ. Perineurioma (localized hypertrophic neuropathy). Arch. Pathol. Lab. Med. 1984;108:557–60.

Birch R. Peripheral Nerve Tumors. In: Dyck PJ, Thomas PK, Griffin J, Low PA, Poduslo JF, eds. Peripheral Neuropathy (3rd ed). Philadelphia: Saunders, 1993;1623–40.

Blumberg AK, Kay S, Adelaar RS. Nerve sheath myxoma of digital nerve. Cancer 1989;63:1215–18.

Bodne D, Quinn SF, Kloss J, Bolton T, Murray WT, Roberts W, Cochran C. Reactive perineural fibroblastic proliferation of the median nerve: MR characteristics. J. Comput. Assist. Tomogr. 1988;12:532–34.

Boren WL, Henry RE Jr., Winch K. MR diagnosis of fibrolipomatous hamartoma of nerve: association with nerve territory-oriented macrodactyly (macrodystrophia lipomatosa). Skeletal Radiol. 1995;24:296–97.

Brodwater BK, Major NM, Goldner RD, Layfield LJ. Macrodystrophia lipomatosa with associated fibrolipomatous hamartoma of the median nerve. Pediatr. Surg. Int. 2000; 16:216–18.

Brooks D. Clinical presentation and treatment of peripheral nerve tumors. In: Dyck PJ, Thomas PK, Lambert EH, Bunge R, eds. Peripheral Neuropathy (2nd ed). Philadelphia: Saunders, 1984;2236–51.

Calder JS, Holten I, Terenghi G, Smith RW. Digital nerve compression by hyperplastic pacinian corpuscles. A case report and immunohistochemical study. J. Hand Surg. 1995;20B:218–21.

Callison JR, Thoms OJ, White WL. Fibro-fatty proliferation of the median nerve. Plast. Reconstr. Surg. 1968;42:403–13.

Cameron S. Two rare cases of nerve entrapment. J. Bone Joint Surg. 1976;58B:266.

Camilleri IG, Milner RH. Intraneural lipofibroma of the median nerve. J. Hand Surg. 1998;23B:120–22.

Canga A, Abascal F, Cerezal L, Bustamante M, Perez-Carro L, Vazquez-Barquero A. Fibrolipomatous hamartoma of the median nerve. Case illustration. J. Neurosurg. 1998;89: 683.

Canovas F, Dereure O, Bonnel F. Apropos of a case of epidermoid carcinoma of the nail bed with intraneural metastasis to the median nerve. Chir. Main. 1998;17:232–35.

Cavallaro MC, Taylor JA, Gorman JD, Haghighi P, Resnick D. Imaging findings in a patient with fibrolipomatous hamartoma of the median nerve. AJR. Am. J. Roentgenol. 1993;161:837–38.

Choi ML, Wey PD, Borah GL. Pediatric peripheral neuropathy in proteus syndrome. Ann. Plast. Surg. 1998;40:528–32.

Coessens B, De Mey A, Lacotte B, Vandenbroeck D. Carpal tunnel syndrome due to an haemangioma of the median nerve in a 12-year-old child. Ann. Chir. Main Memb. Super. 1991;10:255–57.

Cohn I. Epithelial neoplasms of peripheral and cranial nerves. Arch. Surg. 1928;17:117–60.

Das Gupta TK, Brasfield RD. Solitary malignant schwannoma. Ann. Surg. 1970;171:419–28.

Declercq H, De Man R, Van Herck G, Tanghe W, Lateur L. Case report 814: fibrolipoma of the median nerve. Skeletal Radiol. 1993;22:610–13.

De Maeseneer M, Jao Visidha S, Lenchik L, Witte D, Schweitzer ME, Sartoris DJ, Resnik D. Fibrolipomatous hamartoma: MR imaging findings. Skeletal Radiol. 1997; 26:155–60.

Drape JL, Idy-Peretti I, Goettmann S, Wolfram-Gabel R, Dion E, Grossin M, Benacerraf R, Guerin-Surville H, Bittoun J. Subungual glomus tumors: evaluation with MR imaging. Radiology 1995;195:507–15.

Ducatman BS, Scheithauer BW, Piepgras DG, Reiman HM, Ilstrup DM. Malignant peripheral nerve sheath tumors. Cancer 1986;57:2006–21.

Enghardt MH, Jordan SE. Granular cell tumor of a digital nerve. Cancer 1991;68:1764–69.

Ergin MT, Druckmiller WH, Cohen P. Intrinsic hemangiomas of the peripheral nerves report of a case and review of the literature. Conn. Med. 1998;62:209–13.

Evans HA, Donnelly LF, Johnson ND, Blebea JS, Stern PJ. Fibrolipoma of the median nerve: MRI. Clin. Radiol. 1997;52:304–7.

Feyerabend T, Schmitt R, Lanz U, Warmuth-Metz M. CT morphology of benign median nerve tumors. Report of three cases and a review. Acta. Radiol. 1990;31:23–25.

Fornage BD. Peripheral nerves of the extremities: imaging with US. Radiology 1988;167:179–82.

Friedlander HL, Rosenberg NJ, Graubard DJ. Intraneural lipoma of the median nerve. J. Bone Joint Surg. 1969;51A: 352–62.

Frykman GK, Wood VE. Peripheral nerve hamartoma with macrodactyly in the hand: report of three cases and review of the literature. J. Hand Surg. 1978;3:307–12.

Gama C, Franca LCM. Nerve compression by pacinian corpuscles. J. Hand Surg. 1980;5:208–10.

Giele H, Le Viet D. Intraneural mucoid cysts of the upper limb. J. Hand Surg. 1997;22B:805–9.

Giuliano V, Outwater EK, Mitchell DG, Burke MA. Median nerve hamartoma: MR imaging using chemical shift techniques. Magn. Reson. Imaging 1997;15:1091–94.

Guthikonda M, Rengachary SS, Balko MG, van Loveren H. Lipofibromatous hamartoma of the median nerve: case report with magnetic resonance imaging correlation. Neurosurgery 1994;35:127–32.

Harkin JC. Differential Diagnosis of Peripheral Nerve Tumors. In: Omer GE Jr., Spinner M, eds. Management of Peripheral Nerve Problems. Philadelphia: Saunders, 1980;657–68.

Harkin JC, Reed RJ. Tumors of the Peripheral Nervous System. Washington, DC: Armed Forces Institute of Pathology, 1969.

Harkin JC, Reed RJ. Tumors of the Peripheral Nervous System, Supplement. Washington, DC: Armed Forces Institute of Pathology, 1983.

Hart WR, Thompson NW, Hildreth DH, Abell MR. Hyperplastic pacinian corpuscles: a cause of digital pain. Surgery 1971;70:730–35.

Hartwell AS. Cystic tumor of the median nerve, operation and restoration of function. Boston Med. Surg. J. 1901;144: 582–83.

Hems TE, Burge PD, Wilson DJ. The role of magnetic resonance imaging in the management of peripheral nerve tumours. J. Hand Surg. 1997;22B:57–60.

Houpt P, Storm van Leeuwen JB, van den Bergen HA. Intraneural lipofibroma of the median nerve. J. Hand Surg. 1989; 14A:706–9.

Hueston JT, Millroy P. Macrodactyly associated with hamartoma of major peripheral nerves. Aust. N. Z. J. Surg. 1968; 37:394–97.

Iyadomi M, Ohtsubo H, Gotoh Y, Kohda H, Narisawa Y. Neurotropic melanoma invading the median nerve. J. Dermatol. 1998;25:379–83.

Jaradeh S, Sanger JR, Maas EF. Isolated sensory impairment of the thumb due to an intraneural ganglion cyst in the median nerve. J. Hand Surg. 1995;20B:475–78.

Jazayeri MA, Robinson JH, Legolvan DP. Intraneural perineurioma involving the median nerve. Plast. Reconstr. Surg. 2000;105:2089–91.

Johnson RJ, Bonfiglio M. Lipofibromatous hamartoma of the median nerve. J. Bone Joint Surg. 1969;51A:984–90.

Jones NF, Eadie P. Pacinian corpuscle hyperplasia in the hand. J. Hand Surg. 1991;16A:865–69.

Josty IC, Sykes PJ. An unusual schwannoma of the median nerve: effects on the motor branch. Br. J. Plast. Surg. 2001;54:71–73.

Kalisman M, Dolich BH. Infiltrating lipoma of the proper digital nerves. J. Hand Surg. 1982;7:401–3.

Kameh DS, Perez-Berenguer JL, Pearl GS. Lipofibromatous hamartoma and related peripheral nerve lesions. South. Med. J. 2000;93:800–2.

Kline SC, Moore JR, deMente SH. Glomus tumor originating within a digital nerve. J. Hand Surg. 1990;15A:98–101.

Kojima T, Ide Y, Marumo E, Ishikawa E, Yamashita H. Haemangioma of median nerve causing carpal tunnel syndrome. Hand 1976;8:62–5.

Kon M, Vuursteen PJ. An intraneural hemangioma of a digital nerve—case report. J. Hand Surg. 1981;6:357–58.

Levine E, Huntrakoon M, Wetzel LH. Malignant nerve-sheath neoplasms in neurofibromatosis: distinction from benign tumors using imaging techniques. AJR. Am. J. Roentgenol. 1987;149:1059–64.

Lewis RC, Nannini LH, Cocke Jr. WM. Multifocal neurilemomas of median and ulnar nerves of the same extremity—case report. J. Hand Surg. 1981;6:406–8.

Louis DS, Fortin PT. Perineural hemangiomas of the upper extremity: report of four cases. J. Hand Surg. 1992;17A:308–11.

Louis DS, Hankin FM, Greene TL, Dick HM. Lipofibromas of the median nerve: long-term follow-up of four cases. J. Hand Surg. 1985;10A:403–8.

Lowenstein J, Chandnani V, Tomaino MM. Fibrolipoma of the median nerve: a case report and review of the literature. Am. J. Orthop. 2000;29:797–98.

Mackay IR, Barua JM. Perineural tumour spread: an unusual cause of carpal tunnel syndrome. J. Hand Surg. 1990; 15B:104–5.

Mennel HD, Zulch KJ. Morphology of malignant tumors of peripheral nerves. Zentralbl. Neurochir. 1971;32:11–24.

Meyer BU, Roricht S, Schmitt R. Bilateral fibrolipomatous hamartoma of the median nerve with macrocheiria and late-onset nerve entrapment syndrome. Muscle Nerve 1998;21: 656–58.

Mikhail IK. Median nerve lipoma in the hand. J. Bone Joint Surg. 1964;46B:726–30.

Mintz A, Carneiro R. Schwannoma associated with anomalous division of the median nerve: case report. Neurosurgery 1989;25:965–68.

Mirza MA, King ET, Reinhart MK. Carpal tunnel syndrome associated with macrodactyly. J. Hand Surg. 1998;23B: 609–10.

Mitsumoto H, Estes ML, Wilbourn AJ, Culver JE Jr. Perineurial cell hypertrophic mononeuropathy manifesting as carpal tunnel syndrome. Muscle Nerve 1992;15:1364–68.

Mitsumoto H, Wilbourn AJ, Goren H. Perineuroma as the cause of localized hypertrophic neuropathy. Muscle Nerve 1980; 3:403–12.

Moore BH. Macrodactyly and associated peripheral nerve changes. J. Bone Joint Surg. 1942;24:617–31.

Morley GH. Intraneural lipoma of the median nerve in the carpal tunnel. J. Bone Joint Surg. 1964;46B:734–35.

Nagey L, McCabe SJ, Wolff TW. A case of neurofibroma of the palmar cutaneous branch of the median nerve. J. Hand Surg. 1990;15B:489–90.

Nayler SJ, Leiman G, Omar T, Cooper K. Malignant transformation in a schwannoma. Histopathology 1996;29: 189–92.

Nogueira A, Pena C, Martinez MJ, Sarasua JG, Madrigal B. Hyperostotic macrodactyly and lipofibromatous hamartoma of the median nerve associated with carpal tunnel syndrome. Chir. Main. 1999;18:261–71.

Nosanchuk JS, Agostini JC, Georgi M, Posso M. Pork tapeworm of cysticercus involving peripheral nerve. JAMA. 1980;244:2191–92.

Ochoa JL, Marchettini P, Cline M. Lessons from Human Research on the Pathophysiology of Neuropathic Pains in Limbs. In: Wynn Parry CB, ed. Management of Pain in the Hand and Wrist. Edinburgh, U.K.: Churchill Livingstone, 1991;28–33.

Ogose A, Emura I, Iwabuchi Y, Hotta T, Inoue Y, Saito H. Malignant melanoma extending along the ulnar, median, and musculocutaneous nerves: a case report. J. Hand Surg. 1998;23A:875–78.

Paletta FX, Rybka FJ. Treatment of hamartomas of the median nerve. Ann. Surg. 1972;176:217–22.

Pascual-Castroviejo I, Pascual-Pascual SI, Viano J, Martinez V. Generalized nerve sheath tumors in neurofibromatosis type 1 (NF1). A case report. Neuropediatrics 2000;31: 211–13.

Patel CB, Tsai TM, Kleinert HE. Hemangioma of the median nerve: a report of two cases. J. Hand Surg. 1986;11A:76–79.

Patel MR, Naik AN, Mody K, Pollack M. Intraneural mucous cysts of peripheral nerves. Am. J. Orthop. 1997; 26:562–64.

Peckham NH, O'Boynick PL, Meneses A, Kepes JJ. Hypertrophic mononeuropathy. A report of two cases and review of the literature. Arch. Pathol. Lab. Med. 1982; 106:534–37.

Peled I, Iosipovich Z, Rousso M, Wexler MR. Hemangioma of the median nerve. J. Hand Surg. 1980;5:363–65.

Peters WJ, Todd TR. Anterior interosseous nerve compression syndrome: from metastatic bronchogenic carcinoma to the forearm. Plast. Reconstr. Surg. 1983;72:706–7.

Phalen GS. Neurilemmomas of the forearm and hand. Clin. Orthop. 1976;114:219–22.

Phillips LH, Persing JA, Vandenberg SR. Electrophysiological findings in localized hypertrophic mononeuropathy. Muscle Nerve 1991;14:335–41.

Piers W, Terrono AL, Hayek J, Millender LH. Angiomyoma (vascular leiomyoma) of the median nerve. J. Hand Surg. 1996;21A:285–86.

Powers SK, Norman D, Edwards MSB. Computerized tomography of peripheral nerve lesions. J. Neurosurg. 1983;59: 131–36.

Prosser AJ, Burke FD. Haemangioma of the median nerve associated with Raynaud's phenomenon. J. Hand Surg. 1987; 12B:227–28.

Pulvertaft RG. Unusual tumours of the median nerve. J. Bone Joint Surg. 1964;46B:731–33.

Reznik M, Thiry A, Fridman V. Painful hyperplasia and hypertrophy of pacinian corpuscles in the hand: report of two cases with immunohistochemical and ultrastructural studies, and a review of the literature. Am. J. Dermatopathol. 1998;20:203–7.

Rinaldi E. Neurilemomas and neurofibromas of the upper limb. J. Hand Surg. 1983;8:590–93.

Ritt MJPF, Bos KE. A very large neurilemmoma of the anterior interosseous nerve. J. Hand Surg. 1991;16B:98–100.

Rogalski RP, Louis DS. Neurofibrosarcomas of the upper extremity. J. Hand Surg. 1991;16A:873–76.

Rowland SA. Case report: ten-year follow-up of lipofibroma of the median nerve in the palm. J. Hand Surg. 1977;2:316–17.

Rusko RA, Larsen RD. Intraneural lipoma of the median nerve—case report and literature review. J. Hand Surg. 1981;6:388–91.

Sagtas E, Orguc S, Elcin F, Memis A, Menzilcioglu S. Quiz case of the month. Fibrolipomatous hamartoma of the median nerve. Arq. Neuropsiquiatr. 1999;57:903–4.

Salon A, Guero S, Glicenstein J. Fibrolipoma of the median nerve. Review of 10 surgically treated cases with a mean recall of 8 years. Ann. Chir. Main. Memb. Super. 1995; 14:284–95.

Sandzen SC, Baksic RW. Pacinian hyperplasia. Hand 1974;6: 273–74.

Seddon H. Surgical Disorders of the Peripheral Nerves. Baltimore: Williams & Wilkins, 1972.

Silverman TA, Enzinger FM. Fibrolipomatous hamartoma of nerve. A clinicopathologic analysis of 26 cases. Am. J. Surg. Pathol. 1985;9:7–14.

Sone M, Ehara S, Tamakawa Y, Nishida J, Honjoh S. Macrodystrophia lipomatosa: CT and MR findings. Radiat. Med. 2000;18:129–32.

Squarzina PB, Adani R, Cerofolini E, Bagni A, Caroli A. Ancient schwannoma of the motor branch of the median nerve: a clinical case. Chirurgia Degli. Organi. Di. Movimento. 1993;78:19–23.

Steentoft J, Sollerman C. Lipofibromatous hamartoma of a digital nerve. A case report. Acta. Orthop. Scand. 1990;61:181–82.

Stout AP. The peripheral manifestations of the specific nerve sheath tumor (neurilemoma). AJC 1935;24:751–96.

Strickland JW, Steichen JB. Nerve tumors of the hand and forearm. J. Hand Surg. 1977;2:285–91.

Stull MA, Moser J RP, Kransdorf MJ, Bogumill GP, Nelson MC. Magnetic resonance appearance of peripheral nerve sheath tumors. Skeletal Radiol. 1991;20:9–14.

Van Geertruyden J, Lorea P, Goldschmidt D, de Fontaine S, Schuind F, Kinnen L, Ledoux P, Moermans JP. Glomus tumours of the hand. A retrospective study of 51 cases. J. Hand Surg. 1996;21B:257–60.

Vieta JO, Pack GT. Malignant neurilemomas of peripheral nerves. Am. J. Surg. 1951;82:416–31.

Walker CW, Adams BD, Barnes CL, Roloson GJ, FitzRandolph RL. Case report 667. Fibrolipomatous hamartoma of the median nerve. Skeletal Radiol. 1991;20:237–39.

Watson-Jones R. Encapsulated lipoma of the median nerve at the wrist. J. Bone Joint Surg. 1964;46B:736.

Webb JN. The histogenesis of nerve sheath myxoma: report of a case with electron microscopy. J. Pathol. 1979;127:35–37.

Wood MK, Erdmann MW, Davies DM. Malignant schwannoma mistakenly diagnosed as carpal tunnel syndrome. J. Hand Surg. 1993;18B:187–88.

Yeoman PM. Fatty infiltration of the median nerve. J. Bone Joint Surg. 1964;46B:737–39.

Zingale A, Bruno G, Giuffre F, Carpinteri M, Albanese V. Hemangioendothelioma mimicking a median nerve neoplasm. Case report. J. Neurosurg. Sci. 1993;37:119–22.

Zingale A, Consoli V, Tigano G, Pero G, Albanese V. CT morphology of a median nerve neurilemmoma at the arm. Case report and review. J. Neurosurg. Sci. 1993;37:57–59.

Zweig J, Burns H. Compression of digital nerves by pacinian corpuscles. A report of two cases. J. Bone Joint Surg. 1968;50A:999–1001.

Index

Note: Page numbers followed by *f* refer to illustrations; page numbers followed by *t* refer to tables.